D0689131

RAU'S

Respiratory Care
Pharmacology

SEVENTH EDITION

RAU'S
Respiratory Care
Pharmacology

Douglas S. Gardenhire, EdD(c), RRT
Director of Clinical Education
Division of Respiratory Therapy
School of Health Professions
College of Health and Human Sciences
Georgia State University
Atlanta, Georgia

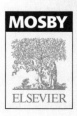

MOSBY

ELSEVIER

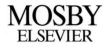

MOSBY
ELSEVIER

11830 Westline Industrial Drive
St. Louis, Missouri 63146

ISBN: 978-0-323-03202-5

RAU'S RESPIRATORY CARE PHARMACOLOGY, SEVENTH EDITION
Copyright © 2008 by Mosby, Inc., an affiliate of Elsevier Inc.

All rights reserved. No part of this publication may be reproduced or transmitted in any form or by any means, electronic or mechanical, including photocopying, recording, or any information storage and retrieval system, without permission in writing from the publisher. Permissions may be sought directly from Elsevier's Health Sciences Rights Department in Philadelphia, PA, USA: phone: (+1) 215 239 3804, fax: (+1) 215 239 3805, e-mail: healthpermissions@elsevier.com. You may also complete your request on-line via the Elsevier homepage (http://www.elsevier.com), by selecting 'Customer Support' and then 'Obtaining Permissions'.

Notice

Knowledge and best practice in this field are constantly changing. As new research and experience broaden our knowledge, changes in practice, treatment, and drug therapy may become necessary or appropriate. Readers are advised to check the most current information provided (i) on procedures featured or (ii) by the manufacturer of each product to be administered, to verify the recommended dose or formula, the method and duration of administration, and contraindications. It is the responsibility of practitioners, relying on their own experience and knowledge of the patient, to make diagnoses, to determine dosages and the best treatment for each individual patient, and to take all appropriate safety precautions. To the fullest extent of the law, neither the Publisher nor the Author assumes any liability for any injury and/or damage to persons or property arising out of or related to any use of the material contained in this book.

The Publisher

Previous editions copyrighted 2002, 1998, 1994, 1989, 1984, 1978

Library of Congress Control Number 2007932318

Managing Editor: Mindy Hutchinson
Associate Developmental Editor: Christina Pryor
Publishing Services Manager: Pat Joiner-Myers
Senior Project Manager: Karen M. Rehwinkel
Designer: Maggie Reid

Printed in China

Last digit is the print number: 9 8 7 6 5 4 3 2 1

Working together to grow
libraries in developing countries

www.elsevier.com | www.bookaid.org | www.sabre.org

ELSEVIER   BOOK AID International   Sabre Foundation

For my girls, Robin, Ali, and Ella.

IN MEMORIAM

Dedicated to the memory of fellow therapist and friend Shawn E. Bond
(May 26, 1973–October 10, 1999)

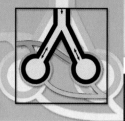

Contributors

Antonia Alafris, BS, PharmD, CGP
Assistant Director of Pharmacotherapy Services and
    Pharmacy Residency Programs
Department of Pharmacy
Kingsbrook Jewish Medical Center
Brooklyn, New York

Teresa Chan, PharmD
Emergency Medicine Clinical Pharmacist
State University of New York Downstate
    Medical Center
Brooklyn, New York

Henry Cohen, PharmD, MS, FCCM, BCPP, CGP
Associate Professor of Pharmacy Practice
Division of Pharmacy Practice
Arnold & Marie Schwartz College of
    Pharmacy and Health Sciences of
    Long Island University
Chief Pharmacotherapy Officer
Director of Pharmacy Residence Programs
    (PGY-1 and PGY-2)
Kingsbrook Jewish Medical Center
Brooklyn, New York

Natalie Erichsen, PharmD
Clinical Pharmacist, Critical Care
Chilton Memorial Hospital
Pompton Plains, New Jersey

Lorena M. Fernandez-Restrepo, MD
Instructor
Department of Pediatrics
Instituto de Ciencias de la Salud (CES)
Medellin, Colombia

James B. Fink, MS, RRT, FAARC
Fellow, Respiratory Science
Nektar Therapeutics
San Carlos, California

Markus O. Henke, MD
Pulmonary Medicine
Philipps University Marburg
Marburg, Germany

Steven B. Levy, BS, PharmD, BCPS, CGP
Clinical Pharmacy Specialist
Internal Medicine and Geriatrics
Department of Pharmacy Service
Kingsbrook Jewish Medical Center
Clinical Assistant Professor of Pharmacy Practice
Arnold & Marie Schwartz College of Pharmacy and
    Health Sciences of Long Island University
Brooklyn, New York

Louis Lovett, MD, FACP, FCCP
Chair, Department of Medicine
Associate Clinical Professor
Atlanta Medical Center
Atlanta, Georgia

Bishoy Luka, PharmD
Clinical Pharmacist, Critical Care
Kingsbrook Jewish Medical Center
Clinical Assistant Professor of Pharmacy Practice
Arnold & Marie Schwartz College of Pharmacy
    and Health Sciences of Long Island University
Adjunct Professor of Pharmacology
State University of New York Downstate College
    of Nursing
Brooklyn, New York

Manjunath P. Pai, PharmD, BCPS
Associate Professor
Department of Pharmacy Practice
College of Pharmacy
University of New Mexico
Albuquerque, New Mexico

Hina N. Patel, PharmD, BCPS
Clinical Pharmacist, Pulmonary/Critical Care Medicine
Department of Pharmacy
Emory Healthcare, Crawford Long Hospital
Atlanta, Georgia

Susan L. Pendland, MS, PharmD
Adjunct Associate Professor
Department of Pharmacy Practice
University of Illinois at Chicago
Chicago, Illinois

Ruben D. Restrepo, MD, RRT
Associate Professor
Department of Respiratory Care
The University of Texas Health Science Center
    at San Antonio
San Antonio, Texas

Bruce K. Rubin, MEngr, MD, MBA, FRCPC
Professor and Vice Chair, Department of Pediatrics
Professor of Physiology and Pharmacology
Wake Forest University School of Medicine
Winston-Salem, North Carolina

Christopher A. Schriever, PharmD, MS
Clinical Pharmacist
Section of Infectious Diseases
Loyola University Medical Center
Maywood, Illinois

Reviewers

Alphonso Baldwin, PhD, RRT, RPFT
Associate Professor
School of Allied Health Sciences
Cardiopulmonary Science
Florida A&M University
Tallahassee, Florida

Clarissa M. Craig, PhD, RRT
Assistant Dean, Science, Health Care & Math Division,
    Respiratory Care Program
Johnson County Community College
Overland Park, Kansas

Tonya Edwards, BSRC, RRT
Program Director, Respiratory Care
Weatherford College
Weatherford, Texas

Bradley H. Franklin, BHS, MEd, RRT, RCP
Professor
Department Chair, Allied Health
Crafton Hills College
Yucaipa, California

William F. Galvin, MSEd, RRT, CPFT
Assistant Professor, School of Allied Health Professions
Program Director, Respiratory Care Program
Gwynedd Mercy College
Gwynedd Valley, Pennsylvania

Donna D. Gardner, MSHP, RRT
Department of Respiratory Care
The University of Texas Health Science Center at
    San Antonio
San Antonio, Texas

George H. Hicks, MS, RRT
Program Director, Respiratory Care and Lecturer,
    Anatomy and Physiology
Allied Health and Science Divisions
Mt. Hood Community College
Gresham, Oregon

Hina N. Patel, PharmD, BCPS
Clinical Pharmacist,
    Pulmonary/Critical Care Medicine
Department of Pharmacy
Emory Healthcare, Crawford Long Hospital
Atlanta, Georgia

Foreword

Thirty years before the 2008 edition of *Rau's Respiratory Care Pharmacology* appeared, the first small version of this text was published in 1978 by Year-Book Medical Publishers, Inc. (Chicago) as *"Respiratory Therapy Pharmacology"*. The book was intended to be a teaching monograph primarily devoted to aerosol and bronchoactive drugs, for the use of respiratory therapy students. The text originated from notes for a course I had been assigned to teach on respiratory therapy pharmacology in the years prior to 1978. At that time, no publication that dealt in suitable detail to serve as a textbook for the students could be found. Students were faced with the challenge of learning general principles of pharmacology as those applied to aerosol drug therapy, and to mastering at least seven categories of aerosolized drugs—adrenergic bronchodilators, anticholinergic bronchodilators, mucolytics, surface-active drugs (e.g., tyloxapol (Alevaire)), inhaled corticosteroids, the single agent cromolyn sodium, and the off-label use of aerosolized antibiotics. Other than chapters on general principles of pharmacology and calculations of drug doses, the only non-aerosol chapters in that edition included neuromuscular blocking agents, prostaglandins (then just being identified and developed as drugs), systems of drug distribution in respiratory therapy, and mathematics of dose calculations.

Respiratory Therapy Pharmacology survived to become the first of six editions. Those editions expanded to include information on non-aerosol drug groups, such as general antibiotic therapy and cardiovascular drugs, and the expertise of additional contributing authors was sought.

The current seventh edition continues the tradition of the previous six under the new authorship of Douglas S. Gardenhire, with expert material from contributing authors. The goal of the new edition remains the same as that stated in the Acknowledgments section of the very first edition: to serve "students . . . whose inquiring minds and need for knowledge have constantly inspired a continuing effort to organize the material presented". I am grateful to Doug Gardenhire and his fellow authors for their work in the service of those who provide respiratory care.

Joseph L. Rau, Jr., PhD, RRT, FAARC
Professor Emeritus
Georgia State University, Atlanta, Georgia

Rau's Respiratory Care Pharmacology, Seventh Edition, provides the most exhaustive and up-to-date information pertaining to the field of respiratory care pharmacology. The importance of this text stems from the ever-changing nature of the field. The improvement of existing drugs and the creation of new drugs that utilize the direct access the lungs provide to the human body have expanded the types of drugs respiratory therapists will be utilizing today and in the future. This book will provide the respiratory therapy student with a strong foundation of the drugs presently used in respiratory care; however, it will also serve as a great bridge for the respiratory care practitioner.

ORGANIZATION

The text is organized into three specific sections to allow the reader easy access to a particular section of interest. The first section covers the basics of respiratory care pharmacology, including the principles of drug action, the basic methods of drug administration, the standard drug calculations, and the effects of drugs on body systems. Fully referenced and comprehensive, the second section covers the drugs most frequently delivered to patients by respiratory therapists, and the third section covers the drugs used to treat critical care and cardiovascular patients.

DISTINCTIVE FEATURES

- The seventh edition marks the 30th year *Respiratory Care Pharmacology* has been in print as the preeminent respiratory care pharmacology text.
- The up-to-date material reflects changes in the field and prepares students for careers as Respiratory Therapists (RTs) in today's healthcare environment.
- Comprehensive coverage provides the most thorough explanations of any respiratory care pharmacology text on the market.
- Pharmacokinetic principles are discussed as they relate to respiratory agents, drug administration, and a range of specific drugs used in respiratory care and their effects on body systems.

- Updated drug information will be routinely posted to the Evolve website, providing the reader with the most current information.
- Student Workbook provides extra opportunities for review and self-assessment.

NEW TO THIS EDITION

- A new author—Douglas S. Gardenhire is an instructor and director of clinical education at Georgia State University and worked with Joe Rau for several years. Joe's legacy will continue with Douglas working on the book.
- Improved readability increases the reader's ability to understand and comprehend this difficult material.
- Full-color illustrations throughout highlight special features and draw out relevant details.
- Learning Objectives that parallel the levels tested by the NBRC exams help identify important information that goes beyond memorization and recall.
- Key Terms with definitions provide easy access to the definitions associated with this topic.
- Boxed Key Points highlight concepts the reader should become familiar with.
- On the inside back cover is a list of websites readers may find useful in the search for additional drug information.
- A new expanded glossary aids in the comprehension of the terminology associated with pharmacology.
- Evolve Resources allow instructors to further customize their course and learning experience, and important drug updates will be posted on a regular basis.

PEDAGOGICAL FEATURES

- Measurable Objectives, Chapter Outlines, and Key Terms with definitions open each chapter and identify the key information covered.
- Key Point boxes are located throughout each chapter, highlighting key concepts the reader should become familiar with while working through the material.
- Finally, each chapter ends with a series of self-assessment questions and clinical scenarios to help

readers assess their comprehension of the material. An answer key is found at the back of the book, along with several appendixes and an extensive glossary.

ANCILLARIES

For the Instructor

- *Evolve Learning Resource* is an interactive learning environment designed to work in coordination with Rau's Respiratory Care Pharmacology, seventh edition. ***Important drug updates will be posted to Evolve on a regular basis.*** Evolve also includes an instructor's manual, a test bank of approximately 550 questions, an image collection of all of the illustrations, a PowerPoint presentation of approximately 500 slides, and weblinks. Instructors may use Evolve to provide an Internet-based course component that reinforces and expands the concepts presented in class. Evolve may be used to publish the class syllabus, outlines, and lecture notes; set up "virtual office hours" and e-mail communication; share important dates and information through the online class calendar; and encourage student participation through chat rooms and discussion boards. Evolve allows instructors to post exams and manage their grade books online. For more information, visit **http://evolve.elsevier.com/Gardenhire/Rau_respiratory/** or contact an Elsevier sales representative.

For the Student

- The **Workbook** contains a variety of exercises for each of the 22 chapters in the book. Examples include NBRC-type questions, critical thinking exercises, case studies, definitions, and appropriate content review to help break down the difficult concepts in the textbook. The workbook creates a more complete learning package for students and allows the student more exposure to different questions in addition to what is available in the text. The answers for the exercises are located in the back of the workbook.

The continuing developments in respiratory drugs, as well as in related critical care drug groups, challenge practitioners, students, and authors alike with increasing complexity and scope of material. In this edition, contributing authors have been sought for their expertise in cardiovascular agents, neuromuscular blocking agents, anti-infective drug groups, and drugs affecting the central nervous system.

Every effort has been made to ensure the accuracy of information on drugs in this text. However, practitioners are urged to review the manufacturer's detailed literature when administering a drug and to keep informed of new information on drug therapy.

Acknowledgments

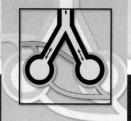

The seventh edition of *Respiratory Care Pharmacology* brings with it a greater debt of acknowledgment than any previous edition. Unlike the previous editions, this edition benefits greatly from the generous contribution of individuals who are each experts in various areas of pharmacology. Their names and affiliations, too numerous to list here, are found in the list of Contributors and in the chapters they have authored. They have willingly, and at times under duress, provided invaluable material for a new revision of the text. In particular, I am extremely grateful to Joseph L. Rau, PhD, RRT; without his expertise and 30 years of contributions to the field the creation of this textbook would not be possible. Dr. Rau mentored me for a number of years and is a great friend. To name this book in his honor signals his accomplishments in respiratory care. Joe, thank you for everything!

I would like to thank Connie Crooks, BS, RRT, Respiratory Care Program Director, Labette Community College, for giving me my first opportunity to learn and to educate respiratory care students. I owe a great deal of gratitude to Greg Belcher, PhD, Associate Professor; Mark L. Johnson, Professor, Pittsburg State University; and Jay W. Rojewski, PhD, Professor, University of Georgia for not only giving me the tools to become a better educator and researcher, but showing me how to properly use each of them. I am deeply indebted to Lynda T. Goodfellow, EdD, RRT, Director, School of Health Professions, Georgia State University, and the entire GSU respiratory therapy faculty for fostering an environment conducive for writing a textbook; without your support this would not be possible. Ultimately, I must give thanks to my wife Robin for her unwavering support during the writing of this text; her ability to take care of the children and me is something many can only dream of...thank you!

Christina Pryor and Mindy Hutchinson provided much-needed editorial and personal support during the development of this text. I am indebted to Meryl Sheard for assistance with the illustrations that are new to this edition. I also wish to thank the reviewers for their valuable suggestions for improvement.

Finally, I would like to thank the students of respiratory care; without you there would be no book!

Douglas S. Gardenhire, EdD(c), RRT

"Education is what survives when what has been learned has been forgotten."

(B. F. Skinner (1904 - 1990),
New Scientist, May 21, 1964)

Contents

RAU'S

Respiratory Care Pharmacology

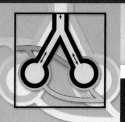

Chapter 1

Introduction to Respiratory Care Pharmacology

DOUGLAS S. GARDENHIRE

CHAPTER OUTLINE

Pharmacology and the Study of Drugs
Naming Drugs
Sources of Drug Information
Sources of Drugs
Process of Drug Approval in the United States
  Chemical Isolation and Identification
  Animal Studies
  Investigational New Drug Approval
  New Drug Application

Food and Drug Administration New Drug
    Classification System
Orphan Drugs
The Prescription
  Over-the-counter Drugs
  Generic Substitution in Prescriptions
Respiratory Care Pharmacology: An Overview
  Aerosolized Agents Given by Inhalation
  Related Drug Groups in Respiratory Care

CHAPTER OBJECTIVES

After reading this chapter, the reader will be able to:
1. Define *pharmacology*
2. Define *drugs*
3. Describe how drugs are named
4. List the various sources of drug information
5. List the various sources used to manufacture drugs
6. Describe the process for drug approval in the United States
7. Define *orphan drugs*
8. Differentiate between prescription drugs and over-the-counter drugs
9. Apply the various abbreviations and symbols used in prescribing drugs
10. Describe the therapeutic purpose of each of the major aerosolized drug groups

KEY TERMS AND DEFINITIONS

Acute respiratory distress syndrome (ARDS) — A respiratory disorder characterized by respiratory insufficiency. This may occur as a result of trauma, pneumonia, oxygen toxicity, gram-negative sepsis, and systemic inflammatory response.

Airway resistance (R_{aw}) — A measure of the impedance to ventilation caused by the movement of gas through the airway.

Chemical name — The name indicating the chemical structure of a drug.

Chronic obstructive pulmonary disease (COPD) — Disease process characterized by airflow limitation that is not fully reversible, is usually progressive, and is associated with an abnormal inflammatory response of the lung to noxious particles or gases. Diseases that cause this include chronic bronchitis, emphysema, asthma, and bronchiectasis.

Code name — A name assigned by a manufacturer to an experimental chemical that shows potential as a drug. An example is aerosol SCH 1000, which was the code name for ipratropium bromide, a parasympatholytic bronchodilator (see Chapter 7).

Cystic fibrosis (CF) — An inherited disease of the exocrine glands, affecting the pancreas, respiratory system, and apocrine glands. Symptoms usually begin in infancy and are characterized by increased electrolytes in the sweat, chronic respiratory infection, and pancreatic insufficiency.

Drug administration — The method by which a drug is made available to the body.

Generic name — The name assigned to a chemical by the United States Adopted Name (USAN) Council when the chemical appears to have therapeutic use and the manufacturer wishes to market the drug.

Nonproprietary name — The name of a drug other than its trademarked name.

Official name — In the event that an experimental drug becomes fully approved for general use and is admitted to the United States Pharmacopeia–National Formulary (USP–NF), the generic name becomes the official name.

Pharmacodynamics — The mechanisms of drug action by which a drug molecule causes its effect in the body.

Pharmacogenetics — The study of the interrelationship of genetic differences and drug effects.

Pharmacognosy — The identification of sources of drugs, from plants and animals.

Pharmacokinetics — The time course and disposition of a drug in the body, based on its absorption, distribution, metabolism, and elimination.

Pharmacology — The study of drugs (chemicals), including their origin, properties, and interactions with living organisms.

Pharmacy — The preparation and dispensing of drugs.

Pneumocystis carinii (jiroveci) — The organism causing *Pneumocystis* pneumonia in humans, seen in immunosuppressed individuals such as those infected with human immunodeficiency virus (HIV).

Pseudomonas aeruginosa — A gram-negative organism, primarily a nosocomial pathogen. It causes urinary tract infections, respiratory system infections, dermatitis, soft tissue infections, bacteremia, bone and joint infections, gastrointestinal infections, and a variety of systemic infections, particularly in patients with severe burns and in patients who are immunosuppressed (e.g., patients with cancer or acquired immunodeficiency syndrome [AIDS]).

Respiratory care pharmacology — The application of pharmacology to the treatment of cardiopulmonary disease and critical care.

Respiratory syncytial virus (RSV) — A virus that causes the formation of syncytial masses in cells. This leads to inflammation of the bronchioles, which may cause respiratory distress in young infants.

Therapeutics — The art of treating disease with drugs.

Toxicology — The study of toxic substances and their pharmacological actions, including antidotes and poison control.

KEY POINT

Key terms in the study of pharmacology are introduced, including *drug* and *pharmacology*. The study of *respiratory care pharmacology* is broadly defined as the application of pharmacology to cardiopulmonary disease and critical care.

Respiratory care pharmacology represents the application of pharmacology to the treatment of pulmonary disorders and, more broadly, critical care. Chapter 1 introduces and defines basic concepts and selected background information useful in the pharmacological treatment of respiratory disease and critical care patients.

PHARMACOLOGY AND THE STUDY OF DRUGS

The many complex functions of the human organism are regulated by chemical agents. Chemicals interact with an organism to alter its function, providing methods of diagnosis, treatment, or prevention of disease. Such

Box 1-1	Legislation Affecting Drugs

1906 The first Food and Drugs Act is passed by Congress; the United States Pharmacopeia (USP) and the National Formulary (NF) were given official status.

1914 The Harrison Narcotic Act is passed to control the importation, sale, and distribution of opium and its derivatives, as well as other narcotic analgesics.

1938 The Food, Drug, and Cosmetic Act becomes law. This is the current Federal Food, Drug, and Cosmetic Act to protect the public health and to protect physicians from irresponsible drug manufacturers. This act is enforced by the Food and Drug Administration (FDA).

1952 The Durham-Humphrey Amendment defines the drugs that may be sold by the pharmacist only on prescription.

1962 The Kefauver-Harris Amendment is passed as an amendment to the Food, Drug, and Cosmetic Act of 1938. This law requires proof of the safety and efficacy of all drugs introduced since 1938. Drugs in use before that time have not been reviewed but are under study.

1971 The Controlled Substances Act becomes effective; this act lists requirements for the control, sale, and dispensation of narcotics and dangerous drugs. Five schedules of controlled substances have been defined. Schedule I to Schedule V generally define drugs of decreasing potential for abuse, increasing medical use, and decreasing physical dependence. Examples of each schedule are as follows:

Schedule I: All nonresearch use is illegal; examples: heroin, marijuana, LSD, peyote, and mescaline

Schedule II: No telephone prescriptions, no refills; examples: opium, morphine, certain barbiturates, amphetamines

Schedule III: Prescription must be rewritten after 6 months or five refills; examples: certain opioid doses, anabolic steroids, and some barbiturates

Schedule IV: Prescription must be rewritten after 6 months or five refills; penalties for illegal possession differ from those for Schedule III drugs; examples: phenobarbital, barbital, chloral hydrate, meprobamate (Equanil, Miltown), and zolpidem (Ambien)

Schedule V: As for any nonopioid prescription drug; examples: narcotics containing nonnarcotics in mixture form, such as cough preparations or Lomotil (diphenoxylate [narcotic; 2.5 mg] and atropine sulfate [nonnarcotic])

For more information, access the FDA website at www.fda.gov

chemicals are termed *drugs*. A drug is any chemical that alters the organism's functions or processes. Examples include oxygen, alcohol, lysergic acid diethylamide (LSD), heparin, epinephrine, and vitamins. The study of drugs is the subject of pharmacology, which may be defined as follows:

Pharmacology: The study of drugs (chemicals), including their origin, properties, and interactions with living organisms

Respiratory care pharmacology, broadly defined, represents the application of pharmacology to the treatment of cardiopulmonary disease and critical care. Pharmacology can be subdivided into the following more specialized topics:

Pharmacy: The preparation and dispensing of drugs
Pharmacognosy: The identification of sources of drugs, from plants and animals
Pharmacogenetics: The study of the interrelationship of genetic differences and drug effects
Therapeutics: The art of treating disease with drugs
Toxicology: The study of toxic substances and their pharmacological actions, including antidotes and poison control

The principles of drug action from dose administration to effect and clearance from the body are the subject of processes known as **drug administration, pharmacokinetics,** and **pharmacodynamics**. These processes are defined and presented in detail in Chapter 2. A summary of key developments in the regulation of drugs in the United States is given in Box 1-1.

NAMING DRUGS

KEY POINT

Each drug has five different names: *chemical, code, official, generic,* and *trade* (or *brand*). *Sources of drug information* include references such as the *Physician's Desk Reference* (PDR), the *United States Pharmacopeia–National Formulary* (USP–NF), and texts such as *Goodman & Gilman's The Pharmacological Basis of Therapeutics*, as well as subscription services such as *Drug Facts and Comparisons*.

A manufacturer of a drug or pharmacological agent must complete numerous steps set forth by the U.S.

Food and Drug Administration (FDA). Along the way, each agent picks up a variety of labels rather than a single name. An agent that becomes officially approved for general clinical use in the United States will have accumulated at least five different names: a chemical name, code name, generic name, official name, and trade (or brand) name.

Chemical name: The name indicating the drug's chemical structure.

Code name: A name assigned by a manufacturer to an experimental chemical that shows potential as a drug. An example is aerosol SCH 1000, which was the code name for ipratropium bromide, a parasympatholytic bronchodilator (see Chapter 7).

Generic name: The name assigned to a chemical by the United States Adopted Name (USAN) Council when the chemical appears to have therapeutic use and the manufacturer wishes to market the drug. Instead of a numerical or alphanumerical code, as in the code name, this name often is loosely based on the drug's chemical structure. For example, isoproterenol has an isopropyl group attached to the terminal nitrogen on the amino side chain, whereas metaproterenol is the same chemical structure as isoproterenol except that a dihydroxy attachment on the catechol nucleus is now in the so-called meta position (carbon-3,5 instead of carbon-3,4). The generic name is also known as the **nonproprietary** name, in contrast to the brand name.

Official name: In the event that an experimental drug becomes fully approved for general use and is admitted to the *United States Pharmacopeia–National Formulary (USP–NF),* the generic name becomes the official name. Because an officially approved drug may be marketed by many manufacturers under different names, it is recommended that clinicians use the official name, which is nonproprietary, and not brand names.

Trade (or brand) name: This is the brand, or proprietary name, given by a particular manufacturer. For example, the generic drug named albuterol is currently marketed by Schering-Plough as Proventil and by GlaxoSmithKline as Ventolin.

The following is an example of the various names for the drug zafirlukast, an agent intended to control asthma:

Chemical name: 4-(5-Cyclopentyloxy-carbonylamino-1-methyl-indol-3-ylmethyl)-3-methoxy-*N-o*-tolylsulfonylbenzamide

Code name: ICI 204,219

Generic name: Zafirlukast

Official name: Zafirlukast

Trade (or brand) name: Accolate (AstraZeneca International)

SOURCES OF DRUG INFORMATION

The *United States Pharmacopeia–National Formulary* (USP–NF) is a book of standards containing information about medications, dietary supplements, and medical devices. The FDA considers this book the official standard for drugs marketed in the United States.

Another source of drug information is the *Physician's Desk Reference* (PDR). Although prepared by manufacturers of drugs, and therefore potentially lacking the objectivity of the preceding source, this annual volume provides useful information, including descriptive color charts for drug identification, names of manufacturers, and general drug actions.

A comprehensive and in-depth discussion of general pharmacological principles and drug classes can be found in several texts. Examples of two of these are the following, with a complete listing in the references:

• *Goodman & Gilman's The Pharmacological Basis of Therapeutics,* eleventh edition[1]
• *Basic & Clinical Pharmacology,* ninth edition[2]

An excellent way to obtain information on drug products and new releases is the monthly subscription service provided as *Drug Facts and Comparisons,* published by Facts and Comparisons.[3]

SOURCES OF DRUGS

Although the source of drugs is not a crucial area of expertise for the respiratory care clinician, it can be extremely interesting. Recognition of naturally occurring drugs dates back to Egyptian papyrus records, to the ancient Chinese, and to the Central American civilizations, and is still seen in remote regions of modern America, such as Appalachia.

For example, the prototype of cromolyn sodium was khellin, found in the eastern Mediterranean plant *Ammi visnaga,* and the plant was used in ancient times as a muscle relaxant. Today its synthetic derivative is used as an antiasthmatic agent. Another example is curare, derived from *Chondrodendron tomentosum* (a large vine) and used by South American Indians to coat their arrow tips for lethal effect. Its derivative is now used as a neuromuscular blocking agent. Digitalis is obtained from the foxglove plant *(Digitalis purpurea),* and was reputedly used by the Mayans for relief of angina. Today this cardiac glycoside is used to treat heart conditions. The notorious poppy seed *(Papaver somniferum)* is the source of the opium alkaloids, immortalized in *Confessions of an English Opium Eater.*[4]

Today, the most common source of drug preparation is chemical synthesis. However, plants, minerals, and animals have often contributed to the synthesis of drug preparation. Examples of these sources include the following:

- *Animal:* Thyroid hormone, insulin, pancreatic dornase
- *Plant:* Khellin *(Ammi visnaga),* atropine (belladonna alkaloid), digitalis (foxglove), reserpine *(Rauwolfia serpentina),* volatile oils of eucalyptus, pine, anise
- *Mineral:* Copper sulfate, magnesium sulfate (Epsom salts), mineral oil (liquid hydrocarbons)

PROCESS OF DRUG APPROVAL IN THE UNITED STATES

KEY POINT

The *process of drug approval* in the United States is lengthy and expensive, involving multiple phases.

The process by which a chemical moves from the status of a promising potential drug to one fully approved by the FDA for general clinical use is, on the average, long, costly, and complex. Cost estimates vary, but in the 1980s it took an average of 13 to 15 years from chemical synthesis to marketing approval by the FDA, with a cost of $350 million in the United States.[5] In a more recent study by DiMasi and associates, it was calculated that companies spend almost $900 million on research and development and on pre- and postclinical trials of a new drug in today's market.[6]

The major steps in the drug approval process have been reviewed by Flieger[7] and by Hassall and Fredd.[8] Box 1-2 outlines the major steps of the process.

Chemical Isolation and Identification

Because a drug is a chemical, the first step in drug development is to identify a chemical with the potential for useful physiological effects. This step is exemplified by the plant product paclitaxel, which is derived from the needles and bark of the western yew tree *(Taxus brevifolia).* Paclitaxel demonstrated antitumor activity, making it attractive for investigation as an anticancer drug. As the first step in the process of drug approval, the exact structure and physical and chemical characteristics of paclitaxel were established. Paclitaxel was subsequently developed and marketed as Taxol by Bristol-Myers Squibb.

Box 1-2	Major Steps in the Process of Marketing a Drug in the United States

ISOLATION AND IDENTIFICATION OF THE CHEMICAL
Animal studies
General effects
- Special effects on organ systems
- Toxicology studies

INVESTIGATIONAL NEW DRUG (IND) APPROVAL
Phase 1 studies: Small number, healthy subjects
Phase 2 studies: Small number, subjects with disease
Phase 3 studies: Large, multicenter studies

NEW DRUG APPLICATION (NDA)
Reporting system for first 6 months

Animal Studies

Once an active chemical is isolated and identified, a series of animal studies examines its general effect on the animal and effects on specific organs such as the liver or kidneys. Toxicology studies to examine mutagenicity, teratogenicity, effect on reproductive fertility, and carcinogenicity are also performed.

Investigational New Drug Approval

At this point an Investigational New Drug (IND) application is filed with the FDA for the chemical being examined. This application includes all the information previously gathered, as well as plans for human studies. These studies proceed in three phases and usually require about 3 years to complete.

Phase 1: The drug is investigated in a small group of healthy volunteers to establish its activity. This is the basis for the pharmacokinetic description of the drug (rates of absorption, distribution, metabolism, and elimination).

Phase 2: The drug is next investigated as a treatment for a small number of individuals with the disease the drug is intended to treat.

Phase 3: The drug is investigated in large, multicenter studies to establish safety and efficacy.

New Drug Application

After a successful IND process, a New Drug Application (NDA) is filed with the FDA, and, on approval, the drug is released for general clinical use. A detailed reporting system is in place for the first 6 months to track any problems that arise with the drug's use. The drug is no longer experimental (investigational) and can be

TABLE 1-1

Examples of Orphan Drugs of Interest to Respiratory Care Clinicians*

Drug	Proposed Use
Acetylcysteine	Intravenous administration for moderate to severe acetaminophen overdose
α_1-Proteinase inhibitor (Prolastin)[†]	Replacement therapy for congenital α_1-proteinase (α_1-antitrypsin) deficiency
Beractant (Survanta)[†]	Prevention or treatment of RDS in newborns
Cystic fibrosis transmembrane conductance regulator	Treatment of cystic fibrosis
Dornase alfa (Pulmozyme)[†]	Treatment of cystic fibrosis: reduction of mucus viscosity and increase in airway secretion clearance
Nitric oxide gas (INOmax)[†]	Treatment of persistent pulmonary hypertension of newborns, or of acute respiratory distress in adults
Tobramycin solution for inhalation (TOBI)[†]	Treatment of **Pseudomonas aeruginosa** in cystic fibrosis or bronchiectasis
Pentamidine isethionate	Prevent **Pneumocystis carinii** (*jiroveci*) pneumonia in high risk patients
Respiratory syncytial virus immune globulin intravenous (human)[†]	Prophylaxis of **respiratory syncytial virus** lower respiratory tract infections in infants and young children at high risk of RSV.

RDS, Respiratory distress syndrome.
*Compiled from *Drug Facts and Comparisons,* St. Louis, Mo, 2006, Facts and Comparisons, Wolters Kluwer Health.
[†]Use has been approved by the Food and Drug Administration.

prescribed for treatment of the general population by physicians.

Because of the involved, lengthy, and expensive process of obtaining approval through the FDA to market a new drug in the United States, there is often criticism of the process.

Food and Drug Administration New Drug Classification System

Because some drugs are simply released in new forms, or are similar to previously approved agents, the FDA has a classification system to help identify the significance of new products.[9] An alphanumeric code is given to provide this information.

Chemical/pharmaceutical standing

1 = New chemical entity   4 = New combination
2 = New salt form   5 = Generic drug
3 = New dosage form   6 = New indication

Therapeutic potential

A = Important (significant) therapeutic gain over other drugs
AA = Important therapeutic gain, indicated for a patient with AIDS; fast-track
B = Modest therapeutic gain
C = Important options; little or no therapeutic gain

Orphan Drugs

An *orphan drug* is a drug or biological product for the diagnosis or treatment of a rare disease. *Rare* is defined as a disease that affects fewer than 200,000 persons

KEY POINT

Certain drugs used for rare diseases, which may not return the cost of their development, are termed *orphan drugs.*

in the United States. Alternatively, a drug may be designated as an orphan if used for a disease that affects more than 200,000 persons but there is no reasonable expectation of recovering the cost of drug development. Table 1-1 lists several orphan drugs of interest to respiratory care clinicians.

THE PRESCRIPTION

KEY POINT

The selling of many drugs requires a physician's order, known as the *prescription,* and involves Latin terms and abbreviations.

The *prescription* is the written order for a drug, along with any specific instructions for compounding, dispensing, and taking the drug. This order may be written by a physician, osteopath, dentist, veterinarian, and others, but not by chiropractors or opticians. The detailed parts of a prescription are shown in Figure 1-1. It should be noted that Latin and English, as well as metric and apothecary measures, are used for drug orders.

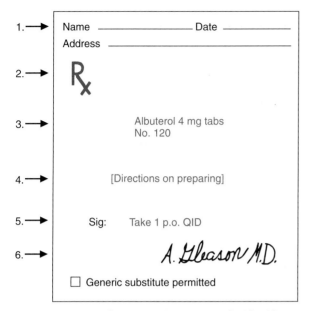

1. →
2. →
3. →
4. →
5. →
6. →

Name ——————— Date ———————

Address —————————————————

Albuterol 4 mg tabs
No. 120

[Directions on preparing]

Sig: Take 1 p.o. QID

 A. Gleason M.D.

☐ Generic substitute permitted

FIGURE 1-1 Parts of a prescription (see text for identification of elements).

The directions (*4* in Figure 1-1) to the pharmacist for mixing or compounding drugs have become less necessary with the advent of the large pharmaceutical firms and their prepared drug products. However, the importance of these directions is in no way diminished, because misinterpretation is potentially lethal when dealing with drugs.

Since passage of the Controlled Substances Act of 1971, physicians must include their registration number provided by the Drug Enforcement Administration (DEA) (usually termed a DEA registration number) when prescribing narcotics or controlled substances. Any licensed physician may apply for a DEA registration number.

The following parts of the prescription are indicated in Figure 1-1:

1. Patient's name and address, and the date the prescription was written.
2. ℞ (meaning "recipe" or "take thou") directs the pharmacist to take the drug listed and prepare the medication. This is referred to as the *superscription*.
3. The *inscription* lists the name and quantity of the drug being prescribed.
4. When applicable, the physician includes a *subscription*, that is, directions to the pharmacist on how to prepare the medication. For example, a direction to make an ointment would be "ft ung," which might be appropriate for certain medications. In many cases, with precompounded drugs, counting out the correct number is the only requirement.

5. *Sig (signa)* means "write." The *transcription* or *signature* is the information the pharmacist writes on the label of the medication as instructions to the patient.
6. *Name of the prescriber:* Note that although the physician signs the prescription, the word "signature," as described in part 5, denotes the directions to the patient, not the physician's name.

A list of the most common abbreviations seen with prescriptions is provided in Table 1-2.

Over-the-counter Drugs

KEY POINT

An *over-the-counter* (OTC) drug does not require a prescription for purchase.

Many drugs are available to the general population without a prescription; these are referred to as *over-the-counter (OTC)* products. Although the strength and amount per dose may be less than with a prescription formulation, OTC drugs can be hazardous in normal amounts if their effects are not understood. In addition, taken in large quantities, OTC products may increase the risk of hazard to the consumer.

Example

Consider OTC preparations containing epinephrine. For example, for patients with mild asthma, epinephrine is available OTC as an inhalation solution known as Primatene Mist. However, epinephrine can provoke cardiac arrhythmia or hypertension and, in particular, can exacerbate these conditions if they preexist in a patient. Dependence on OTC preparations may encourage "self-treatment" that could mask or complicate a serious medical condition.

Generic Substitution in Prescriptions

A physician can indicate to the pharmacist that generic substitution is permitted in the filling of a prescription. In such a case the pharmacist may provide any manufacturer's version of the prescribed drug, and not a specific brand. This is intended to save money, because the manufacturer of the generic substitute has not invested the considerable time and money in developing the original drug product, and presumably the generic substitute will be less expensive to the consumer than the original proprietary brand.

TABLE 1-2

Abbreviations and Symbols Used in Prescriptions*

Abbreviation	Meaning	Abbreviation	Meaning
$\bar{a}$	before	ol	oil
$\overline{aa}$	of each	OS	left eye
ac	before a meal	OU	both eyes
ad lib	as much as desired	$\bar{p}$	after
alt hor	every other hour	part aeq	equal parts
aq dest	distilled water	pc	after meals
bid	twice daily	pil	pill
C, cong	gallon	placebo	I please (inert substitute)
$\bar{c}$	with	po	per os (by mouth)
cap	capsule	prn	as needed
cc	cubic centimeter	pr	rectally
	(another term for mL)	pulv	powder
dil	dilute	q	every
dtd	give such doses	qh	every hour
elix	elixir	qid	four times daily
emuls	emulsion	qod	every other day
et	and	qd	every day
ex aq	in water	q2h	every 2 hours
ext	extract	q3h	every 3 hours
fld	fluid	q4h	every 4 hours
ft	make	qs	as much as required
gel	a gel, jelly		(quantity sufficient)
g	gram	qt	quart
gr	grain	Rx, ℞	take
gtt	a drop	$\bar{s}$	without
hs	at bedtime	sig	write
IM	intramuscular	sol	solution
IV	intravenous	solv	dissolve
L	liter	sos	if needed (for one time)
lin	liniment	spt	spirit
liq	liquid, solution	sp frumenti	whiskey
lot	lotion	$\overline{ss}$	half
M	mix	stat	immediately
mist, mixt	mixture	syr	syrup
ml	milliliter	tab	tablet or tablets
nebul	a spray	tid	three times daily
non rep	not to be repeated	tr, tinct	tincture
npo	nothing by mouth	ung	ointment
O, $\bar{o}$	pint	ut dict	as directed
OD	right eye	vin	wine

*Not all of these abbreviations are considered safe practice; however, they may still be seen on occasion.

RESPIRATORY CARE PHARMACOLOGY: AN OVERVIEW

Helping people with pulmonary diseases such as **cystic fibrosis (CF)** or pulmonary derangements such as **acute respiratory distress syndrome (ARDS)** defines a spectrum of pharmacological care from maintenance support of a person with stable disease through intervention for a critically ill patient. The respiratory system cannot

KEY POINT

Central to the respiratory care of pulmonary disease are *aerosolized agents*. This group of drugs includes adrenergic, anticholinergic, mucoactive, corticosteroid, antiasthmatic, and antiinfective agents, as well as surfactants instilled directly into the trachea. Other drug groups important in respiratory care include cardiovascular, antiinfective, neuromuscular blocking, and diuretic agents.

TABLE 1-3

Aerosolized Agents

Drug Group	Therapeutic Purpose	Agents
Adrenergic agents	*β-Adrenergic:* Relaxation of bronchial smooth muscle and bronchodilation, to reduce R_{aw} and to improve ventilatory flow rates in airway obstruction resulting from, e.g., COPD, asthma, CF, acute bronchitis	Albuterol Arformoterol Formoterol Isoetharine Levalbuterol Metaproterenol Pirbuterol Salmeterol
	α-Adrenergic: Topical vasoconstriction and decongestion	Epinephrine
Anticholinergic agents	Relaxation of cholinergically induced bronchoconstriction to improve ventilatory flow rates in **COPD** and asthma	Ipratropium bromide Tiotropium bromide
Mucoactive agents	Modification of the properties of respiratory tract mucus; current agents lower viscosity and promote clearance of secretions	Acetylcysteine Dornase alfa
Corticosteroids	Reduction and control of airway inflammatory response usually associated with asthma (lower respiratory tract) or with seasonal or chronic rhinitis (upper respiratory tract)	Beclomethasone dipropionate Budesonide Ciclesonide Flunisolide Fluticasone propionate Mometasone furoate Triamcinolone acetonide
Antiasthmatic agents	Prevention of the onset and development of the asthmatic response, through inhibition of chemical mediators of inflammation	Cromolyn sodium Montelukast Nedocromil sodium Zafirlukast Zileuton
Antiinfective agents	Inhibition or eradication of specific infective agents, such as *Pneumocystis carinii (jiroveci)* (pentamidine), respiratory syncytial virus (ribavirin), *Pseudomonas aeruginosa* in CF or influenza A and B	Pentamidine Ribavirin Tobramycin Zanamivir
Exogenous surfactants	Approved clinical use is by direct intratracheal instillation, for the purpose of restoring more normal lung compliance in respiratory distress syndrome of newborns	Beractant Calfactant Poractant alfa

CF, Cystic fibrosis; *COPD,* chronic obstructive pulmonary disease; R_{aw}, airway resistance.

be dissociated from the cardiac and vascular systems, given the interlinked function of these systems. As a result, respiratory care pharmacology involves a relatively broad area of drug classes.

Aerosolized Agents Given by Inhalation

Drugs delivered by oral inhalation or nasal inhalation are intended to provide a local topical treatment of the respiratory tract. The following are advantages of this method and route of delivery:

- Aerosol doses are smaller than those used for the same purpose and given systemically.
- Side effects are usually fewer and less severe with aerosol delivery than with oral or parenteral delivery.
- The onset of action is rapid.

- Drug delivery is targeted to the respiratory system, with lower systemic bioavailability.
- The inhalation of aerosol drugs is painless, relatively safe, and may be convenient depending on the specific delivery device used.

The classes of aerosolized agents (including surfactants, which are directly instilled into the trachea), their uses, and individual agents are summarized in Table 1-3.

Related Drug Groups in Respiratory Care

Additional groups of drugs important in critical care are the following:

- *Antiinfective agents,* such as antibiotics or antituberculous drugs

- *Neuromuscular blocking agents,* such as curariform agents and others
- *Central nervous system agents,* such as analgesics and sedatives/hypnotics
- *Antiarrhythmic agents,* such as cardiac glycosides and lidocaine
- *Antihypertensive and antianginal agents,* such as β-blocking agents or nitroglycerin
- *Anticoagulant and thrombolytic agents,* such as heparin or streptokinase
- *Diuretics,* such as the thiazides or furosemide

SELF-ASSESSMENT QUESTIONS

1. What is the definition of the term drug?
2. What is the difference between the generic name and trade name of a drug?
3. What part of a prescription contains the name and amount of the drug being prescribed?
4. A physician's order reads as follows: "gtts iv of racemic epinephrine, c̄ 3 cc of normal saline, q4h, while awake." What has been ordered?
5. The drug salmeterol was released for general clinical use in the United States in 1994. Where would you look to find information about this drug, such as the available dosage forms, doses, properties, side effects, and action?

Answers to Self-Assessment Questions are found in Appendix A.

CLINICAL SCENARIO

A 24-year-old male played golf on a newly mown course. He had exhibited allergies in the past few years and was diagnosed as having asthma. He did not have a regular physician or medical treatment site, nor was he taking any medications to control his asthma and allergies. He began to experience difficulty breathing later in the day, with wheezing and some shortness of breath on mild exertion. He visited his local drugstore and purchased Primatene Mist. On use, he obtained immediate relief for his breathing but his heart rate increased from 66 to 84 beats/min and he felt shaky. By midnight, his wheezing had returned. He continued using the Primatene Mist through the next morning. The relief he experienced with the drug diminished during the afternoon, and a friend found him later that evening with audible wheezing, gasping for air, and in severe respiratory distress. He was rushed to a local emergency room, where he went into respiratory arrest approximately 5 minutes after arrival.

Where could you find information on the drug, Primatene Mist, which he was taking?

In general, what is the fundamental error this person displayed?

Answers to Clinical Scenario questions are found in Appendix A.

References

1. Brunton LL, Lazo JS, Parker KL, editors: *Goodman & Gilman's The Pharmacological Basis of Therapeutics*, digital edition, ed 11, New York, 2006, McGraw-Hill Medical Publishing.
2. Katzung BG, editor: *Basic & Clinical Pharmacology*, ed 9, New York, 2004, Lange Medical Books/McGraw-Hill.
3. *Drug Facts and Comparisons*, St. Louis, Mo, 2006, Facts and Comparisons, Wolters Kluwer Health.
4. De Quincey T, *Confessions of an English Opium-Eater* (Dover Thrift Editions). Mineola, NY, 1995, Dover Publications.
5. Gale EA, Clark A: A drug on the market? *Lancet* 355:61, 2000.
6. DiMasi JA, Hansen RW, Grabowski HG: The price of innovation: new estimates of drug development costs, *J Health Econ* 22:151, 2003.
7. Flieger K: How experimental drugs are tested in humans, *Pediatr Infect Dis J* 8:160, 1989.
8. Hassall TH, Fredd SB: A physician's guide to information available from the FDA about new drug approvals, *Am J Gastroenterol* 84:1222, 1989.
9. Covington TR: The ABCs of new drugs, *Facts and Comparisons Newsletter* 10:73, 1991.

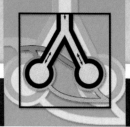

Chapter 2

Principles of Drug Action

DOUGLAS S. GARDENHIRE

CHAPTER OUTLINE

The Drug Administration Phase
  Drug Dosage Forms
  Routes of Administration
The Pharmacokinetic Phase
  Absorption
  Distribution
  Metabolism
  Elimination
  Pharmacokinetics of Inhaled Aerosol Drugs

The Pharmacodynamic Phase
  Structure–Activity Relations
  Nature and Type of Drug Receptors
  Dose–Response Relations
Pharmacogenetics

CHAPTER OBJECTIVES

After reading this chapter, the reader will be able to:

1. Define the *drug administration phase*
2. Describe the various routes of administration available
3. Define the *pharmokinetic phase*
4. Discuss the key factors in the pharmokinetic phase (e.g., absorption, distribution, metabolism, and elimination)
5. Describe the first-pass effect
6. Differentiate between systemic and inhaled drugs in relation to the pharmokinetic phase
7. Explain the L/T ratio
8. Define the *pharmacodynamic phase*
9. Discuss the importance of structure–activity relations
10. Discuss the role of drug receptors
11. Discuss the importance of dose–response relations
12. Describe the importance of pharmogenetics

KEY TERMS AND DEFINITIONS

Agonist — A chemical or drug that binds to a receptor and creates an effect on the body

Antagonist — A chemical or drug that binds to a receptor but does not create an effect on the body; it actually blocks the receptor site from accepting an agonist

Bioavailability — Amount of drug that reaches the systemic circulation

Drug administration — Method by which the drug is made available to the body

Enteral — Use of the intestine

First-pass effect — Initial metabolism in the liver of a drug taken orally before the drug reaches the systemic circulation

Hypersensitivity — An allergic or immune-mediated reaction to a drug, which can be serious, requiring airway maintenance or ventilatory assistance

Idiosyncratic effect — An abnormal or unexpected reaction to a drug, other than an allergic reaction, as compared with the predicted effect

Inhalation — Taking a substance, typically in the form of gases, fumes, vapors, mists, aerosols, or dusts, into the body by breathing in

Local effect — Limited to the area of treatment (e.g., inhaled drug to treat constricted airways)

Lung availability/systemic availability (L/T ratio) — Amount of drug that is made available to the lung out of the total available to the body

Parenteral — Any way other than the intestine, most commonly an injection (e.g., intravenous, intramuscular, or subcutaneous)

Pharmacodynamics — The mechanisms of drug action by which a drug molecule causes its effect in the body

Pharmacogenetics — The study of genetic factors and their influence on drug response

Pharmacokinetics — The time course and disposition of a drug in the body, based on its absorption, distribution, metabolism, and elimination

Receptor — A cell component that combines with a drug to change or enhance the function of the cell

Structure–activity relation (SAR) — Relationship between a drug's chemical structure and the outcome it has on the body

Synergism — A drug interaction that occurs from combined drug effects that are greater than if the drugs were given alone

Systemic effect — Pertains to the whole body, whereas the target for the drug is not local, possibly causing side effects (e.g., capsule of acetaminophen for a headache)

Tachyphylaxis — A rapid decrease in response to a drug

Therapeutic index (TI) — Difference between the minimal therapeutic and toxic concentrations of a drug; the smaller the difference the greater chance the drug will be toxic

Tolerance — Describes a decreasing intensity of response to a drug over time

Topical — Use of the skin or mucous membrane (e.g., lotion)

Transdermal — Use of the skin (e.g., patch)

KEY POINT

Principles of drug action encompass three major topic areas: drug administration, pharmacokinetics, and pharmacodynamics.

The entire course of a drug's action, from *dose* to *effect*, can be understood in three phases of action: the *drug administration phase*, the *pharmacokinetic phase*, and the *pharmacodynamic phase*. This useful conceptual framework, based on the principles offered by Ariëns and Simonis,[1] organizes the steps of a drug's action from drug administration through effect and ultimate elimination from the body. This framework is illustrated in Figure 2-1, and provides an overview of the interrelationship of the three phases of drug action, each of which is discussed.

THE DRUG ADMINISTRATION PHASE

KEY POINT

The *drug administration phase* identifies drug dosage forms and routes of administration. The *pharmacokinetic phase* describes the factors determining drug absorption, distribution in the body, metabolism, and breakdown of the active drug to its metabolites and elimination of active drug and inactive metabolites from the body.

Drug administration: The method by which a drug dose is made available to the body.

Drug Dosage Forms

The drug administration phase entails the interrelated concepts of drug formulation (e.g., compounding a tablet for particular dissolution properties) and drug delivery

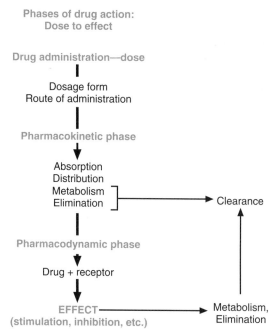

Phases of drug action:
Dose to effect

Drug administration—dose

Dosage form
Route of administration

Pharmacokinetic phase

Absorption
Distribution
Metabolism
Elimination ──────────► Clearance

Pharmacodynamic phase

Drug + receptor

EFFECT ──────────► Metabolism,
(stimulation, inhibition, etc.)   Elimination

FIGURE 2-1 A conceptual scheme illustrating the major phases of drug action in sequence, from dose administration to effect in the body. (Modified from Ariëns EJ, Simonis AM: Drug action: target tissue, dose–response relationships, and receptors. In Teorell T, Dedrick RL, Condliffe PG, editors: *Pharmacology and pharmacokinetics,* New York, 1974, Plenum Press.)

(e.g., designing an inhaler to deliver a unit dose). Two key topics of this phase are the drug dosage form and the route of administration. The *drug dosage form* is the physical state of the drug in association with nondrug components. Tablets, capsules, and injectable solutions are common examples of drug dosage forms. The *route of administration* is the portal of entry for the drug into the body, such as oral (enteral), injection, or inhalation. The form in which a drug is available must be compatible with the route of administration desired. For example, the injectable route, such as intravenously, requires a liquid solution of a drug, whereas the oral route is possible with capsules, tablets, or liquid solutions. Some common

drug formulations are listed in Box 2-1 for each of the common routes of drug administration.

Drug Formulations and Additives

A drug is the active ingredient in a dose formulation, but it is usually not the only ingredient in the total formulation. For example, in a capsule of an antibiotic, the capsule itself is a gelatinous material that allows the drug to be swallowed. The capsule material then disintegrates in the stomach, and the active drug ingredient is released for absorption. The rate at which the active drug is liberated from a capsule or tablet can be controlled during the formulation process, for example, by altering drug particle size or by using a specialized coating or formulation matrix. Aerosolized agents for inhalation and treatment of the respiratory tract also contain ingredients other than the active drug. These include preservatives, propellants for metered dose inhaler (MDI) formulations, dispersants (surfactants), and carrier agents with dry powder inhalers (DPIs). An example of various formulations with different ingredients for the β-adrenergic bronchodilator albuterol is given in Table 2-1. In the nebulizer solution, the benzalkonium chloride is a preservative and sulfuric acid adjusts the pH of the solution. In the CFC-MDI, the chlorofluorocarbons are propellants and oleic acid is a dispersing agent. In the HFA MDI, a hydrofluoroalkane is used in place of the chloroflurocarbon.

Routes of Administration

Advances in drug formulation and delivery systems have yielded a wide range of routes by a which a drug can be administered. In the discussion below, routes of administration have been divided into five broad categories: enteral, parenteral, transdermal, inhalation, and topical.

Enteral

The term **enteral** refers literally to the small intestine, but the enteral route of administration is more broadly applicable to administration of drugs intended for absorption anywhere along the gastrointestinal tract.

Box 2-1	Common Drug Formulations for Various Routes of Administration			
Enteral	**Parenteral**	**Inhalation**	**Transdermal**	**Topical**
Tablet	Solution	Gas	Patch	Powder
Capsule	Suspension	Aerosol	Paste	Lotion
Suppository	Depot			Ointment
Elixir				Solution
Suspension				

TABLE 2-1		
Three Different Dosage Forms for the Bronchodilator Drug Albuterol, Indicating Ingredients Other Than Active Drug		
Dosage Form	**Active Drug**	**Ingredients**
Nebulizer solution	Albuterol sulfate	Benzalkonium chloride, sulfuric acid
MDI CFC	Albuterol	Trichloromono-fluoromethane, dichlorodifluoro-methane, oleic acid
Tablets	Albuterol sulfate	Lactose, butylparaben, sugar
MDI HFA	Albuterol	1,1,1,2-Tetrafluoroethane, ethanol, oleic acid

CFC, Chlorofluorocarbons; *HFA,* Hydrofluoroalkane; *MDI,* metered dose inhaler

The most common enteral route is by mouth (oral) because it is convenient, is painless, and offers flexibility in possible dosage forms of the drug, as seen in Table 2-1. The oral route requires the patient to be able to swallow; therefore, airway-protective reflexes should be intact. If the drug is not destroyed or inactivated in the stomach and can be absorbed into the bloodstream, distribution throughout the body and a **systemic effect** can be achieved. Other enteral routes of administration include suppositories inserted in the rectum, tablets placed under the tongue (sublingual), and drug solutions introduced though an indwelling gastric tube.

Parenteral (Injectable)

Technically, the term **parenteral** means "besides the intestine," which implies any route of administration other than enteral. However, the parenteral route is commonly taken to mean injection of a drug. Various options are available for injection of a drug, the most common of which are the following:

- *Intravenous (IV):* Injected directly into the vein, allowing nearly instantaneous access to the systemic circulation. Drugs can be given as a bolus, in which case the entire dose is given rapidly, leading to a sharp rise in the plasma concentration, or a steady infusion can be used to avoid this precipitous rise.
- *Intramuscular (IM):* Injected deep into a skeletal muscle. Because the drug must be absorbed from the muscle into the systemic circulation, the drug effects occur more gradually than with intravenous injection, although typically more rapidly than by the oral route.
- *Subcutaneous (SC):* Injected into the subcutaneous tissue beneath the epidermis and dermis.

Box 2-2	Devices for Inhaled Administration of Drugs

- Vaporizer (anesthetic gases)
- Atomizer
- Nebulizer, small or large
- Metered dose inhaler (MDI), with/without spacer
- Dry powder inhaler (DPI)
- Ultrasonic nebulizer (USN)

Transdermal

An increasing number of drugs are being formulated for application to the skin (i.e., **transdermal**) to produce a systemic effect. The advantage of this route is that it can supply long-term continuous delivery to the systemic circulation. The drug is absorbed percutaneously, obviating the need for a hypodermic needle and decreasing the fluctuations in plasma drug levels that can occur with repeated oral administration.

Inhalation

Drugs can be given by **inhalation** for either a systemic effect or a local effect in the lung. Two of the most common drug formulations given by this route are gases, which usually are given by inhalation for anesthesia (a systemic effect), and aerosolized agents intended to target the lung or respiratory tract in the treatment of respiratory disease **(local effect)**. The technology and science of aerosol drug delivery to the respiratory tract continue to develop and are described in detail in Chapter 3. A summary of devices commonly used for inhaled aerosol drug delivery is given in Box 2-2. The general rationale for aerosolized drug delivery to the airways for treating respiratory disease is the local delivery of the drug to the target organ, with reduced or minimal body exposure to the drug and, it is hoped, reduced prevalence or severity of possible side effects.

Topical

Drugs can be applied directly to the skin or mucous membranes to produce a local effect. Such drugs are often formulated to minimize systemic absorption. Examples of **topical** administration include the application of corticosteroid cream to an area of contact dermatitis (e.g., poison ivy), administration of an eye drop containing a β-adrenergic antagonist to control glaucoma, and instillation of nasal drops containing an α-adrenergic agonist to relieve congestion.

THE PHARMACOKINETIC PHASE

Pharmacokinetic phase: The time course and disposition of a drug in the body, based on its absorption, distribution, metabolism, and elimination.

Once presented to the body, as described in the drug administration phase, a drug crosses local anatomical barriers to varying extents depending on its chemical properties and the physiological environment of the body compartment it occupies. For a systemic effect it is desirable for the drug to get into the bloodstream for distribution to the body; for a local effect this is not desirable and can lead to unwanted side effects throughout the body. Absorption, distribution, metabolism, and elimination describe the factors influencing and determining the course of a drug after it is introduced to the body. In essence, **pharmacokinetics** describes what the body does to a drug and **pharmacodynamics** describes what the drug does to the body.

Absorption

When given orally for a systemic effect, a pill must first dissolve to liberate the active ingredient. The free drug must then reach the epithelial lining of the stomach or intestine and traverse the lipid membrane barriers of the gastric and vascular cells before reaching the bloodstream for distribution into the body. The lining of the lower respiratory tract also presents barriers to drug absorption. This mucosal barrier consists of the following five identifiable elements:
1. Airway surface liquid
2. Epithelial cells
3. Basement membrane
4. Interstitium
5. Capillary vascular network

After traversing these layers a drug can reach the smooth muscle or glands of the airway. The mechanisms by which drugs move across membrane barriers are briefly outlined and include aqueous diffusion, lipid diffusion, active or facilitated diffusion, and pinocytosis. In general, a drug must be sufficiently water soluble to reach a lipid (cell) membrane and sufficiently lipid soluble to diffuse across the cell barrier. Figure 2-2 illustrates these basic mechanisms, which are briefly discussed.

Aqueous Diffusion

Aqueous diffusion occurs in the aqueous compartments of the body, such as the interstitial spaces or within a cell. Transport across epithelial linings is restricted because of small pore size; capillaries have

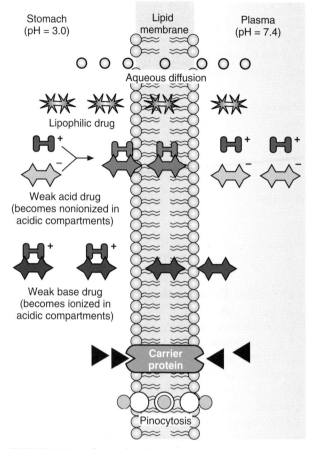

FIGURE 2-2 Pathways by which drugs can traverse lipid membranes and enter the circulation. A membrane separating an acidic compartment (stomach) and a neutral compartment (plasma) is shown to illustrate that only the nonionized form of weak acids or weak bases substantially cross these lipophilic barriers.

larger pores, allowing passage of most drug molecules. Diffusion occurs by a concentration gradient.

Lipid Diffusion

Lipid diffusion is an important mechanism for drug absorption because of the many epithelial membranes that must be crossed if a drug is to distribute in the body and reach its target organ. Epithelial cells have lipid membranes, and a drug must be lipid soluble to diffuse across such a membrane. Lipid-insoluble drugs tend to be ionized, or have positive and negative charges separated on the molecule (polar).

Lipid insoluble: Ionized, polar, water-soluble drug
Lipid soluble: Nonionized, nonpolar drug

Many drugs are weak acids or weak bases, and the degree of ionization of these molecules is dependent on the pK_p (the pH at which the drug is 50% ionized and 50% nonionized), the ambient pH, and whether the drug is a weak acid or base. The direction of increasing ionization is opposite for weak acids and weak bases, as ambient pH changes.

Weak acid: Because an acid contributes protons (H^+ ions), the protonated form is neutral, or nonionized.

Drug	$\Leftrightarrow$	Drug$^-$	$+$	H^+
neutral		anion		proton (protonated)

Weak base: Because a base accepts protons (H^+ ions), the unprotonated form is neutral, or nonionized.

Drug$^+$	$\Leftrightarrow$	Drug	$+$	H^+
cation		neutral		proton (protonated)

- The protonated weak acid is neutralized by the addition of H^+ ions in an acidic environment, is nonionized, and is lipid soluble.
- The protonated weak base gains a charge by adding H^+ ions in an acidic environment, is ionized, and is not lipid soluble.

Figure 2-2 conceptually illustrates the principle of lipid diffusion and absorption for weak acids and bases.

Some drugs, such as ethanol, are neutral molecules and are always nonionized. They are well absorbed into the bloodstream and across the blood–brain barrier. Other drugs, such as ipratropium bromide and *d*-(+)-tubocurarine, are quaternary amines, have no unshared electrons for reversible binding of H^+ ions, and are permanently positively charged. Ipratropium is not lipid soluble, and does not absorb and distribute well from the mouth or the lung with oral inhalation. A secondary or tertiary amine, such as atropine, can give up its H^+ ion, and become nonionized, increasing its absorption and distribution, and consequent side effects, in the body.

Carrier-Mediated Transport

Special carrier molecules embedded in the membrane can transport some substances, such as amino acids, sugars, or naturally occurring peptides and the drugs that resemble these substances. In some instances a drug can compete with the endogenous substance normally transported by the carrier.

Pinocytosis

Pinocytosis describes the incorporation of a substance into a cell by a process of membrane engulfment and transport of the substance to the cell interior in vesicles, thereby allowing translocation across a membrane barrier.

Factors Affecting Absorption

The route of administration determines which barriers to absorption must be crossed by a drug. This can affect the drug's time to onset and time to peak effect. Intravenous administration bypasses the need for absorption from the gastrointestinal tract seen with oral administration, generally gives a very rapid onset and peak effect, and provides 100% availability of the drug in the bloodstream. The term **bioavailability** is used to indicate the proportion of a drug that reaches the systemic circulation. For example, the bioavailability of oral morphine is 0.24 because only about a quarter of the morphine ingested actually arrives in the systemic circulation. Bioavailability is influenced not only by absorption but also by inactivation caused by stomach acids and by metabolic degradation, which can occur before the drug reaches the main systemic compartment. Another important variable governing absorption and bioavailability is blood flow to the site of absorption.

Distribution

To be effective at its desired site of action, a drug must have a certain concentration. For example, an antibiotic is investigated for its *minimal inhibitory concentration (MIC)*, that is, the lowest concentration of a drug at which a microbial population is inhibited. *Drug distribution* is the process by which a drug is transported to its sites of action, eliminated, or stored. When given intravenously, most drugs distribute initially to organs that receive the most blood flow. After this brief initial distribution phase, subsequent phases of distribution occur on the basis of the principles of diffusion and transport just outlined, as well as the drug's physical/chemical nature and ability to bind to plasma proteins. The initial distribution phase is clinically important for lipophilic anesthetics (e.g., propofol and thiopental) because they produce rapid onset of anesthesia as a function of the high blood flow to the brain and their effects are quickly terminated during redistribution to other tissues. The binding of drugs to plasma proteins can also be clinically relevant in rare instances, such as when a large portion of a drug is inactive because it is bound to plasma proteins but subsequently becomes displaced (and thus active) by a second drug that binds to the same proteins.

The plasma concentration of a drug is partially determined by the rate and extent of absorption versus the rate of elimination for a given dose amount. In addition, the volume in which the drug is distributed

TABLE 2-2

Volumes (approximate) of Major Body Compartments

Compartment	Volume (L)
Vascular (blood)	5
Interstitial fluid	10
Intracellular fluid	20
Fat (adipose tissue)	14-25

also determines the concentration achieved in plasma. Those compartments and their approximate volumes in a 70-kg adult are given in Table 2-2.

Volume of Distribution

Suppose a certain drug that distributes exclusively in the plasma compartment is administered intravenously. If a 10-mg bolus of the drug is given, and the volume of the patient's plasma compartment is 5 L, then (barring degradation or elimination) the concentration in the plasma would be 2 mg/L. In this simple example, the *volume of distribution (V_D)* is the same as the volume of the plasma compartment. In practice, drug distribution is usually more complex and the actual tissue compartments occupied by the drug are not known. Nonetheless, volume of distribution describes a useful mathematical equation relating the total amount of drug in the body to the plasma concentration.

Volume of distribution (V_D) =

$$\text{Drug amount/plasma concentration}$$

Example

If 350 mg of theophylline results in a concentration in the plasma of 10 mg/L (equivalent to 10 µg/mL), then the volume of distribution is calculated as:

$$V_D = 350 \text{ mg}/(10 \text{ mg}/L)$$
$$V_D = 35 \text{ L}$$

The drug can be absorbed and distributed into sites other than the vascular compartment, which is only approximately 5 L, and therefore the calculated volume of distribution can be much larger than the blood volume, as in the case of theophylline, which has a V_D of 35 L in a 70-kg adult. For this reason the volume of distribution is referred to as the *apparent volume of distribution* to emphasize that V_D does not necessarily refer to an actual physiological space. In fact, drugs such as fluoxetine (an antidepressant) and inhaled anesthetics are sequestered in peripheral tissues, and therefore can have apparent volumes of distribution many times greater than the entire volume of the body.

In a clinical setting, V_D is rarely measured but is nonetheless important for estimating the dose needed for a given therapeutic level of drug. By rearranging the equation for V_D, the drug amount should equal the V_D multiplied by the concentration.

Example

To achieve a concentration of theophylline of 15 mg/L with a V_D of 35 L, we calculate a dose of

$$\text{Drug amount (drug dose)} = \text{plasma concentration} \times V_D$$
$$\text{Dose} = 15 \text{ mg}/L \times 35 \text{ L}$$
$$\text{Dose} = 525 \text{ mg}$$

Several points should be noted:
- The preceding calculation assumes that the dose is completely available to the body. This may be true if a dose is given intravenously, but there may be less than 100% bioavailability if given orally.
- This is a *loading dose,* and subsequent doses to maintain a level of concentration will depend on the rate of absorption versus the rates of metabolism and excretion (discussed in the next sections).
- The volume of distribution may change as a function of age or disease state.
- The concept of the volume of distribution is not directly helpful in topical drug administration and delivery of aerosolized drugs intended to act directly on the airway surface. The volume of distribution for topical deposition in the airway is not measured, and the drug is deposited locally in the respiratory tract, with some drugs absorbed from the airway into the blood.

Metabolism

KEY POINT

The liver is a primary site of drug metabolism and biotransformation, and the kidneys are the site of primary drug excretion, although drug and metabolites can be excreted in the feces as well.

The processes by which drug molecules are metabolized, or biotransformed, constitute a complex area of biochemistry, which is beyond the scope of this text. Common pathways for the biotransformation of drugs are listed in Box 2-3. In general, phase 1 biochemical reactions convert the active drug to a more polar (water-soluble) form, which can be excreted by the kidney. Drugs that are transformed in a phase 1 reaction also may be further transformed in a phase 2 reaction, which combines (conjugates) a substance (e.g., glucuronic acid)

Box 2-3	Common Pathways for Drug Metabolism

PHASE 1
- Oxidative hydroxylation
- Oxidative dealkylation
- Oxidative deamination
- N-Oxidation
- Reductive reactions
- Hydrolytic reactions (e.g., esterase enzymes)

PHASE 2
- Conjugation reactions (e.g., glucuronide or sulfate)

TABLE 2-3

Drugs Causing Induction or Inhibition of Cytochrome P450 (CYP) Enzymes

Cytochrome P450 Isoenzyme	Inducers	Inhibitors
CYP1A2	Phenytoin Rifampin	Ciprofloxacin Diltiazem
CYP2D6		Ranitidine Fluoxetine
CYP3A4	Carbamazepine Corticosteroids Rifampin	Diltiazem Fluoxetine Erythromycin

with the metabolite to form a highly polar conjugate. For some drugs, biotransformation is accomplished by just phase 1 or phase 2 metabolism without prior transformation by the other phase. Metabolites are often less biologically active than the parent drug. Nevertheless, some drugs are inactive until metabolized (e.g., enalapril) or produce metabolites that are more toxic than their progenitors (e.g., breakdown products of acetaminophen).

Site of Drug Biotransformation

The liver is the principal organ for drug metabolism, although other tissues, including the lung, intestinal wall, and endothelial vascular wall, can transform or metabolize drugs. For example, epinephrine, a weak base, will be absorbed into the intestinal wall, where sulfatase enzymes inactivate it as the drug diffuses into the circulation. The liver contains intracellular enzymes that usually convert lipophilic (lipid-soluble) drug molecules into water-soluble metabolites that are more easily excreted. The major enzyme system in the liver is the cytochrome P450 oxidase system. There are many forms of cytochrome P450, which are hemoproteins with considerable substrate versatility and the ability to metabolize new drugs or industrial compounds. The various forms of cytochrome P450 have been divided into about a dozen subcategories, termed *isoenzyme families*. The four most important isoenzyme families for drug metabolism have been designated CYP1, CYP2, CYP3, and CYP4. A given drug may be metabolized predominantly by only one member of an isoenzyme family, whereas another drug may be metabolized by multiple enzymes in the same family or even by several distinct enzymes across families. Knowing which particular CYP enzyme(s) metabolizes a drug can be important for predicting drug interactions, as described further below.

Enzyme Induction and Inhibition

Chronic administration or abuse of drugs that are metabolized by the enzyme systems in the liver can induce (increase) or inhibit the levels of the enzymes (enzyme induction and inhibition, respectively). Some examples of drugs or agents that can induce or inhibit CYP enzymes are listed in Table 2-3.

Enzyme induction can affect the therapeutic doses of drugs required. For example, rifampin can induce CYP enzymes and increase the metabolism of several drugs, including warfarin and oral contraceptives. Likewise, cigarette smoking can increase the breakdown of theophylline in patients with chronic lung disease, shortening the half-life of the drug from approximately 7.0 to 4.3 hours. Dosages would need to be adjusted accordingly to maintain a suitable plasma level of theophylline. Conversely, a substantial portion of drug interactions involves inhibition of CYP enzymes. A given drug is not likely to inhibit all the CYP isoenzymes equally. For example, the antibiotic ciprofloxacin is a potent inhibitor of an enzyme in the CYP family that also metabolizes theophylline. Thus coadministration of ciprofloxacin with theophylline can raise theophylline levels, the opposite effect of cigarette smoking.

First-Pass Effect

Another clinically important effect of the liver on drug metabolism is referred to as the **first-pass effect** of elimination. When a drug is taken orally and absorbed into the blood from the stomach or intestine, the portal vein drains this blood directly into the liver. This is illustrated in Figure 2-3. The blood from the liver is then drained by the right and left hepatic veins directly into the inferior vena cava and on into the general circulation.

If a drug is highly metabolized by the liver enzymes and is administered orally, most of the drug's activity

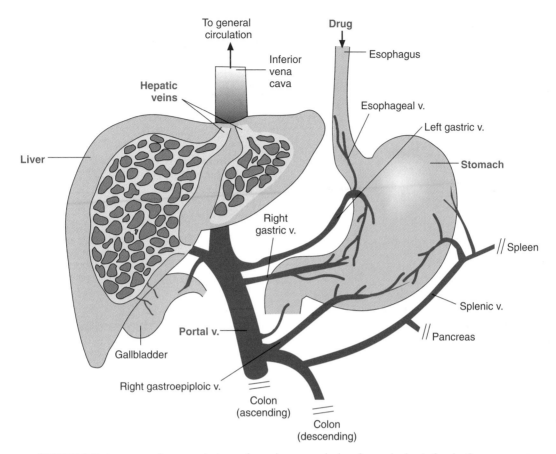

FIGURE 2-3 Anatomy of venous drainage from the stomach that forms the basis for the first-pass effect of orally administered drugs.

will be terminated in its passage through the liver before it ever reaches the general circulation and the rest of the body. This is the first-pass effect. Examples of drugs with a high first-pass effect are propranolol, nitroglycerin (sublingual is preferred to oral), and fluticasone propionate, an aerosolized corticosteroid. The first-pass effect causes difficulties with oral administration that must be overcome by increasing the oral dose (compared with the parenteral dose) or by using a delivery system that circumvents first-pass metabolism. The following routes avoid first-pass circulation through the liver: injection, buccal or sublingual tablets, the transdermal (e.g., patch) or rectal (e.g., suppositories) route, and the inhalation route. These routes of administration bypass the liver's portal venous circulation, allowing drugs to be generally distributed in the body before being circulated through the liver and ultimately metabolized. They also bypass metabolic degradation occurring in the gut as a result of specific metabolic enzymes (e.g., CYP3) or bacterial flora.

Elimination

The primary site of drug excretion in the body is the kidney, just as the liver is the site of much drug metabolism. The kidney is important for removing drug metabolites produced by the liver. Some drugs are not metabolized and are eliminated from the circulation entirely by the kidney. The route of elimination becomes important when choosing between alternative therapies, because liver or kidney disease can alter the clearance of a drug by these organs. In general terms, *clearance* is a measure of the body's ability to rid itself of a drug. Most often, clearance is expressed as *total systemic* or *plasma clearance* to emphasize that all of the various mechanisms by which a given drug is cleared (metabolism, excretion, etc.) are taken into account.

Plasma Clearance

Just as the term V_D is an abstraction that does not usually correspond to any real physiological volume, so the term *plasma clearance (Cl_p)* refers to a hypothetical volume of plasma that is completely cleared of all drug over a given period. Consequently, plasma clearance is usually expressed as liters per hour (L/hr), or if body weight is taken into account, liters per hour per kilogram. Because Cl_p gives an indication of the quantity of drug removed from the body over a given time, it can be used to estimate the rate at which a drug must be replaced to maintain a steady plasma level.

Maintenance Dose

To achieve a steady level of drug in the body, dosing must equal the rate of elimination.

$$\text{Dosing rate (mg/hr)} = (Cl_p)(L/hr) \times$$
$$\text{plasma concentration (mg/L)}$$

Example

The clearance of theophylline is given as 2.88 L/hr/70 kg. For a 70-kg ideal adult, to maintain a plasma drug level of 15 mg/L (equivalent to 15 μg/mL), calculate the dosing rate:

$$\text{Dosing rate} = 2.88 \, \text{L/hr} \times 15 \, \text{mg/L} = 43.2 \, \text{mg/hr}$$

The preceding simplified calculation assumes total bioavailability of the drug, which may not be true for some routes of administration, and is intended for conceptual illustration only. Actual patient treatment must take other factors into account. The drug could be given by constant infusion or divided into dosing intervals (e.g., where half the daily dose is given every 12 hours). When deciding on a dosing interval, it is desirable to know the *plasma half-life*.

Plasma Half-life

Plasma half-life ($T_{1/2}$): The time required for the plasma concentration of a drug to decrease by one-half.

The plasma half-life is a measure of how quickly a drug is eliminated from the body. However, more pertinent to dosing schedules, the plasma half-life indicates how quickly a drug can accumulate and reach steady-state plasma levels. Drugs with a short half-life (e.g., amoxicillin) reach steady-state levels quickly and must be given more frequently to maintain plasma levels, whereas the opposite is true of drugs with a long half-life, such as digoxin. Table 2-4 lists selected drugs in common use, with their plasma half-lives.

Time–Plasma Curves

The concentration of a drug in the plasma over time can be graphed as a time–plasma curve (Figure 2-4). The shape of this curve describes the interplay of the kinetic factors

TABLE 2-4	
Plasma Half-lives of Common Drugs	
Drug	**Half-life (hr)**
Acetaminophen	2
Amoxicillin	1.7
Azithromycin	40
Digoxin	39
Gabapentin	6.5
Morphine	1.9
Paroxetine	17
Terbutaline	14

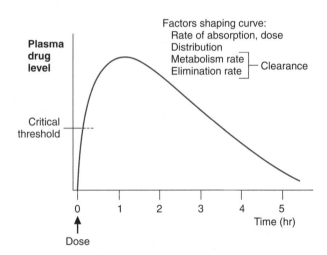

FIGURE 2-4 Plasma concentration of a drug over time. The critical threshold is the minimal level of drug concentration needed for a therapeutic effect.

of absorption, distribution, metabolism, and elimination. These curves can indicate whether the dose given is sufficient to reach and maintain a critical threshold of concentration needed for the desired therapeutic effect. Such a curve can also be plotted for concentrations of an aerosol drug in respiratory tract secretions. However, the duration of the *clinical effect* rather than the concentration of the drug is often represented in studies of aerosol drugs, particularly bronchodilators. This is more helpful than a blood level in describing the pharmacokinetics of inhaled aerosols, which rely on topical delivery with a local effect in the airway. Figure 2-5 illustrates hypothetical curves for the peak effect and duration of effect of three bronchodilator drugs on expiratory flow rates. The short-acting curve could represent a drug such as isoetharine, a catecholamine bronchodilator. On the basis of its time curve, this agent is too short-acting for maintenance therapy but could be useful for a before-and-after pulmonary function evaluation, where rapid peak

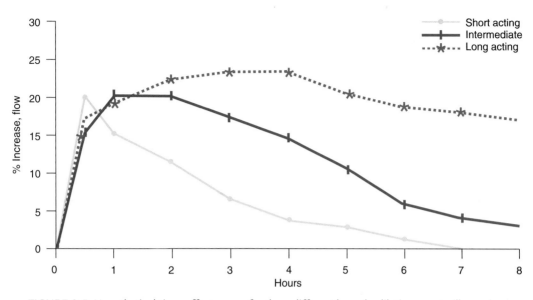

FIGURE 2-5 Hypothetical time–effect curves for three different bronchodilating agents, illustrating onset, peak effect, and duration.

effect and short duration would be desirable. The intermediate curve could represent an agent such as albuterol, with a peak effect of 30 to 60 minutes by inhalation and a duration of action of approximately 4 to 6 hours. These kinetics are useful for as-required bronchodilation or for maintenance therapy if a subject uses the drug four times daily. The kinetics indicate that bronchodilation with albuterol, an intermediate-acting drug, would not necessarily be maintained during an entire night. Finally, a long-acting agent such as the bronchodilator salmeterol could provide a 12-hour duration of effect, although time to peak effect is slower (>2 hours). These kinetics are useful for convenient twice-daily dosing and around-the-clock bronchodilation. This example illustrates how pharmacokinetics of an inhaled aerosol can help determine the choice of a particular drug for a given clinical application, as well as the dosing schedule needed for the therapeutic effect. Other factors in the choice of a drug, whether inhaled aerosol or oral/injectable, include the side effect profile, the individual's reaction to the drug, allergies, and compliance factors (patient adherence to dosing instructions) such as delivery formulations and dose timing.

Pharmacokinetics of Inhaled Aerosol Drugs

The inhalation route used for inhaled therapeutic aerosols, together with the physical/chemical nature of the drug, will determine the absorption, distribution, metabolism, and elimination of the aerosol drug.

Local Versus Systemic Effect

Inhaled aerosols are deposited on the surface of the upper or lower airway and thus are a form of topically administered drug. As topically deposited agents, inhaled aerosols can be intended for either a local effect in the upper or lower airway or a systemic effect as the drug is absorbed and distributed in the blood. A *local effect* is exemplified by a nasally inhaled vasoconstricting agent (decongestant), such as oxymetazoline (Afrin), or by an inhaled bronchodilator aerosol, such as albuterol (Proventil, Ventolin), to dilate the lower airways. A systemic effect might be exemplified by the administration of inhaled zanamivir (Relenza) to treat influenza, inhaled morphine for pain control, or inhaled insulin aerosol for systemic control of diabetes.[2]

Inhaled Aerosols in Pulmonary Disease

Inhaled aerosols used in the treatment of respiratory diseases such as asthma, chronic obstructive pulmonary disease (COPD), or cystic fibrosis (CF) are intended for a local, targeted effect in the lung and airway. The rationale for the inhalation route in therapy of the lung is to maximize lung deposition while minimizing body (systemic) exposure and unwanted side effects. If the ratio of drug in the lung is high relative to the amount of drug in the body overall (systemic drug level), the inhalation route offers an advantage over direct systemic administration (oral, intravenous) in treating the lung.

Distribution of Inhaled Aerosols

KEY POINT

The inhaled route of administration can involve both gastrointestinal and lung distribution. The systemic level of an inhaled drug and possible extrapulmonary side effects depend on both gastrointestinal and lung absorption of active drug.

Because a portion of an inhaled aerosol is swallowed, the inhalation route leads to gastrointestinal absorption, as well as lung absorption of the drug, as illustrated in Figure 2-6. Early work by Davies[3] on the distribution of isoproterenol, an older bronchodilator, elucidated the basic paths of distribution for an inhaled drug.

After inhalation of an aerosol, by a spontaneously breathing patient with no artificial airway, a proportion of the aerosol impacts in the oropharynx and is swallowed, and a proportion is inhaled into the airway. The traditional percentages given for stomach and airway proportions, based on Stephen Newman's classic measures[4] in 1981 with an MDI, are approximately 90 and 10%, respectively. Similar percentages have been found with other aerosol delivery devices. Approximately 50 to 60% of the drug impacts in the mouth or oropharynx and contributes to the 90% reaching the stomach. These amounts are used in discussing the pathways of metabolism for an inhaled drug. Although the remaining 10% is traditionally accepted as the proportion of inhaled drug reaching the lower respiratory tract with current delivery devices, the exact percentage can vary with different delivery devices or techniques of patient use from 10 to 30%. For example, lung deposition with an inhaled corticosteroid, budesonide (Pulmicort), has been reported as 15% with a pressurized MDI (pMDI) and 32% with a DPI (Pulmicort Turbuhaler; AstraZeneca International).[5] Use of reservoir devices with MDIs or delivery through endotracheal tubes (ETTs) can significantly change oropharyngeal impaction or airway delivery (see Chapter 3).

Oral Portion (Stomach). The swallowed aerosol drug is subject to gastrointestinal absorption, distribution, and metabolism as with an orally administered drug. The aerosol drug can be absorbed from the stomach and metabolized in the liver (see Figure 2-6), producing a first-pass effect. The drug may also be inactivated in the intestinal wall as it is absorbed into the portal circulation. The site of absorption in the gastrointestinal tract is determined by the principles governing diffusion of drugs through lipid membranes. In general, if the first-pass metabolism is high, systemic levels will be due only to lung absorption; if the first-pass metabolism is low and drug is swallowed, there will be a higher systemic level from gastrointestinal tract absorption, which may increase side effects in the body. The first-pass metabolism of two common inhaled aerosol drugs is as follows:
- Albuterol: 50%
- Budesonide: 90%
- Terbutaline: 90%

Inhaled Portion. It is thought that aerosol drugs interact with the site of action in the airway: secretions in the lumen, nerve endings, cells (e.g., mast cells), or the bronchial smooth muscle in the airway wall. The drug may be subsequently absorbed into the bronchial circulation, which drains into both the right and left atria of the heart, and then into the systemic circulation. The exact mechanism by which an aerosol drug, such as a bronchodilator, reaches the appropriate receptors to exert an effect is not well known. If the inhaled drug is not removed by mucociliary action or locally inactivated, the drug may be absorbed and this will increase the systemic availability of the drug.

Lung Availability/Total Systemic Availability Ratio

KEY POINT

The sources of the total systemic level of a drug are quantified in the *L/T ratio*—the higher the ratio, the more the systemic drug level is from the lung, as a result of efficient lung delivery, high first-pass metabolism, or both.

The lung availability/total systemic availability ratio (L/T ratio) quantifies the efficiency of aerosol drug delivery to the lung and is based on the distribution to the airway and gastrointestinal tract just described.

Lung availability/total systemic availability ratio (L/T ratio): For an aerosol drug (e.g., a bronchodilator, or corticosteroid, that targets the respiratory tract, the L/T ratio can be defined as the proportion of drug available from the lung, out of the total systemically available drug.

The *clinical* or *therapeutic effect* of a bronchoactive aerosol comes from the inhaled drug deposited in the airways. The *systemic* or *extrapulmonary side effects* come from the total amount of drug absorbed into the system. The total systemic drug level is due to airway absorption plus the amount absorbed from the gastrointestinal tract. As a lung/total systemic ratio, the ratio can quantify and compare the efficiency of drug

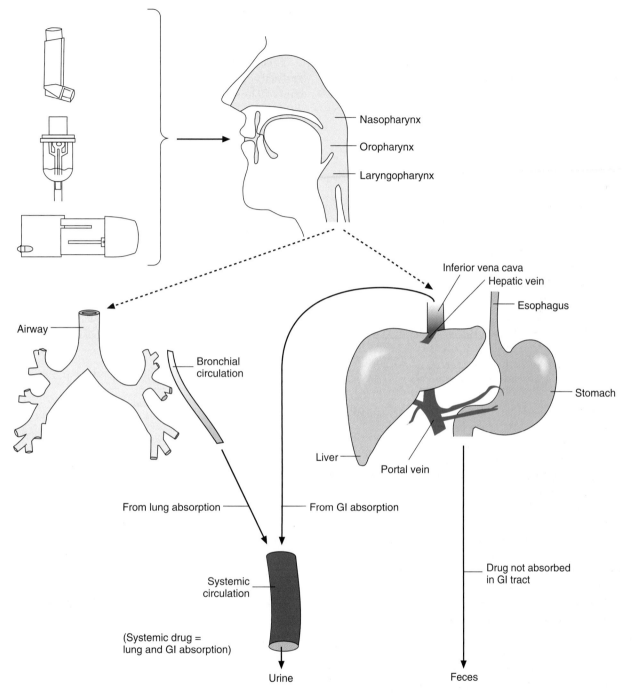

Nasopharynx
Oropharynx
Laryngopharynx

Inferior vena cava
Hepatic vein
Esophagus

Airway

Bronchial
circulation

Stomach

Liver
Portal vein

From lung absorption — — From GI absorption

Systemic
circulation

Drug not absorbed
in GI tract

(Systemic drug =
lung and GI absorption)

Urine

Feces

FIGURE 2-6 Orally inhaled aerosol drugs distribute to the respiratory tract and to the stomach through swallowing of oropharyngeally deposited drug. *Top left:* The inhalation devices shown include a metered dose inhaler *(top)*, a nebulizer *(middle)*, and a dry powder inhaler *(bottom)*. *GI,* Gastrointestinal.

delivery systems targeting the respiratory tract. Any action that reduces the swallowed portion of the inhaled drug, such as a reservoir device (spacer, holding chamber), or high first-pass metabolism, can increase the L/T ratio. Factors that can increase the L/T ratio are summarized in Box 2-4. A perfectly efficient inhalation device would deliver all of the drug to the lung and none to the oropharynx or gastrointestinal tract, thus giving a ratio of 1 (lung availability = total systemic availability; all systemic drug comes only from the lung absorption).

This concept was proposed in 1991 by Borgström[6] and elaborated by Thorsson.[7] An example, based on the data of Thorsson for albuterol inhalation using two different delivery devices, is given in Figure 2-7. Using an MDI, approximately 30% of the inhaled drug reaches the lung, with 70% going to the stomach. With complete absorption from the stomach, half of this 70% is broken down in the liver, so that 35% reaches the systemic circulation. The total amount of the original 100% dose reaching the circulation is 65% (lung, 30%; stomach and liver, 35%). Because 30% of the 65% comes from the lung, this gives an L/T ratio of 30/65 = 0.46.

The data for the DPI, using a Rotahaler, which is no longer available, (Allen & Hanburys/GlaxoSmithKline), gives an L/T ratio of 0.23 (lung, 13%; stomach and liver, 44%). On the basis of these ratios, inhalation of albuterol via an MDI gives more efficient lung delivery with less systemic availability compared with inhalation via a DPI

Box 2-4	Factors Increasing the Lung Availability/Total Systemic Availability (L/T) Ratio With Inhaled Drugs

- Efficient delivery devices (high airway and low gastrointestinal delivery)
- Inhaled drugs with high first-pass metabolism
- Mouthwashing, including rinsing and spitting
- Use of a reservoir device (spacer, holding chamber) to decrease oropharyngeal deposition and swallowed drug amount

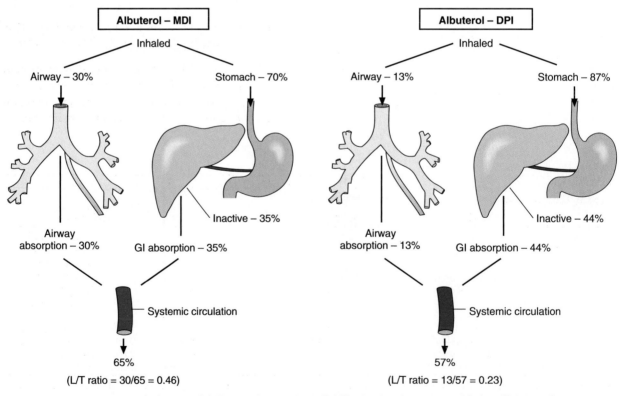

FIGURE 2-7 The lung availability/total systemic availability (L/T) ratio can quantify the efficiency of aerosol drug delivery to the respiratory tract by partitioning relative amounts from the gastrointestinal tract and from the respiratory tract (see text for explanation). (Data from Thorsson L: Influence of inhaler systems on systemic availability, with focus on inhaled corticosteroids, *J Aerosol Med* 8[suppl 3]: S29, 1995.)

such as the Rotahaler. With the MDI, 46% of the systemic exposure is due to the lung, whereas with the DPI, 23% is due to the lung. A high L/T ratio is desired; to indicate this, Table 2-5 gives examples of various L/T ratios, along with lung deposition for several drugs and delivery devices.

The L/T ratio is determined by the rate of first-pass metabolism and the efficiency of the inhalation device in placing drug in the airway. Note that a high L/T ratio can be achieved even with poor lung delivery and efficient stomach absorption if there is a high first-pass effect on the swallowed drug. Comparisons of L/T ratios must be between the *same* drugs with different delivery devices. Two drugs with different first-pass metabolism rates can have different L/T ratios even if the airway deposition or delivery device is the same. A good example is provided in Table 2-5 by comparing albuterol and terbutaline, both administered with a Turbuhaler (DPI). Albuterol and terbutaline have first-pass metabolism rates of 50 and 90%, respectively. With approximately the same lung delivery of 22 to 23% for both drug–device systems, the L/T ratio is 0.45 for albuterol but 0.79 for terbutaline. The improved L/T ratio of terbutaline compared with albuterol is not caused by a difference in device efficiency, but by the higher rate of metabolism of terbutaline that reduces systemic blood levels from gastrointestinal absorption. The L/T ratio also suggests that aerosol delivery devices should be evaluated together with the drug to be used. "Each combination of active drug and device is a unique pharmaceutical formulation, as both the drug itself and the device can influence the overall properties of the formulation."[6] The L/T ratio does not determine whether systemic toxicity or side effects will occur. First, systemic effects depend on the amount of active drug absorbed into the system, whether from the lung or gastrointestinal tract. An inhaled corticosteroid such as flunisolide, is rapidly metabolized in a first-pass effect. As a result, the swallowed portion will give minimal systemic levels. However, good absorption of the aerosol drug from the lungs in sufficiently high doses could cause systemic effects. Second, delivery to the oropharynx and gastrointestinal tract by a less efficient aerosol delivery device or method may be irrelevant if the drug is largely inactivated when taken orally and causes no local oropharyngeal effects. The catecholamine bronchodilators would be examples of such a drug. The L/T ratio indicates clearly how close an aerosol drug delivery system comes to the ideal of having all of the systemic drug exposure come from only the lung dose.

THE PHARMACODYNAMIC PHASE

Pharmacodynamic phase: The mechanisms of drug action by which a drug molecule causes its effect in the body.

Most drugs exert their effects by binding to protein targets and subsequently modulating the normal function of these proteins, usually inducing physiological changes that affect multiple tissues and organ systems.

TABLE 2-5				
Lung Availability/Total Systemic Availability (L/T) Ratios for Several Inhaled Drugs With Various Aerosol Delivery Devices*				
Drug	**Device**	**Lung Deposition (%)**	**L/T Ratio**	**Subjects**
Albuterol	pMDI	18.6	0.36	Patients—good coordinators
		7.2	0.17	Patients—poor coordinators
	BAI (pMDI)	20.8	0.41	Patients—poor coordinators
	Turbuhaler	23.2	0.45	Healthy volunteers
Budesonide	pMDI (CFC)	15.0	0.66	Healthy subjects
	Turbuhaler	32.0	0.87	Healthy subjects
	MDI (HFA)†	59.0	0.92	Patients

Data from Borgström L: Local versus total systemic bioavailability as a means to compare different inhaled formulations of the same substance, *J Aerosol Med* 11:55, 1998.
BAI, Breath-actuated inhaler; *CFC,* chlorofluorocarbon; *HFA,* hydrofluoroalkane; *pMDI,* pressurized metered dose inhaler.
*All drug amounts are expressed as percentages of metered or nominal dose.
†Harrison LI: Local versus total systemic bioavailability of beclomethasone dipropionate CFC and HFA metered dose inhaler formulations, *J Aerosol Med* 15:401, 2002 [erratum in: *J Aerosol Med* 2003;16:97].

KEY POINT

Pharmacodynamics describes the mechanism of activity by which drugs cause their effects in the body. The principal concept is the *drug target protein* (e.g., drug receptor).

The relevant protein targets include **receptors,** enzymes, ion channels, and carrier molecules. In addition, some drugs exert their main therapeutic effect by interacting with DNA rather than by binding directly to proteins. For example, the chemotherapeutic agent cisplatin inhibits cell division by binding to and disrupting cancer cell DNA, and the antiviral drug ganciclovir inhibits herpesvirus replication by insinuating itself in the viral DNA and stopping further transcription.

Structure–Activity Relations

The matching of a drug molecule with a receptor or enzyme in the body is based on a structural similarity between the drug and its binding site. The relationship between a drug's chemical structure and its clinical effect or activity is termed the **structure–activity relation (SAR).** Isoproterenol and albuterol are examples of two aerosol bronchodilators whose differing structures cause different pharmacokinetic activity and tissue responses. The drugs' structures are illustrated in Figure 2-8, with a summary of two critical differences in their pharmacokinetic profile and one critical difference in their side effects (heart rate increase). Although the two structures are very similar, and both are in the same family of β-adrenergic bronchodilators (see Chapter 6 for a discussion of

this class of drugs), they are different. Isoproterenol is a catecholamine, which is metabolized rapidly as it is absorbed in the airway by the enzyme catechol *O*-methyltransferase (COMT), giving it a short duration of action. Albuterol, a saligenin, is not a substrate for the enzyme COMT, but is instead metabolized through sulfate conjugation, a slower process. This difference is caused by the substitution of $HOCH_2$ for the OH group at the carbon-3 position. In addition, the structures of the two side chains are sufficiently different to change their receptor selectivity. Isoproterenol matches to receptors found in the airway (β_2 receptors), as well as the heart (β_1 receptors), whereas albuterol is more selective for receptors in the airway only. In recommended doses, albuterol has little or no effect on heart rate; however, isoproterenol usually will cause an increase in heart rate.

Nature and Type of Drug Receptors

KEY POINT

Two mechanisms of drug receptor action form the basis for the effects of two drug classes in respiratory care: intracellular receptor binding and modified gene transcription by lipid-soluble drugs (glucocorticoids) and receptors linked to their effector systems by G proteins (β-adrenergic bronchodilators).

At present, drugs having the greatest relevance to respiratory therapy act through receptor proteins, although enzymes are important targets for some antibiotics,

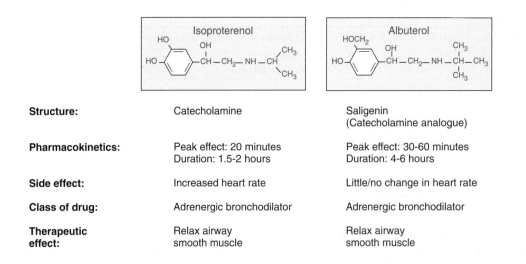

	Isoproterenol	Albuterol
Structure:	Catecholamine	Saligenin (Catecholamine analogue)
Pharmacokinetics:	Peak effect: 20 minutes Duration: 1.5-2 hours	Peak effect: 30-60 minutes Duration: 4-6 hours
Side effect:	Increased heart rate	Little/no change in heart rate
Class of drug:	Adrenergic bronchodilator	Adrenergic bronchodilator
Therapeutic effect:	Relax airway smooth muscle	Relax airway smooth muscle

FIGURE 2-8 Structure–activity relations (SARs) for two drugs representing the same class of bronchodilator. Both isoproterenol and albuterol are β-adrenergic agents, with minor structural differences leading to significantly different clinical effects.

antiviral drugs, and antihypertensive drugs. Receptors for many drugs have been biochemically purified and directly characterized, whereas in the past such receptors were only indirectly inferred from drug action and differences of action between similar drugs.

Drug Receptors

Most drug receptors are proteins, or polypeptides, whose shape and electric charge provide a match to a drug's corresponding chemical shape or charge. Drug receptor proteins include receptors on cell surfaces and within the cell.

The process by which attachment of a drug to its receptor results in a clinical response involves complex molecular mechanisms. This process sends a signal from the drug chemical into an intracellular sequence that controls cell function. Usually the drug attaches to a receptor protein that spans the cell membrane, and so the process is one of "transmembrane signaling." Four mechanisms for transmembrane signaling are well understood. Each mechanism can transduce signals for a group of different drug receptors and therefore for different drugs. The four mechanisms are as follows:

1. Lipid-soluble drugs cross the cell membrane and act on intracellular receptors, to initiate the drug response. Examples: Corticosteroids, vitamin D, thyroid hormone.
2. The drug attaches to the extracellular portion of a protein receptor, which projects into the cell cytoplasm (a "transmembrane protein") and activates an enzyme system, such as tyrosine kinase, in the intracellular portion to initiate an effect. Examples: Insulin, platelet-derived growth factor (PDGF).
3. The drug attaches to a surface receptor, which regulates the opening of an ion channel. Examples: Acetylcholine receptors on skeletal muscle; γ-aminobutyric acid (GABA).
4. The drug attaches to a transmembrane receptor that is coupled to an intracellular enzyme by a G protein (guanine nucleotide–regulating protein). Examples: β-Adrenergic agents, acetylcholine at parasympathetic nerve endings.

The first, third, and fourth mechanisms are reviewed in more detail, because these are the basis for the activity of drugs commonly used in respiratory care.

Lipid-Soluble Drugs and Intracellular Receptor Activation

Intracellular receptor activation by lipid-soluble drugs is the basis on which corticosteroids, an important class of drugs in respiratory care, cause a cell response. Examples of

corticosteroid drugs are inhaled beclomethasone and flunisolide and oral prednisone. In this drug–receptor mechanism, the drug is sufficiently lipid soluble to cross the lipid bilayer of the cell membrane, diffuse into the cytoplasm, and attach to an intracellular polypeptide receptor. The drug–receptor complex translocates to the cell nucleus and binds to specific DNA sequences termed *hormone response elements*, which can either stimulate or repress the transcription of genes in the nucleus. An example of such drug–receptor signaling is illustrated in Figure 2-9 for glucocorticoid drugs, such as inhaled flunisolide or oral prednisone. The glucocorticoid diffuses across the cell membrane and attaches to a receptor in the cytoplasm. Attachment of the drug to the receptor causes displacement of certain proteins, termed heat shock proteins,

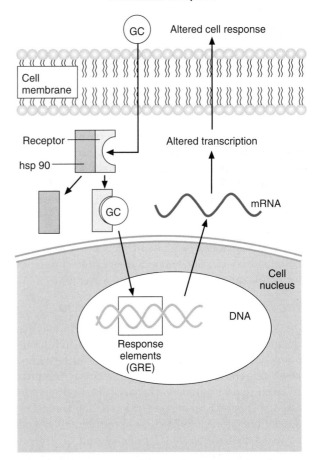

FIGURE 2-9 A diagram of the mechanism of action for lipid-soluble drugs such as glucocorticoids, which bind to intracellular receptors and then modify cell nuclear transcription. *GC,* Glucocorticoid; *GRE,* glucocorticoid response element; *hsp 90,* heat shock protein 90.

and a change in the receptor configuration to an active state. The newly coupled drug–receptor then moves or *translocates* to the nucleus of the cell, where it pairs with other drug–receptor complexes, which then bind to a glucocorticoid response element (GRE) of the cell's DNA. This initiates or represses transcription of target genes and cell response (see Chapter 11 for a discussion of the mechanism and effects of glucocorticoids).

Drugs that act by diffusing into the cell and regulating gene responses have longer periods for observed responses, from 30 minutes to several hours. Typically there is also a persistence of effect for hours or days, even after the drug has been eliminated from the body.

Drug-Regulated Ion Channels

Another process of drug signal transduction regulates the flow of ions such as sodium or potassium through cell membrane channels. This can be seen in Figure 2-10. The drug binds to a receptor on the cell membrane surface. The receptor has a portion above or on the surface of the cell membrane and extends through the membrane into the cytoplasm of the cell. When activated by the drug (or by an endogenous ligand), the receptor opens an ion channel to allow increased transmembrane conductance of an ion. An example of such a receptor is that for acetylcholine, a neurotransmitter, on skeletal muscle. This acetylcholine receptor is termed a *nicotinic receptor* because it responds to the substance nicotine, as well as acetylcholine. Attachment of acetylcholine or nicotine opens an ion channel and allows the high sodium (Na^+) concentration in extracellular fluid to flow into the lower concentration of the cell. This produces a reversal of voltage, or *depolarization*, and a corresponding muscle twitch. Acetylcholine is the neurotransmitter for voluntary muscle contraction and movement, and stimulation by nicotine can increase skeletal muscle tremor.

Receptors Linked to G Proteins

G protein–linked receptors mediate both bronchodilation and bronchoconstriction in the airways, in response to endogenous stimulation by neurotransmitters epinephrine and acetylcholine. These same airway responses can be elicited by adrenergic bronchodilator drugs (discussed in Chapter 6) or blocked by acetylcholine-blocking (anticholinergic) agents such as ipratropium bromide (discussed in Chapter 7). G proteins and G protein–linked receptors also mediate the effects of other chemicals, including those of histamine and glucagon, and the phototransduction of light in retinal rods and cones. Drug receptor signaling with G protein–linked receptors involves three main components: the *drug receptor,* the

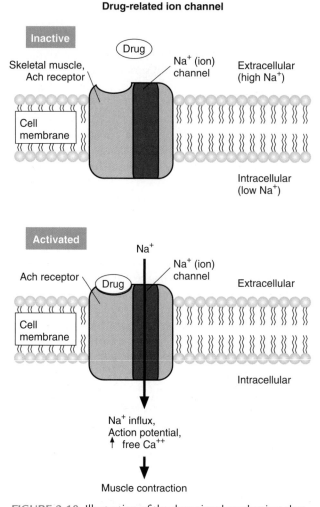

FIGURE 2-10 Illustration of the drug signal mechanism that regulates ion channel flow to cause a drug response, such as that of acetylcholine *(Ach)* or nicotine in stimulating skeletal muscle fibers to contract.

G protein, and the *effector system.* When a drug attaches to a G protein–linked receptor, these three components interact to cause a cellular response to the drug. The effector system triggers the cell response ultimately by activating or inhibiting a *second messenger* within the cell. A diagram showing the main elements of a G protein–linked receptor is given in Figure 2-11. Each of the major elements in this signaling mechanism complex is described briefly, along with the dynamics of their interaction.

Receptors that couple with G proteins have been well characterized and show a similar structure, in which there is a polypeptide chain that crosses the cell membrane seven times, giving a serpentine appearance to the receptor. The polypeptide chain has an amino (NH_2, or N)-terminal site outside the cell membrane and a carboxyl

G protein-linked receptor

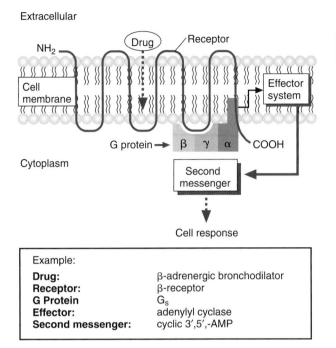

FIGURE 2-11 Simplified diagram of the components by which a G protein-linked receptor causes a cell response: the drug, the receptor, the G protein, the effector system, and the second messenger. Each of these components is identified in this example of a β-adrenergic bronchodilator drug and the β receptor, which is a G protein-linked receptor. G_s, Stimulatory G protein.

(COOH, or C) terminus inside the cell. Although the seven transmembrane segments of the receptor are illustrated in Figure 2-12 as side by side, the receptor appears to form a cylindrical structure if viewed perpendicular to the surface of the cell membrane, with the transmembrane loops forming the sides of the cylinder. The drug usually couples to the receptor at a site surrounded by the transmembrane regions of the receptor protein, that is, within the interior of the cylinder. The receptor then activates a G protein on the cytoplasmic (inner) surface of the cell membrane. The site of the G protein's interaction with the receptor polypeptide is thought to be at the third cytoplasmic loop of the receptor chain.

G proteins are so termed because they are a family of guanine nucleotide–binding proteins with a three-part, or *heterotrimeric,* structure. The three subunits of the G protein are designated by the Greek letters alpha (α), beta (β), and gamma (γ). The α subunit differentiates members of the G protein family. On the basis of the α subunit, the G protein is classified into subgroups, such as G_s, which *stimulates* an effector system, and G_i, which *inhibits*

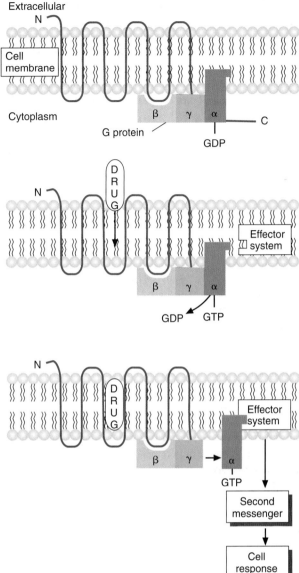

FIGURE 2-12 A sequential diagram of G protein-linked receptor activation and G protein function in linking a drug signal to a cell response.

the effector system. Other types of G proteins have been identified as well; they are not reviewed in this chapter.

The activated G protein changes the activity of an *effector system,* which may be either an enzyme, which in turn catalyzes the formation of a *second messenger,* or an ion channel, which allows the outflow of K^+ ions from the cell. One of the second messengers is the well-known cyclic adenosine 3',5'-monophosphate (cyclic AMP [cAMP]). The effector enzyme for increasing cAMP is adenylyl cyclase (previously termed adenyl cyclase), which converts ATP to cAMP. The G protein that stimulates adenylyl cyclase is the G_s (for *stimulatory*) protein. β Receptors, which couple with β-adrenergic bronchodilators, activate G_s proteins. Another G protein, G_i (for *inhibitory*), inhibits the activation of adenylyl cyclase; G_i proteins are activated by cholinergic (muscarinic) agonists such as acetylcholine or the drug methacholine.

The dynamics of cell signaling by G protein-linked receptors are illustrated schematically in Figure 2-12. When there is no drug attached to the receptor site, the α subunit of the G protein is bound to guanosine diphosphate (GDP) and the G protein is in an inactive state. When a drug attaches to the receptor, there is a change in the receptor conformation that causes the release of GDP and the binding of guanosine triphosphate (GTP) to the α subunit. This is the active state for the G protein. The GTP-bound α subunit dissociates, or *unlinks,* from the β–γ portion, and couples with the effector system to stimulate or inhibit a second messenger within the cell. The GTP bound to the α subunit is then hydrolyzed by a GTPase enzyme, dissociates from the effector, and reassociates with the β–γ dimer. The G protein-linked receptor is then ready for reactivation.

Details on specific G proteins, their effector systems, and their second messengers are presented for neurotransmitters such as epinephrine and acetylcholine in the nervous system (Chapter 5), and for those classes of drugs that link to such receptors, such as adrenergic bronchodilators (Chapter 6) and anticholinergic bronchodilators (Chapter 7).

Dose–Response Relations

KEY POINT

A variety of terms describe the *dose–response relation* of drugs, as they combine with their corresponding receptors, and drug interactions. These include *potency, maximal effect, therapeutic index, agonists* and *antagonists, synergism, additivity, potentiation,* and reactions such as *idiosyncratic, hypersensitivity, tolerance,* and *tachyphylaxis.*

The response to a drug is proportional to the drug concentration. As drug concentration increases, the number of receptors occupied increases, and the drug effect also increases up to a maximal point. This is graphed as a dose–response, or concentration–effect, curve, as seen in Figure 2-13. Increasing amounts of drug will increase the response in a fairly direct fashion; however, the rate of response usually diminishes as the dose increases, until a plateau of maximal effect is reached. Such a convex, or *hyperbolic,* curve is normally transformed mathematically by using the logarithm of the dose, so that a sigmoid curve is obtained. The linear midportion of a sigmoid curve allows easier comparison of the dose–response for different drugs. In particular, the dose at which 50% of the response to the drug occurs is indicated in Figure 2-13 and is referred to as the ED_{50}, the dose of drug that produces 50% of the maximal effect. This may also be denoted as the EC_{50}, for effective concentration giving 50% of maximal response.

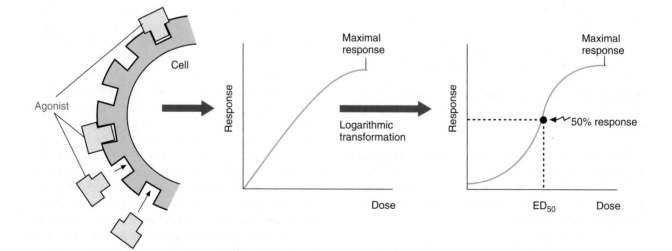

FIGURE 2-13 Illustration of the dose-response curve *(left)*, showing an increasing effect that ultimately plateaus, and its logarithmic transformation to produce a sigmoid curve *(right)*. ED_{50}, drug dose that produces 50% of the maximal effect.

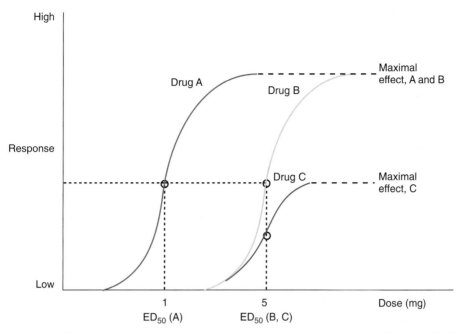

FIGURE 2-14 The potency of a drug is defined as the dose producing 50% of the drug's maximal effect. Drug A is more potent than drug B; however, drugs B and C are equally potent, although drug C has less maximal effect than drug B.

Potency Versus Maximal Effect

Dose–response curves are the basis for defining and illustrating several concepts used to characterize and compare drugs. Two concepts that allow comparison of drugs are potency and maximal effect, both illustrated in Figure 2-14.

Potency: Refers to the concentration (EC_{50}) or dose (ED_{50}) of a drug producing 50% of that drug's maximal response. The potency of two drugs, A and B, can be compared on the basis of the ED_{50} values of the two drugs: relative potency, A and B = ED_{50} (B)/ED_{50} (A).

Maximal effect: The greatest response that can be produced by a drug, a dose above which no further response can be elicited.

The lower the ED_{50} for a given drug, the more potent the drug is, as seen in Figure 2-14. Curves for drugs A and B show different potencies. If the ED_{50} for drug B is 5 mg and for drug A is 1 mg, then drug A is five times more potent than drug B.

$$ED_{50} \text{ (B)}/ED_{50} \text{ (A)} = 5 \text{ mg}/1 \text{ mg} = 5$$

Drug B requires five times the amount of drug A to produce 50% of its maximal effect. Note that potency is not the same as maximal effect, also illustrated in Figure 2-14. Potency is relatively defined using the ED_{50} values of two drugs, whereas maximal effect is absolutely defined as a physiological or clinical response. The curves indicate that drugs B and C have the same potency; that is, the same dose produces 50% of the maximal response. However, drug B has a greater maximal effect than drug C. Because the ED_{50} is the dose causing a response that is half the maximal response of the *same* drug, two drugs can have different maximal responses but the same ED_{50} (and therefore the same potency), as seen in Figure 2-14.

Therapeutic Index

The therapeutic index is also based on the dose-response curve of a drug. However, instead of a graded clinical or physiological response such as an increase in heart rate, we substitute an all-or-nothing response of improvement for each subject, or toxicity/death for each subject. In this case the ED_{50} represents the dose of the drug at which half of the test subjects improve. Similarly, the LD_{50} will be the lethal dose for 50% of the test population. Doses are established for a test population of animals (as illustrated in Figure 2-15). The therapeutic index can then be defined as follows:

Therapeutic index (TI): The ratio of the LD_{50} to the ED_{50} for a given drug, with ED_{50} and LD_{50} indicating half of the test subjects rather than a 50% clinical response.

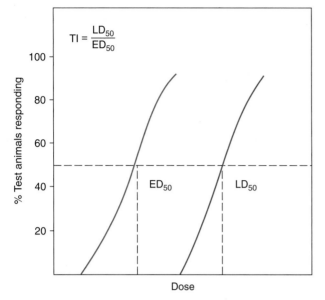

FIGURE 2-15 The therapeutic index (TI), defined as the ratio of the dose that is lethal for 50% of the test animals (LD_{50}) to the dose causing improvement in 50% of the test animals (ED_{50}).

The ratio of the dose that is toxic to 50% of test subjects to the dose that provides relief to 50% of the subjects is the clinical therapeutic index. This index represents the safety margin of the drug. The smaller the TI, the greater is the possibility of crossing from a therapeutic effect to a toxic effect. Theophylline is an example of a drug used in respiratory care that has a narrow therapeutic margin. As a result, toxic side effects can be seen at close to therapeutic dose levels in some individuals.

Agonists and Antagonists

An **agonist** is a drug or chemical that binds to a corresponding receptor (has affinity) and *initiates* a cellular effect or response (has efficacy). An **antagonist** is a drug or chemical that is able to bind to a receptor (has affinity) but causes no response (zero efficacy). Because the antagonist drug is occupying the receptor site, it can prevent other drugs or an endogenous chemical from reaching and activating the receptor site. By so doing, an antagonist *inhibits* or *blocks* the agonist at the receptor. Agonists are further divided into *full* and *partial agonists*. A full agonist is a drug that gives a higher maximal response than a partial agonist. The dose–response curves for a partial agonist and a full agonist are represented in Figure 2-16. Both have receptor affinity, but a partial agonist has less efficacy than a full agonist.

Drug Interactions

The concept of drug antagonism just discussed is an example of a drug interaction in which one drug can block the effect of another. There are several mechanisms of drug antagonism, as follows:

Chemical antagonism: A direct chemical interaction between drug and biologic mediator, which inactivates the drug. An example is chelation of toxic metals by a chelating agent.

Functional antagonism: Can occur when two drugs each produce an effect, and the two effects cancel each other. For example, methacholine can stimulate parasympathetic (muscarinic) receptors in the airways, causing bronchoconstriction; epinephrine can stimulate β_2 receptors in the airways, causing bronchodilation.

Competitive antagonism: Occurs when a drug has affinity for a receptor, but no efficacy, and at the same time blocks the active agonist from binding to and stimulating the receptor. For example, fexofenadine is a competitive antagonist to histamine on specific receptors (H_1) on bronchial smooth muscle and the nasopharynx and therefore is used to treat allergies to pollens.

In addition to antagonistic drug interactions, several terms are used to describe positive interactions between two drugs.

Synergism: Occurs when two drugs act on a target organ by different mechanisms of action, and the effect of the drug pair is greater than the sum of the separate effects of the drugs.

Additivity: Occurs when two drugs act on the same receptors and the combined effect is the simple linear sum of the two drugs' effects, up to a maximal effect.

Potentiation: A special case of synergism in which one drug has no effect but can increase the activity of the other drug.

Terms for Drug Responsiveness

Individuals exhibit variation in their responses to drugs, and the dose–response curves previously illustrated represent an average of an entire group. The following terms are encountered in pharmacology to describe individual reactions to drugs.

Idiosyncratic effect: An effect that is the opposite of, or unusual, or an absence of effect, compared with the predicted usual effect in an individual.

Hypersensitivity: An allergic or immune-mediated reaction to a drug, which can be serious, requiring airway maintenance or ventilatory assistance.

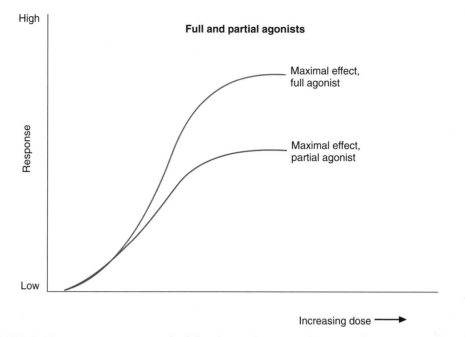

FIGURE 2-16 Dose–response curves for full and partial agonists, illustrating the greater maximal effect of the full agonist.

Tolerance: Describes a decreasing intensity of response to a drug over time.

Tachyphylaxis: Describes a rapid decrease in responsiveness to a drug.

PHARMACOGENETICS

KEY POINT

Pharmacogenetics refers to hereditary differences in the way the body handles specific drugs.

The well-described variations between patients in their responses to drugs are being increasingly traced to hereditary differences. The study of these hereditary or genetic differences is referred to as **pharmacogenetics.** These genetic variations may not be manifested as an "abnormality" until the patient is challenged with a drug, at which time the irregularity in the pharmacokinetic or pharmacodynamic response is revealed. Genetic differences affecting drug metabolism have been most extensively studied, although variation in target proteins may be equally important.

Several examples can be given from drugs commonly seen in respiratory and critical care.

Isoniazid: An antituberculosis drug that varies in its rate of metabolism and inactivation among individuals, with rapid and slow inactivators seen. The proportion of rapid versus slow inactivators is about 50/50 among white and black individuals, but Inuit and some Asian populations tend to be rapid inactivators.

Succinylcholine: A neuromuscular paralyzing agent used during surgery, succinylcholine is normally metabolized by a butyrylcholinesterase enzyme (pseudocholinesterase). Approximately 1 in 3000 individuals has a genetically determined variant of this enzyme. As a result, a patient may take several hours to recover from the drug and begin to breathe spontaneously, rather than the several minutes usually seen. Mechanical ventilatory support will be required until spontaneous breathing is adequate.

Isoflurane: An inhalation anesthetic that (like several other, related anesthetics) can cause malignant hyperthermia in genetically susceptible individuals. Patients with an atypical variant of a calcium release channel can succumb to this serious complication of general anesthesia, which involves a rapid rise in body temperature and increased oxygen consumption.

SELF-ASSESSMENT QUESTIONS

1. If a drug is in liquid solution, what routes of administration are available for its delivery, considering only its dosage form?
2. Although generic drug equivalents all have the same amount of active drug, will formulations of the same drug from different manufacturers all have the same ingredients?
3. If 200 mg of a drug results in a plasma concentration of 10 mg/L, what is the calculated volume of distribution (V_D)?
4. If the V_D of a drug such as phenobarbital is 38 L/70 kg and an effective concentration is 10 mg/L, what loading dose would be needed for an average adult (assuming total bioavailability)?
5. If an inhaled aerosol has zero gastrointestinal absorption of active drug and only lung absorption, what is the L/T ratio?
6. True or False: A patient uses a reservoir device with an inhaled aerosol and there is no swallowed portion of the drug; therefore there will be no systemic side effects.
7. Which receptor system signal mechanism is responsible for the effects caused by β-receptor activation, such as those seen with adrenergic bronchodilators (e.g., albuterol)?

Answers to Self-Assessment Questions are found in Appendix A.

CLINICAL SCENARIO

A resident orders isoetharine (Bronkosol), a bronchodilator, to be given qid, for a 67-year-old male. The patient has been diagnosed for the past 10 years with chronic obstructive pulmonary disease (COPD) and was admitted to the hospital the previous evening with a respiratory infection. At 8:00 AM, you administer the prescribed aerosol treatment by nebulizer, with the usual recommended dose. After the treatment, the patient's respiratory rate is reduced from 22 to 14 breaths/min and there is less use of accessory muscles. Wheezing on auscultation is also decreased, although you hear adequate breath sounds bilaterally. He seems less short of breath. At 10:30 AM, he is exhibiting moderate respiratory distress, using accessory muscles, complaining of dyspnea, and has increased wheezing on auscultation. His next aerosol treatment is due at noon. He admits to no chest pain; both wheezes and breath sounds can be auscultated over the entire thorax. You review the pharmacokinetics of isoetharine and find the following:

Onset: 1-3 minutes

Peak effect: Approximately 20 minutes

Duration: Approximately 3 hours or less

What may be a likely cause of the patient's respiratory symptoms? What solutions could you offer?

Answers to Clinical Scenario Questions are found in Appendix A.

References

1. Ariëns EJ, Simonis AM: Drug action: target tissue, dose–response relationships, and receptors. In Teorell T, Dedrick RL, Condliffe PG, editors: *Pharmacology and pharmacokinetics*, New York, 1974, Plenum Press.
2. Laube BL, Benedict W, Dobs AS: The lung as an alternative route of delivery for insulin in controlling postprandial glucose levels in patients with diabetes, *Chest* 114:1734, 1998.
3. Davies DS: Pharmacokinetics of inhaled substances, *Postgrad Med J* 51(suppl 7):695, 1975.
4. Newman SP, Pavia D, Moren F, Sheahan NF, Clarke SW: Deposition of pressurized aerosols in the human respiratory tract, *Thorax* 36:52, 1981.
5. Thorsson L, Edsbäcker S, Conradson T-B: Lung deposition of budesonide from Turbuhaler is twice that from a pressurised metered-dose inhaler P-MDI, *Eur Respir J* 7:1839, 1994.
6. Borgström L: A possible new approach of comparing different inhalers and inhaled substances, *J Aerosol Med* 4:A13, 1991 (abstract).
7. Thorsson L: Influence of inhaler systems on systemic availability, with focus on inhaled corticosteroids, *J Aerosol Med* 8(suppl 3):S29, 1995.

Suggested Readings

Chilvers ER, Sethi T: How receptors work: mechanisms of signal transduction, *Postgrad Med J* 70:813, 1994.
Katzung BG, editor: *Basic & Clinical Pharmacology*, ed 9, New York, 2004, Lange Medical Books/McGraw-Hill.

Chapter 3

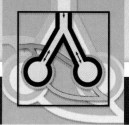

Administration of Aerosolized Agents

DOUGLAS S. GARDENHIRE

CHAPTER OBJECTIVES

After reading this chapter, the reader will be able to:
1. Define aerosol therapy
2. Be able to select an appropriate aerosol medication
   nebulizer on the basis of particle size distributions
3. Discuss aerosol particle size and deposition in the
   lungs
4. Differentiate between the types of aerosol devices
5. Describe the clinical applications of aerosol devices
6. Recommend the use of various aerosol devices

KEY TERMS AND DEFINITIONS

Aerodynamic diameter of a particle — The diameter of a unit-density (1 g/cc) spherical particle having the same terminal settling velocity as the measured particle.

Aerosol — Suspension of liquid or solid particles, between 0.001 and 100 microns (μm) in diameter, in a carrier gas

Aerosol therapy — Delivery of aerosol particles to the lungs

Cascade impactor — A device that uses multiple steps in determining aerosol particles' sizes

Chlorofluorocarbons (CFCs) — A liquefied gas (e.g., Freon) propellant used to administer medication from a metered dose inhaler

Dead volume — The amount of solution that remains in the reservoir of a small volume nebulizer once sputtering begins, causing a decrease in aerosolization

Deposition — Process of particles depositing out of suspension to remain in the lung

Heterodisperse — In reference to the size of particles in an aerosol, meaning the particles are of different sizes

Hydrofluoroalkane (HFA) — A nontoxic liquefied gas propellant used to administer medication from a metered dose inhaler

In vitro — Mechanically simulating the clinical setting; testing in a laboratory.

In vivo — Testing done on animals or humans; clinical testing

Monodisperse — In reference to the size of particles in an aerosol, meaning all particles are the same size

Nebulizer — A device used for making a fine spray or mist, also know as an *aerosol generator*

Penetration — Refers to the depth within the lung reached by particles

Polydisperse — In reference to the size of particles in an aerosol, meaning many different particle sizes

Reservoir device — Global term describing or referring to extension, auxiliary, add-on devices attached to metered dose inhalers (MDIs) for administration. This term could include both "spacer" and "valved holding chamber," defined below

Spacer — Denotes a simple tube or extension device, with no one-way valves to contain the aerosol cloud; its purpose is simply to extend the MDI spray away from the mouth

Stability — Describing the tendency of aerosol particles to remain in suspension

Valved holding chamber — Denotes a spacer device with the addition of one-way valve(s) to contain and hold the aerosol cloud until inspiration occurs

---

The term **aerosol therapy** may be defined as the delivery of aerosol particles to the respiratory tract. At present there are three main uses of aerosol therapy in respiratory care, as follows:

- Humidification of dry inspired gases, using bland aerosols
- Improved mobilization and clearance of respiratory secretions, including sputum induction, using bland aerosols of water, and hypertonic or hypotonic saline
- Delivery of aerosolized drugs to the respiratory tract

This last use of aerosol therapy is the subject of the current chapter, which offers a comprehensive consideration of the delivery of inhaled therapeutic aerosol drugs. As outlined in Chapter 2, the first prerequisite for a drug to exert a therapeutic effect at the target organ is an effective dosage form and route of administration for the target organ. Aerosol generation and delivery to the lung is a complex topic. There is ongoing development of both the technology and the scientific basis of inhaled aerosol administration. This chapter reviews physical principles of aerosol delivery to the airways and aerosol-generating devices for inhalation of drugs. Research findings on aerosol delivery devices and methods of administration are summarized. The general advantages supporting the use of aerosolized drug therapy in respiratory care and the disadvantages with this method of drug delivery are summarized in Box 3-1.

PHYSICAL PRINCIPLES OF INHALED AEROSOL DRUGS

KEY POINT

An *aerosol* is a suspension of solid or liquid particles whose *deposition* in the respiratory tract is determined by *inertial impaction, gravitational settling (sedimentation),* and perhaps less importantly, *diffusion (Brownian motion).*

The term *aerosol* has been used for almost all of the last century; however, inhaled agents use for medicinal purposes date as far back as 4000 years ago.[1] The following definitions apply to inhaled therapeutic aerosols:

Aerosol: Suspension of liquid or solid particles between 0.001 and 100 microns (μm) in diameter in a carrier gas.[2] For pulmonary diagnostic and therapeutic

Box 3-1	Advantages and Disadvantages Seen With the Aerosol Delivery of Drugs

ADVANTAGES
- Aerosol doses are smaller than those for systemic treatment
- Onset of drug action is rapid
- Drug delivery is targeted to the respiratory system for local pulmonary effect
- Systemic side effects are fewer and less severe than with oral or parenteral therapy
- Inhaled drug therapy is painless and relatively convenient
- The lung provides a portal to the body for inhaled aerosol agents intended for systemic effect (e.g., pain control, insulin)

DISADVANTAGES
- The number of variables affecting the dose of aerosol drug delivered to the airways
- Difficulties in dose estimation and dose reproducibility
- Difficulty in coordinating hand action and breathing with metered dose inhalers
- Lack of physician, nurse, and therapist knowledge of device use and administration protocols
- Lack of standardized technical information for practitioners on aerosol-producing devices
- Number of device types and variability of use is confusing to patients and practitioners

KEY POINT

A major factor in lung *penetration* by aerosols is particle size, which is best characterized by the *mass median aerodynamic diameter (MMAD)* for inhaled drugs, because particle mass is a function of the third power of the particle radius. The particle size of interest for pulmonary applications is in the range of 1 to 10 μm, and the *fine particle fraction* is considered to include particles less than 5 μm.

Count mode: The most frequently occurring particle size in the distribution

Count median diameter (CMD): The particle size above and below which 50% of the particles is found (i.e., the size that evenly divides the number of particles in the distribution)

Mass median diameter (MMD) or Mass Median Aerodynamic Diameter (MMAD): The particle size above and below which 50% of the mass of the particles is found (i.e., the size that evenly divides the mass of the particles in the distribution)

Geometric standard deviation (GSD): A measure of the dispersion of a distribution (i.e., the scattering of values from the average), calculated as the ratio of particle size below which 84% of the particles occur to the particle size below which 50% occur, in a lognormal distribution. This will allow you to determine how spread out the particles are in relationship to their size

applications, the particle size range of interest is 1 to 10 μm. Particles in this size range are small enough to exist as a suspension and to enter the lung, and large enough to deposit and contain the required amount of an agent[3,4]

Stability: Describing the tendency of aerosol particles to remain in suspension

Penetration: Referring to the depth within the lung reached by particles

Deposition: Describing the process by which particles deposit out of suspension to remain in the lung

Aerosol-generating devices for orally inhaled drugs have typically had an efficiency of 10% to 15%; that is, only 10% to 15% of a given dose from a device usually reaches the lower respiratory tract, regardless of the device type. Newer aerosol-generating devices are proving exceptions to this lack of efficiency, with 30 to 50% or more of the dose reaching the lungs.

Aerosol Particle Size Distributions

Aerosol particles produced for inhalation into the lungs by inhalant devices such as the metered dose inhaler (MDI), small volume nebulizer (SVN), or dry powder inhaler (DPI) include a range of sizes (**polydisperse** or **heterodisperse**) rather than a single size (**monodisperse**).

The mass median diameter (MMD) or mass median aerodynamic diameter (MMAD), indicates where the mass of drug is centered in a distribution of particle sizes. Aerosol particles are three-dimensional and have volume. Aerosol particles are assumed to be roughly spherical, and the relation of volume (or mass, if all particles have equal densities) to diameter in a sphere is given by

$$V = (4/3)\pi r^3$$

where V = volume and r = radius.

The volume increases or decreases as the third power of the radius of the particle, as seen in the preceding formula. As a result, the bulk of drug mass will be centered in the larger particle sizes. Because it is the mass of the drug entering the lung on which the therapeutic effect is based, it is necessary to know where the mass is centered in a range of particle sizes, in order to know whether that distribution will be efficient for penetration into the respiratory tract and delivery of an adequate dose.

Example

Two hypothetical SVNs, A and B, have the following specifications from the manufacturer:

A	B
CMD = 1.9 μm	CMD = 1.7 μm
MMAD = 3.4 μm	MMAD = 7.9 μm
GSD = 1.2	GSD = 1.6

Although nebulizer B has a smaller CMD compared with nebulizer A, which appears to indicate that it gives smaller particles, it is evident from the respective MMADs that nebulizer B has more particles in a larger size range (>5 μm) compared with nebulizer A. Nebulizer A produces particles whose mass centers within a lower size range (1 to 5 μm), and would be the better nebulizer for treatment of the lower respiratory tract. Inspect aerosol products for their MMAD, as this will be the best way to determine whether the nebulizer will be better suited for the upper or lower airway.

Aerosol generators should be characterized using the MMD for the center of distribution and either the standard deviation or geometric standard deviation to indicate the range of variability of particle size.

Measurement of Particle Size Distributions

Several physical methods are used to measure aerosol particle size distributions, including *cascade impaction* and less commonly *laser scattering*. The **cascade impactor** measures what is termed the *aerodynamic diameter of aerosols*, because the measurement is based on the aerodynamic behavior (sedimentation velocity and impaction characteristics) of the particles in the cascade impactor. Measuring particle size with the *laser scattering method*, the instrument determines the relationship between the intensity and the angle of light scattered from a particle, then calculates the particle size based on the Mie-scattering theory.

Aerodynamic diameter of a particle: The diameter of a unit-density (1 g/cc) spherical particle having the same terminal settling velocity as the measured particle.[1,5]

The principle by which a cascade impactor measures the particle size distribution of an aerosol cloud is illustrated in a simplified diagram in Figure 3-1.

The cascade impactor consists of a series of stages, each of which has progressively smaller orifices through

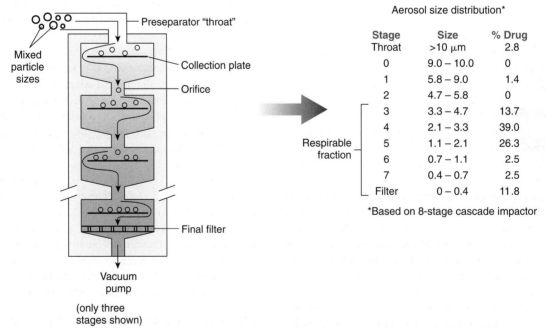

Multistage cascade impactor

Preseparator "throat"
Mixed particle sizes
Collection plate
Orifice
Final filter
Vacuum pump
(only three stages shown)

Aerosol size distribution*

Stage	Size	% Drug
Throat	>10 μm	2.8
0	9.0 – 10.0	0
1	5.8 – 9.0	1.4
2	4.7 – 5.8	0
3	3.3 – 4.7	13.7
4	2.1 – 3.3	39.0
5	1.1 – 2.1	26.3
6	0.7 – 1.1	2.5
7	0.4 – 0.7	2.5
Filter	0 – 0.4	11.8

Respirable fraction (stages 3–7 bracketed)

*Based on 8-stage cascade impactor

FIGURE 3-1 The principle of aerodynamic particle size measurement, using multistage cascade impaction. A series of successively smaller orifices and collection plates separate large and smaller particle sizes. Drug amounts (% drug) shown are actual measures of particle sizes for a sample of albuterol (Ventolin) through a Volumatic reservoir. (Data courtesy J.P. Mitchell, Trudell Medical International Aerosol Laboratory, London, ON, Canada.)

which the aerosol particles must pass. A constant flow draws the particles through the stages. The largest particles are collected on the first stage, and particles not impacting out at this stage move on to the subsequent stages with smaller orifices in the air stream. By means of successively smaller filtration stages, the particles are separated, or *fractionated,* on the basis of size. Any particles leaving the last stage are then collected on a final filter. The amount of aerosol on each stage is then measured by weight or, preferably, by spectrophotometry or high-performance liquid chromatography (HPLC). HPLC measurement is considered the most sensitive technique for quantifying the amount of aerosol on each stage. Because each stage is calibrated for a unit-density sphere of specific diameter, the distribution of aerodynamic diameters can be calculated as the percentage of drug on each stage. The mass median aerodynamic diameter can be determined as the particle size dividing the drug in half. Sources of error in aerodynamic measures include particle bounce, interstage impaction, possible fragmentation of particles, and particle evaporation/condensation.[5] In addition, **in vitro** methods of aerosol measurement may not reflect conditions in the human lung, such as temperature, humidity, inspiratory flow rates, and exhalation phase. Dolovich[6] has reviewed *in vitro* measures used with MDI and auxiliary devices. Feddah and associates found that MDI formulations did better *in vitro* than did DPI formulations with respect to inhaled dose.[7] The same method of aerosol characterization is not necessarily useful or accurate for different methods of aerosol production because of differences in the physical nature of their generation.

Particle Size and Lung Deposition

One of the major factors influencing aerosol deposition in the lung is particle size. The effect of particle size on deposition in the respiratory tract is illustrated in Figure 3-2.

The upper airway (nose and mouth) is efficient in filtering particulate matter, so that generally there is 100% deposition in the nose and mouth of particles larger than 10 and 15 μm, respectively. Particle sizes in the 5- to 10-μm range tend to deposit out in the upper airways and the early airway generations, whereas 1- to 5-μm sizes have a greater probability of reaching the lower respiratory tract from the trachea to the lung periphery. Larger or coarser aerosol particles (>5 μm) may be useful for treating the upper airway (nasopharynx and oropharynx). It is not possible to specify exactly where a given size of particle will deposit in the lung. Particle deposition is a function of several mechanisms, including

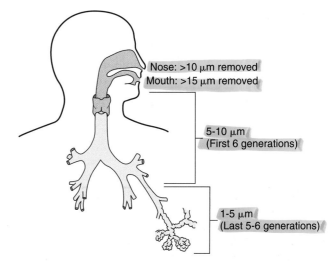

FIGURE 3-2 The effect of aerosol particle size on area of preferential deposition within the airway.

the breathing pattern, so that the site of penetration is treated. For example, tables are often seen listing the percentage of droplets of a given size that will deposit in the lung at each bronchial level.[8] Yu and colleagues[9] observed that optimal deposition in the normal human lung is achieved for particles of 3 μm inhaled with low inspiratory flows of less than 1 L/sec (60 L/min) and tidal volumes of 1 L; total lung deposition is divided almost equally throughout the 23 lung generations.

Fine Particle Fraction

The labels *respirable fraction* and *respirable dose* previously were used to refer to the percentage or fraction of aerosol drug mass in a particle size range with a high probability of penetrating into the lower respiratory tract. These generally have been considered to be in the particle size range of less than 5 or 6 μm. There is rarely an absolute correspondence of lower respiratory tract deposition to this particle size range because of age, disease, and breathing patterns, all of which can affect lung deposition. The more descriptive terms *fine particle fraction (FPF)* and *fine particle dose (FPD)* were proposed for use in place of respirable fraction and respirable dose.[10] Agreement was not reached on what size fraction represents the FPF. These terms may be restricted to particles in the size range of 1 to 3 μm, rather than those less than 5 or 6 μm.

Particle Size and Therapeutic Effect

Because the respiratory tract appears to function as a progressive filter of successively smaller particles from the upper airway to the periphery, specific areas of the respiratory tract may be targeted by various aerosol particle sizes. On the basis of the preceding considerations, the respiratory tract might be segmented according to the following particle size ranges.

Particles Greater Than 10 μm. Particles that are greater than 10 μm are useful to treat the nasopharyngeal and oropharyngeal regions. An example might be a nasal spray for perennial rhinitis, such as a corticosteroid.

Particles 5 to 10 μm. Particles in the range of 5 to 10 μm may shift deposition to the more central airways, although significant oropharyngeal deposition is expected. An example may be a nasal spray, as described above, but there is no one standard device that creates this specific particle size. Most of the aerosol devices use a smaller particle size, which is discussed below.

Particles 2 to 5 μm. As particle size decreases below 5 μm, deposition shifts from the oropharynx and large airways to the overall lower respiratory tract (large airways to periphery).[11] This size range is considered useful for the bronchoactive aerosols currently in use. For example, β-adrenergic receptors have been identified throughout the airway, but with greater density in bronchioles. An interesting study by Clay and colleagues[12] showed greater improvement in midmaximal expiratory flow rates among subjects using a β-adrenergic bronchodilator with an MMAD of 1.8 μm than with an MMAD of 4.6 or 10.3 μm. This was confirmed subsequently by Johnson and associates,[13] who found a greater response to the β-adrenergic bronchodilator albuterol (see Chapter 6) with an MMD of 3.3 μm compared with 7.7 μm. Leach[14] found similar results with a chlorofluorocarbon (CFC)-MDI of albuterol, where particles averaged 3.5–4.0 μm; however, when testing a hydrofluoroalkane (HFA)-MDI, particle size dropped to an average of 1.1 μm. In contrast, cholinergic receptors are numerous in proximal bronchial smooth muscle, but rare in distal bronchioles.[15]

Particles 0.8 to 3.0 μm. Increased delivery of an aerosol to the lung parenchyma, including the terminal airways and alveolar region, could be achieved with particles less than 3 μm.[11] For example, an MMAD of 1 to 2 μm is suggested for peripheral deposition of the antiinfective drug pentamidine, to minimize deposition in and irritation of larger airways and to maximize intraalveolar deposition.[16] However, with the introduction of HFA-MDIs into the market a finer particle size is seen.[14]

Mechanisms of Deposition

Three physical mechanisms usually are considered for aerosol particle deposition in the human lung: *inertial impaction, gravitational settling (sedimentation),* and *diffusion (Brownian motion).*

Inertial Impaction

Inertial impaction is a function of particle size (mass) and velocity, and increases with larger size and higher velocities. In the upper airway and early bronchial generations, particle velocity is highest, airflow tends to be turbulent, and total cross-sectional area of the airway is smallest. These factors favor inertial impaction on the airway wall, especially at airway bifurcations, for larger, fast-moving particles. Deposition by inertial impaction is expected to occur in the first 10 airway generations.[4]

Gravitational Settling

Gravitational settling, or *sedimentation,* is a function of particle size and time. Settling will be greater for larger particles with slow velocities, under the influence of gravity. As particles small enough to escape inertial impaction in earlier airway generations reach the periphery, velocity probably slows and airflow is less turbulent. There is also a shorter distance to the airway wall in smaller, peripheral airways, favoring impaction resulting from settling. The probability of deposition by sedimentation is highest in the last five or six airway generations.[4] Because the process of sedimentation is time dependent, the end-inspiratory breath-hold should maximize deposition in the periphery. The rate of settling is proportional to the square of the particle size. For a 5-μm-diameter particle, the settling rate is reported to be 0.7 mm/sec.[17] The encouragement of a breath-hold can increase settling of particles; however, depending on particle size, a particle may not fall out of suspension.

Diffusion (Brownian Motion)

Diffusion (Brownian motion) affects particles of less than 1 μm and is a function of time and random molecular motion. Particles between 0.1 and 1.0 μm may remain suspended or even exhaled, because the time required to diffuse to the airway surface tends to be greater than the inspiratory time of a normal breath.[18] The importance of diffusion for lung deposition of therapeutic aerosols is debatable, because the size range involved contains so little drug mass and gives such stability.

Effect of Temperature and Humidity

Prediction of particle deposition with therapeutic aerosols is further complicated by the fact that the aerosol is generated under relatively dry ambient conditions and then taken into the airway, where temperature and humidity rapidly increase to saturation at 37° C. Inhaled aerosol drugs are not only heterodisperse in size but are also *hygroscopic* (i.e., readily absorbing moisture). For example, between ambient and BTPS conditions, the MMAD of cromolyn sodium powder particles from an MDI increases from 2.31 to 3.02 µm.[19,20] Fuller and colleagues[21] measured 50% less aerosol for ventilator delivery through an endotracheal tube when using an *in vitro* model based on a jet nebulizer in warm, humidified air compared with warm, nonhumidified air.

AEROSOL DEVICES FOR DRUG DELIVERY

KEY POINT

Common devices for the delivery of inhaled aerosol drugs include *nebulizers, metered dose inhalers,* and *dry powder inhalers. Reservoir devices,* such as spacers and holding chambers, can reduce oropharyngeal deposition of drug and simplify hand–breathing coordination with MDIs. Proper use of these aerosol-generating devices is absolutely necessary to ensure adequate lung delivery, and correct use should be understood by practitioners. Traditional aerosol-generating devices all deliver about 10 to 15% of the dose produced to the lung, although different types of devices vary in their loss patterns.

Several important questions arise concerning aerosol devices. How should they be quantitatively described for clinicians? Are there differences in clinical effect with different devices, including spacer and reservoir accessories? What is the correct or optimal use of different types of devices? With all aerosol delivery devices, respiratory care personnel should carefully review instructional materials and package inserts to train patients in their correct use. Knowledge of aerosol delivery devices by medical personnel, together with the ability to teach patients in their correct use, is necessary for effective drug delivery. Respiratory care practitioners have been shown to receive formal education in the use of various aerosol devices more often than nursing staff or physicians. Both knowledge and demonstration scores with MDIs, a reservoir device, and a DPI were higher for respiratory therapists than for registered nurses or physicians in a study by Hanania and associates.[22] Dolovich and colleagues give eight questions that should be asked when selecting an aerosol device.[23]

1. In what devices is the desired drug available?
2. What device is the patient likely to be able to use properly, given age and clinical setting (e.g., home, hospital)?
3. For which device and drug combination is reimbursement available?
4. Which device is least expensive?
5. Can you use the same device for all inhaled drugs that the patient is taking?
6. Which device is the most convenient for the patient or family?
7. How durable is the device?
8. Does the patient or practitioner have a specific device preference?

Ultrasonic Nebulizers

The term **nebulizer** encompasses a variety of devices that operate on different physical principles to generate an aerosol from a drug solution. Ultrasonic nebulizers (USNs) are electric-powered devices operating on the piezoelectric principle and capable of high output. Particle sizes vary by brand. A generic illustration of a USN is given in Figure 3-3. Although these devices have not been used as routinely for aerosolization of drugs as others (described below), they have been reintroduced as portable, small units that can operate on direct current (DC) voltage. Such units have several advantages and some disadvantages, as listed in Box 3-2.

At the frequencies used in medical devices, there are several effects with the potential for altering drug activity of the nebulizer solution. Most of the energy produced during ultrasonic nebulization is dissipated as heat. Protein and other heat-sensitive (or *thermolabile*) formulations can be denatured by heat, especially if the melting temperature of the protein is reached. For example, insulin was shown to be inactivated by USN delivery.[24] Most currently available inhaled drugs are stable with use of a USN.[25] However, the breakdown of a drug can be a cumulative effect of surface denaturation, heat, cavitation, and direct pressure effects in a USN.[25] Drug solutions must be tested by ultrasonic delivery to determine that activity is preserved, particularly when proteins or liposomes are nebulized. Refer to the manufacturer's directions to help determine which device should be used for each drug.

Small Particle Aerosol Generator

The small particle aerosol generator (SPAG) device is a large reservoir nebulizer, capable of holding 300 mL of solution for long periods of nebulization. It operates on a jet-shearing principle. The device was used during the clinical trials of the aerosolized antiviral drug ribavirin (Virazole) and is marketed for delivery of that drug by its manufacturer (Valeant Pharmaceuticals International,

Ultrasonic Nebulizer

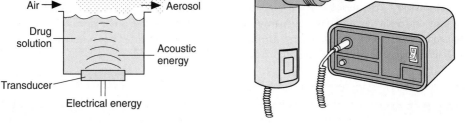

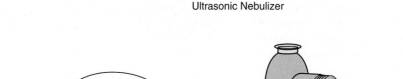

FIGURE 3-3 Illustration of the principle of ultrasonic nebulization, with an example of a portable device used to aerosolize medications.

Box 3-2	Advantages and Disadvantages of Portable Ultrasonic Drug Nebulizers

ADVANTAGES
- Small size
- Rapid nebulization with shorter treatment times
- Smaller drug amounts with no diluent for filling volume
- Can be used during car travel or camping

DISADVANTAGES
- Expense
- Fragility, lack of durability
- Requires electrical source (either AC or DC)
- Possible degrading effect on drug must be determined

Aliso Viejo, CA). The SPAG unit is described more fully when ribavirin is discussed in Chapter 13.

Small Volume Nebulizers

> **KEY POINT**
>
> Most of the loss with an SVN occurs in the device, whereas an MDI and a DPI lose drug in the mouth and gastrointestinal tract. Addition of a reservoir device to an MDI shifts loss from the throat to the reservoir.

Small volume nebulizer (SVN) devices are small reservoir, gas-powered (pneumatic) aerosol generators, also referred to as *handheld nebulizers (HHNs)* or as *updraft nebulizers* or *unit dose nebulizers (UDNs)*. A generic illustration is given in Figure 3-4. They use a jet-shearing principle for creation of an aerosol from the drug solution. An external source of compressed gas is directed

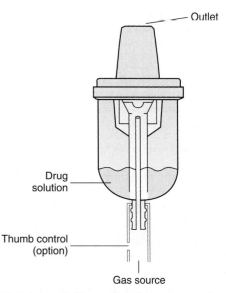

FIGURE 3-4 A generic illustration of a gas-powered small volume nebulizer with a thumb control attachment to allow for inspiratory nebulization only when the control port is occluded.

through a narrow orifice inside the reservoir cup. The expanding gas creates a localized negative pressure, drawing the drug solution up feeder tubes. As the liquid enters the gas stream, droplets are formed from gas turbulence and impaction on baffles. Smaller particle sizes are emitted after the baffling process. Larger liquid particles are recirculated back to the reservoir. There is significant evaporation of the aqueous solution with gas-powered nebulization. Nebulizer temperatures can fall from ambient to approximately 10° C within minutes because of the latent heat of vaporization. With evaporation and constant recirculation, drug solute becomes increasingly concentrated, up to 150 to 300% of the original concentration.[26] Box 3-3 summarizes the advantages and disadvantages of these types of nebulizing devices.

Because SVNs are often used with infants or with patients in acute respiratory distress, slow breathing and an inspiratory pause may not be feasible or obtainable. One of the main advantages of SVNs is that dose delivery occurs over 60 to 90 breaths, rather than in one or two inhalations. Thus a single ineffective breath will not destroy the efficacy of the treatment. Several factors must be considered with gas-powered nebulizers: residual or "dead volume," flow rate, filling volume, temperature, output rate, continuous versus inspiratory nebulization, type of power gas, length of treatment time, and physical nature of the solution to be nebulized. Some of these factors are reviewed in greater detail below. Recommendations for the use of SVNs, based on the considerations reviewed and the studies available, are summarized in Appendix C.

Dead Volume

Gas-powered nebulizers do not aerosolize below a minimal volume, termed the **dead volume,** which is the amount of drug solution remaining in the reservoir when the device begins to sputter, and aerosolization ceases. This volume can vary with the brand of nebulizer, but is on the order of 0.5 to 1.0 mL. This is the primary reason why diluent, which is effectively additional volume, is added to 0.5 mL of a bronchodilator solution. One-half of one milliliter does not nebulize well, although the needed dose is present. Adding diluent does not alter the amount of drug (dose) in the nebulizer, but simply "expands" the solution volume. The concentration of the solution is less, not the amount of drug (see Chapter 4 for further discussion). Drug loss with nebulization can also occur into the ambient air. As a result of these factors, the amount of dose available from a nebulizer is considerably less than the dose placed into the reservoir. Kradjan and Lakshminarayan[27] found that under clinical conditions of nebulization until sputter, approximately 35 to 60% of a drug solution was delivered from the nebulizer. Even with vigorous agitation, this amount increased to only 53 to 72%. A study by Shim and Williams[28] found that only 40 to 52% of the total dose was delivered from gas-powered nebulizers. In a positive-pressure circuit, this efficiency may decrease further, to approximately 30% of the total dose.[29] Evaporation of an aqueous solution will not only cause cooling of the nebulizer and liquid but can also increase

Box 3-3	Advantages and Disadvantages of Small Volume Nebulizers (SVNs)

ADVANTAGES
- Ability to aerosolize many drug solutions
- Ability to aerosolize drug mixtures (i.e., more than one drug) with suitable testing of drug activity
- Minimal coordination required for inhalation
- Useful in very young or very old, debilitated patients or those in acute distress
- Effective with low inspiratory flows or volumes
- Inspiratory pause (breath hold) not required for efficacy
- Drug concentrations can be modified if desired

DISADVANTAGES
- The equipment required for use is expensive and cumbersome.
- Treatment times are somewhat lengthy for traditional nebulizers compared with other aerosol devices and other routes of administration.
- There is variability in performance characteristics among different brands.
- Contamination is possible with inadequate cleaning.
- A wet, cold spray occurs with mask delivery.
- An external power source, either electricity or compressed gas, is needed.

the concentration of solute in the residual (dead) volume. If this dead volume is not discarded and the nebulizer rinsed, an increasingly concentrated solution and drug dose could be administered with subsequent treatments.

Filling Volume and Treatment Time

Figure 3-5 demonstrates the relation of volume and flow rate to the time of nebulization, based on the work of Hess and associates,[30] presented as the pooled average performance of 17 nebulizer brands. Increasing the volume will increase the time of effective nebulization, at any given flow rate. Below 2 mL, most pneumatic nebulizers do not perform well because the volume is close to the dead volume, that is, the residual amount that does not nebulize. At 6 mL, an excessively long time is required for treatment (>10 minutes) with most brands. Although 5 minutes seems to be a short time, even this can be inconveniently long as a way of taking medication three or four times a day; some patients have difficulty in taking a pill four times a day, an approximately 2- to 3-second activity. Patient compliance is directly proportional to convenience. Given the volume requirements of nebulizers for efficient operation and the need for relatively brief treatments, a volume between 3 and 5 mL of solution is recommended. Increasing the volume will also decrease the concentration of drug remaining in the dead volume when nebulization ceases.[30] This will

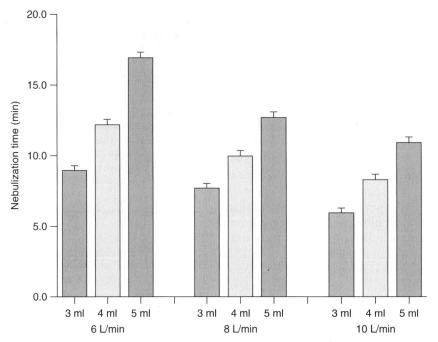

FIGURE 3-5 The relationship of volume and flow rate to time of nebulization averaged for 17 gas-powered nebulizers. (From Hess D, Fisher D, Williams P, Pooler S, Kacmarek RM: Medication nebulizer performance: effects of diluent volume, nebulizer flow, and nebulizer band, *Chest* 110:498, 1996.)

increase the dose of drug available to the patient, although treatment times do increase also, at any given flow rate.

Effect of Flow Rate

A second practical question concerns the flow rate at which to power pneumatic nebulizers. The flow rate affects two variables: the length of treatment time and the size of the particles produced. Figure 3-5 illustrates the interaction between volume and flow rate in determining time of nebulization. At a flow rate of 6 L/min, a volume of 3 mL requires less than 10 minutes; at 10 L/min, a volume of 5 mL can be nebulized in approximately 10 minutes. Figure 3-6 demonstrates the effect of flow rates on particle size of the aerosol produced, averaged for the 17 nebulizers studied by Hess and associates.[30] With pneumatically powered nebulizers, increasing the flow rate will decrease the particle size and shift the MMAD lower. On the basis of results of Hess and colleagues in Figures 3-5 and 3-6, an average optimal volume and flow rate for many nebulizers is a volume of 5 mL with a 10-L/min flow rate. Treatment time is kept to approximately 10 minutes or less, available drug is maximized, and the MMAD is minimized. It must be emphasized that variability among different brands will affect nebulizer performance with these recommendations.

Type of Power Gas

Use of gases other than oxygen or air can change the performance characteristics of a nebulizer. Hess and associates[30] showed that the use of heliox (a mixture of helium and oxygen) to nebulize albuterol caused particle size and inhaled drug mass to decrease, along with a more than twofold increase in nebulization time. Increasing the flow of heliox returned output to that seen with air.[31] Selecting the appropriate gas to power a nebulizer will need to be done by the practitioner on the basis of patient data, or policy and procedure set by the institution. Oxygen has always been used because of its availability; however, with newer constructions air is becoming standard at the bedside. Using air to control the oxygen a patient receives may be of importance to practitioners.

Type of Solution

Droplet size of nebulized solutions is related to surface tension and viscosity of the solution, and is partially determined as well by the baffles in the device.[32] Recommended filling volumes and flow rates are suitable for the aqueous bronchodilator solutions usually administered with these devices. However, the volumes and flow rates suggested may require modification for

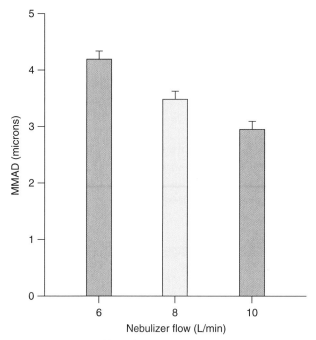

FIGURE 3-6 The effect of power gas flow rate on the mass median aerodynamic diameter (MMAD) of aerosol particles produced on average by 17 gas-powered nebulizers. (From Hess D, Fisher D, Williams P, Pooler S, Kacmarek RM: Medication nebulizer performance: effects of diluent volume, nebulizer flow, and nebulizer band, *Chest* 110:498, 1996.)

TABLE 3-1	
Representative Drug–Device Combinations Tested for Nebulizer Drug Delivery	
Drug	**Nebulizer**
Tobramycin	PARI LC PLUS (with DeVilbiss Pulmo-Aide compressor)
Dornase alfa	Hudson T Updraft II, Acorn II, PARI LC JET PLUS (with Pulmo-Aide or PARI compressors)
Levalbuterol	PARI LC PLUS
Pentamidine	RESPIRGARD
Ribavirin	Small particle aerosol generator

some drug solutions, such as pentamidine, or antibiotics, which have different physical characteristics and viscosities. Administration by SVN is described when these drugs are discussed. For example, higher viscosity antibiotic solutions of gentamicin or carbenicillin require 10- to 12-L/min power gas flow rates to produce suitably small aerosol particles for inhalation with some jet nebulizers.[33] Some disposable nebulizers may exhibit greater variability in performance or not achieve adequate output characteristics with new or nonbronchodilator drug solutions. The performance of an SVN should be tested with various drug solutions, and newly introduced nebulizer drugs should be tested with an intended nebulizer system to ensure adequate performance. It must be noted that it is best to nebulize only drugs that have been manufactured for nebulization; however, it is not uncommon to nebulize agents intended for a different route of administration. Nebulizers not tested for performance with a new or unknown drug solution cannot be assumed to produce adequate output and particle sizes. As indicated in Chapter 2 in the review of L/T ratios and the pharmacokinetics of inhaled aerosol drugs, efficiency of lung delivery is a function of *both*

drug and device. The drug–device combination should be tested before clinical use. Table 3-1 lists some tested and adequate drug–device combinations for nebulizer delivery. Additives to the drug solution can also affect aerosol characteristics and drug delivery.

Development of Various Nebulizer Designs

The traditional jet nebulizer or SVN, as commonly used, exhibits a large amount of drug wastage, especially within the device itself. For a traditional SVN, the typical emitted dose and loss pattern is as follows[34]:

- Lung deposition, 12.4 (4.5)
- Oropharynx, 1.5 (0.9)
- Device loss, 66.3 (8.6)
- Exhaled, 19.7 (3.9)

The data represented are for an Inspiron MiniNeb powered by compressed air at 8 L/min, using radiolabeled human serum albumin in saline. It should be noted that the overall efficiency in lung deposition of 10 to 15% of the total drug dose is not significantly better than with most MDI or DPI devices used clinically in the past, as discussed subsequently in the section on clinical application and equivalence of various devices. Nebulizers, as well as MDIs and DPIs, are undergoing an evolutionary transition to greater efficiency. The spectrum of gas-powered nebulizer design and operation has been conceptualized into three categories by Dennis[26] and is illustrated in Figure 3-7.

1. *Constant output:* This is the traditional nebulizer, in which aerosol is produced constantly during inspiration and exhalation. Emitted aerosol is lost to the environment during exhalation or breath hold. This loss is the basis for using 6 inches of expiratory reservoir tubing, which reduces but does not eliminate ambient contamination.

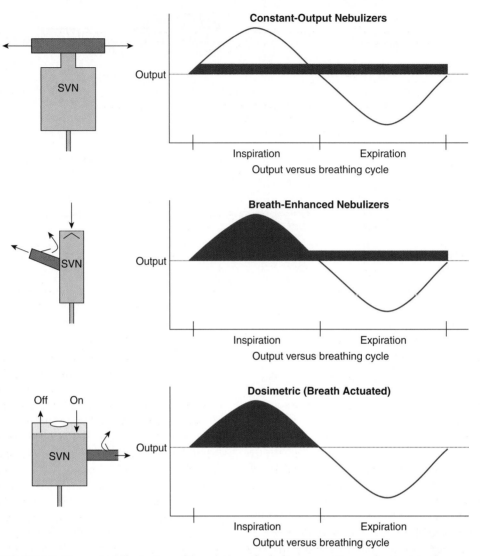

FIGURE 3-7 Conceptual illustration of the relation of nebulizer generation and output to the inspiratory and expiratory phases. (Based on concept introduced by Dennis JH: A review of issues relating to nebulizer standards, *J Aerosol Med* 11[suppl 1]:S73, 1998.)

2. *Breath enhanced:* Nebulizer operation allows more aerosol release during inspiration with decreased output during exhalation or breath hold. The PARI LC nebulizers are an example of this type. Aerosol is produced during inspiration and exhalation, but expired gas is routed through a one-way valve in the mouthpiece, with containment of aerosol in the reservoir and reduced ambient loss. Inspired gas comes through the reservoir via another one-way valve.

3. *Dosimetric:* Aerosol is released only during inspiration and all released aerosol is available for patient inhalation. In some designs, such as the AeroEclipse or the Circulaire, aerosol is generated and released only during inspiration. In these designs, no aerosol is lost during expiration and there is usually substantial reduction in the dead volume loss of drug. On the basis of the concept of dosimetric described by Dennis,[26] any constant-output nebulizer could be a dosimetric nebulizer if a thumb control was used, so that dose delivery occurs only on inspiration, with no nebulization during expiration.

The newest technology is *vibrating plate technology*. These devices use a vibrating plate or mesh with multiple apertures (small holes), which allow the liquid to generate an aerosol. These devices are battery powered

TABLE 3-2			

Examples of Newer Nebulizer Designs* With Selected Features and Solutions Tested

Nebulizer	Design Features	Drug(S) Studied	Lung Deposition (% of emitted dose)
AeroEclipse	Gas powered, breath actuated; aerosol generated only during inspiratory effort	Various, including β agonists	39%
AERx	Battery powered, unit-dose drug blister packs; microprocessor-controlled delivery based on inspiratory flow, volumes	Insulin, morphine	Up to 75–80%
Respimat Soft Mist	Spring-powered, button-actuated multidose device, with single-breath unit drug dose delivery and "soft mist" plume	Fenoterol, flunisolide	30–40%
iNeb	Battery powered, breath-actuated adaptive aerosol delivery, specific metering chambers for unit dose delivery	Iloprost	82-100%

Data from Dolovich M: New propellant-free technologies under investigation, *J Aerosol Med* 12(suppl 1):S9, 1999.
DTPA, Diethylenetriaminepentaacetic acid.
*All the devices would be categorized as dosimetric.

and do not require a gas source, making them portable. The device creates a fine mist with no internal baffling system by way of the vibrating element and about 1000 holes on an electroformed sheet. Another benefit of this technology is that it leaves very little if any dead volume in the nebulizer. Some of the manufacturers have developed the technology to be used with mechanical ventilation. Another device developed for use with mechanical ventilation is an intratracheal catheter that allows targeted aerosol delivery via an endotracheal tube or bronchoscope. A description of both can be found in the review by Dhand.[35]

It is evident that the direction of development in nebulizer design is toward higher efficiency in dose release and shorter treatment times, while preserving the ease of patient use traditionally seen. Greater efficiency may lessen the required drug dose in the device, similar to what is seen with MDIs when compared with traditional nebulizers. In effect, a dosimetric or breath-controlled nebulizer becomes a "metered dose liquid inhaler," a term used by Dolovich.[36] Newer nebulizer devices are described briefly in Table 3-2 and include both devices in development and those available commercially. Comparisons have been made by Rau and associates and can be reviewed further in the literature.[37]

Metered Dose Inhalers

Metered dose inhalers (MDIs) have been used in respiratory therapy for the past 60 years.[38] These devices are small, pressurized canisters for oral or nasal inhalation of aerosol drugs and contain multiple doses of accurately metered drug.

Technical Description

There are five major components found in an MDI: drug, propellant/excipient mixture, canister, metering valve, and mouthpiece/actuator. Figure 3-8 illustrates this device. The drug in an MDI is either a suspension of micronized powder in a liquefied propellant or a solution of the active ingredient in a cosolvent (usually ethanol) mixed with the propellant. Dispersing agents, or *surfactants,* are added to prevent aggregation of drug particles and to lubricate the valve mechanism, thereby maintaining suitable particle sizes in the aerosol plume produced in **chlorofluorocarbon (CFC)** (e.g., Freon) devices. These surfactants are not soluble in hydrofluoroalkane (HFA) devices.[39] Surfactants currently used include oleic acid, sorbitan trioleate (also termed *Span 85*), or soya lecithin. The use of ethanol as a cosolvent in HFA formulations makes the surfactants more soluble; however, they have been found to make the drug itself more soluble. Flavoring agents also may be added. A detailed technical description of the complexities involved in producing an MDI is offered by Newman.[40]

When the canister is depressed into the actuator (see Figure 3-8), the drug-propellant mixture in the metering valve is released under pressure. The liquid propellant rapidly expands and vaporizes, or "flashes," as it ejects from the pressurized valve into ambient pressure. This expansion and vaporization shatters the liquid stream into an aerosol. The initial vaporization of propellant causes cooling of the liquid–gas aerosol suspension, which can be felt if discharged onto the skin; however,

Metered Dose Inhaler

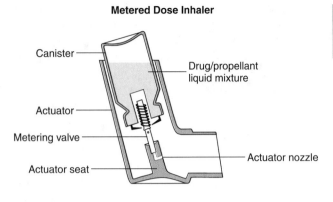

Metering Valve Function

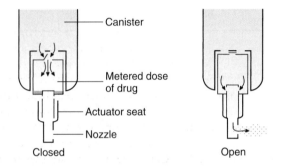

FIGURE 3-8 The major components of a metered dose inhaler, with an illustration of the function of the metering valve. Both oral and nasal adapters are shown.

HFA versions have a much "warmer" spray temperature. The cold mist from a CFC spray may cause users to stop inhaling as the cold aerosol hits the oropharynx. On release, the metering valve refills with the mixture of drug and propellant from the bulk of the canister and is ready for the next discharge. The metering valve varies from 25 to 100 μL in volume.[40]

The propellants originally used as a power source with MDIs to create an aerosol are blends of liquefied gas (CFCs) (e.g., Freon). However, because of the ban on CFCs after the year 2008, HFAs will be the power source used. Advantages and disadvantages of drug delivery by MDI are listed in Box 3-4.

Correct Use of a Metered Dose Inhaler

The effectiveness of treatment with an aerosolized drug delivered by an MDI depends on correct use of the device. The major problem with MDI devices is the difficulty of patient use.[41] The most common error noted is the failure to coordinate inhalation and actuation

---

Box 3-4	Advantages and Disadvantages of Metered Dose Inhaler (MDI) Aerosol Devices

ADVANTAGES
- MDIs are portable and compact.
- Drug delivery is efficient.
- Treatment time is short.
- They are easy to use.
- More than 100 doses are available.
- Fine particle sizes are available in HFA formulations.

DISADVANTAGES
- Complex hand–breathing coordination is required.
- Drug concentrations are fixed.
- Canister depletion is difficult to determine accurately.
- Reactions to the propellants may occur in a small percentage of patients.
- High oropharyngeal impaction and loss occur if an extension device is not used.
- Foreign body aspiration of coins and debris from the mouthpiece can occur.*
- CFCs are released into the environment until replacement by non-CFC propellants.

*Data from Hannan SE, Pratt DS, Hannan JM, Brienza LT: Foreign body aspiration associated with the use of an aerosol inhaler, *Am J Respir Dis* 129:1205, 1984; Schultz CH, Hargarten SW, Babbitt J: Inhalation of a coin and a capsule from a metered-dose inhaler [letter], *N Engl J Med* 325:432, 1991.
CFCs, Chlorofluorocarbons; *HFA,* hydrofluoroalkane.

---

of the inhaler (hand–breathing incoordination). Other problems include a too-rapid inspiratory flow rate, inadequate or missing breath-hold after inhalation, failure to shake and mix canister contents, cessation of inspiration as the aerosol strikes the throat, actuation of the MDI at total lung capacity, inhaling through the nose, and exhaling during actuation. Evidence indicates that 50 to 70% of patients do not use MDIs correctly.[23] In addition, physician, nurse, and respiratory therapist knowledge of correct MDI use is often inadequate for patient education.[23]

Recommendations on use of MDIs are provided in Appendix C.

Factors Affecting Metered Dose Inhaler Performance

The accuracy and consistency of dose from MDIs may be more sensitive to handling practices than previously thought. Research on the drug content of sprays of albuterol by MDI has shown that various factors affect dose consistency.

Loss of Dose. *Loss of dose* refers to the loss of drug content in the valve even though propellant may seem to discharge a normal dose. A dose with less than the nominal amount of drug has been noted to occur on first actuating an albuterol MDI when the canister is stored in the valve-down position, even after only a few hours and with shaking before discharge. The loss of dose ranged from 25% to more than 50% in the studies referenced.[42,43] This was not observed with storage in a valve-up position. Other drug formulations may increase or decrease drug concentration in the first discharge, after standing unused; this would need to be determined for each product. These findings suggest that the canister be stored valve-up between uses and that a waste dose be discharged if more than 4 hours have elapsed with the valve down, when using albuterol by MDI. However, the new HFA formulation does not suffer from loss of dose.[14]

Shaking the Canister. Many of the drugs in MDI formulation are suspensions that can separate from the propellants on standing *(creaming)*.[43] This should not affect the dose in the valve, which was filled after the previous actuation. However, if the suspended drug is either lighter or heavier than the propellant and separation occurs, a second actuation could deliver more or less concentrated drug if the canister is not shaken to mix the propellant and drug suspension thoroughly. The MDI should be shaken *before* the first actuation after standing, so that the metering valve refills with adequately mixed suspension from the canister. Everard and colleagues[43] found that not shaking an albuterol canister before use and after the canister has been standing upright overnight led to a 26% reduction in total dose and a 36% reduction in particles less than 6.8 µm. This occurred despite wasting two discharges before the measurement. Rubin and Durotoye[44] found similar results with CFC inhalers, but HFA beclomethasone did not seem to be influenced by shaking of the canister.

Timing of Actuation Intervals. A pause of 1 to 5 minutes has been advocated between each puff of a bronchodilator from an MDI, in an attempt to improve distribution of the inhaled drug in the lung.[45] The study by Everard and colleagues[43] found that two actuations of albuterol MDI 1 second apart caused no change in total drug output, although there was a 15.8% decrease in the amount of particles below 6.8 µm. However, four actuations 1 second apart led to significant reductions in dose output. Concern over cooling of the MDI valve with rapid actuations does not seem to be supported by the results presented by Everard and colleagues. Loss of dose probably occurs as a result of turbulence and coalescence of particles with more than two rapid actuations. Clinically, a pause between puffs from an MDI

has not been found to be beneficial in routine maintenance therapy. Pedersen[46] showed no difference in forced expiratory volume in 1 second (FEV_1) with a 3- and 10-minute divided dose under nonacute basic maintenance conditions. This was found to be the case for both a β agonist (terbutaline) and a corticosteroid (budesonide) in preadolescents.[47] However, during asthma exacerbations with acute wheezing, a pause between puffs resulted in significantly improved bronchodilation, with greater effect using a 10-minute pause.[45]

There is no consensus on any of the preceding information covered. It is best to educate the healthcare practitioner and patient to apply a systematic approach when using an MDI. The better the routine and consistency in using this device, the more likely it is that patients will benefit.

Open-Mouth Versus Closed-Mouth Use of a Metered Dose Inhaler. Actuating the MDI several centimeters in front of the open mouth theoretically allows for slowing of the particle velocity and evaporation of aerosol droplets, resulting in less oropharyngeal impaction and loss. This maneuver further complicates the use of the MDI. Studies with both children and adults have shown no difference in lung function between an open-mouth and a closed-mouth technique in use of a bronchodilator.[48,49] Consequently, the simpler technique should be preferred. If oropharyngeal impaction is undesirable, as in the case of inhaled corticosteroids, or if accurate timing between actuations is a problem, as is sometimes the case for older patients, an extension device (spacer or holding chamber) should be used. It should be noted that more drug will be inhaled from the MDI with the use of an extension device and is as good as a standard small volume nebulizer.[23]

Loss of Prime. *Loss of prime* refers to the loss of propellant from the metering valve of the MDI.[50] When this occurs, little or no drug will be discharged on actuation; this can be felt and heard by a user. Loss of prime usually takes days or weeks to occur; regular use of the MDI should prevent this. Shaking of the canister and discharge of a waste dose are suggested after long periods of no use, to prime the valve with propellant and drug.

Storage Temperature. Data indicate that dose delivery from CFC-propelled MDIs of albuterol decreases at lower temperatures. A significant decrease of 65 to 70% of the usual dose has been observed at 10° C. An even greater drop was observed in a fine particle mass (<4.7 µm), with approximately 75% of the usual dose at 10° C and only 25% at 10° C. No medication was delivered at −20° C.[51] In contrast, HFA-propelled albuterol remained constant in total dose over the range of −20 to 20° C.

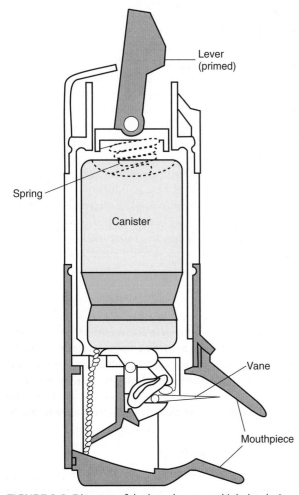

FIGURE 3-9 Diagram of the breath-actuated inhaler device marketed for pirbuterol (Maxair).

The fine particle mass of the CFC-free formulation decreased significantly only at $-20°$ C, delivering approximately 60% of the initial fine particle dose. Temperature effects such as these are likely to be relevant only for outdoor use of MDI canisters in extreme weather.

Breath-actuated Inhalers

A type of device to simplify MDI use is a breath-actuated adapter (Figure 3-9). In the United States the adrenergic bronchodilator pirbuterol (Maxair; see Chapter 6) is marketed as a breath-actuated inhaler. Breath-actuated inhalers offer an alternative for individuals who find it difficult to coordinate MDI actuation with inhalation. The device is described by Newman,[40] Newman and associates,[52] and Baum and Bryant.[53]

The Autohaler. A conventional pressurized MDI (pMDI) canister is fitted within the Autohaler actuator, as seen in Figure 3-9. The MDI canister is triggered by a spring, through a triggering mechanism activated when the patient inhales. To use, the device is primed, or "cocked," by raising the lever on top of the adapter. This applies pressure to the canister. The canister cannot move downward because of a vane in the mouthpiece. As the patient inhales at flow rates of 22 to 26 L/min, the vane lifts, the spring forces the canister downward, and a metered dose is released. The device is reset by lowering the lever to its resting position, which allows the MDI valve to refill.

Other Devices. There are a number of other devices on the market, or that are currently being brought to market, in the United Sates. These devices include Easi-Breathe, K-Haler, MD Turbo, Xcelovent, and SmartMist. All these devices are similar to the Autohaler in that they assist the patient in actuating a dose of drug for inhalation. More detailed information can be found in the article by Newman.[40]

Hydrofluoroalkane (Nonchlorofluorocarbon) Propellants

The potential for damage to the protective ozone layer in the earth's atmosphere by CFCs has been noted since 1974. One CFC molecule can destroy 100,000 molecules of stratospheric ozone. The U.S. Food and Drug Administration (FDA) has set the date of December 31, 2008 for the removal of single-ingredient albuterol CFC-MDIs. There is a medical exemption for MDIs that is renewable on a yearly basis. Hydrofluorocarbons (HFCs), also termed **hydrofluoroalkanes (HFAs)**, have been identified as propellants that are nontoxic to the atmosphere and to the patient, and that have properties suitable for MDI aerosol generation. In particular, HFA 134a has a vapor pressure similar to that of CFC 12, the CFC propellant most commonly used. The structure of HFA 134a is illustrated in Figure 3-10 and compared with that of CFC 12. Replacement of CFC propellants has led to overall reengineering of MDI components (valve, seals, exit orifice, and drug formulation), which has improved MDI performance. Some of the differences, such as the lower plume force (Figure 3-11) and warmer plume temperature, cause patients who have used CFC-propelled MDI formulations to think there is reduced or no drug delivery occurring with the HFA formulation of albuterol.[14]

Equivalence and Safety. The efficacy and safety of all reformulated HFA drugs have been studied. It should be noted that the amount of drug may have changed from the CFC form; however, many companies have reformulated with the same strength and dose.

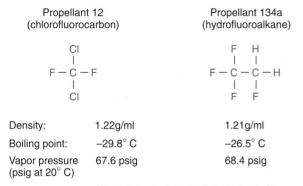

Propellant 12
(chlorofluorocarbon)

Propellant 134a
(hydrofluoroalkane)

Density:	1.22g/ml	1.21g/ml
Boiling point:	−29.8° C	−26.5° C
Vapor pressure (psig at 20° C)	67.6 psig	68.4 psig

FIGURE 3-10 Structure and properties of a CFC propellant, CFC 12, and a non-CFC propellant, HFA 134a, used in pressurized metered dose inhaler drug formulations.

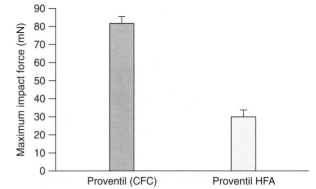

FIGURE 3-11 Measures of plume force exiting a metered dose inhaler for CFC- and HFA-propelled albuterol (Proventil and Proventil HFA). (Data from Ross DL, Gabrio BJ: Advances in metered dose inhaler technology with the development of a chlorofluorocarbon-free drug delivery system, *J Aerosol Med* 12:151, 1999.)

Improved Drug Delivery With Hydrofluoroalkane Formulation. Although equivalent drug amounts and effects were found with the drugs, the reengineering of the MDI for HFA propellant can result in significant improvements in performance and in particular in lung deposition of the aerosol drug. The traditional amount of 10% for lung deposition has been increased more than fivefold with some HFA formulations.[54] Figure 3-12 illustrates a comparison of lung delivery between HFA-based and CFC-based MDI systems. Notice the increase in lung delivery when using the HFA formulation.

Metered Dose Inhaler Reservoir Devices

Figure 3-13 is an illustration of a generic reservoir device. Extension, or reservoir, devices were introduced primarily to simplify the complex coordination of aiming, actuation, and breathing with an MDI. Reservoir devices can modify the aerosol discharged from an MDI in the following three ways:

1. Such devices allow space and time for more vaporization of the propellants and evaporation of initially large particles to smaller sizes.
2. Reservoirs allow the high initial velocity of particles released from an MDI to slow before reaching the oropharynx. Particles discharged from the actuator nozzle have velocities exceeding 30 m/sec. By holding the actuator 4 cm in front of the mouth or by using an extension device, this velocity is allowed to slow.[55]
3. As holding chambers for the aerosol cloud released, reservoir devices separate the actuation of the canister from the inhalation and simplify the coordination required for good use.

The combined effect of the first two advantages reduces oropharyngeal deposition. This will reduce the amount of drug swallowed and thereby absorbed from the gastrointestinal tract and also reduce any local oropharyngeal side effects, such as those seen with inhaled corticosteroids. The advantages and disadvantages of reservoir devices are summarized in Box 3-5.

Reservoir Devices

More than a dozen varieties of reservoir devices are now available, and the size ranges from 70–80 to 750 mL for some European brands; some are available with a mask. Numerous terms are used to refer to such devices, including *spacer, reservoir, auxiliary device, extension device, holding chamber,* and *add-on device.* Some distinction of terms may be useful to denote significant design differences among these devices. The following terminology is offered, partially based on Dolovich[56]:

Reservoir device: Global term describing or referring to extension, auxiliary, and add-on devices attached to MDIs for administration. This term could include both "spacer" and "holding chamber," defined as follows.

Spacer: Denotes a simple tube or extension device, with no one-way valves to contain the aerosol cloud; its purpose is simply to extend the MDI spray away from the mouth.

Valved holding chamber: Denotes a spacer device with the addition of one-way valve(s) to contain and hold the aerosol cloud until inspiration occurs.

Deposition Pattern of Inhaled Beclomethasone

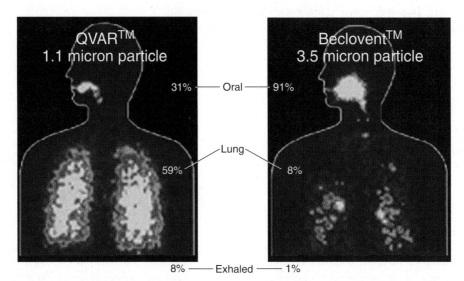

FIGURE 3-12 Comparison of lung deposition between CFC *(right)* and HFA *(left)* formulations of beclomethasone dipropionate by metered dose inhaler. (Scintigraph and data courtesy of C. Leach, Lovelace Respiratory Research Institute, Albuquerque, NM.)

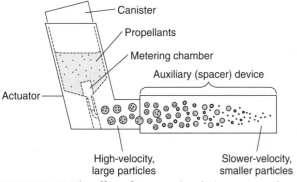

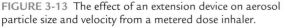

FIGURE 3-13 The effect of an extension device on aerosol particle size and velocity from a metered dose inhaler.

Design Variables

Spacers are simple devices that extend the distance and space between the MDI and the patient. MDIs with spacers do provide more drug to the patient than do those without. However, valved holding chambers can increase drug delivery, decrease oropharyngeal deposition, and help with coordination. Valves in the holding chamber do two important things: they act as a baffle reducing particle size, which in turn reduces oropharyngeal impaction, and they allow the patient to exhale without disrupting the aerosol inside the chamber. Valved holding chambers are superior to simple spacers.

Box 3-5	Advantages and Disadvantages of Reservoir Devices

ADVANTAGES
- Reduced oropharyngeal drug loss
- Separation of MDI actuation and inhalation
- Allows use of MDI during acute airflow obstruction with dyspnea
- Available with mask for children

DISADVANTAGES
- Large and cumbersome (some brands)
- Additional expense compared with MDI alone
- Some assembly required
- Possible source of bacterial contamination with inadequate cleaning

MDI, Metered dose inhaler.

Reservoir devices have several design variables, including volume, shape, direction of MDI spray, presence of one-way valves, inspiratory flow rate indicators, and presence or absence of an integral (built-in) MDI actuator. Table 3-3 summarizes these design variables for some reservoir devices available in the United States. Figure 3-14 illustrates differences in the size and design of several units.

TABLE 3-3

Characteristics of Selected Reservoir Devices Used in the United States, Exemplifying Design Variable Differences

Brand	Volume (approximate)	Inspiratory Valve	Spray Direction*	Flow Indicator	Integral Actuator
AeroChamber Plus	198 mL	One way	Forward	Yes	No†
OptiChamber Advantage	218 mL	One way	Forward	No	No†
ACE	175 mL	One way	Reverse	Yes	Yes
InspirEase	600 mL	No	Reverse	Yes	Yes
OptiHaler	70 mL	No	Reverse	No	Yes
MediSpacer	160 mL	No	Reverse	Yes	Yes

*Relative to mouth.
†Accepts mouthpiece actuator of drug brand.

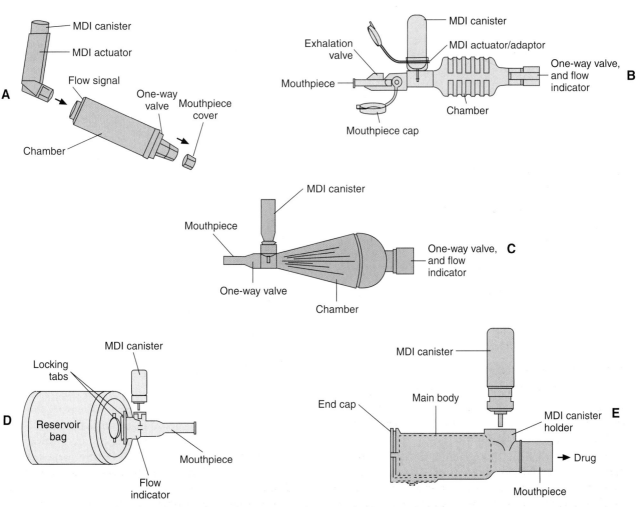

FIGURE 3-14 Representative metered dose inhaler auxiliary reservoir devices. **A,** AeroChamber Plus. **B,** MediSpacer. **C,** Aerosol Cloud Enhancer (ACE). **D,** InspirEase. **E,** OptiHaler. (**A** courtesy Monaghan Medical; **B** courtesy Cardinal Health; **C** courtesy DHD Healthcare/Smiths Medical; **D** courtesy Schering-Plough; **E** courtesy Respironics.)

Electrostatic Charge

> **KEY POINT**
>
> Reducing electrostatic charge in a reservoir device can significantly increase drug delivery.

An electrostatic charge is inherent on most plastic holding chambers. It has been discovered that by reducing the electrostatic charge, an increase in drug delivery will occur. Simply washing the chamber with water and standard household detergent reduces the electrostatic charge, and the effects can last as long as 30 days. Manufacturers have begun making chambers that are "antistatic." Louca and associates[57] found that the AeroChamber MAX, a valved holding chamber made from antistatic plastic, performed better than those that were washed and rinsed to reduce the electrostatic charge. Reducing electrostatic charge can increase delivery of the aerosolized drug by up to 70%.[58]

Size

The size of a spacer or holding chamber can affect the amount of drug made available to the patient: the larger the spacer, the more drug available. Most spacers in the United States are less than 200 mL. Larger chambers, as large as 750 mL, are available outside the United States. There is a tradeoff with inconvenience, as the larger and bulkier devices are less likely to be used or taken on travel.

Other Metered Dose Inhaler Auxiliary Devices

The market is saturated with various inventions that can make it easier to actuate an MDI, from counters that indicate the number of actuations the MDI has performed, to apparatuses that allow easier actuation. These devices may help some patients, but ultimately it is best that respiratory therapists educate themselves on MDI use and be able to properly instruct patients. Proper instruction about the MDI and holding chamber may be all that is needed for successful use.

Dry Powder Inhalers

A dry powder inhaler (DPI) is similar to an MDI, except that the drug is in powdered form. The main advantage is that the DPI is breath actuated, meaning that hand–breathing coordination is not needed. The main disadvantage is that it requires a high inspiratory flow rate from the patient to dispense the drug. The flow rate needed is usually between 30 and 90 L/min. Children

Box 3-6	Advantages and Disadvantages of Dry Powder Inhaler Devices

ADVANTAGES
- Small and portable
- Short preparation and administration times
- Breath actuation; no need for hand–breathing coordination
- No inspiratory hold or head tilt needed
- No CFC propellants (environmentally friendly)
- No "cold, Freon effect" to cause bronchoconstriction or inhibit full inspiration
- Simple determination of remaining drug doses

DISADVANTAGES
- Only a limited range of drugs is available to date.
- Patients are not as aware of the dose inhaled as with an MDI and may distrust delivery.
- Moderate to high inspiratory flow rates are needed for powder dispersion.
- Relatively high oropharyngeal impaction and deposition can occur.
- A device such as the Rotahaler is single-dose and must be loaded before each use.

CFC, Chlorofluorocarbon; *MDI,* metered dose inhaler.

and patients with respiratory disease may not be able to generate the flow needed to use such a device. A list of advantages and disadvantages can be seen in Box 3-6.

The basic principle of a DPI has been carried out in two different designs. Figure 3-15 diagrammatically illustrates two common devices on the market. Note that one (the Turbuhaler) is tall and slender, whereas the other (the Diskus inhaler) is round and flat. Other devices on the market allow for a "pill" or "blister" (e.g., formoterol or tiotropium) to be placed, one at a time, into a specialized compartment, which on closure punctures the pill and releases a powder for inhalation. Generic recommendations for the use of DPI devices are provided in Appendix C.

Inspiratory Flow Rate

Dispersal of drug powder depends on the energy of the inspiratory flow. A moderate to high inspiratory flow is needed with DPIs to obtain an optimal dose. This affects the use of these devices by young children, especially those less than 5 years of age, and by any patient with an acute wheezing episode associated with airflow reduction. Figure 3-16 illustrates the effect of various inspiratory flows with three DPI devices. The Turbuhaler, illustrated in Figure 3-15, was found effective at flow rates of approximately 30 L/min, which can be achieved by many children between 3 and 6 years of age, in a study

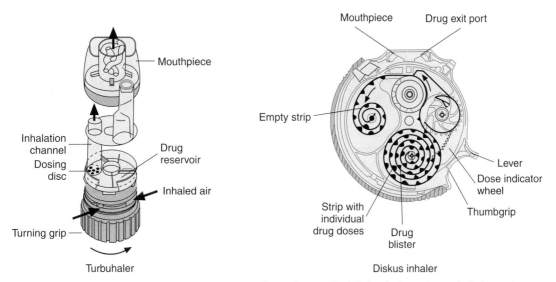

FIGURE 3-15 Diagrammatic representation of two dry powder inhaler devices, the Turbuhaler and the Diskus inhaler.

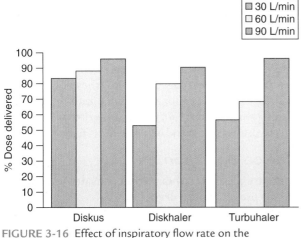

FIGURE 3-16 Effect of inspiratory flow rate on the percentage of nominal dose delivered by three DPI devices. Data were derived *in vitro* for albuterol. (Modified from Prime D, Grant AC, Slater AL, Woodhouse RN: A critical comparison of the dose delivery characteristics of four alternative inhalation devices delivering salbutamol: pressurized MDI, Diskus inhaler, Diskhaler, and Turbuhaler, *J Aerosol Med* 12:75, 1999.)

by Pedersen and colleagues.[59] In this study, Pedersen and colleagues reported the Turbuhaler to be approximately 30% effective even with inspiratory flows as low as 13 L/min. It appears that most devices on the market are effective with an inspiratory flow of about 30 L/min.[58]

Humidity

Another factor that can affect dose delivery from a DPI is humidity and moisture, which can reduce the fine particle mass in the dose. With the Turbuhaler, which has a bulk reservoir of drug powder, fine particle mass has been seen to decrease in approximately 2 weeks, under humid conditions (30° C, 75% relative humidity).[60] In contrast, the Diskus, in which each drug dose is protected inside a blister on the foil strip, showed no change in 8 weeks under such conditions. With any DPI, it is absolutely essential that patients not exhale into the device before inhaling; in all devices, including the Diskus, the drug powder is exposed once the device is activated.[58,61]

Clinical Efficacy

DPIs have been shown to be equivalent in efficacy to pressurized MDIs.[62,63] The need to replace CFC-propelled MDIs has given renewed impetus to the development of DPI technology. In evidence-based guidelines, Dolovich and associates recommend that a DPI is just as good as an MDI when selecting a device for inhaled medication in the outpatient setting. However, it is stressed that selection should be based on the patient's knowledge and understanding of the device's use.[23]

CLINICAL APPLICATION OF AEROSOL DELIVERY DEVICES

At times it seems that with so much information available, it is difficult to decide what is best for patients. Dolovich and colleagues[23] conducted an overview of all pertinent literature to develop recommendations for the clinical use of aerosol devices. The following sections summarize their findings. Refer to their paper for more detailed analysis.

Recommendations Based on Clinical Evidence

Aerosol Delivery of Short-acting β₂ Agonists in the Emergency Department

Both an MDI with a holding chamber and a nebulizer were equally effective in the treatment of adult and pediatric patients in the emergency room. Both modes of delivery improved symptoms and lung function. There is little information to show that a DPI is as effective as an MDI with a holding chamber or a nebulizer.

Aerosol Delivery of Short-acting β₂ Agonists in the Hospital

Again, there was no significant difference in lung function among inpatients treated with either an MDI with a holding chamber or a nebulizer. Reliable studies examining outcomes among inpatients treated with DPIs are lacking. At present it is better to use an MDI with a holding chamber or a nebulizer to deliver short-acting β agonists.

Intermittent Versus Continuous Nebulizer Delivery of β₂ Agonists

There is no difference in effect between intermittent and continuous nebulizer delivery of short-acting bronchodilators. Specifically, there is no change in lung function, asthma scores, or incidence of adverse effects when comparing the two delivery methods. It has been noted that the time required for staff to maintain and administer a continuous aerosol is less than that required with an intermittent nebulizer.

Aerosol Delivery of β₂ Agonists to Patients Receiving Mechanical Ventilation

The quality of evidence concerning the administration of bronchodilators to patients receiving mechanical ventilation is fair. It appears there is no difference in effect regardless of whether a nebulizer, or an MDI with a holding chamber, is used to deliver bronchodilators to adults or children being mechanically ventilated. Concerning patients receiving noninvasive ventilation, there is little evidence to suggest which formulation is superior. In any case, with both invasive and noninvasive ventilation the technical factors for delivering an aerosolized agent have changed dramatically.

Aerosol Delivery of Short-acting β₂ Agonists for Asthma in the Outpatient Setting

Among outpatients using either an MDI (with or without a holding chamber) or a DPI, there appears to be no difference in effect on lung function and asthma symptoms. However, the need for a holding chamber is evident; the literature favors the use of this device. Little research has been done on the use of nebulizers in the outpatient setting. Selection of the most appropriate aerosol device for outpatients must be made on a case-by-case basis.

Delivery of Inhaled Corticosteroids for Asthma

Whether an MDI with a holding chamber or a DPI is used, symptom scores and lung function remain the same among adult patients with asthma treated with inhaled corticosteroids.

Delivery of β₂ Agonists and Anticholinergic Agents for Chronic Obstructive Pulmonary Disease

Evidence gathered in the treatment of patients with chronic obstructive pulmonary disease (COPD) shows no difference in effect, whether a nebulizer, an MDI with or without a holding chamber, or a DPI is used. Selection of the proper aerosol device will depend on numerous factors.

Device Selection

There are a number of factors to consider when selecting the proper aerosol device:
• Patient or clinical preference
• Convenience of device
• Practicality of device
• Durability of device
• Cost and reimbursement
• Drug availability
• Ability of all prescribed drugs to be delivered by same device

Once these factors have been addressed and selection has taken place, it is important to properly educate the patient. Education of the patient cannot take place until proper education of the respiratory therapist has been completed.

Lung Deposition and Loss Patterns With Traditional Aerosol Devices

Aerosol devices that have traditionally been used in respiratory care deliver approximately 10 to 15% of the total drug dose to the lung. The pattern of loss to the mouth,

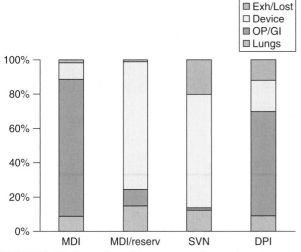

FIGURE 3-17 Illustration of the patterns of aerosol loss for four drug delivery systems. Exh, Exhaled; OP/GI, oropharynx/gastrointestinal. [Data for each device are based on the following studies (see References): *DPI,* Zainudin and co-workers (1990)[71]; *MDI,* Newman and co-workers (1991)[52]; *MDI/reserve,* Newman and co-workers (1981)[68]; *SVN,* Lewis and Fleming (1985).[34]]

KEY POINT

A traditional aerosol device delivers approximately 10 to 15% of the total dose to the airway. Because total dose amounts differ among the various types of devices for the same drug, these devices do not necessarily deliver equivalent amounts of drug. Newer aerosol devices, and some still being developed, are more efficient, with resultant lung depositions of 30 to 50% or greater. This improved efficiency in lung delivery will necessitate dose modifications.

stomach, and digestive apparatus and through exhalation differs among the device types. Figure 3-17 illustrates both the percentage of dose deposited in the lung and the pattern of loss with drug delivery systems that have traditionally been used in respiratory care, that is, an MDI, an MDI with a spacer, an SVN, and a DPI.

Some of the lung deposition data presented in Figure 3-17 are summarized in the following list, along with information from additional studies, including one comparing CFC and HFA formulations. It is clear that with the HFA formulation the percentage of lung deposition is much greater.

- MDI (CFC, ^{99m}Tc-labeled Teflon): 8.8%[64]
- MDI (HFA, ^{99m}Tc label): 53%[65]
- MDI and spacer (CFC, ^{99m}Tc-labeled Teflon and InspirEase): 14.8%[66]
- SVN (Inspiron Mini-Neb, ^{99m}Tc label): 12.4%[34]
- DPI (Turbuhaler): 14.8–27.7%[67]

The MDI and the SVN show the greatest contrast in the loss pattern of aerosol drug. Most of the loss with an MDI occurs in the mouth and stomach (approximately 80%). The loss with an SVN is primarily in the delivery apparatus (66%), with most of that remaining in the nebulizer, whereas an MDI loses approximately 10% in the actuator.

Adding a spacer or holding chamber to an MDI lowers the amount of drug lost in the oropharynx and stomach.[68] The DPI is similar to the MDI in its pattern of aerosol loss.

Equivalent Doses Among Device Types

If traditional MDI, SVN, and DPI devices all deliver approximately the same percentage of total device dose to the lungs, with the exception of HFA formulations, and the nominal dose in the devices differs, then different amounts of drug are placed within the lung. For example, the dose of albuterol, a β-adrenergic bronchodilator, by MDI versus nebulizer is as follows:

- MDI: 2 puffs, or 0.2 mg (200 µg)
- SVN: 0.5 cc, or 2.5 mg (2500 µg)

The ratio of MDI to SVN dose is approximately 1:12. If approximately 10% of the dose reaches the lungs, very different doses are being delivered from these aerosol devices. For example, if we assume that 10% of an albuterol dose reaches the lungs when administered by MDI and SVN, then a lung dose of 20 µg would be given by MDI versus a lung dose of 250 µg from an SVN (10% of 200 µg versus 10% of 2.5 mg). Several studies have examined this question of equipotent doses between delivery devices.

Equipotent dose: The dose by each delivery method that produces an equivalent degree of effect (for bronchodilators, this would be bronchodilation).

The standard difference in dose between the MDI and SVN delivery methods for albuterol is in the ratio of 1:12. However, at least two studies suggest MDI:SVN dose ratios of 1:3 and 1:4 to achieve equal bronchodilation or equivalent amounts of drug delivery to the lung.[69,70] An equipotent dose ratio of 1:3 or 1:4 is achieved by increasing the number of puffs from the MDI to 7 and 10, respectively, in the two studies.

One of the clearest statements on the question of delivery efficiency among traditional aerosol devices resulted from the study by Zainudin and colleagues.[71] The study examined drug delivery by pMDI (CFC propellants), DPI (Rotahaler), and gas-powered SVN (Acorn). The results are particularly helpful because the investigators used the same dose of 400 µg of albuterol (salbutamol)

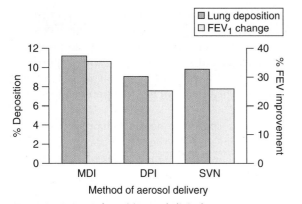

FIGURE 3-18 Lung deposition and clinical response: a comparison of three bronchodilator delivery methods. Shown are lung deposition (as a percentage of total dose) and clinical response (percent improvement in FEV_1) following aerosol delivery of the same dose of albuterol (400 μg) from three types of aerosol devices. (Data from Zainudin BM, Biddiscombe M, Tolfree SE, Short M, Spiro SG: Comparison of bronchodilator responses and deposition patterns of salbutamol inhaled from a pressurized metered dose inhaler, as a dry powder, and as a nebulized solution, *Thorax* 45:469, 1990.)

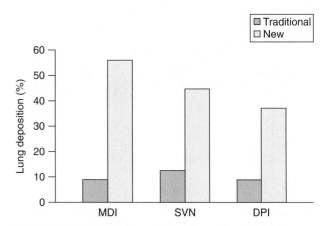

FIGURE 3-19 Comparison of lung deposition with older, traditional aerosol devices (*traditional MDI,* CFC-MDI; *traditional SVN,* Inspiron MiniNeb; *traditional DPI,* Rotahaler) and with newer devices (*new MDI,* HFA-beclomethasone[75]; *new SVN,* Respimat[74]; *new DPI,* Spiros[36]). (See References for further detail.)

in each of the device types. This allowed a direct microgram-for-microgram comparison of the dose from the devices. The percentage of lung deposition is shown in Figure 3-18, with an MDI delivery of 11.2%, a DPI delivery of 9.1%, and an SVN delivery of 9.9%.

The clinical response, measured as the improvement in FEV_1, is also similar, although the change with the MDI (35.6%) is statistically significantly greater than that seen with the DPI (25.2%) or the SVN (25.8%), a result not well explained in the study. These results support the view that the amount of aerosol drug delivered to the lung is similar with any of the three device types, and the clinical response is similar. *The amount of bronchodilation obtained is a reflection of the dose of drug given and not the method of delivery.*[72,73] As discussed in the following section, the development of aerosol devices that are highly efficient for lung delivery of drug is likely to lead to changes in recommended doses. For example, the increased efficiency of MDI HFA-propelled beclomethasone, cited in the section on HFA propellants, has resulted in the use of half the dose normally found with MDI CFC-propelled beclomethasone, with equivalent effects. These changes will in turn affect what constitutes equivalent doses between different types of devices.

Lung Deposition With Newer Aerosol Devices

The development of increasingly efficient devices compared with older MDIs, SVNs, and DPIs will cause the traditional figures of 10 to 15% for lung deposition to be revised upward. Unless newer devices completely replace the older, traditional aerosol generators used clinically, there will be a wide variety of lung depositions seen rather than a single range of 10 to 15%. The amount of lung delivery will depend on which device is used. Figure 3-19 graphically compares lung deposition with traditional devices (MDIs, SVNs, and DPIs) with that from newer devices. These data are compiled from several studies and for various drugs.[36,74,75]

One implication of changing and increasing lung deposition amounts is that the total dose from a device must be reduced. With a greater percentage reaching the lung, a lower total dose is needed from the device. Without proportional reduction in total device dose, toxic effects would be possible. Ultimately, the important factor is not the device per se but rather the amount of drug reaching the lungs when treating pulmonary disease.

Clinical Equivalence of Metered Dose Inhalers and Nebulizers

It is still relatively common in clinical practice to use an SVN instead of an MDI in emergent acute situations requiring aerosol bronchodilator delivery. However, a large and growing body of evidence indicates that an MDI with a spacer or holding chamber is as effective as an SVN in acute airway obstruction. Further, an MDI with a reservoir has been shown to be as effective as an SVN in the treatment of all age groups, from nonventilated preterm infants (with addition of a face mask) to adult patients in emergency departments. Table 3-4

TABLE 3-4

Studies Showing Equivalence of a Metered Dose Inhaler (MDI), With Reservoir or Face Mask, to a Small Volume Nebulizer (SVN) for Bronchodilator Administration in Acute Airflow Obstruction for Various Age Groups

Age Group	Drug	Dose	Outcome Variables	Reference*
Preterm infants, 47 ± 4.8 d	Albuterol†	MDI/spacer/mask: 2 puffs (200 µg) q4h SVN/mask: 0.2 mL (200 µg) q4h	Lung compliance, resistance	Fok et al.[87]
Infants, 16 ± 15 mo	Albuterol	MDI/HC/mask: 4 puffs (400 µg) q20min × 3 SVN: 2.5 mg q20min × 3	Respiratory rate, clinical scores, admissions	Mandelberg et al.[88]
Children, 5–16 yr	Terbutaline	MDI/HC/mask: 3 puffs (0.75 mg) × 1 SVN/mouthpiece: 0.5 mL (2.5 mg) × 1	Lung function, clinical scores	Lin and Hsieh[89]
Adults, 64.6 ± 13.3 yr	Albuterol	MDI/HC: 2 puffs (200 µg) q15min × 3 SVN: 0.5 mL (2.5 mg) q15min × 3	Spirometry, asthma scores	Mandelberg et al.[90]

*First author and year of publication are given, with full citation in references.
†Albuterol is also known as salbutamol outside the United States.
HC, Holding chamber (valved reservoir); *spacer*, nonvalved reservoir.

summarizes selected studies supporting the clinical equivalence of either an MDI or SVN in emergency treatment for various age groups. Amirav and Newhouse[76] offer a comprehensive review of studies on this issue. A meta-analysis of studies comparing bronchodilator administration by MDI or "wet nebulizer" (SVN) concluded that either method was equivalent in the treatment of acute airflow obstruction in adults.[77]

Age Guidelines for the Use of Aerosol Devices

It cannot be assumed that every patient will correctly use each type of delivery device. However, the differences, and in particular the relative advantages and disadvantages of the available devices, can be used as the basis for choosing which type of device best matches a patient's needs. Age is an important factor to consider when selecting an aerosol delivery system. Age guidelines have been provided in the National Asthma Education and Prevention Program Expert Panel Report 2 (NAEPP EPR 2) and are listed in Table 3-5.[78] A consideration that applies to the final decision is discussed by Dolovich and colleagues.[23]

Patient–Device Interface

Most aerosol drug administration is by oral inhalation; that is, the subject inhales the aerosol through the open mouth. However, other types of interface occur in clinical practice and raise questions concerning

TABLE 3-5

Age Guidelines for Use of Aerosol Delivery Devices

Aerosol System	Age
SVN	≤2 yr
MDI	>5 yr
MDI with reservoir	>4 yr
MDI with reservoir/mask	≤4 yr
MDI with ETT	≥neonate
Breath-actuated MDI	>5 yr
DPI	≥5 yr

Data from National Asthma Education and Prevention Program, National Heart, Lung, and Blood Institute, National Institutes of Health: National Asthma Education and Prevention Program, Expert Panel Report 2: *Guidelines for the diagnosis and management of asthma,* NIH Publication 97-4051. Bethesda, Md, 1997, National Institutes of Health.
DPI, Dry powder inhaler; *ETT,* endotracheal tube; *MDI,* metered dose inhaler; *SVN,* small volume nebulizer.

KEY POINT

The *patient–device interface* is another variable in aerosol delivery to the lung and includes *intermittent positive-pressure breathing administration, face mask administration,* and *delivery to intubated, ventilated patients,* which is complicated by numerous variables.

efficacy and drug delivery. These include positive-pressure aerosol administration with a face mask and administration of aerosolized drugs through endotracheal tubes (ETTs).

Administration by Intermittent Positive-pressure Breathing

Although administration by intermittent positive-pressure breathing (IPPB) has been a popular form of aerosol therapy, the consensus of research on this method of delivery is that IPPB delivery of aerosolized medication is no more clinically effective than simple spontaneous, unassisted inhalation from SVNs.[79-81] As a result, the use of IPPB for delivery of aerosolized drugs is not supported for general clinical or at-home use, if the patient is able to breathe spontaneously without machine support.

Face Mask Administration

Use of a face mask with an aerosol generator usually occurs with infants and young children or with debilitated, unresponsive patients. The clinical efficacy of a face mask in a pediatric application has been demonstrated by Conner and associates[82] and by Kraemer and co-workers.[83] A study published by Lowenthal and Kattan[84] compared face mask and mouthpiece delivery of nebulized albuterol in children and adolescents ages 6 to 19 years for emergency department treatment of acute asthma. Their study found that face mask administration did not significantly improve lung function measures, even in subjects with nasal congestion. They speculated that congested nasal passages caused mouth breathing while using the mask. Greater tremor was observed with the face mask group, implying a higher systemic level of drug compared with patients using a mouthpiece.

Lung deposition of drug has also been measured for both mouthpiece and face mask administration of aerosol drugs. Most of the available data are for infants and children, because this age group is most likely to be treated with a face mask for aerosol delivery.

Endotracheal Tube Administration

Aerosolized drug delivery commonly occurs with intubated subjects, both neonatal and adult. Data quantifying the efficiency of aerosol administration with this interface are well summarized in a review by Duarte.[85] Evaluation of aerosol delivery in this way is complicated by the number of variables introduced if the patient is receiving mechanical ventilation and by the difficulty in quantifying drug delivery accurately. Box 3-7 lists the many variables with administration of aerosol drug through an endotracheal

---

Box 3-7 | **Summary of Variables Present in Aerosol Delivery to Intubated, Mechanically Ventilated Critical Care Patients**

VENTILATOR
- Nebulizer power system
- Duty cycle (flow, volume, rate)
- Inspiratory flow pattern
- Mode of ventilation
- Breath modifications (PEEP, inflation hold)
- Spontaneous, assisted, or controlled breaths
- Humidification and temperature
- Position of generator in circuit
- Size of endotracheal tube

AEROSOL GENERATOR

SVN
- Volume of fill
- Type of solution
- Brand of SVN
- Intraproduct reliability
- Continuous versus intermittent
- Power flow rate

MDI
- Timing of actuation
- Use and design of reservoir device
- Type of drug used

MDI, Metered dose inhaler; *PEEP,* positive end-expiratory pressure; *SVN,* small volume nebulizer.

---

tube (ETT) to ventilated subjects. The effect of some of these variables, with either SVN or MDI aerosol administration, has been investigated. The following list summarizes the state of knowledge presented by Duarte:

- Both an MDI and nebulizer can be effectively used in administering inhaled agents to a patient receiving mechanical ventilation.
- The diameter of the tube plays a role in the impaction of aerosol particles. The narrower the tube (such as in pediatrics), the lower the percentage of drug that is delivered to the patient.
- The literature makes note that a reduction in humidity may increase the number of inhaled particles, but because some nebulizers require a longer time to nebulize, disconnecting a circuit to bypass the humidifier could lead to increased risk of ventilator-associated pneumonia.
- A heat and moisture exchanger (HME) should be bypassed when delivering aerosolized agents.
- The use of a less dense gas, such as a helium–oxygen mixture (heliox), can increase particle deposition.

- To improve aerosol delivery, place the nebulizer 30 cm from the ETT, instead of between the circuit Y and the ETT.
- When using an MDI, timing the actuation of the aerosol device with precise inspiration by the ventilator may increase drug delivery by 30%.

The use of HFA-MDIs may increase the amount of drug to the intubated patient. Mitchell and colleagues[86] found that the emitted dose of an HFA-MDI was almost six times more than that of its CFC counterpart.

SELF-ASSESSMENT QUESTIONS

1. What are the three most common aerosol-generating devices used to deliver inhaled drugs?
2. Describe the inspiratory pattern you would instruct a patient to use with an MDI.
3. What are three advantages offered by a reservoir device used with an MDI?
4. Would a DPI be appropriate for a 3-year-old child with asthma?
5. What is meant by the term *dead volume* in an SVN?
6. What is the optimal filling volume and power gas flow rate to use with an SVN?
7. How does the electrostatic charge affect an MDI when utilized with a holding chamber?
8. Which device would be better to deliver a β agonist to an adult patient in the emergency department, SVN, MDI, or DPI?

Answers to Self-Assessment Questions are found in Appendix A.

CLINICAL SCENARIO

A 17-year-old adolescent male with a history of allergic asthma is given a prescription for MDI albuterol, a bronchodilator used as a rescue agent. The HFA formulation of albuterol (Proventil HFA) is prescribed. After using the MDI a few times, the patient complains to you that he can feel drug in the canister when he shakes it before using, but it feels as if "very little spray" is coming out when he inhales a puff. He believes the MDI is not functioning properly and that he is not getting the regular inhaled dose.

What would you do to analyze this situation and ensure that the MDI is functioning properly?

Assuming the MDI appears functional based on the preceding check, how would you explain the situation with HFA albuterol to the patient?

Answers to Clinical Scenario Questions are found in Appendix A.

References

1. Morrow PE: An evaluation of the physical properties of monodisperse and heterodisperse aerosols used in the assessment of bronchial function, *Chest* 80(suppl 6):809, 1981.
2. Kohler D, Fleischer W: Established facts in inhalation therapy: a review of aerosol therapy and commonly used drugs, *Lung Respir* VI:1, 1989.
3. Morrow PE: Aerosol characterization and deposition, *Am Rev Respir Dis* 110:88, 1974.
4. Lourenco RV, Cotromanes E: Clinical aerosols. I. Characterization of aerosols and their diagnostic uses, *Arch Intern Med* 142:2163, 1982.
5. Hiller C, Mazumder M, Wilson D, Bone R: Aerodynamic size distribution of metered-dose bronchodilator aerosols, *Am Rev Respir Dis* 118:311, 1978.
6. Dolovich M: *In vitro* measurements of delivery of medications from MDIs and spacer devices, *J Aerosol Med* 9(suppl 1):S49, 1996.
7. Feddah MR, Brown KF, Gipps EM, Davies NM: *In-vitro* characterisation of metered dose inhaler versus dry powder inhaler glucocorticoid products: influence of inspiratory flow rates, *J Pharm Pharm Sci* 3:318, 2000.
8. Lippman M: Regional deposition of particles in the human respiratory tract. In Lee DHK, Falk HL, Murphy SD, editors: *Handbook of physiology*, section 9 Bethesda, MD, 1977, American Physiological Society.
9. Yu CP, Nicolaides P, Soong TT: Effect of random airway sizes on aerosol deposition, *Am Ind Hyg Assoc J* 40:999, 1979.
10. Clark AR, Gonda I, Newhouse MT: Towards meaningful laboratory tests for evaluation of pharmaceutical aerosols, *J Aerosol Med* 11(suppl 1):S1, 1998.
11. Consensus Conference on Aerosol Delivery: Aerosol consensus statement, *Chest* 100:1106, 1991.
12. Clay MM, Pavia D, Clarke SW: Effect of aerosol particle size on bronchodilation with nebulised terbutaline in asthmatic subjects, *Thorax* 41:364, 1986.
13. Johnson MA, Newman SP, Bloom R, Talaee N, Clarke SW: Delivery of albuterol and ipratropium bromide from two nebulizer systems in chronic stable asthma: efficacy and pulmonary deposition, *Chest* 96:6, 1989.
14. Leach CL: The CFC to HFA transition and its impact on pulmonary drug development, *Respir Care* 50:1201, 2005.
15. Barnes PJ, Basbaum CB, Nadel JA: Autoradiographic localization of autonomic receptors in airway smooth muscle, *Am Rev Respir Dis* 127:758, 1983.
16. Corkery KJ, Luce JM, Montgomery AB: Aerosolized pentamidine for treatment and prophylaxis of *Pneumocystis carinii* pneumonia: an update, *Respir Care* 33:676, 1988.
17. Newman SP: Aerosol deposition considerations in inhalation therapy, *Chest* 88(suppl 2):152S, 1985.
18. Dolovich M: Physical principles underlying aerosol therapy, *J Aerosol Med* 2:171, 1989.
19. Smith G, Hiller C, Mazumder M, Bone R: Aerodynamic size distribution of cromolyn sodium at ambient and airway humidity, *Am Rev Respir Dis* 121:513, 1980.

20. Hiller FC, Mazumder MK, Smith GM, Bone RC: Physical properties, hygroscopicity and estimated pulmonary retention of various therapeutic aerosols, *Chest* 77 (suppl 2):318, 1980.

21. Fuller HD, Dolovich MB, Chambers C, Newhouse MT: Aerosol delivery during mechanical ventilation: a predictive *in-vitro* lung model, *J Aerosol Med* 5:251, 1992.

22. Hanania NA, Wittman R, Kesten S, Chapman KR: Medical personnel's knowledge of and ability to use inhaling devices: metered-dose inhalers, spacing chambers, and breath-actuated dry powder inhalers, *Chest* 105:111, 1994.

23. Dolovich MB, Ahrens RC, Hess DR, Anderson P, Dhand R, Rau JL, Smaldone GC, Guyatt G; American College of Chest Physicians; American College of Asthma, Allergy, and Immunology: Device selection and outcomes of aerosol therapy: evidence-based guidelines, *Chest* 127:335, 2005.

24. Wigley FW, Londono JH, Wood SH, Shipp JC, Waldman RH: Insulin across respiratory mucosae by aerosol delivery, *Diabetes* 20:552, 1971.

25. Niven RW, Ip AY, Mittelman S, Prestrelski SJ, Arakawa T: Some factors associated with the ultrasonic nebulization of proteins, *Pharm Res* 12:53, 1995.

26. Dennis JH: A review of issues relating to nebulizer standards, *J Aerosol Med* 11(suppl 1):S73, 1998.

27. Kradjan WA, Lakshminarayan S: Efficiency of air compressor-driven nebulizers, *Chest* 87:512, 1985.

28. Shim CS, Williams MH Jr: Effect of bronchodilator therapy administered by canister versus jet nebulizer, *J Allergy Clin Immunol* 73:387, 1984.

29. Rau JL Jr, Harwood RJ: Comparison of nebulizer delivery methods through a neonatal endotracheal tube: a bench study, *Respir Care* 37:1233, 1992.

30. Hess D, Fisher D, Williams P, Pooler S, Kacmarek RM: Medication nebulizer performance: effects of diluent volume, nebulizer flow, and nebulizer brand, *Chest* 110:498, 1996.

31. Hess DR, Acosta FL, Ritz RH, Kacmarek RM, Camargo CA Jr: The effect of heliox on nebulizer function using a β agonist bronchodilator, *Chest* 115:184, 1999.

32. O'Callaghan C, Barry PW: The science of nebulised drug delivery, *Thorax* 52(suppl 2):S31, 1997.

33. Newman SP, Pellow PG, Clay MM, Clarke SW: Evaluation of jet nebulisers for use with gentamicin solution, *Thorax* 40:671, 1985.

34. Lewis RA, Fleming JS: Fractional deposition from a jet nebulizer: how it differs from a metered dose inhaler, *Br J Dis Chest* 79:361, 1985.

35. Dhand R: New frontiers in aerosol delivery during mechanical ventilation, *Respir Care* 46:666, 2004.

36. Dolovich M: New propellant-free technologies under investigation, *J Aerosol Med* 12(suppl 1):S9, 1999.

37. Rau JL, Ari A, Restrepo RD: Performance comparison of nebulizer designs: constant-output, breath-enhanced, and dosimetric, *Respir Care* 49:174, 2004.

38. Freedman T: Medihaler therapy for bronchial asthma: a new type of aerosol therapy, *Postgrad Med* 20:667, 1956.

39. Varvaet C, Byron PR: Drug-surfactant-propelled interaction in HFA formulations, *Int J Pharm* 186:13, 1999.

40. Newman SP: Principles of metered-dose inhaler design, *Respir Care* 50:1177, 2005.

41. McFadden ER Jr: Improper patient techniques with metered dose inhalers: clinical consequences and solutions to misuse, *J Allergy Clin Immunol* 96:278, 1995.

42. Cyr TD, Graham SJ, Li KY, Lovering EG: Low first-spray drug content in albuterol metered-dose inhalers, *Pharm Res* 8:658, 1991.

43. Everard ML, Devadason SG, Summers QA, Le Souef PN: Factors affecting total and "respirable" dose delivered by a salbutamol metered dose inhaler, *Thorax* 50:746, 1995.

44. Rubin BK, Durotoye L: How do patients determine their metered-dose inhaler is empty? *Chest* 126:1134, 2004.

45. Heimer D, Shim C, Williams MH Jr: The effect of sequential inhalation of metaproterenol aerosol in asthma, *J Allergy Clin Immunol* 66:75, 1980.

46. Pedersen S: The importance of a pause between the inhalation of two puffs of terbutaline from a pressurized aerosol with a tube spacer, *J Allergy Clin Immunol* 77:505, 1986.

47. Pedersen S, Steffensen G: Simplification of inhalation therapy in asthmatic children, *Allergy* 41:296, 1986.

48. Unzeitig JC, Richards W, Church JA: Administration of metered-dose inhalers: comparison of open- and closed-mouth techniques in childhood asthmatics, *Ann Allergy* 51:571, 1983.

49. Chhabra SK: A comparison of "closed" and "open" mouth techniques of inhalation of a salbutamol metered-dose inhaler, *J Asthma* 31:123, 1994.

50. Schultz RK: Drug delivery characteristics of metered-dose inhalers, *J Allergy Clin Immunol* 96:284, 1995.

51. Ross DL, Gabrio BJ: Advances in metered dose inhaler technology with the development of a chlorofluorocarbon-free drug delivery system, *J Aerosol Med* 12:151, 1999.

52. Newman SP, Weisz AW, Talaee N, Clarke SW: Improvement of drug delivery with a breath actuated pressurized aerosol for patients with poor inhaler technique, *Thorax* 46:712, 1991.

53. Baum EA, Bryant AM: The development and laboratory testing of a novel breath-actuated pressurized inhaler, *J Aerosol Med* 1:219, 1988.

54. Donnell D: Development of a CFC-free glucocorticoid metered-dose aerosol system to optimize drug delivery to the lung, *Pharm Sci Technolo Today* 3:183, 2000.

55. Dolovich M, Ruffin RE, Roberts R, Newhouse MT: Optimal delivery of aerosols from metered dose inhalers, *Chest* 80(suppl 6):911, 1981.

56. Dolovich M: Spacer design II: holding chambers and valves. Oral presentation at the International Symposium on Spacer Devices, Horsham, PA, 1995, Drug Information Association.

57. Louca E, Leung K, Coates AL, Mitchell JP, Nagel MW: Comparison of three valved holding chambers for the delivery of fluticasone propionate–HFA to an infant face model, *J Aerosol Med* 19:160, 2006.

58. Rau RL: Practical problems with aerosol therapy in COPD, *Respir Care* 51:158, 2006.

59. Pedersen S, Hansen OR, Fuglsang G: Influence of inspiratory flow rate upon the effect of a Turbuhaler, *Arch Dis Child* 65:308, 1990.

60. Fuller R: The Diskus: a new multi-dose powder device—efficacy and comparison with Turbuhaler, *J Aerosol Med* 8(suppl 2):S11, 1995.

61. Rubin DK, Fink JB: Optimizing aerosol delivery by pressurized metered-dose inhalers, *Respir Care* 50:1191, 2005.

62. Ram FSF, Wright J, Brocklebank D, White JE: Systematic review of clinical effectiveness of pressurised meted dose inhalers versus other hand held inhaler devices for delivering β₂ agonist bronchodilators in asthma, *BMJ* 323:901, 2001.

63. Chapman KR, Friberg K, Balter MS, Hyland RH, Alexander M, Abboud RT, Peters S, Jennings BH: Albuterol via Turbuhaler versus albuterol via pressurized metered-dose inhaler in asthma, *Ann Allergy Asthma Immunol* 78:59, 1997.

64. Newman SP, Pavia D, Garland N, Clarke SW: Effects of various inhalation modes on the deposition of radioactive pressurized aerosols, *Eur J Respir Dis Suppl* 119:57, 1982.

65. Leach CL, Davidson PJ, Hasselquist BE, Boudreau RJ: Lung deposition of hydrofluoroalkane-134a beclomethasone is greater than that of chlorofluorocarbon fluticasone and chlorofluorocarbon beclomethasone: a cross over study in healthy volunteers, *Chest* 122:510, 2002.

66. Kim CS, Eldridge MA, Sackner MA: Oropharyngeal deposition and delivery aspects of metered-dose inhaler aerosols, *Am Rev Respir Dis* 135:157, 1987.

67. Newman SP, Busse WW: Evolution of dry powder inhaler design, formulation and performance, *Respir Med* 96:293, 2002.

68. Newman SP, Moren F, Pavia D, Little F, Clarke SW: Deposition of pressurized suspension aerosols inhaled through extension devices, *Am Rev Respir Dis* 124:317, 1981.

69. Tarala RA, Madsen BW, Paterson JW: Comparative efficacy of salbutamol by pressurized aerosol and wet nebulizer in acute asthma, *Br J Clin Pharmacol* 10:393, 1980.

70. Blake KV, Hoppe M, Harman E, Hendeles L: Relative amount of albuterol delivered to lung receptors from a metered-dose inhaler and nebulizer solution, *Chest* 101:309, 1992.

71. Zainudin BM, Biddiscombe M, Tolfree SE, Short M, Spiro SG: Comparison of bronchodilator responses and deposition patterns of salbutamol inhaled from a pressurised metered dose inhaler, as a dry powder, and as a nebulised solution, *Thorax* 45:469, 1990.

72. Mestitz H, Copland JM, McDonald CF: Comparison of outpatient nebulized vs metered dose inhaler terbutaline in chronic airflow obstruction, *Chest* 96:1237, 1989.

73. Newhouse M, Dolovich M: Aerosol therapy: nebulizer vs metered dose inhaler [editorial], *Chest* 91:799, 1987.

74. Newman SP, Brown J, Steed KP, Reader SJ, Kladders H: Lung deposition of fenoterol and flunisolide delivered using a novel device for inhaled medicines: comparison of RESPIMAT with conventional metered-dose inhaler with and without spacer devices, *Chest* 113:957, 1998.

75. Leach CL, Davidson PJ, Boudreau RJ: Improved airway targeting with the CFC-free HFA-beclomethasone metered-dose inhaler compared with CFC-beclomethasone, *Eur Respir J* 12:1346, 1998.

76. Amirav I, Newhouse MT: Metered-dose inhaler accessory devices in acute asthma: efficacy and comparison with nebulizers: a literature review, *Arch Pediatr Adolesc Med* 151:876, 1997.

77. Turner MO, Patel A, Ginsburg S, FitzGerald JM: Bronchodilator delivery in acute airflow obstruction: a meta-analysis, *Arch Intern Med* 157:1736, 1997.

78. National Asthma Education and Prevention Program, National Heart, Lung, and Blood Institute, National Institutes of Health: Expert Panel Report 2: *Guidelines for the diagnosis and management of asthma,* NIH Publication 97–4051. Bethesda, Md, 1997, National Institutes of Health. (Available at http://www.nhlbi.nih.gov/guidelines/asthma/asthgdln.pdf; accessed February 2007.)

79. Chester EH, Racz I, Barlow PB, Baum GL: Bronchodilator therapy: comparison of acute response to three methods of administration, *Chest* 62:394, 1972.

80. Dolovich MB, Killian D, Wolff RK, Obminski G, Newhouse MT: Pulmonary aerosol deposition in chronic bronchitis: intermittent positive pressure breathing versus quiet breathing, *Am Rev Respir Dis* 115:397, 1977.

81. Loren M, Chai H, Miklich D, Barwise G: Comparison between simple nebulization and intermittent positive-pressure in asthmatic children with severe bronchospasm, *Chest* 72:145, 1977.

82. Conner WT, Dolovich MB, Frame RA, Newhouse MT: Reliable salbutamol administration in 6- to 36-month-old children by means of a metered dose inhaler and Aerochamber with mask, *Pediatr Pulmonol* 6:263, 1989.

83. Kraemer R, Frey U, Sommer CW, Russi E: Short-term effect of albuterol, delivered via a new auxiliary device, in wheezy infants, *Am Rev Respir Dis* 144:347, 1991.

84. Lowenthal D, Kattan M: Facemasks versus mouthpieces for aerosol treatment of asthmatic children, *Pediatr Pulmonol* 14:192, 1992.

85. Duarte A: Inhaled bronchodilator administration during mechanical ventilation, *Respir Care* 49:623, 2004.

86. Mitchell JP, Nagel MW, Wiersema KJ, Doyle CC, Migounov VA: The delivery of chlorofluorocarbon-propelled versus hydrofluoroalkane-propelled beclomethasone dipropionate aerosol to the mechanically ventilated patient: a laboratory study, *Respir Care* 48:1025, 2003.

87. Fok TF, Lam K, Ng PC, Leung TF, So HK, Cheung KL, Wong W: Delivery of salbutamol to nonventilated preterm infants by metered-dose inhaler, jet nebulizer, and ultrasonic nebulizer, *Eur Respir J* 12:159, 1998.

88. Mandelberg A, Tsehori S, Houri S, Gilad E, Morag B, Priel IE: Is nebulized aerosol treatment necessary in the pediatric emergency department? Comparison with a metal spacer device for metered-dose inhaler, *Chest* 117:1309, 2000.

89. Lin YZ, Hsieh KH: Metered dose inhaler and nebuliser in acute asthma, *Arch Dis Child* 72:214, 1995.

90. Mandelberg A, Chen E, Noviski N, Priel IE: Nebulized wet aerosol treatment in emergency department: is it essential? Comparison with large spacer device for metered-dose inhaler, *Chest* 112:1501, 1997.

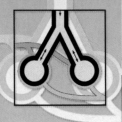

Chapter 4

Calculating Drug Doses

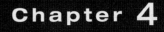

DOUGLAS S. GARDENHIRE

CHAPTER OBJECTIVES

After reading this chapter, the reader will be able to:
1. Use the metric system
2. Calculate drug doses, using proportions
3. Calculate drug doses, using percentage-strength
   solutions
4. Calculate intravenous infusion rates for drugs

KEY TERMS AND DEFINITIONS

Percentage — Amount of solute that is in a solution containing 100 parts

Schedule — Amount of drug that is needed, based on a patient's weight

Solute — A substance that is dissolved in a solution

Solution — Physically homogeneous mixture of two or more substances

Solvent — A substance, usually a liquid, that is used to make a solution

Strength — Amount of solute in a solution, usually expressed as a percentage

---

Chapter 4 presents calculations of drug doses. Systems of measure are reviewed briefly. Dose calculations from prepared-strength formulations such as liquids, tablets, and capsules are presented with examples. Calculations of doses from solutions whose concentrations are expressed as a percentage strength, along with intravenous dose calculations, are presented with examples. Practice problems and answers are included.

SYSTEMS OF MEASURE

The Metric System

KEY POINT

Drug calculations use the metric system of measurement.

Table 4-1 provides metric units of measures for length, volume, and weight. Primary units in the metric system are as follows:

Length: Meter
Volume: Liter
Mass: Gram

Fractional parts, or multiples of these primary (base) units, are expressed by adding Latin prefixes for sizes smaller than the primary unit, and Greek prefixes for sizes larger than the primary unit. Examples of both Latin and Greek prefixes found in Table 4-1 are as follows:

Increasing prefixes—Latin:
   Micro = 1/1,000,000
   Milli = 1/1000
   Centi = 1/100
   Deci = 1/10

Increasing prefixes—Greek:
   Deca = 10
   Hecto = 100
   Kilo = 1000

In calculating drug doses, the metric units for volume and mass (weight) are needed. A commonly encountered unit of volume in respiratory care pharmacology is the milliliter (ml), or 0.001 L. Common units of weight are the kilogram (kg), the gram (g), the milligram (mg), and, with aerosolized drugs, the microgram (μg). Blood levels of drug amounts within the body may be in nanograms per milliliter (ng/ml). Conversions within the metric system should be familiar, such as converting 1 mg to 0.001 g, 500 ml to 0.5 L, or 0.4 mg to 400 μg. Familiarity with decimal fractions and with the other basic rules of arithmetic are necessary for drug dose calculations.

The gram is defined as the weight of 1 milliliter of distilled water at 4° C *in vacuo.* Under these conditions, 1 g of water and 1 ml of water are equal. This should not be used to convert from weight to volume, however, because a gram of liquid is not always equal to a milliliter of liquid, depending on the temperature, pressure, and nature of the substance.

Appendix B provides a summary of scientific notation, metric and SI *(Système International)* units, and temperature scales with conversions. Although three different systems of measure have been used in drug calculations, metric units of measure are currently employed with formulations in the United States. Therefore all of the examples in this chapter are based on the metric system.

The International System of Units

KEY POINT

Volume and weight measures are commonly encountered in pharmacology.

The International System of Units, or *Système International d'Unités (SI),* was adopted in 1960 and is the modern metric system (see Appendix B). The SI system is well presented by Chatburn,[1] with conversion factors between older metric units for volume and the English system of measurement units. The SI system is based on

| TABLE 4-1 | | | | |

The Metric System of Length, Volume, and Mass (Weight)

Length

1 Kilometer (km)	=	10^3 meters	=	1000 meters
1 Hectometer (hm)	=	10^2 meters	=	100 meters
1 Decameter (dam)	=	10^1 meters	=	10 meters
1 Meter (m)		**Base unit**		
1 Decimeter (dm)	=	10^{-1} meter	=	0.1 meter
1 Centimeter (cm)	=	10^{-2} meter	=	0.01 meter
1 Millimeter (mm)	=	10^{-3} meter	=	0.001 meter
1 Micrometer (μm)	=	10^{-6} meter	=	0.000001 meter

Volume (Capacity)

1 Kiloliter (kl)	=	10^3 liters	=	1000 liters
1 Hectoliter (hl)	=	10^2 liters	=	100 liters
1 Decaliter (dal)	=	10^1 liters	=	10 liters
1 Liter (L)		**Base unit**		
1 Deciliter (dl)	=	10^{-1} liter	=	0.1 liter
1 Centiliter (cl)	=	10^{-2} liter	=	0.01 liter
1 Milliliter (ml)	=	10^{-3} liter	=	0.001 liter
1 Microliter (μl)	=	10^{-6} liter	=	0.000001 liter

Mass

1 Kilogram (kg)	=	10^3 grams	=	1000 grams
1 Hectogram (hg)	=	10^2 grams	=	100 grams
1 Decagram (dag)	=	10^1 grams	=	10 grams
1 Gram (g)		**Base unit**		
1 Decigram (dg)	=	10^{-1} gram	=	0.1 gram
1 Centigram (cg)	=	10^{-2} gram	=	0.01 gram
1 Milligram (mg)	=	10^{-3} gram	=	0.001 gram
1 Microgram (μg)	=	10^{-6} gram	=	0.000001 gram
1 Nanogram (ng)	=	10^{-9} gram	=	0.000000001 gram
1 Picogram (pg)	=	10^{-12} gram	=	0.000000000001 gram

the meter–kilogram–second (MKS) system, with volume as a derived unit of length. The primary units of interest in pharmacology calculations are as follows:

Mass: Kilogram (kg)

Volume: Cubic meter (m³)

Although the base unit of measure in the SI system for volume is the cubic meter (m³), the liter (L) and its fractions or multiples are currently accepted in measures of liquid volume.

$$\text{Equivalence}: 10^{-3}\ m^3 = 1\ \text{liter (L)}$$

Drops as Units of Volume

Orders in respiratory care may often involve *drops,* such as 4 drops of racemic epinephrine, with 2.5 cubic centimeters (cc) of distilled water. The following equivalence is used:

$$16\ \text{drops (gtts)} = 1\ \text{milliliter (ml)}$$

In this example, then, 4 drops would equal 1/4 milliliter (1 ml/16 drops × 4 drops = 4/16 ml). Therefore 1/4 ml is

drawn up into a small accurate syringe, such as a tuberculin syringe, to obtain the 4 drops.

One cubic centimeter (cc) is equivalent to

$$1\ \text{milliliter (ml)}: 1\ cc = 1\ ml$$

It should be noted that drops are not standardized and can vary in size because of the physical properties of the particular fluid (e.g., specific gravity and viscosity) and the orifice of the dropper. Because drops can vary in amount delivered, physicians should be diplomatically cautioned to prescribe in metric units (cubic centimeters or milliliters) unless a dropper calibrated specifically for the particular medication is supplied by the manufacturer.

Household Units of Measure

Household units of measure are useful when instructing patients to take medications at home, and are based on common kitchen measures, such as the teaspoon, tablespoon, and cup. Metric equivalents to these household

KEY POINT

Household measures (cup, teaspoon, etc.) are also used in administering medication.

measures are given in Appendix B. Although the teaspoon is equivalent to 5 ml, not every teaspoon used for eating will actually equal 5 ml. However, measuring spoons and cups will more accurately give the volumes indicated, such as 5 ml per teaspoon, 15 ml per tablespoon, or 240 ml per cup.

KEY POINT

The three types of drug calculations include prepared-strength doses, doses from solutions with a concentration expressed as a percentage, and intravenous dose calculations.

CALCULATING DOSES FROM PREPARED-STRENGTH LIQUIDS, TABLETS, AND CAPSULES

Once the clinician is able to freely convert within the metric system, it is possible to begin calculating drug doses. In general, such calculations will be of the following three types:
1. Those involving fluids, tablets, or capsules of a given strength (e.g., 5 mg/ml)
2. Those involving solutions of a percentage strength (e.g., 0.5 ml of a 0.5% solution)
3. Those involving intravenous infusion rates (e.g., 10 μg/min)
  Each type of dose calculation is treated separately.

Calculating With Proportions

When using a prepared-strength liquid, tablet, or capsule, you are always trying to determine how much liquid or how many tablets or capsules are needed to give the amount, or dose, of the drug ordered. For example, if one tablet of a drug contains 5 mg and you want to give 2.5 mg, you immediately realize that half a tablet must be given. The simplest and therefore probably the most accurate, error-free method of calculation when using a vial of a prepared-strength drug (or a tablet or capsule) involves two steps at most, as follows:
1. Convert to consistent units of measure
2. Set up a straightforward proportion:

$$\frac{\text{Original dose}}{\text{Per amount}} = \frac{\text{desired dose}}{\text{per amount}}$$

or, original dose:per amount :: desired dose:per amount.

In step 1, this conversion may be from grams to milligrams within the metric system, or even from apothecary to metric, if an apothecary dosage strength has been ordered. In step 2, either format for the proportion is correct. In the second form, the extremes and means are each multiplied together. If one arrangement is intuitively clearer, that should be preferred by the user.

Example 1

You have oxytetracycline tablets, each 250 mg in strength. If the patient needs 0.5 g of the drug, how many tablets should be administered?

Solution: If you need 0.5 g of the drug, either convert 250 mg to 0.25 g, or 0.5 g to 500 mg (preferred). Once the units are consistent, set up the proportion to find the unknown, that is, the number of tablets needed to deliver the desired dose to the patient. Using the preceding formula,

Original drug dose = 250 mg
Per amount = per tablet
Desired drug dose = 0.5 g = 500 mg
Per amount = unknown

$$\frac{250\text{ mg}}{1\text{ tab}} = \frac{500\text{ mg}}{x\text{ tab}}$$
$$\frac{250 \times x}{250} = \frac{500 \times 1}{250}$$
$$x\text{ tab} = \frac{500}{250}$$
$$x = 2\text{ tablets}$$

Answer

The amount required is 2 tablets.

Whereas this calculation is trivially clear and can be performed mentally, others may require calculation for the sake of accuracy.

Example 2

You have 120 mg of phenobarbital in 30 ml of phenobarbital elixir. How many milliliters of elixir will you use to give a 15-mg dose?

Solution:

$$\frac{120\text{ mg (original dose)}}{30\text{ ml (per amount)}} = \frac{15\text{ mg (desired dose)}}{x\text{ (per amount)}}$$

Cross-multiplying:

$$\frac{120 \text{ mg} \times x}{120 \text{ mg}} = \frac{15 \text{ mg} (30 \text{ ml})}{120 \text{ mg}}$$

$$\frac{120x}{120} = \frac{450}{120}$$

$$x \text{ ml} = 3.75 \text{ ml}$$

Answer

The amount required is 3.75 ml.

Simplification is possible, such as reducing 120 mg/30 ml to 4 mg/ml. Then, knowing that there are 4 mg in every milliliter, simply divide 4 mg/ml into 15 mg, to determine how many milliliters are needed. Often, reducing a liquid to its dosage strength per 1 ml allows quick mental computation of the dose. Caution and care should be observed in the initial reduction, however. An error at that point causes a subsequent dosage error. *Do not hesitate to write out a calculation:* In a busy clinical setting, a patient's well-being should take precedence over a practitioner's mathematical pride.

KEY POINT

Prepared-strength doses involve calculating how many tablets, capsules, or milliliters of a liquid are needed to administer a given amount of drug and are most easily solved using a proportion, after units are made consistent, as follows:

$$\frac{\text{Original dose}}{\text{Per amount}} = \frac{\text{desired dose}}{\text{per amount}}$$

Drug Amounts in Units

It should be noted that some drugs are manufactured in units (U) rather than in grams or milligrams. Examples are penicillin, insulin, and heparin. Solving dose problems for these drugs is exactly the same as for the other dosage units previously mentioned.

Example 3

A brand of sodium heparin is available as 1000 U/ml. How many milliliters do you need for 500 U of the drug?

Solution: Using the second form of the proportion (extremes and means), we set up the following:

Original dose:per amount :: desired dose:per amount.

1000 U:1 ml :: 500 U: x ml

By multiplying the extremes and the means, we obtain

$$\frac{1000(x)}{1000} = \frac{500}{1000}$$

$$x \text{ ml} = 0.5 \text{ ml}$$

Answer

The amount required for 500 U, given the prepared-strength liquid, is 0.5 ml.

There is no universal equivalence between units as a measure of amount and the metric weight system. Units are used with biological standardization and are defined for each drug by a standard preparation of that drug, when the drug is measured in units. For example, there is a standard preparation of digitalis, consisting of dried, powdered digitalis leaves, and 100 mg of this preparation equals 1 United States Pharmacopeia (USP) unit of activity. In this way, when drugs are extracted from animals, plants, or minerals, there is a standard reference preparation. Note that 100 mg is not 1 U for every drug with units; for example, insulin has a standard preparation of 0.04 mg = 1 U. When a drug is isolated as a pure chemical form, either extracted as the active substance in a natural source or synthesized in the laboratory, biological standardization based on a standard preparation from the natural source is no longer necessary. The specific chemical amount is given in metric weight or volume measure.

Calculations With a Dosage Schedule

There are times when the dose of a drug must be obtained from a **schedule,** which may be based on the size of a person. For example, a suggested schedule for albuterol syrup in children 2 to 6 years old is 0.1 mg/kg of body weight. This means that the *dose* must first be calculated after the body weight is obtained, and then the amount of the drug preparation needed for treatment can be calculated.

Example 4

Using a schedule of 0.1 mg/kg for albuterol syrup, and a prepared-strength mixture of 2 mg/5 ml, how much of the syrup is needed for a 20-kg child?

Solution:

Calculate the dose needed:

$$\text{Dose} = 0.1 \text{ mg/kg} \times 20 \text{ kg} = 2.0 \text{ mg}$$

or

$$\frac{0.1 \text{ mg}}{1 \text{ kg}} = \frac{x}{20 \text{ kg}}$$

$$x = (0.1)(20) = 2.0 \text{ mg}$$

Next, calculate the amount of the preparation:

$$\frac{2 \text{ mg}}{5 \text{ ml}} = \frac{2 \text{ mg}}{x \text{ ml}}$$

Simplifying,

$$2(x) = 10$$
$$x \text{ ml} = 5 \text{ ml}$$

Answer

This 20-kg child needs 5 ml of albuterol syrup.

Additional Examples of Calculations With Prepared-strength Drugs

Example 5

An injectable solution of glycopyrrolate with a prepared strength of 0.2 mg/ml is used for nebulization. How many milliliters are needed for a 1.5-mg dose?

Solution:

Original dose per amount: 0.2 mg/ml
Desired dose: 1.5 mg
Amount needed: x ml

Substituting:

$$\frac{0.2 \text{ mg}}{1 \text{ ml}} = \frac{1.5 \text{ mg}}{x \text{ ml}}$$

Using cross-multiplication to simplify:

$$0.2 \text{ mg}(x) = 1.5 \text{ mg} (1 \text{ ml})$$
$$x = 1.5/0.2$$
$$x \text{ ml} = 7.5 \text{ ml}$$

Answer

An amount of 7.5 ml will contain the desired dose of 1.5 mg, using the prepared strength given.

Example 6

You have terbutaline, 1 mg/ml in an ampoule for injection. How much do you need, to give a 0.25-mg dose subcutaneously?

Solution:

Original dose per amount: 1 mg/ml
Desired dose: 0.25 mg
Amount needed: x ml

Substituting:

$$\frac{1 \text{ mg}}{1 \text{ ml}} = \frac{0.25 \text{ mg}}{x \text{ ml}}$$

Solving for x:

$$1 \text{ mg} (x \text{ ml}) = 0.25 \text{ mg}(1 \text{ ml})$$
$$x = 0.25 \text{ ml}$$

Answer

Give 0.25 ml for the desired dose of 0.25 mg.

Example 7

A dosage schedule for a surfactant calls for 5 ml/kg of body weight. If a premature infant weighs 1200 g, how many milliliters are needed?

Solution:

Convert body weight to kilograms:

$$1 \text{ kg}/1000 \text{ g} \times 1200 \text{ g} = 1.2 \text{ kg}$$

Multiply the weight in kilograms by the schedule of 5 ml/kg:

$$x \text{ ml} = 1.2 \text{ kg} \times 5 \text{ ml}/\text{kg} = 6 \text{ ml}$$

Answer

Based on the dosage schedule and weight, 6 ml should be given.

Example 8

The prepared strength of a drug is 100 mg/4 ml. The dosage schedule is 100 mg/kg of birth weight. A premature newborn weighs 1100 g. Based on the weight of the newborn, what dose is needed? How many milliliters of the drug should be given to achieve this dose?

Solution: To determine the dose that is needed, perform two steps:

Convert the birth weight to kilograms:

$$1 \text{ kg}/1000 \text{ g} \times 1100 \text{ g} = 1.1 \text{ kg}$$

Multiply the birth weight by the dosage schedule to find the dose required:

$$x \text{ mg} = 100 \text{ mg}/\text{kg} \times 1.1 \text{ kg} = 110 \text{ mg}$$

The dose needed is 110 mg of drug.

Solution: To find the number of milliliters required to achieve this dose:

Original dose per amount: 100 mg/4 ml
Desired dose: 110 mg
Amount needed: x ml

Substituting:

$$\frac{100\ \text{mg}}{4\ \text{ml}} = \frac{110\ \text{mg}}{x\ \text{ml}}$$

$$100\ \text{mg}\,(x) = 110\ \text{mg}\,(4\ \text{ml})$$

$$x = \left[110\ \text{mg}\,(4\ \text{ml})\right]/100\ \text{mg}$$

$$x = 4.4\ \text{ml}$$

Answer

Based on the dosage schedule, the weight of the newborn, and the prepared strength, 4.4 ml will give the needed dose of 110 mg.

CALCULATING DOSES FROM PERCENTAGE-STRENGTH SOLUTIONS

KEY POINT

Calculating doses based on a percentage-strength concentration of a solution can be done with the following equation:

$$\text{Percent strength (in decimals)} = \frac{\text{solute (in grams or cubic centimeters)}}{\text{total amount (solute and solvent)}}$$

Because an area of expertise for respiratory therapists is solutions for aerosolization, solutions and percentage strengths will often be needed to calculate a drug dose. A **solution** contains a **solute,** which is dissolved in a **solvent,** giving a homogeneous mixture. The **strength** of a solution is expressed as the percentage of solute relative to total solvent and solute. **Percentage** means parts of the active ingredient (solute) in a preparation contained in 100 parts of the total preparation (solute *and* solvent).

Types of Percentage Preparations
Weight to Weight

Percent in weight (W/W) expresses the number of grams of a drug or active ingredient in 100 g of a mixture:

W/W: Grams per 100 g of mixture

Weight to Volume

Percent may be expressed as the number of grams of a drug or active ingredient in 100 ml of a mixture:

W/V: Grams per 100 ml of mixture

Volume to Volume

Percent volume in volume (V/V) expresses the number of milliliters of drug or active ingredient in 100 ml of a mixture:

V/V: Milliliters per 100 ml of mixture

Solutions by Ratio

Frequently when diluting a medication for use in an aerosol or intermittent positive-pressure breathing (IPPB) treatment, a solute-to-solvent ratio is given (e.g., isoproterenol 1:200 or epinephrine 1:100).

Ratio by Grams to Milliliters

In the preceding isoproterenol example, the following is indicated:

$$1\ \text{g per 200 ml of solution} = \frac{1\ \text{g}}{200\ \text{ml}} = 0.005 \times 100 = 0.5\%$$

(multiplying by 100 is the same as moving the decimal *two* places to the *right*).

This is what is indicated with traditional examples such as epinephrine 1:100, which is a 1% strength solution:

$$\frac{1\ \text{g}}{100\ \text{ml}} = 0.01 \times 100 = 1\%$$

Ratio by Simple Parts

In the parts to parts example below, actual parts medication to parts solvent are indicated, as follows:

1:8 = 1 part to 8 parts, which is the same as: 1/4 cc to 2 cc

However, part-to-part ratios do not indicate actual amounts or specific units, although usually milliliters to milliliters are meant. It is assumed you know that 1/4 or 1/2 cc of an agent is given as the usual dose, and not 1 cc. An order such as 1:8 is not precise, without further specifications, about the amount of drug (whether 0.25 ml, 0.5 ml, etc.) to be given.

Solving Percentage-strength Solution Problems

For solutions in which the active ingredient itself is pure (undiluted, 100% strength), the following equation can be used:

EQUATION 1

Percent strength (in decimals) =

$$\frac{\text{solute (in grams or cubic centimeters)}}{\text{total amount (solute and solvent)}}$$

Alternatively, a ratio format can be used:

EQUATION 2

$$\frac{\text{Amount of solute}}{\text{Total amount}} = \frac{\text{amount of solute}}{100 \text{ parts (grams or cubic centimeters)}}$$

When the active ingredient, or solute, is already diluted and less than pure, the following equation can be used:

EQUATION 3

Percent strength (in decimals) =

$$\frac{(\text{dilute solute}) \times (\text{percent strength of solute})}{\text{total amount (solution)}}$$

In equation 3 the solute (active ingredient) multiplied by the percent strength gives the amount of pure active ingredient in the dilute solution. This equation adds only one modification to the formula given in equation 1. This is to multiply the dilute solute by its actual percentage strength, with the result indicating the amount of active ingredient at a 100% (pure) strength. For example, 10 ml of 10% solute means you have 1 ml of pure (100%) solute. Put another way, you would need 10 ml of dilute solute to have 1 ml of pure solute (active ingredient). When used in equation 3, the unknown is usually how much of the dilute solute, or active ingredient, is needed in the total solution to give the desired strength. The preceding equations are illustrated in the following two examples.

KEY POINT

Move the decimal point to easily convert between grams, percent strength, and milligrams per milliliter. If beginning with percent strength, for example 1%, move the decimal *one* place to the *right* to convert to milligrams per milliliter (1% = 1.0% = 10 mg/ml). If beginning with percent strength, for example 10%, move the decimal *two* places to the *left* to convert to grams (10% = 10.0% = 0.10 g).

Example 9

Undiluted active ingredient: How many milligrams of active ingredient are there in 2 cc of 1:200 isoproterenol?

Solution:
Percent strength: 1:200 = 0.5% = 0.005
Total amount of solution: 2 cc
Active ingredient: x

Substituting in equation 1:

$$0.005 = x \text{ g} / 2 \text{ cc}$$
$$x \text{ g} = 0.005 \times 2$$
$$x \text{ g} = 0.01 \text{ g}$$

Answer

Converting 0.01 g to milligrams gives 10 mg. In 2 cc of 1:200 solution there are 10 mg of isoproterenol.

Alternative Solution:

Percent strength : 1 : 200

$$\frac{1}{200} = 0.005 \text{ g}$$

Move the decimal point *two* places to the *right* (i.e., mathematically multiply by 100) and add a percent sign. At this point it changes from grams to a percent solution:

$$0.005 \text{ g} = 000.5 = 0.5\%$$

or

$$0.005 \text{ g} = 0.005 \times 100 = 0.5\%$$

Move the decimal point an additional *one* place (for a total of *three* places, i.e., mathematically multiply by 1000) to convert from percent strength to milligrams per milliliter:

$$0.5\% = 5 = 5 \text{ mg} / \text{ml}$$

or

$$0.005 \text{ g} = 0.005 \times 1000 = 5 \text{ mg} / \text{ml}$$

Answer

The question asks how many milligrams of active ingredients are in 2 cc. If we remember that 1 cc = 1 ml and we know there are 5 mg in every 1 ml, we then multiply by 2 cc to obtain the answer: 10 mg/2 cc. (If you need to set up the equation, refer to the earlier section, Calculating With Proportions.)

Example 10

Diluted active ingredient: How much 20% Mucomyst (a brand of acetylcysteine) is needed to prepare 5 cc of 10% Mucomyst?

Solution: Using the equation for dilute active ingredients (here the acetylcysteine is only 20% strength, not pure), the following is obtained:

Desired percent strength (in decimals): 10% = 0.10
Total amount of solution: 5 cc
Percent strength of solute (active ingredient):
20% = 0.20

Dilute solute (i.e., amount of active ingredient needed): x

Substituting in equation 3:

$$0.10 = x(0.20)/5 \text{ cc}$$
$$x = 5(0.10)/0.20$$
$$x = 2.5 \text{ cc of 20\% Mucomyst}$$

Answer

The 2.5 cc of 20% Mucomyst is then mixed with 2.5 cc of normal saline to give a total of 5 cc of solution. This 5 cc will be a 10% strength solution.

Although diluting a 20% solution to a 10% solution is obviously a "half-and-half" procedure and does not require the use of an equation, less intuitive dilutions may need to be calculated. The reader might try diluting 20% Mucomyst to obtain 5 cc of a 5% strength solution, using the preceding approach.

Alternative Solution to Example 10: Convert 10% to 100 mg/ml by moving the decimal *one* place to the *right* (think of it as 10.0%, move one place, drop the percent sign and add mg/ml, and it becomes 100 mg/ml; or change the percent to a decimal and multiply by 1000 (10% = 0.10 × 1000 = 100 mg/ml). The question really asks how many milligrams are in 5 cc of 10% Mucomyst? That is easy: we already know there are 100 mg for every 1 cc of drug, so multiply 100 mg × 5 cc, equaling 500 mg. This is the desired dose, and the original dose is 20% or 200 mg/ml. Set up the proportions equation (refer to the earlier section, Calculating With Proportions):

Original dose per amount: 200 mg/1 ml
Desired dose: 500 mg
Amount desired: x ml

Substituting:

$$\frac{200 \text{ mg}}{1 \text{ ml}} = \frac{500 \text{ mg}}{x \text{ ml}}$$

Cross-multiply:

$$\frac{200 \text{ mg} (x \text{ ml})}{200 \text{ mg}} = \frac{500 \text{ mg} (1 \text{ ml})}{200 \text{ mg}}$$
$$x = 2.5 \text{ cc of 20\% Mucomyst}$$

Answer

The 2.5 cc of the 20% Mucomyst is then mixed with 2.5 cc of normal saline to give a total solution volume of 5 cc. This 5 cc will be a 10% strength solution. The key is to know the amount of milligrams of drug that is ordered. So, there is no difference between 5 cc of 10% strength solution and 2.5 cc of 20% solution. They both equal what is ultimately desired, 500 mg of drug.

Summary

Calculations with solutions of drugs, using percentage strengths, can be summarized as follows:

1. Convert to metric units and decimal expressions.
2. Substitute knowns in the appropriate equation (undilute or dilute active ingredient).
3. Use grams or milliliters in the percentage equation.
4. Express the answer in the units requested.

Note on Mixing Solutions

In mixing solutions, determine the amount of active ingredient needed for the percent strength desired, and then add enough solvent to "top off" to the total solution amount needed. When ordering a solution this is indicated by *quantity sufficient (qs),* for the total needed. For example, to obtain 30 cc of 3% procaine HCl, we calculate 0.9 cc of the active ingredient, and water qs for 30 cc of solution. Do not merely give the difference between solute and total solution (30 cc − 0.9 cc = 29.1 cc), because certain solutes can change volume (e.g., alcohol "shrinks" in water).

Percentage Strengths in Milligrams per Milliliter

The basic definition of percentage strength in solutions involves grams or milliliters. However, the amount of active ingredient in most nebulized drug solutions is in milligrams. It may be a useful clinical reference, and one that is easily remembered, to define percentage strengths in terms of milligrams per single milliliter, using a 1% strength reference point. Recall that 1% strength is 1 g/100 ml. Using equation 1 for percentage strength, you have:

$$0.01 = \frac{1 \text{ g}}{100 \text{ ml}}$$

For 1 ml of a 1% strength solution, you would have:

$$0.01 = \frac{x \text{ g}}{1 \text{ ml}}$$
$$x \text{ g} = 0.01 \text{ g}$$

and 0.01 g × 1000 mg/g = 10 mg. Because 0.01 g equals 10 mg, you then have 10 mg/ml in a 1% solution. The 1% strength is an easily learned reference point. Table 4-2 lists some common percentage strengths, giving amounts in milligrams per milliliter, in reference to the 1% concentration.

Note the relationship of 1% to 10%: If there are 10 mg/ml in a 1% solution, there would be 10 times that amount in a 10% solution, or 100 mg/ml. Likewise, a 0.5% solution has one-half as much active ingredient as

TABLE 4-2

Drug Amounts in Milligrams per Milliliter for Common Percentage Strengths

Percentage Strength (%)	Drug Amount (mg/ml)
20	200
10	100
5	50
1	**10**
0.5	5
0.1	1
0.05	0.5

NOTE: Starting with percentage strength, move the decimal *one* place to the *right* and it becomes a drug amount.

a 1% solution: one-half of 10 mg/ml would be 5 mg/ml. This amount of 5 mg/ml could have been used to solve example 9, an undiluted active ingredient percentage problem. In example 9, it was found that a 1:200 solution (a 0.5% strength solution) has 10 mg in 2 ml, which is the same as 5 mg in 1 ml.

KEY POINT

An easy reference point for the amount of drug contained in a solution, in milligrams per milliliter, is 1% strength, which is 10 mg/ml.

Equations 1 and 3 should be known and represent a more general statement of percentage strengths for solving any problem. However, knowledge of milligrams per milliliters for a 1% solution can be very helpful in many problems, to know how many milligrams of the active ingredient are being given. Examples of drug solutions with the strengths listed in Table 4-2 can be given. Metaproterenol is available as a 5% solution or 50 mg/ml, and an ampoule of terbutaline (1 mg/cc) is a 0.1% strength solution.

Remember, you can easily convert from gram to percent strength to milligrams per milliliter by simply moving the decimal point—no math is needed. *Or,* mathematically, multiply the amount of grams by 1000 to achieve milligrams (0.001 g × 1000 = 1 mg). This will work for any drug expressed as grams, percent strength, or milligrams per milliliter. Using the preceding example:

$$0.001 \text{ g} = 0.1\% = 1 \text{ mg/ml}$$

Move the decimal point *two* places to the *right* to convert from grams to percent strength. From a percent strength, move the decimal *one* place to the *right* to convert to milligrams per milliliter. This process can be reversed:

$$50 \text{ mg/ml} = 5\% = 0.05 \text{ g}$$

If you begin with milligrams per milliliter, move the decimal point *one* place to the *left* to convert to percent strength. From a percent strength move the decimal point *two* places to the *left* to convert to grams.

Diluents and Drug Doses

A common misconception persists that the amount of diluent added to a liquid drug to be aerosolized by nebulization is intended to "weaken" the dose or strength delivered to the patient. This is not necessarily the case. One-half cubic centimeter of a 1% drug solution has the same amount (5 mg) of active ingredient, whether it is diluted with 2 or 10 cc of normal saline. The amount of diluent affects the time required to nebulize a given solution but not the amount of active ingredient in a nebulizer reservoir. Practicality dictates that 2.5 cc of solution nebulizes in a reasonable time limit of 10 minutes or so, whereas 10 cc may take much longer. The diluent also is needed because disposable nebulizers cannot create an aerosol with less than approximately 1 ml of solution in the reservoir (the "dead volume"). Theoretically, given a suitable nebulizing device, there is no reason that the original 0.5 cc of 1% drug could not be nebulized undiluted in order to deliver the dose of 5 mg. It is the amount of the active ingredient, determined by the percentage strength and quantity in cubic centimeters of the drug, that gives a dose amount. Although technically the percentage strength of the resulting solution in the reservoir is weaker, the dose remains unchanged at 5 mg. It is the dose in milligrams that should be of concern to the clinician.

Additional Examples of Calculations With Solutions

Example 11

How many milligrams of active ingredient are in 3 cc of a 2% solution of procaine HCl?

Solution: Use the percentage formula of equation 1, pure-strength ingredient:

$$\text{Percent strength (in decimals)} = \frac{\text{solute}}{\text{total amount}}$$

Convert the percentage to decimals and substitute the known values:

$$0.02 = \frac{x \text{ g}}{3 \text{ cc}}$$
$$0.02(3 \text{ cc}) = x \text{ g}$$
$$x \text{ g} = 0.06 \text{ g}$$

In milligrams:

$$0.06 \text{ g} \times 1000 \text{ mg} / \text{g} = 60 \text{ mg}$$

Answer

Sixty milligrams of active ingredient is in 3 cc of a 2% solution of procaine HCl.

Alternative Solution to Example 11: Moving the decimal can easily convert to milligrams per milliliter. If we think of 2% as 2.0% and move the decimal *one* place to the *right* we convert the percent to 20 mg/ml. Remember that 1 ml = 1 cc, so if we need to find how many milligrams of active ingredient are in 3 cc of solution we simply multiply 3 cc by 20 mg/ml to equal 60 mg. The reader can use the proportions equation to confirm:

$$\frac{20 \text{ mg}}{1 \text{ ml}} = \frac{x}{3 \text{ cc}}$$

Solve for x:

$$x(1 \text{ ml}) = 20 \text{ mg}(3 \text{ cc})$$
$$x = 60 \text{ mg}$$

Example 12

A resident wants to dilute 20% acetylcysteine to a strength of 6% for a research study. How many milliliters of 20% drug solution are needed to have 10 ml of 6% strength?

Solution: Use the modified equation 3 for dilute active ingredient:

Percent strength (decimals) =

$$\frac{(\text{dilute solute}) \times (\text{percent strength of solute})}{\text{total amount (solution)}}$$

Percent strength desired: 6% = 0.06
Dilute solute: unknown = x ml
Percent strength: 20% = 0.20
Total amount of solution: 10 ml

Substituting and solving:

$$0.06 = \frac{(x \text{ ml}) \times (0.20)}{10 \text{ ml}}$$
$$0.06 \ (10 \text{ ml}) = x \text{ ml} \ (0.20)$$
$$x = 0.06(10) / 0.20$$
$$x \text{ ml} = 3 \text{ ml}$$

Answer

Draw up 3 ml of the 20% strength and add saline, quantity sufficient, for a total of 10 ml. Check your calculation for correctness: 3 ml of 20% strength

solution has 600 mg of active ingredient (20% = 200 mg/ml); 600 mg is 0.6 g and 0.6 g/10 ml (or 6 g/100 ml) is in fact a 6% strength. So you obtained the needed amount of drug with 3 ml of the 20% solution.

Alternative Solution to Example 12: First, we convert the needed amount of drug. The resident asks for 10 ml at 6% strength, so we convert 6% to 60 mg/ml by moving the decimal *one* place to the *right*. If we need 10 ml then we multiply 10 ml × 60 mg, which equals 600 mg. We now know the resident needs 600 mg of drug. How do we know how much of the 20% strength is needed? We convert 20% to 200 mg/ml and set up the equation as a proportion (original dose: per amount :: desired dose: per amount).

$$\frac{200 \text{ mg}}{1 \text{ ml}} = \frac{600 \text{ mg}}{x}$$

Cross-multiply and solve for x:

$$\frac{200 \text{ mg} \ (x)}{200 \text{ mg}} = \frac{600 \text{ mg} \ (1 \text{ ml})}{200 \text{ mg}}$$
$$x = 3 \text{ ml}$$

Example 13

The usual dose of albuterol sulfate is 0.5 ml of a 0.5% strength solution. How many milligrams is this?

Solution: Using equation 1 for percentage strength:

Percentage in decimals: 0.5% = 0.005
Active ingredient: unknown (x)
Total solution: 0.5 ml

Substituting:

$$0.005 = \frac{x \text{ g}}{0.5 \text{ ml}}$$
$$x \text{ g} = 0.005(0.5) = 0.0025 \text{ g}$$

Converting:

$$0.0025 \text{ g} = 2.5 \text{ mg}$$

Answer

There is 2.5 mg of active ingredient in the usual dose.

Alternative Solution to Example 13: First we need to convert the percent solution to milligrams per milliliter. To do this, move the decimal one place to the right to convert to milligrams per milliliter (0.5% = 5 mg/ml). If we know that there are 5 mg in 1 ml and we need 0.5 ml, all we need to do is halve 5 mg, which is 2.5 mg.

Example 14

Albuterol sulfate is also available as a unit dose of 3 ml at a percentage strength of 0.083%. If the entire amount of 3 ml is given, is this the same as the usual dose of 2.5 mg?

Solution: Using equation 1 for percentage strength:

Percent strength (in decimals): 0.083% = 0.00083
Active ingredient: unknown = x
Total amount of solution: 3 ml

Substituting:

$$0.00083 = \frac{x \text{ g}}{3 \text{ ml}}$$
$$x \text{ g} = 3(0.00083) = 0.00249 \text{ g}$$

and

$$0.00249 \text{ g} = 2.49 \text{ mg}$$

Answer

The result is approximately 2.5 mg, the usual dose.

Alternative Solution to Example 14: First, we need to convert 0.083% to milligrams per milliliter. To do this we move the decimal *one* place to the *right* to convert to milligrams per milliliter (0.083% = 0.83 mg/ml). Set up the proportions equation and solve for x:

$$\frac{0.83 \text{ mg}}{1 \text{ ml}} = \frac{x}{3 \text{ ml}}$$
$$0.83(3) = x$$
$$2.49 = x$$

Rounding up, we obtain 2.5 mg.

Example 15

Terbutaline sulfate is available as 1 mg per 1 ml of solution. What percentage strength is this?

Solution: Convert 1 mg to 0.001 g (1 mg × 1 g/1000 mg = 0.001 g). Then,

$$x = \frac{0.001 \text{ g}}{1 \text{ ml}}$$
$$x = 0.001 = 0.1\%$$

Answer

The percentage strength is 0.1%.

Alternative Solution to Example 15: This is straightforward; all we need to do is remember to move the decimal *one* place to the *left*. This will convert to percent strength (1 mg/ml = 0.1%).

CALCULATING INTRAVENOUS INFUSION RATES

The previous knowledge of prepared-strength drug units and solutions allows relatively straightforward calculation of intravenous (IV) infusion rates. IV infusion incorporates calculation of the *rate* of drug administration per unit time (e.g., milligrams per minute). Ultimately an infusion rate in drops per minute will be needed on the IV infusion set. This requires knowing the standard drop factor for that IV administration set, which gives the number of drops that equal 1 ml in the drip chamber. This information can be found when the IV set is opened. The following formulas can be used, depending on the type of order to be followed.

Total Solution Over Time

The simplest IV infusion calculation involves administering a volume of solution over a period of time. In this case, the flow rate is expressed as milliliters per minute, using the solution amount in milliliters and time in minutes.

$$\text{Flow rate (ml/min)} = \frac{\text{total solution (ml)}}{\text{time (min)}}$$

The flow rate can be converted into drops per minute, using the standard drop factor, which gives the number of drops in each milliliter.

EQUATION 4

$$\text{Flow rate (ml/min)} = \frac{\text{total solution (ml)}}{\text{time (min)}}$$

$$\text{Flow rate (drops/min)} = \frac{\text{drops}}{\text{milliliter}} \times \frac{\text{milliliter}}{\text{minute}}$$

Example 16

You wish to give 1 L of solution in a 3-hour period. What is the flow rate in drops per minute, if the standard drop factor for your IV set is 15 drops per milliliter?

Solution:

1 L of solution = 1000 ml
3 hr = 180 min

Calculate the flow rate in milliliters per minute, based on the volume of solution and the time given:

$$\text{Flow rate (ml/min)} = \frac{1000 \text{ ml}}{180 \text{ min}} = 5.56 \text{ ml/min}$$

Calculate the flow rate as drops per minute, using equation 4:

Flow rate (in drops/min)=

$$15\,\text{drops/ml} \times 6\,\text{ml/min} = 90\,\text{drops/min}$$

Answer

An infusion rate of 90 drops/min should deliver the desired 1 L in about 3 hours.

Amount of Drug per Unit of Time

An IV drug may be administered as an amount per unit of time (usually minutes). For example, epinephrine can be given as micrograms per minute (μg/min). The drug amount per minute must be converted into a drip rate of drops per minute, for proper drug infusion. In this case the concentration of the drug solution is used to calculate the drug amount in 1 ml.

EQUATION 5

$$\text{Concentration (in amount/ml)} = \frac{\text{total drug amount}}{\text{total solution (in milliliters)}}$$

The rate of flow in milliliters per minute can then be calculated from the needed drug amount per minute and the concentration of drug per milliliter.

EQUATION 6

$$\text{Flow rate (in ml/min)} = \frac{\text{amount}}{\text{minute}} \times \frac{\text{milliliter}}{\text{amount}}$$

The flow rate can then be converted from milliliters per minute to drops per minute needed to give the desired amount of drug per unit of time, as before, using the standard drop factor, as shown in equation 4.

Flow rate (in drops/min)=

$$\text{drop factor (in drops/ml)} \times \text{ml/min}$$

The last two equations can be combined to allow direct calculation of drops per minute, from the known concentration in amount per milliliter and the desired delivery rate in amount per unit of time.

EQUATION 7

$$\text{Flow rate (in drops/min)} = \frac{\text{amount}}{\text{minute}} \times \frac{\text{milliliters}}{\text{amount}} \times \frac{\text{drops}}{\text{milliliter}}$$

Example 17

What infusion rate is needed to deliver 10 μg/min of a drug that comes in a solution of 500 μg/250 ml? The standard drop factor for the IV administration set is 15 drops/ml.

Solution:
Concentration of drug (in μg/ml) = 500 μg/250 ml
$$= 2\,\text{μg/ml}$$
Rate of flow (in ml/min) = 10 μg/min × 1 ml/2 μg
$$= 5\,\text{ml/min}$$
Rate of flow (in drops/min) = 15 drops/ml × 5 ml/min
$$= 75\,\text{drops/min}$$

Answer

An infusion rate of 75 drops/min will deliver the desired drug dose of 10 μg/min.

The maximal dose of drug to be delivered will determine how long the infusion continues. For example, if the maximal dose is 1 mg, this dose would be reached in 100 minutes at the infusion rate of 10 μg/min:

$$1\,\text{mg} = 1000\,\text{μg}$$
$$\text{Time (min)} = 1000\,\text{μg} \times 1\,\text{min}/10\,\text{μg}$$
$$\text{Time} = 100\,\text{minutes } or\ 1\,\text{hour and 40 minutes}$$

The rate of drug administration, expressed as amount per minute, is used to calculate how long it will take to deliver a set amount of drug. In general, equations 4, 5, and 6 or 7 can be used to solve for any unknown factor in IV drug administration, as shown in the following examples.

Additional Examples of Intravenous Dose Calculations

Example 18

In advanced cardiac life support (ACLS), dopamine is given IV to increase cardiac output. If you add a 200-mg ampoule of dopamine to 250 ml of 5% dextrose in water (D_5W), what drip rate is needed to deliver a dose of 10 μg/kg/min for the average adult of 70 kg? Assume that the drop factor is 15 drops/ml.

Dose needed (in μg/min):
70 kg x 10 μg/kg/min = 700 μg/min

Concentration available:
200 mg/250 ml, or 0.8 mg/ml = 800 μg/ml

KEY POINT

Intravenous (IV) drug dose calculations are based on solutions and solution concentrations. Given the concentration of the drug solution in milliliters per amount of drug, calculate how many milliliters per minute are needed. Convert this flow rate of milliliters per minute into drops per minute, using the standard drop factor obtained from the IV administration set.

$$\text{Flow rate (in drops/min)} =$$
$$\frac{\text{amount}}{\text{minute}} \times \frac{\text{milliliters}}{\text{amount}} \times \frac{\text{drops}}{\text{milliliter}}$$

Using the combined equation 7 for amount per minute, milliliters per amount, and drops per milliliter (drop factor), we would calculate

Flow rate (in drops/min)
$$= \frac{700 \text{ mug/min}}{\text{minute}} \times \frac{1 \text{ ml}}{800 \text{ mug}} \times \frac{15 \text{ drops}}{1 \text{ ml}}$$
$$= 13.125 \text{ drops/min}$$

Answer

A drip rate of 13 drops/min will deliver approximately 693 µg/min total, *or* about 10 µg/kg/min to the patient.

Example 19

Phenobarbital may be given in status epilepticus as an IV infusion, with a dose of 10 mg/kg. The rate of infusion should not exceed 50 mg/min. The drop factor is 15 drops/ml, and you have a solution of 650 mg in 10 ml. What is the total dose for a 65-kg adult?

Solution:

$$\text{Total dose} = 10 \text{ mg/kg} \times 65 \text{ kg} = 650 \text{ mg}$$

How long will it take for the dose to be given, using the maximal allowed rate of infusion (50 mg/min)?

Solution:

$$\text{Time (in min)} = 650 \text{ mg} \times 1 \text{ min/50 mg} = 13 \text{ min}$$

What is the maximal rate of drip (drops per minute) allowed?

Solution: First calculate the drug concentration available in milligrams per milliliter, using equation 5:

$$\text{Concentration (in mg/ml)} = 650 \text{ mg/10 ml} = 65 \text{ mg/ml}$$

Then you can use the combined equation 7 to calculate flow rate in milliliters per minute and convert to drops per minute, using the drop factor:

Flow rate (drops/min)
$$= 50 \text{ mg/min} \times 1 \text{ ml/65 mg} \times 15 \text{ drops/ml}$$
$$= 750 \text{ drops/65 min}$$

or

$$\text{Flow rate (drops/min)} = 11.5 \text{ drops/min}$$

Example 20

If a drug concentration is 500 µg/250 ml, and the standard drop factor is 15 drops/ml, how long will it take to deliver the 500 µg at a drip rate of 30 drops/min?

Solution: Calculate the drug concentration in a single milliliter:

$$\text{Concentration (in µg/ml)} = 500 \text{ µg/250 ml} = 2 \text{ µg/ml}$$

Convert the flow rate from drops per minute to milliliters per minute, using the drop factor and the given drip rate of 30 drops/min:

$$\text{Flow rate (in ml/min)} = 30 \text{ drops/min} \times 1 \text{ ml/15 drops}$$
$$= 2 \text{ ml/min}$$

Convert this flow rate into a drug amount per unit of time, using the concentration (amount per milliliter):

$$\text{Drug amount (per min)} = 2 \text{ ml/min} \times 2 \text{ µg/ml}$$
$$= 4 \text{ µg/min}$$

and

$$\text{Time (in min)} = 1 \text{ min/4 µg} \times 500 \text{ µg}$$
$$= 125 \text{ min, } or \text{ 2 hours and 5 minutes}$$

Or, more simply, the flow rate in milliliters per minute and the total amount of solution (250 ml) could be used to calculate the time the infusion would take:

$$\text{Time (in min)} = 250 \text{ ml} \times 1 \text{ min/2 ml} = 125 \text{ min}$$

Answer

It would take 2 hours and 5 minutes to deliver 500 µg at a drip rate of 30 drops/min.

Example 21

If an IV dose is ordered at 5 µg/min, how long will it take to reach a maximal dose of 0.375 mg?

Solution: Convert 0.375 mg to micrograms:
$$0.375 \text{ mg} = 375 \text{ µg}$$

Calculate the total time for delivery, based on the rate of delivery and the total amount of drug:

$$\text{Time (in min)} = 1\,\text{min} / 5\,\mu g \times 375\,\mu g = 75\,\text{min}$$

Answer

It would take 75 min to reach a maximal dose of 0.375 mg.

Example 22

If an IV dose is given at 30 drops/min and the drug solution is 100 µg/2 ml, how much drug in micrograms per minute is being given? The standard drop factor is 15 drops/ml.

Solution:

$$\text{Concentration (in amount/ml)} =$$
$$100\,\mu g / 2\,\text{ml} = 50\,\mu g / \text{ml}$$

Calculate the flow rate in milliliters per minute, from the drop factor and the drops per minute:

$$\text{Flow rate (in ml/min)} = \frac{30\,\text{drops}}{1\,\text{min}} \times \frac{1\,\text{ml}}{15\,\text{drops}}$$
$$= 2\,\text{ml/min}$$

The drug amount per minute is obtained from the flow rate in milliliters per minute and the concentration in µg/ml:

$$x\,\mu g / \text{min} = 2\,\text{ml/min} \times 50\,\mu g / \text{ml} = 100\,\mu g / \text{min}$$

Answer

The drug is being administered at 100 µg/min.

SELF-ASSESSMENT QUESTIONS

Answers to Self-assessment Questions are found in Appendix A, where the solution to each problem is set up and the answer given. Details of the algebraic solution are not given.

Prepared-Strength Dose Calculations

1. A bottle is labeled Demerol (meperidine) 50 mg/cc. How many cubic centimeters are needed to give a 125-mg dose?
2. Promazine HCl comes as 500 mg/10 ml. How many milliliters are needed to give a 150-mg dose?
3. Hyaluronidase comes as 150 U/cc. How many cubic centimeters are needed for a 30-U dose?

SELF-ASSESSMENT QUESTIONS —cont'd

4. Morphine sulfate 4 mg is ordered. You have a vial with 10 mg/ml. How much do you need?
5. A dosage schedule for the surfactant poractant calls for 2.5 ml/kg birth weight. How much drug will you need for a 800-g baby?
6. Diphenhydramine (Benadryl) elixir contains 12.5 mg of diphenhydramine HCl in each 5 ml of elixir. How many milligrams are there in a one-half teaspoonful dose (1 tsp = 5 ml)?
7. A pediatric dose of oxytetracycline 100 mg is ordered. The dosage form is an oral suspension containing 125 mg/5 cc. How much of the suspension contains a 100-mg dose?
8. How many units (U) of heparin are found in 0.2 ml, if you have 1000 U/ml?
9. Albuterol syrup is available as 2 mg/5 ml. If a dose schedule of 0.1 mg/kg is used, how much syrup is needed for a 30-kg child? How many teaspoons is this?
10. Terbutaline is available as 2.5-mg tablets. How many tablets do you need for a 5-mg dose?
11. If Tempra is available as 120 mg/5 ml, how much dose is there in 1/2 tsp?
12. Theophylline is available as 250 mg/10 ml and is given intravenously at 6 mg/kg body weight. How much solution do you give for a 60-kg woman?
13. Terbutaline sulfate is available as 1 mg/ml in an ampoule. How many milliliters are needed for a 0.25-mg dose?
14. A patient is told to take 4 mg of albuterol four times daily. The medication comes in 2-mg tablets. How many tablets are needed for one 4-mg dose?
15. Metaproterenol is available as a syrup with 10 mg/5 ml. How many teaspoons should be taken for a 20-mg dose?
16. If you have *d*-(+)-tubocurarine at 3 mg/ml, how many milliliters are needed for a dose of 9 mg?
17. If a dosage schedule requires 0.25 mg/kg of body weight, what dose is needed for an 88-kg person?
18. If theophylline is available as 80 mg/15 ml, how much is needed for a 100-mg dose?
19. How much drug is needed for a 65-kg adult, using 0.5 mg/kg?
20. The pediatric dosage of an antibiotic is 0.5 g/20 lb of body weight, not to exceed 75 mg/kg/24 hr.
    a. What is the dose for a 40-lb child?
    b. If this dose is given twice in 1 day, has the maximal dose been exceeded?

Percentage-Strength Solutions

1. How many grams of calamine are needed to prepare 120 g of an ointment containing 8% calamine?

SELF-ASSESSMENT QUESTIONS —cont'd

2. One milliliter of active enzyme is found in 147 ml of solution. What is the percentage strength of active enzyme in the solution?
3. If theophylline is available in a 250-mg/10 ml solution, what percentage strength is this?
4. You have epinephrine 1:100. How many milliliters of epinephrine would be needed to contain 30 mg of active ingredient?
5. A dose of 0.4 ml of epinephrine HCl 1:100 is ordered. This dose contains how many milligrams of epinephrine HCl (the active ingredient)?
6. If you administer 3 ml of a 0.1% strength solution, how many milligrams of active ingredient have you given?
7. A drug is available as a 1:200 solution and the maximal dose that may be given by aerosol for a particular patient is 3 mg. What is the maximal amount of solution (in milliliters) that may be used?
8. Epinephrine 1:1000 contains how many milligrams per milliliter?
9. How many milligrams per milliliter are there in 0.3 ml of 5% strength metaproterenol?
10. How many milligrams of sodium chloride are needed for 10 ml of a 0.9% solution?
11. If you have lidocaine (Xylocaine) at 5 mg/ml, what percentage strength is this?
12. A 0.5% strength solution contains how many milligrams in 1 ml?
13. Cromolyn sodium contains 20 mg in 2 ml of water. What is the percentage strength?
14. How much active ingredient of acetylcysteine (Mucomyst) have you given with 4 cc of a 20% solution?
15. You have 20% acetylcysteine; how many milliliters of this do you need to form 4 ml of an 8% solution?
16. The recommended dose of metaproterenol 5% is 0.3 cc. How many milligrams of solute are there in this amount?
17. The Mucomyst brand of acetylcysteine was marketed as 10% acetylcysteine with 0.05% isoproterenol. How many milligrams of each ingredient were in a 4-cc dose of solution?
18. Which contains more drug: 1/2 cc of a 1% drug solution with 2 ml of saline, or 1/2 cc of a 1% drug solution with 5 ml of saline?
19. How many milligrams per milliliter are in a 20% solution?

Intravenous Infusion Rates
Assume a drop factor of 15 drops = 1 ml.

1. You wish to give a solution of 500 mg/L of dobutamine, at a rate of 10 μg/kg/min, to a 50-kg woman. What drip rate will you need?

SELF-ASSESSMENT QUESTIONS —cont'd

2. If you have 2 mg of isoproterenol in 500 ml of solution, and you wish to deliver 5 μg/min intravenously, what drip rate is needed?
3. You have 250 mg of dobutamine in 1 L of solution. You want to deliver 5 μg/kg/min to a 60-kg man. What infusion rate in milliliters per minute and in drops per minute is needed?
4. You have 250 ml of D_5W and a drip rate of 15 drops/min. How long will the bag of solution last?
5. You have an epinephrine solution, 1 mg/250 ml. What drip rate is needed to deliver 4 μg/min?
6. If you wish to deliver 500 ml of a solution in 1 hour and 40 minutes, what drip rate should you set?
7. A recommended dose of epinephrine IV is 15 ml/hr, using a solution of 4 μg/ml. What drip rate is needed to achieve the recommended infusion rate?

Answers to Self-Assessment Questions are found in Appendix A.

CLINICAL SCENARIO

You have a 1 normal (N) solution of saline (NaCl), and you need isotonic saline 0.9%, also called "normal saline," for diluent in a nebulizer solution.

Can you use the 1 N solution as diluent, unchanged?

Answers to Clinical Scenario Questions are found in Appendix A.

Reference

1. Chatburn RL: Measurement, physical quantities, and le Système International d'Unités (SI units), *Respir Care* 33:861, 1988.

Suggested Reading

Fitch GE, Larson MA, Mooney MP: *Basic arithmetic review and drug therapy,* ed 4, New York, 1977Macmillan,

Richardson LI, Richardson JK: *The mathematics of drugs and solutions with clinical applications,* New York, 1976, McGraw-Hill.

Saxton DF, Walter JF: *Programmed instruction in arithmetic, dosages and solutions,* ed 3, St. Louis, Mo, 1974, Mosby.

Chapter 5

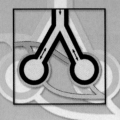

The Central and Peripheral Nervous Systems

DOUGLAS S. GARDENHIRE

CHAPTER OBJECTIVES

After reading this chapter, the reader will be able to:
1. Classify the branches of the nervous system
2. Differentiate between the *central, peripheral,* and
   autonomic nervous systems
3. Discuss the use of *neurotransmitters*
4. Explain in detail the difference between the
   parasympathetic and *sympathetic* branches of the
   nervous system
5. Differentiate the effects of *cholinergic* and
   anticholinergic agents on the nervous system
6. Differentiate the effects of *adrenergic* and
   antiadrenergic agents on the nervous system
7. Discuss the various receptors in the airways
8. Differentiate between *nonadrenergic, noncholinergic
   inhibitory* and *excitatory* nerves

KEY TERMS AND DEFINITIONS

Acetylcholine (ACh) — A chemical produced by the body that is used in the transmission of nerve impulses. It is destroyed by the enzyme cholinesterase

Adrenergic (adrenomimetic) — Refers to a drug stimulating a receptor for norepinephrine or epinephrine

Afferent — Signals that are transmitted to the brain and spinal cord

Antiadrenergic — Refers to a drug blocking a receptor for norepinephrine or epinephrine

Anticholinergic — Refers to a drug blocking a receptor for acetylcholine

Central nervous system (CNS) — A system that includes the brain and spinal cord, controlling voluntary and involuntary acts

Cholinergic (cholinomimetic) — Refers to a drug causing stimulation of a receptor for acetylcholine

Efferent — Signals that are transmitted from the brain and spinal cord

Norepinephrine — A naturally occurring catecholamine, produced by the adrenal medulla, that has properties similar to those of epinephrine. It is used as a neurotransmitter in most sympathetic terminal nerve sites

Parasympatholytic — An agent blocking or inhibiting the effects of the parasympathetic nervous system

Parasympathomimetic — An agent causing stimulation of the parasympathetic nervous system

Peripheral nervous system (PNS) — Portion of the nervous system outside the CNS, including sensory, sympathetic, and parasympathetic nerves

Sympatholytic — An agent blocking or inhibiting the effect of the sympathetic nervous system

Sympathomimetic — An agent causing stimulation of the sympathetic nervous system

---

*T*he goal of Chapter 5 is to provide a clear introduction to and understanding of the peripheral nervous system; its control mechanisms, especially neurotransmitter functions; and its physiological effects in the body. The control mechanisms and physiological effects form the basis for a subsequent understanding of drug actions and drug effects, both for agonists and antagonists that act at various points in the nervous system. The chapter concludes with a summary of autonomic and other neural control mechanisms and their effects in the pulmonary system.

THE NERVOUS SYSTEM

KEY POINT

One of the major control systems in the body is the *nervous system,* comprising *sensory* afferent nerves, *motor* efferent nerves, and the *autonomic nervous system,* which is further divided into the *sympathetic* and *parasympathetic* branches.

There are two major control systems in the body: the *nervous system* and the *endocrine system.* Both systems of control can be manipulated by drug therapy, which either mimics or blocks the usual action of the control system, to produce or inhibit physiological effects. The endocrine system is considered separately in Chapter 11, which discusses the corticosteroid class of drugs. The nervous system is divided into the **central nervous system** and the **peripheral nervous system**, both of

which offer sites for drug action. The overall organization of the nervous system may be outlined as follows:

I. Central nervous system
  A. Brain
  B. Spinal cord
II. Peripheral nervous system
  A. Sensory (afferent) neurons
  B. Somatic (motor) neurons
  C. Autonomic nervous system
    1. Parasympathetic branch
    2. Sympathetic branch

Figure 5-1 indicates a functional, but not anatomically accurate, diagram of the central and peripheral nervous systems. The *sensory* branch of the nervous system consists of afferent neurons from heat, light, pressure, and pain receptors in the periphery, to the central nervous system. The *somatic* portion (or motor branch) of the nervous system is under voluntary, conscious control and innervates skeletal muscle for motor actions such as lifting, walking, or breathing. This portion of the nervous system is manipulated by neuromuscular blocking agents, to induce paralysis in surgical procedures or during mechanical ventilation. The *autonomic nervous system* is the involuntary, unconscious control mechanism of the body, sometimes said to control vegetative or visceral functions. For example, the autonomic nervous system regulates heart rate, pupillary dilation and contraction, glandular secretion such as salivation, and smooth muscle in blood vessels and the airway. It is divided into the *parasympathetic* and *sympathetic* branches.

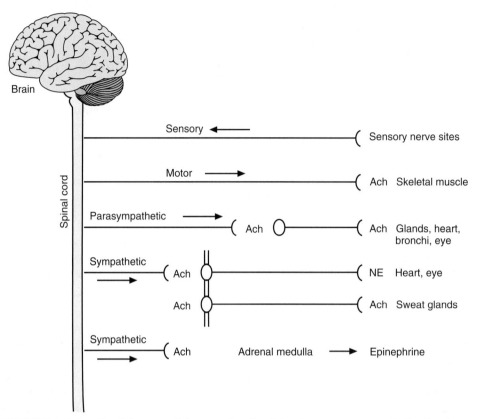

FIGURE 5-1 A functional diagram of the central and peripheral nervous systems, indicating the somatic branches (sensory, motor) and the autonomic branches (sympathetic, parasympathetic), with their neurotransmitters. *ACh,* Acetylcholine; *NE,* norepinephrine.

Anatomical Description of the Autonomic Branches

Neither motor nor sensory branch neurons have synapses outside of the spinal cord before reaching the muscle or sensory receptor site. The motor neuron extends without interruption from the CNS to the skeletal muscle, and its action is mediated by a neurotransmitter, **acetylcholine**. This is in contrast to the synapses occurring in the sympathetic and parasympathetic divisions of the autonomic system. The multiple synapses of the autonomic system offer potential sites for drug action, in addition to the terminal neuroeffector sites.

The parasympathetic branch arises from the craniosacral portions of the spinal cord and consists of two types of neuron—a preganglionic fiber leading from the vertebrae to the ganglionic synapse outside the cord and a postganglionic fiber from the ganglionic synapse to the gland or smooth muscle being innervated. The parasympathetic branch has good specificity, with the postganglionic fiber arising very near the effector

site (e.g., a gland, or smooth muscle). As a result, stimulation of a parasympathetic preganglionic neuron causes activity limited to individual effector sites, such as the heart or the eye. Figure 5-2 illustrates the portions of the spinal cord where the parasympathetic and sympathetic nerve fibers originate.

KEY POINT

Nerve impulses are conducted by both electrical and chemical means; the chemical portion of nerve transmission is referred to as a *neurotransmitter.* The neurotransmitter is *acetylcholine* at the *myoneural (neuromuscular)* junction, at *ganglia,* and at *parasympathetic end sites.* The neurotransmitter at *sympathetic end sites* is generally *norepinephrine,* except at sweat glands and the adrenal medulla, where acetylcholine is the neurotransmitter.

The sympathetic branch arises from the thoracolumbar portion of the spinal cord, and consists of short preganglionic fibers and long postganglionic fibers.

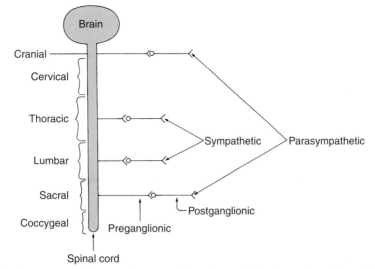

FIGURE 5-2 Parasympathetic nerve fibers arise from the cranial and sacral portions of the spinal cord, whereas sympathetic fibers leave the cord primarily from the thoracic and lumbar regions.

Sympathetic neurons from the spinal cord terminate in ganglia that lie on either side of the vertebral column. In the *ganglia*, or the *ganglionic chain*, the preganglionic fiber makes contact with postganglionic neurons. As a result, when one sympathetic preganglionic neuron is stimulated, the action passes to many or all of the postganglionic fibers. The effect of sympathetic activation is further widened because sympathetic fibers innervate the adrenal medulla and cause the release of epinephrine into the general circulation. Circulating epinephrine stimulates all receptors responding to **norepinephrine**, even if no sympathetic nerves are present. Where the parasympathetic system allows discrete control, the design of the sympathetic system causes a widespread reaction in the body.

Contrasts Between Parasympathetic and Sympathetic Regulation

There are general differences between the parasympathetic and sympathetic branches of the autonomic nervous system, which can be contrasted. Parasympathetic control is essential to life and is considered a more discrete, finely regulated system than sympathetic control. Parasympathetic effects control the day-to-day bodily functions of digestion, bladder and rectal discharge, and basal secretion of bronchial mucus. Overstimulation of the parasympathetic branch would render the body incapable of violent action, resulting in what is termed the *SLUD syndrome*: *s*alivation, *l*acrimation, *u*rination,

and *defecation*. These reactions are definitely counterproductive to fleeing or fighting!

By contrast, the sympathetic branch reacts as a general alarm system and does not exercise discrete controls. This is sometimes characterized as a "fight-or-flight" system: heart rate and blood pressure increase, blood flow shifts from the periphery to muscles and the heart, blood sugar rises, and bronchi dilate. The organism prepares for maximal physical exertion. The sympathetic branch is not essential to life; sympathectomized animal models can survive but of course are not prepared to cope with violent stress.

KEY POINT

Sympathetic effects are widespread, mediated by norepinephrine at nerve endings, as well as by circulating epinephrine released from the adrenal medulla.

Neurotransmitters

Another general feature of the autonomic nervous system, both sympathetic and parasympathetic branches, is the mechanism of neurotransmitter control of nerve impulses. Nerve propagation is both electrical and chemical (electrochemical). A nerve signal is carried along a nerve fiber by *electrical* action potentials, caused by ion exchanges (sodium, potassium). At gaps in the nerve fiber (synapses), the electrical transmission is replaced by a chemical neurotransmitter. This is the *chemical* transmission of the electrical impulse at the ganglionic synapses and at the end of the nerve fiber, termed the *neuroeffector site*. Identification of the chemical transmitters dates back to Loewi's experiments in 1921, and is fundamental to understanding autonomic drugs and their classifications. The usual neurotransmitters in the peripheral nervous system, including the ganglionic synapses and terminal sites in the autonomic branches, are indicated in Figure 5-1, where *ACh* is acetylcholine and *NE* is norepinephrine.

The neurotransmitter conducting the nerve impulse at skeletal muscle sites is acetylcholine, and this site is referred to as the *neuromuscular junction,* or the myoneural junction. In the parasympathetic branch, the neurotransmitter is also acetylcholine at both the ganglionic synapse and at the terminal nerve site, referred to as the *neuroeffector site*. In the sympathetic branch, acetylcholine is the neurotransmitter at the ganglionic synapse; however, norepinephrine is the neurotransmitter at the neuroeffector site. There are two exceptions to this pattern, both in the sympathetic branch. Sympathetic fibers to sweat glands release acetylcholine instead of norepinephrine, and preganglionic sympathetic fibers directly innervate the adrenal medulla, where the neurotransmitter is acetylcholine. Sympathetic fibers that have acetylcholine at the neuroeffector sites are *cholinergic* (for acetylcholine) *sympathetic* fibers. This would be an apparent contradictory combination of terms if not for the exceptions to the rule of norepinephrine as the sympathetic neurotransmitter. For example, sweating can be caused by giving a cholinergic drug such as pilocarpine, although this effect is under sympathetic control. "Breaking out in a sweat," along with sweaty palms and increased heart rate resulting from circulating epinephrine, are common effects of stress or fright mediated by sympathetic discharge.

Although it is an oversimplification, an easy way to initially learn the various neurotransmitters is to remember that acetylcholine is the neurotransmitter *everywhere* (skeletal muscle, all ganglionic synapses, and parasympathetic terminal nerve sites) *except* at sympathetic terminal nerve sites, where norepinephrine is the neurotransmitter. Then the exceptions provided by sympathetic fibers releasing acetylcholine can be remembered as exceptions to the general rule.

Efferent and Afferent Nerve Fibers

The autonomic system is generally considered an **efferent system**; that is, impulses in the sympathetic and parasympathetic branches travel *from* the brain and spinal cord out *to* the various neuroeffector sites,

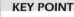

KEY POINT

The neurotransmitter acetylcholine is terminated by the enzyme *cholinesterase,* and norepinephrine and sympathetic transmission are terminated by neurotransmitter *reuptake* into the presynaptic neuron (uptake-1), as well as by the enzymes *catechol O-methyltransferase (COMT)* and *monoamine oxidase (MAO).*

such as the heart, gastrointestinal tract, and lungs. However, **afferent** nerves run alongside the sympathetic and parasympathetic efferent fibers and carry impulses *from* the periphery to the cord. The afferent fibers convey impulses resulting from visceral stimuli and can form a reflex arc of stimulus input–autonomic output analogous to the well-known somatic reflex arcs, such as the knee-jerk reflex. The mechanism of a vagal reflex arc mediating bronchoconstriction is further discussed in Chapter 7, in conjunction with drugs used to block the parasympathetic impulses.

Terminology of Drugs Affecting the Nervous System

KEY POINT

The terms *cholinergic* or *cholinoceptor* and *adrenergic* or *adrenoceptor* are used, respectively, for acetylcholine and norepinephrine/epinephrine receptors in the two autonomic branches.

Terminology of drugs and drug effects on the nervous system can be confusing and may seem inconsistent. The confusion is due to the fact that drugs and drug effects are derived from the type of nerve fiber (parasympathetic or sympathetic) or, alternatively, the type of neurotransmitter and receptor (acetylcholine and norepinephrine). The following terms are based on the anatomy of the nerve fibers, to describe stimulation or inhibition.

Parasympathomimetic: An agent causing stimulation of the parasympathetic nervous system sites
Parasympatholytic: An agent blocking or inhibiting effects of the parasympathetic nervous system
Sympathomimetic: An agent causing stimulation of the sympathetic nervous system
Sympatholytic: An agent blocking or inhibiting effects of the sympathetic nervous system

Additional terms are used, based on the type of neurotransmitter and receptor. Cholinergic refers to acetylcholine, and adrenergic is derived from adrenaline, another term for epinephrine, which is similar to norepinephrine and can stimulate sympathetic neuro-effector sites. Because acetylcholine is the neurotransmitter at more sites than just parasympathetic sites, and because receptors exist on smooth muscle or blood cells without any nerve fibers innervating them, these terms denote a wider range of sites than the anatomically based terms such as parasympathomimetic, defined above. For example, cholinergic can refer to a drug effect at a ganglion, a parasympathetic nerve ending site, or the neuromuscular junction. Adrenergic describes receptors on bronchial smooth muscle or on blood cells, where there are no sympathetic nerves. For this reason, cholinergic and adrenergic are not strictly synonymous with parasympathetic or sympathetic. *Cholinoceptor* and *adrenoceptor* are alternative terms for cholinergic and adrenergic receptors, respectively.

Cholinergic (cholinomimetic): Refers to a drug causing stimulation of a receptor for acetylcholine
Anticholinergic: Refers to a drug blocking a receptor for acetylcholine
Adrenergic (adrenomimetic): Refers to a drug stimulating a receptor for norepinephrine or epinephrine
Antiadrenergic: Refers to a drug blocking a receptor for norepinephrine or epinephrine
Cholinoceptor: An alternative term for cholinergic receptor
Adrenoceptor: An alternative term for adrenergic receptor

KEY POINT

- Parasympathomimetic = Cholinergic
- Parasympatholytic = Anticholinergic
- Sympathomimetic = Adrenergic
- Sympatholytic = Antiadrenergic

PARASYMPATHETIC BRANCH

Cholinergic Neurotransmitter Function

KEY POINT

Parasympathetic effects on the cardiopulmonary system include decreased heart rate, lower blood pressure, bronchoconstriction, and mucous secretion in the airways.

In the parasympathetic branch, the neurotransmitter *acetylcholine* conducts nerve transmission at the ganglionic site, as well as at the parasympathetic effector site at the end of the postganglionic fiber. This action is illustrated in Figure 5-3. The term *neurohormone* has also been used in place of neurotransmitter. Acetylcholine (Ach) is concentrated in the presynaptic neuron (both at the ganglion and the effector site). Acetylcholine is

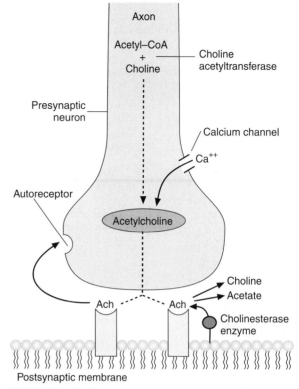

FIGURE 5-3 Cholinergic nerve transmission mediated by the neurotransmitter acetylcholine *(Ach)*. The action of the neurotransmitter is terminated by cholinesterase enzymes; attachment of acetylcholine to presynaptic autoreceptors inhibits further neurotransmitter release.

synthesized from acetyl-CoA and choline, catalyzed by the enzyme choline acetyltransferase. The acetylcholine is stored in vesicles as quanta of 1000 to 50,000 molecules per vesicle. When a nerve impulse *(action potential)* reaches the presynaptic neuron site, an influx of calcium is triggered into the neuron. Increased calcium in the neuron causes cellular secretion of the acetylcholine-containing vesicles from the end of the nerve fiber. After release, the acetylcholine attaches to receptors on the postsynaptic membrane and initiates an effect in the tissue or organ site.

Acetylcholine is then inactivated through hydrolysis by cholinesterase enzymes, which split the acetylcholine molecule into choline and acetate, terminating stimulation of the postsynaptic membrane. In effect the nerve impulse is "shut off." There are also receptors on the presynaptic neuron, termed *autoreceptors,* that can be stimulated by acetylcholine to regulate and inhibit further neurotransmitter release from the neuron. The effects of the parasympathetic branch of the autonomic system on various organs are listed in Table 5-1. Drugs can mimic or

TABLE 5-1

Effects of Parasympathetic Stimulation on Selected Organs or Sites

Organ/Site	Parasympathetic (Cholinergic) Response
Heart	
SA node	Slowing of rate
Contractility	Decreased atrial force
Conduction velocity	Decreased AV node conduction
Bronchi	
Smooth muscle	Constriction
Mucus glands	Increased secretion
Vascular smooth muscle	
Skin and mucosa	No innervation*
Pulmonary	No innervation*
Skeletal muscle	No innervation†
Coronary	No innervation*
Salivary glands	Increased secretion
Skeletal muscle	None
Eye	
Iris radial muscle	None
Iris circular muscle	Contraction (miosis)
Ciliary muscle	Contraction for near vision
Gastrointestinal tract	Increased motility
Gastrointestinal sphincters	Relaxation
Urinary bladder	
Detrusor	Contraction
Trigone sphincter	Relaxation
Glycogenolysis	
Skeletal muscle	None
Sweat glands	None‡
Lipolysis (multiple sites)	None
Renin secretion (kidney)	None
Insulin secretion (pancreas)	Increased

AV, Atrioventricular; *SA,* sinoatrial

*No direct parasympathetic nerve innervation; response to exogenous cholinergic agonists is dilation.

†Dilation occurs as a result of sympathetic cholinergic discharge or as a response to exogenous cholinergic agonists.

‡Sweat glands are under sympathetic control; receptors are cholinergic, however, and the response to exogenous cholinergic agonists is increased secretion.

block the action of the neurotransmitter acetylcholine, to stimulate parasympathetic nerve ending sites (parasympathomimetics) or to block the transmission of such impulses (parasympatholytics). Both categories of drugs affecting the parasympathetic branch are commonly seen clinically. The effects of the parasympathetic system on the heart, bronchial smooth muscle, and exocrine glands should be mentally reviewed before considering parasympathetic agonists or antagonists (blockers).

- Heart: Slows rate (vagus)
- Bronchial smooth muscle: Constriction
- Exocrine glands: Increased secretion

Muscarinic and Nicotinic Receptors and Effects

Two additional terms are used to refer to stimulation of receptor sites for acetylcholine; they are derived from the action in the body of two substances, the alkaloids *muscarine* and *nicotine*. Receptor sites that are stimulated by these two chemicals are illustrated in Figure 5-4.

Muscarinic Effects

KEY POINT

Muscarinic refers to cholinergic receptors at parasympathetic end sites. Muscarinic receptors are distinguished into subtypes: M_1 through M_5, with M_2 receptors in the heart, and M_3 receptors on airway smooth muscle, mediating bronchoconstriction.

Muscarine, a natural product from the mushroom *Amanita muscaria,* stimulates acetylcholine (cholinergic) receptors at the parasympathetic terminal sites: exocrine glands (lacrimal, salivary, and bronchial mucous glands), cardiac muscle, and smooth muscle (gastrointestinal tract). Acetylcholine receptors at these sites, and the effects of parasympathetic stimulation at these sites, are therefore termed *muscarinic.* A muscarinic effect well known to respiratory care clinicians is the increase in airway secretions after administration of acetylcholine-like drugs such as neostigmine. There is also a fall in blood pressure caused by slowing of the heart and vasodilation. *In general, a parasympathomimetic effect is the same as a muscarinic effect, and a parasympatholytic effect is referred to as an* antimuscarinic *effect.*

Nicotinic Effects

KEY POINT

The term *nicotinic* refers to cholinergic receptors on ganglia and at the neuromuscular junction.

Nicotine, a substance in tobacco products, stimulates acetylcholine (cholinergic) receptors at autonomic ganglia (both parasympathetic and sympathetic) and at skeletal muscle sites. Acetylcholine receptors at autonomic ganglia and at the skeletal muscle are termed *nicotinic,* as are the effects on these sites of stimulation. Practical effects of stimulating these nicotinic receptors include a rise in blood pressure resulting from stimulation of sympathetic ganglia, causing vasoconstriction when the postganglionic fibers discharge, and muscle tremor caused by skeletal tissue stimulation.

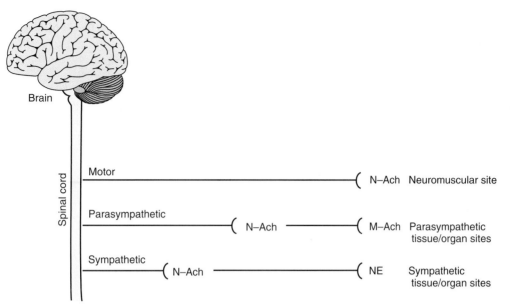

FIGURE 5-4 Location of nicotinic and muscarinic receptor sites in the peripheral nervous system. *M–Ach,* Muscarinic site; *N–Ach,* nicotinic site; *NE,* norepinephrine.

Subtypes of Muscarinic Receptors

Parasympathetic receptors, and cholinergic receptors in general with or without corresponding nerve fibers, are further classified into subtypes. These differences among cholinergic or muscarinic (M) receptors are based on different responses to different drugs, or recognition through use of DNA probes. Five muscarinic receptor subtypes have been identified: M_1, M_2, M_3, M_4, and M_5. They are all G protein linked (see Chapter 2). As G protein–linked receptors, these five subtypes of muscarinic receptors share a structural feature common to such receptors—a long, "serpentine" polypeptide chain that crosses the cell membrane seven times, as previously illustrated for G protein receptors in Chapter 2. Table 5-2 summarizes THE muscarinic receptor subtypes, with their predominant location and the type of G protein with which they are coupled. Additional detail on muscarinic receptor location and function in the pulmonary system is presented in the final section of this chapter, which summarizes nervous control and receptors in the lung.

CHOLINERGIC AGENTS

Cholinergic drugs mimic the action caused by acetylcholine at receptor sites in the parasympathetic system and neuromuscular junction. Such agents can cause stimulation at the terminal nerve site (neuroeffector junction) by two distinct mechanisms, leading to their classification as

TABLE 5-2		
Muscarinic Receptor Subtypes, Location, and G-Protein Linkage		
Muscarinic Receptor Type	**Location**	**G-Protein Subtype**
M_1	Parasympathetic ganglia, nasal submucosal glands	G_q
M_2	Heart, postganglionic parasympathetic nerves	G_i
M_3	Airway smooth muscle, submucosal glands	G_q
M_4	Postganglionic cholinergic nerves, possible effect on CNS	G_i
M_5	Possible effect on CNS	G_q

CNS, Central nervous system

direct or indirect acting. Table 5-3 lists cholinergic agents, categorized as direct or indirect acting, and their clinical uses. The terms *cholinergic, cholinoceptor stimulant,* and *cholinomimetic* are broader than *parasympathomimetic* and denote agents stimulating acetylcholine receptors located in the parasympathetic system (muscarinic) or other sites, such as the neuromuscular junction (nicotinic). A cholinergic drug can activate muscarinic and nicotinic receptors.

Direct-Acting Cholinergic Agents

Direct-acting cholinergic agents are structurally similar to acetylcholine. As shown in Figure 5-3, direct-acting cholinergic agents mimic acetylcholine, binding and

TABLE 5-3

Examples of Direct- and Indirect-Acting Cholinergic Agents, With Their Generic Names, Brand Names, and Clinical Uses

Category	Generic Name	Brand Name	Clinical Uses
Direct Acting			
	Acetylcholine chloride	Miochol-E	Ophthalmic miotic, glaucoma
	Carbachol	Carboptic	Ophthalmic miotic, glaucoma
	Pilocarpine hydrochloride	Pilocar, various	Ophthalmic miotic, glaucoma
	Methacholine	Provocholine	Diagnostic, asthma
	Bethanechol	Urecholine	Treatment of urinary retention
Indirect Acting			
	Echothiophate	Phospholine	Ophthalmic miotic, glaucoma
	Pyridostigmine	Mestinon	Muscle stimulant, myasthenia gravis, Reversal of nondepolarizing muscle relaxants
	Ambenonium	Mytelase	Muscle stimulant, myasthenia gravis
	Neostigmine	Prostigmin	Muscle stimulant, myasthenia gravis, Reversal of nondepolarizing muscle relaxants
	Edrophonium	Tensilon	Diagnostic, myasthenia gravis,

activating muscarinic or nicotinic receptors directly. Examples of this group include methacholine, carbachol, bethanechol, and pilocarpine. Methacholine has been used in bronchial challenge tests by inhalation to assess the degree of airway reactivity in asthmatics and others. The parasympathetic effect is bronchoconstriction. Methacholine is a useful diagnostic agent to detect differences in degree of airway reactivity between asthmatics with hyperreactive airways and nonasthmatic individuals.

Indirect-Acting Cholinergic Agents

KEY POINT

Parasympathomimetic, or cholinergic, agonists are divided into *direct-acting* agents (e.g., methacholine), which resemble acetylcholine and stimulate cholinergic receptors directly, and *indirect-acting* agents (e.g., neostigmine), which inhibit the enzyme cholinesterase, to allow increased acetylcholine transmission. A typical *parasympatholytic*, or *anticholinergic*, agent is atropine.

Indirect-acting cholinergic agonists inhibit the cholinesterase enzyme, as seen in Figure 5-3. Because cholinesterase usually inactivates the acetylcholine neurotransmitter, inhibiting this enzyme results in accumulation of endogenous acetylcholine at the neuroeffector junction of parasympathetic nerve endings or the neuromuscular junction. This makes more acetylcholine available to attach to receptor sites and to stimulate cholinergic responses. If acetylcholine receptors have been blocked, this increase in neurotransmitter can

reverse the blockage by competing with the blocking drug for the receptors. Nerve transmission can then resume, either at the parasympathetic terminal site or the neuromuscular junction.

The drug echothiophate, listed in Table 5-3, stimulates autonomic muscarinic receptors in the iris sphincter and ciliary muscle of the eye, to produce pupillary constriction *(miosis)* and lens thickening. An increase in the neurotransmitter acetylcholine at the neuromuscular junction makes drugs such as neostigmine useful in reversing neuromuscular blockade caused by paralyzing agents such as pancuronium or doxacurium (see Chapter 18). Neostigmine and edrophonium are also useful in increasing muscle strength in a neuromuscular disease such as myasthenia gravis, in which the cholinergic receptor is blocked by autoantibodies. The drug edrophonium (Tensilon) is used in the Tensilon test, to determine whether muscle weakness is caused by overdosing with an indirect-acting cholinergic agent (causing ultimate receptor fatigue and blockade) or undertreatment with insufficient drug. Because edrophonium is short-acting (5 to 15 minutes, depending on the dose), it is useful as a diagnostic agent, rather than as a maintenance treatment in neuromuscular disease.

When using indirect-acting cholinergic agents such as neostigmine to increase nerve function at the neuromuscular junction, acetylcholine activity at parasympathetic sites such as salivary and nasopharyngeal glands also increases. These undesirable muscarinic effects can be blocked by pretreatment with a parasympatholytic or antimuscarinic drug such as atropine or its derivatives.

Cholinesterase Reactivator (Pralidoxime)

Organophosphates such as parathion and malathion, and the drug echothiophate (Phospholine), form an irreversible bond with cholinesterase (also called *acetylcholinesterase*). The organophosphates are used as insecticides, and occasionally patients are seen with toxic exposure and absorption. The effects of these agents can be lethal, and because of this, they have also been used as "nerve gas." Because they affect acetylcholine, they have an effect on neuromuscular function as well as muscarinic receptors; there is initial stimulation, then blockade if a high enough dosage is absorbed. Muscle weakness and paralysis can result.

The bonding of irreversible inhibitors with the cholinesterase is slow, taking up to 24 hours. However, once formed, the duration is limited only by the body's ability to produce new cholinesterase, which takes 1 to 2 weeks. A drug such as pralidoxime (Protopam), a cholinesterase reactivator, can be used in the treatment of organophosphate toxicity, in the first 24 hours. After this time, the bond of cholinesterase and cholinesterase inhibitors cannot be reversed, but atropine (a parasympatholytic) can be used to block the overly available acetylcholine neurotransmitter at the receptor sites. Support of ventilation and airway maintenance would be required for the duration of the effects.

ANTICHOLINERGIC AGENTS

Anticholinergic agents block acetylcholine receptors and act as cholinergic antagonists. Parasympatholytic (antimuscarinic) agents such as atropine, as well as drug classes such as neuromuscular blockers and ganglionic blockers, are all anticholinergic because they all block acetylcholine at their respective sites. However, a neuromuscular or ganglionic blocking agent would *not* be considered a parasympatholytic or antimuscarinic agent, because the site of action is not within the parasympathetic system. The parasympatholytic agents are antimuscarinic because of the limitation to parasympathetic terminal fiber sites.

Atropine as a Prototype Parasympatholytic Agent

Atropine is usually considered the prototype parasympatholytic, and there is renewed interest in the use of aerosolized analogs of atropine in respiratory care. This is discussed more fully in Chapter 7. Atropine occurs naturally as the levo isomer in *Atropa belladonna*,

the nightshade plant, and also in *Datura stramonium*, or jimsonweed. The drug is referred to as a *belladonna alkaloid*. Atropine is a *competitive antagonist* to acetylcholine at muscarinic receptor sites (glands, gastrointestinal tract, heart, and eyes), and can form a reversible bond with these cholinergic receptors. It is nonspecific for muscarinic receptor subtypes and blocks M_1, M_2, and M_3 receptors. Atropine blocks salivary secretion and causes dry mouth. In the respiratory system, atropine decreases secretion by mucous glands, and relaxes bronchial smooth muscle by blocking parasympathetically maintained basal tone. Atropine blocks vagal innervation of the heart to produce increased heart rate. There is no effect on blood vessels because these do not have parasympathetic innervation, only the acetylcholine receptors. Vascular resistance would not increase with atropine. Of course, if a parasympathomimetic *were* given, then atropine would block the dilating effect on blood vessel receptor sites. Pupillary dilation *(mydriasis)* occurs as a result of blockade of the circular iris muscle, and the lens is flattened *(cycloplegia)* by blockade of the ciliary muscle. In the gastrointestinal tract, atropine decreases acid secretion, tone, and mobility. Bladder wall smooth muscle is relaxed and voiding is slowed. Sweating is inhibited by atropine, which blocks acetylcholine receptors on sweat glands. Sweat glands are innervated by sympathetic cholinergic fibers.

At usual clinical doses, atropine exerts a low level of central nervous system stimulation, with a slower sedative effect in the brain. Scopolamine, another classic antimuscarinic agent, can produce drowsiness and even amnesia. In larger doses, atropine can cause toxic effects in the central nervous system, including hallucinations.

The anticholinergic (antimuscarinic) effect on the vestibular system can inhibit motion sickness. Scopolamine was used for this, and antihistamine drugs such as dimenhydrinate (Dramamine) that have anticholinergic effects are commonly used to prevent motion sickness. The dry mouth and drowsiness that also occur with a drug such as dimenhydrinate are typical antimuscarinic effects.

Parasympatholytic (Antimuscarinic) Effects

If the basic effects of the parasympathetic system are known, the effects of an antagonist such as atropine can be deduced. For example, if parasympathetic (vagal) stimulation slows the heart rate, OKa parasympatholytic should increase the heart rate by blocking that innervation. Box 5-1 lists the effects and uses of parasympatholytic agents.

Box 5-1	Uses and Effects of Parasympatholytic (Antimuscarinic) Agents

- Bronchodilation
- Preoperative drying of secretions
- Antidiarrheal agent
- Prevention of bed-wetting in children (increase in urinary retention)
- Treatment of peptic ulcer
- Treatment of organophosphate poisoning
- Treatment of mushroom *(Amanita muscaria)* ingestion
- Treatment of bradycardia

SYMPATHETIC BRANCH

KEY POINT

Sympathetic effects on the cardiopulmonary system include increased heart rate and contractile force, increased blood pressure, bronchodilation, and probable increased secretion from mucous glands in the airway.

As noted in the general description of the parasympathetic and sympathetic branches of the autonomic nervous system, sympathetic (adrenergic) effects are mediated both by neurotransmitter release from sympathetic nerves and by the release of circulating catecholamines, norepinephrine and epinephrine, from the adrenal medulla. Circulating catecholamines stimulate adrenergic receptors throughout the body, not just receptors with nerve fibers present. Sympathetic activation results in stimulation of the heart, increased cardiac output, increased blood pressure, mental stimulation, accelerated metabolism, and bronchodilation in the pulmonary system.

Adrenergic Neurotransmitter Function

In the sympathetic branch of the autonomic nervous system, the usual neurotransmitter at the terminal nerve sites is norepinephrine, with the exceptions described previously (sweat glands and the adrenal medulla). Figure 5-5 illustrates neurotransmitter function with norepinephrine. In the presynaptic neuron, tyrosine is converted to dopa and then to dopamine, which is then converted by dopamine β-hydroxylase to norepinephrine, in the storage vesicles. An action potential in the nerve opens calcium channels, allowing an influx of calcium. Increased intracellular calcium leads to exocytosis of the vesicles containing norepinephrine, which then attaches to receptors on the postsynaptic membrane. The exact physiological effect depends on

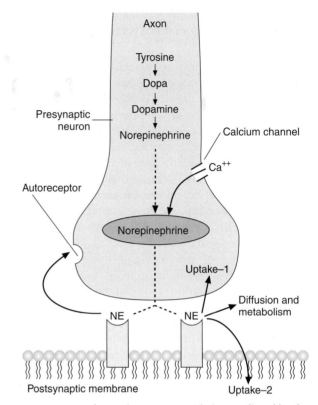

FIGURE 5-5 Adrenergic nerve transmission mediated by the neurotransmitter norepinephrine *(NE)*. The action of the neurotransmitter is terminated primarily by a reuptake mechanism (uptake-1), as well as by enzyme metabolism and a second uptake mechanism into tissue sites (uptake-2). Norepinephrine attaches to autoreceptor sites on the presynaptic neuron to inhibit further neurotransmitter release.

the site of innervation and the type of sympathetic receptor, which can also vary, as described below.

The primary method of terminating the action of norepinephrine at the postsynaptic membrane is through a reuptake process, back into the presynaptic neuron. This is termed *uptake-1*. The neurotransmitter action can be ended by two other mechanisms as well: uptake into tissue sites around the nerve terminal, a process termed *uptake-2* to distinguish it from reuptake into the nerve terminal itself, and diffusion of excess norepinephrine away from the receptor site, to be metabolized in the liver or plasma. In addition, norepinephrine can stimulate *autoreceptors* on the presynaptic neuron, which inhibits further neurotransmitter release. These autoreceptors have been identified as α_2-receptors (discussed later in this chapter).

The distinction between two types of uptake process is due to research published by Iversen in 1965.[1]

TABLE 5-4

Effects of Sympathetic (Adrenergic) Stimulation on Selected Organs or Sites*

Organ/Site	Sympathetic (Adrenergic) Response
Heart	
SA node	Increase in rate
Contractility	Increase in force
Conduction velocity	Increased AV node conduction
Bronchi	
Smooth muscle	Relaxation and dilation of airway diameter
Mucous glands	Increased secretion
Vascular smooth muscle	
Skin and mucosa	Vasoconstriction
Pulmonary	Dilation/constriction (two types of sympathetic receptors)
Skeletal muscle	Dilation (predominantly)
Coronary	Dilation/constriction (two types of sympathetic receptors)
Salivary glands	Decreased secretion
Skeletal muscle	Increased contractility
Eye	
Iris radial muscle	Contraction (mydriasis)
Iris circular muscle	None
Ciliary muscle	Relaxation for far vision[†]
Gastrointestinal tract	Decreased motility
Gastrointestinal sphincters	Contraction
Urinary bladder	
Detrusor	Relaxation
Trigone sphincter	Contraction
Sweat glands	Increased secretion[‡]
Glycogenolysis	
Skeletal muscle	Increased
Lipolysis (multiple sites)	Increased
Renin secretion (kidney)	Increased
Insulin secretion (pancreas)	Decreased

*Effects of sympathetic activation are mediated by direct innervation of nerve fibers, as well as by circulating epinephrine released from the adrenal medulla.
[†]Relaxes as a result of circulating epinephrine, with sympathetic activation.
[‡]Innervated by sympathetic nerves with *acetylcholine* neurotransmitter (cholinergic receptors); response to exogenous cholinergic agent is increased sweating.

The uptake-2 process is a mediated uptake of exogenous amines (chemicals such as norepinephrine) in *nonneuronal* tissues; for example, cardiac muscle cells. Iversen distinguished the following details of the uptake-2 process[2]:

- It is a mediated transport system.
- It is a low-affinity but high-capacity system.
- It is not as stereochemically specific as uptake-1.
- It is specific to catecholamines.
- The order of affinity for uptake of specific agents, in *decreasing* order, is as follows: isoproterenol > epinephrine > norepinephrine.
- Certain corticosteroids can inhibit the uptake-2 process, thereby potentiating catecholamines.

The last effect of uptake-2 inhibition by corticosteroids is discussed more fully in Chapter 11. The physiological effects of sympathetic activation are listed in Table 5-4. The effects in Table 5-4 are given for the same organs as those listed in Table 5-1 for the parasympathetic system, for comparison.

Enzyme Inactivation

The enzymes that metabolize norepinephrine, epinephrine, and chemicals similar to these neurotransmitters are important for understanding differences in the action of the adrenergic bronchodilator group. Chemicals structurally related to epinephrine are termed *catecholamines,* and their general structure is outlined in Chapter 6 in the discussion of sympathomimetic (adrenergic) bronchodilators. Two enzymes are available that can inactivate catecholamines such as epinephrine. These are catechol *O*-methyltransferase (COMT) and monoamine oxidase (MAO). The action of both enzymes on epinephrine (Figure 5-6) is of importance because COMT is responsible for ending the action of catecholamine bronchodilators.

Sympathetic (Adrenergic) Receptor Types

The effects of adrenergic receptors are mediated by coupling with G proteins, and they are identified as G protein–linked receptors. A summary of adrenergic receptor subtypes, with examples of their location and the type of G protein with which they are coupled, is given in Table 5-5.

α and β Receptors

KEY POINT

Receptors at sympathetic end sites are subdivided into α and β receptors, with α receptors mediating excitatory effects (e.g., vasoconstriction) and β receptors mediating inhibitory effects (e.g., smooth muscle relaxation).

In 1948, Ahlquist distinguished *alpha (α)* and *beta (β)* sympathetic receptors on the basis of differing responses to a variety of adrenergic drugs, all of which

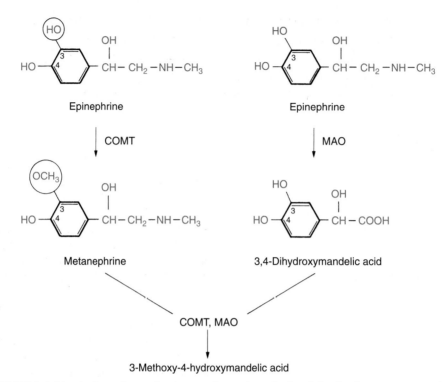

FIGURE 5-6 Metabolic pathways for the transformation of epinephrine by the enzymes catechol O-methyltransferase *(COMT)* and monoamine oxidase *(MAO)* to an inactive form.

were similar to norepinephrine, with minor structural differences.[3] These drugs included phenylephrine, norepinephrine, epinephrine, and isoproterenol. The two types of sympathetic receptors were distinguished as follows:

α Receptors: Generally *excite,* with the exception of the intestine and central nervous system receptors, where inhibition or relaxation occurs

β Receptors: Generally inhibit or *relax,* with the exception of the heart, where stimulation occurs

TABLE 5-5

Adrenergic Receptor Subtypes: Location and G-Protein Linkage

Receptor Type	Location	G-Protein Subtype
Alpha-1 (α_1)	Peripheral blood vessels	G_q
Alpha-2 (α_2)	Presynaptic sympathetic neurons (autoreceptor), CNS	G_i
Beta-1 (β_1)	Heart	G_s
Beta-2 (β_2)	Smooth muscle (including bronchial), cardiac muscle	G_s
Beta-3 (β_3)	Lipocytes	G_s

CNS, Central nervous system.

α-Sympathetic receptors are found on peripheral blood vessels, and stimulation results in vasoconstriction. α-Adrenergic agonists are frequently used for topical vasoconstriction of the nasal mucosa, to treat symptoms of nasal congestion caused by the common cold. β-Adrenergic receptors are found on airway smooth muscle and in the heart. Drug activity of adrenergic stimulants (sympathomimetics) ranges along the spectrum seen in Figure 5-7.

As illustrated in Figure 5-7, phenylephrine is one of the purest α stimulants, and isoproterenol is an almost pure β stimulant. It is stressed that "pure" reactions do not occur with any drug; that is, even phenylephrine may affect other sites. Epinephrine stimulates both α and β sites equally, but norepinephrine has more of an α than β effect.

β_1 and β_2 Receptors

In 1967, Lands further differentiated β receptors into β_1 and β_2 subtypes.[4] β_1 receptors are found in cardiac muscle, and β_2 receptors (which encompass all other β receptors) include those found in bronchial, vascular, and skeletal muscle. The distinction among types of β receptors is as follows:

β_1 Receptors: Increases the rate and force of cardiac contraction

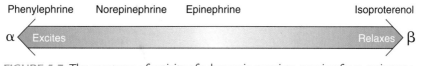

FIGURE 5-7 The spectrum of activity of adrenergic agonists, ranging from excitatory effects to inhibitory effects, by which α and β receptors are distinguished.

β₂ Receptors: Relaxes bronchial smooth muscle and vascular beds of skeletal muscle

> **KEY POINT**
>
> The β receptors are subdivided into β₁ receptors, which are excitatory and found in the heart, and β₂ receptors, which are found elsewhere and mediate inhibitory responses.

The β₁ receptors constitute the exception to the general rule that β receptors cause relaxation. The β₂ receptors form the basis for the class of adrenergic bronchodilators, which act to relax bronchial smooth muscle by stimulation of these receptors. The β receptor, briefly characterized as an example of a G protein-linked receptor in Chapter 2 in the introduction to *pharmacodynamics* (drug–receptor interaction), is discussed in more detail in Chapter 6, which discusses β-adrenergic bronchodilators. A third type of β receptor, the β₃ receptor, has also been distinguished as a β-receptor type found on lipocytes (fat cells) and whose stimulation results in lipolysis.

α₁ and α₂ Receptors

The α receptors have also been differentiated into α₁ and α₂ receptor types. This classification has been made on a *morphological* basis (location of the receptors) and a *pharmacological* basis (differences in response to various drugs). The pharmacological differentiation of α₁ and α₂ receptors is similar to the distinction between α and β receptors (Figure 5-8). This differentiation is based on a

> **KEY POINT**
>
> The α receptors are subdivided into α₁ receptors, which are excitatory, and α₂ receptors, which are inhibitory are found on the presynaptic neuron to inhibit further neurotransmitter release.

response continuum ranging from excitation (α₁) to inhibition (α₂) as different drugs are administered. For example, phenylephrine causes vasoconstriction, as previously mentioned, whereas clonidine (Catapres) causes a lowering of blood pressure and sympathetic activity. *Both* agents are considered α-receptor agonists. Other agents such as prazosin (Minipress) or labetalol (Normodyne) cause a lowering of blood pressure, but yohimbine causes a rise in blood pressure. Yet these agents are *all* considered α-receptor antagonists. However, blockade of α₁-excitatory receptors by prazosin would prevent vasoconstriction and lower blood pressure, whereas blockade of α₂-inhibitory receptors by yohimbine would prevent vasodilation and increase blood pressure. Because different α agonists can cause opposite effects, and different α blockers do the same, α receptors were subdivided into the two types given. The location-based, or morphologic, differentiation of α₁ and α₂ receptors is more complex. In *peripheral* nerves, α₁ receptors are located on postsynaptic sites such as vascular smooth muscle and α₂ receptors are presynaptic (Figure 5-9). Stimulation of these peripheral α₁ receptors causes excitation and vasoconstriction; activation of peripheral (presynaptic) α₂ receptors causes inhibition of further neurotransmitter release. Peripheral α₂ receptors thereby perform a negative feedback control

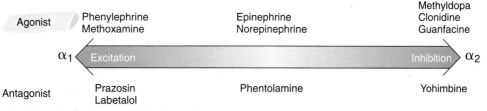

FIGURE 5-8 The spectrum of activity of α-receptor agonists and antagonists, from excitatory to inhibitory. Epinephrine and norepinephrine can stimulate both α₁- and α₂-receptor sites. A drug such as phenylephrine stimulates α₁ receptors and causes vasoconstriction, whereas methyldopa stimulates α₂ receptors and can lower blood pressure, although both are α-receptor agonists. Prazosin is a selective α₁-blocking agent, and yohimbine is a selective α₂-blocking agent.

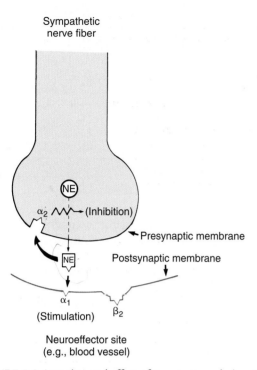

Sympathetic
nerve fiber

(NE)

α_2 ∿∿∿ (Inhibition)

← Presynaptic membrane

NE

Postsynaptic membrane →

α_1
(Stimulation) β_2

Neuroeffector site
(e.g., blood vessel)

FIGURE 5-9 Location and effect of α_2 receptors, designated *autoreceptors*. Stimulation of α_2 receptors by norepinephrine on the presynaptic neuron inhibits further neurotransmitter release and nerve action.

mechanism, referred to as *autoregulation,* which has been demonstrated with sympathetic (adrenergic) neurons; they are referred to as *autoreceptors* (see Figure 5-5).[5] Norepinephrine released from the nerve ending can activate both α_1 (postsynaptic) and α_2 (presynaptic) receptors. The postsynaptic stimulation causes the cell response such as vasoconstriction, but the presynaptic stimulation leads to inhibition of further neurotransmitter release. In the central nervous system, α_2 receptors are generally considered to be on postsynaptic sites; this is the reverse of their location peripherally, where they are presynaptic. These central postsynaptic α_2 receptors are the site of action for antihypertensive agents such as clonidine (Catapres) or methyldopa (Aldomet). These are further discussed and illustrated in Chapter 20.

To summarize, α_1 and β_1 receptors *excite,* and α_2 and β_2 receptors *inhibit.* This consistency of subscripts for excitation (1) versus inhibition (2) aids in remembering their effects.

Dopaminergic Receptors

There are other receptors in the central nervous system (brain) that respond to dopamine, a chemical precursor of norepinephrine, and are therefore termed *dopaminergic.* Because dopamine is chemically similar to epinephrine and stimulates α and β receptors, dopaminergic receptors are classified as a type of adrenergic receptor.

SYMPATHOMIMETIC (ADRENERGIC) AND SYMPATHOLYTIC (ANTIADRENERGIC) AGENTS

Drugs that stimulate the sympathetic system and produce adrenergic effects (sympathomimetics) and drugs that block adrenergic effects (sympatholytics) are discussed in greater detail in separate chapters. In this book, emphasis is placed on β-adrenergic agonists used for bronchodilation (see Chapter 6) and on adrenergic agonists used for cardiovascular effects such as cardiac stimulation (see Chapter 19) or vasoconstriction (Chapter 20). Adrenergic blocking agents are considered for their antihypertensive and antianginal effects (see Chapter 20). To exemplify both sympathomimetic and sympatholytic agents, Table 5-6 provides selected examples of drugs categorized as agonists or antagonists of the sympathetic system, with generic names, brand names, and common clinical uses.

NEURAL CONTROL OF LUNG FUNCTION

Both branches of the autonomic nervous system, sympathetic and parasympathetic, exert control of lung function. At present, the two branches form the basis for two classes of respiratory care drugs that modify airway smooth muscle tone: the adrenergic bronchodilator group and the anticholinergic bronchodilator group.

Lung function includes more than just airway smooth muscle tone. Multiple sites and tissues are involved in lung function, as follows:
- Airway smooth muscle
- Submucosal and surface secretory cells
- Bronchial epithelium
- Pulmonary and bronchial blood vessels

In addition to autonomic nerve fibers and the receptors associated with them, sites in the lung (smooth muscle, glands, and vascular beds) may be affected by release of mediators from inflammatory cells, such as mast cells and platelets, or by release of epithelial factors, such as a relaxant factor, which can reduce airway contractility in response to spasmogens such as histamine, serotonin, or even acetylcholine.[6] Receptors in

TABLE 5-6

Examples of Adrenergic Agonists and Antagonists, With Their Generic Names, Brand Names, and Common Clinical Uses

Category	Generic Name	Brand Name	Uses
Sympathomimetic			
	Epinephrine	Adrenalin	Bronchodilator, cardiac stimulant, vasoconstrictor
	Ephedrine	Sudafed, various	Nasal decongestant
	Amphetamine	Dexedrine	CNS stimulant
	Dopamine	Intropin	Vasopressor, Shock syndrome
	Albuterol	Proventil, Ventolin	Bronchodilator
	Salmeterol	Serevent	Bronchodilator
	Ritodrine	Yutopar	Uterine relaxation in preterm labor
Sympatholytic			
	Phentolamine	Regitine	Vasodilator, Pheochromocytoma
	Prazosin	Minipress	Antihypertensive
	Labetalol	Normodyne, Trandate	Antihypertensive
	Metoprolol	Lopressor	Antihypertensive, antianginal
	Propranolol	Inderal	Antiarrhythmic (PAT)
	Timolol	Betimol	Ophthalmic solution, Treat IOP in patients with glaucoma
	Esmolol	Brevibloc	Antiarrhythmic

CNS, Central nervous system; *PAT,* paroxysmal atrial tachycardia; *IOP,* interoccular pressure.

the lung and airways for mediators released by inflammatory cells include the following:

- *Histamine receptors:* Especially the H_1 type
- *Prostaglandin receptors:* Such as prostacyclin, prostaglandin D_2 (PGD$_2$), prostaglandin $F_2\alpha$ (PGF$_2\alpha$), and thromboxane A_2
- *Leukotriene receptors:* Such as B_4 and the C_4-D_4-E_4 series that comprise what was formerly termed *slow-reacting substance of anaphylaxis (SRS-A)*
- *Platelet-activating factor (PAF) receptors*
- *Adenosine receptors:* Such as A_1 and A_2
- *Bradykinin receptors*

The mediators of inflammation and their receptors (e.g., histamine and prostaglandins) are discussed in the review of corticosteroids (Chapter 11) and other antiasthmatic drugs (Chapter 12) intended to inhibit or prevent an inflammatory response in the lung.

Sympathetic Innervation and Effects

The sympathetic nervous system exerts its effects by both direct and indirect means, as outlined in previous sections. *Direct effects* refer to direct innervation of tissue sites by nerve fibers. *Indirect effects* are mediated by the release of circulating catecholamines epinephrine and norepinephrine.

Sympathetic nerve fibers form ganglionic synapses outside the lung. Postganglionic sympathetic nerve fibers from the cervical and upper thoracic ganglia form plexuses at the hilar region of the lung and enter the lung mingled with parasympathetic nerves. Histochemical and ultrastructural studies show a relatively high density of sympathetic nerve fibers to submucosal glands and bronchial arteries, but few or no nerve fibers to airway smooth muscle in human lung.[7] Figure 5-10 illustrates sympathetic innervation and effects mediated by direct nerve action, and indirectly by circulating epinephrine, in the human lung.

Airway Smooth Muscle

There is little or no direct sympathetic innervation of airway smooth muscle in the human lung.[8] The sympathetic nervous system controls bronchial smooth muscle tone by circulating epinephrine and norepinephrine, which act on α and β receptors on airway smooth muscle. Recall that epinephrine stimulates both α and β receptors, whereas norepinephrine acts primarily on α receptors.

β **Receptors.** The β receptors mediate relaxation of airway smooth muscle. This action is mimicked by the class of β-adrenergic bronchodilators, introduced in Chapter 6. The β receptors are distributed from the trachea to the terminal bronchioles, and the density of these receptors increases as airway diameter becomes smaller. The β agonists can therefore cause relaxation of small airways.

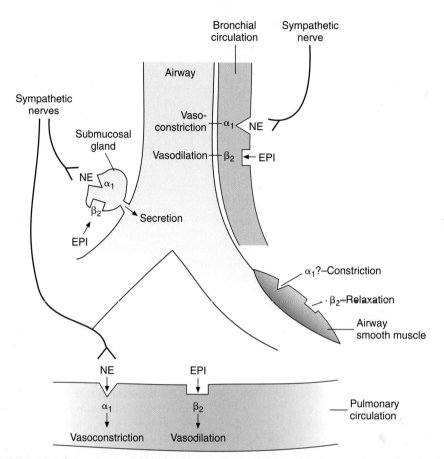

FIGURE 5-10 Adrenergic control mechanisms, including adrenergic receptor subtypes and effects in the pulmonary system. Sites of direct sympathetic nerve innervation, such as the pulmonary vasculature, are indicated. Other sites such as airway smooth muscle lack nerve innervation but respond to circulating epinephrine released by the adrenal medulla with sympathetic activation, and can also respond to exogenous catecholamines. *EPI,* Epinephrine; *NE,* norepinephrine.

The β_2 receptors traditionally have been identified as the β-receptor subtype on the airway smooth muscle. This has been further verified for human lung by autoradiographic studies and molecular gene studies.[9] There is species variation for the presence of β-receptor subtypes, however, with β_1 and β_2 receptors present in guinea pig and dog airways.

The β_1 and β_2 receptors in the lung have also been distinguished as *neuronal* and *hormonal* receptors, respectively. This is based on the concept that β_1 receptors are β receptors for sites where norepinephrine is released from sympathetic nerve terminal fibers (neuronal); β_2 receptors are β receptors responsive to circulating epinephrine (hormonal). Both cause airway smooth muscle relaxation when stimulated, either by sympathetic nerve release of norepinephrine or by circulating epinephrine, in species such as the dog or guinea pig, which have β_1 receptors on airway smooth muscle.[10] In

the human lung, which has no sympathetic innervation of the airway smooth muscle, adrenergic receptors are all of the β_2 type; β_1 receptors have been identified by radioligand binding and autoradiographic studies of alveolar walls in the lung periphery.[9] Using this terminology, relaxation of human airway smooth muscle would be accomplished by stimulation of hormonal β receptors, by circulating or exogenous catecholamines. The β_3 receptors, which have also been identified on lipocytes, have no known function in the human airway.[11]

α Receptors. The α receptors exist in human lung in less quantity than β receptors and with no difference in distribution between large and small airways. Norepinephrine stimulates α receptors, but their effect in the airway appears to be minor. Evidence of sympathetic-induced bronchoconstriction has been provided by studies in which lung tissue was treated with a β blocker, or antagonist, such as propranolol, and then exposed to epinephrine, which stimulates both α and β receptors.[12] Because β receptors were blocked, the epinephrine attached to the free α receptors, and the result was contraction of the smooth muscle, thus providing evidence of the existence of α receptors and showing a contractile effect. The clinical use of α receptor–blocking agents such as dibenamine, thymoxamine, and phentolamine in cases of status asthmaticus has been reported for more than 40 years, lending support to the role of α receptors in bronchial contraction.[13] The role of α receptors in controlling airway smooth muscle remains the subject of investigation.

Lung Blood Vessels

Blood flow in the lung is made up of two different systems: the *pulmonary* and the *bronchial* circulations. The pulmonary circulation receives the body's venous return from the right heart and is critical for gas exchange. The bronchial circulation is an arterial supply and perfuses lung tissue, to supply nutrients and remove metabolic by-products.

The pulmonary circulation is innervated by both parasympathetic and sympathetic nerves. Sympathetic nerves release norepinephrine to stimulate α receptors and cause vascular contraction. The β receptors on pulmonary blood vessels cause relaxation and are stimulated by circulating epinephrine. An exogenous catecholamine can cause vasoconstriction, dilation, or no effect, depending on the relative stimulation of receptor types.

The bronchial circulation is innervated predominantly by sympathetic nerves. Activation of sympathetic nerves causes vasoconstriction, mediated by α receptors. Stimulation of β receptors by circulating epinephrine causes relaxation and vasodilation of bronchial blood vessels.

Mucus Glands

Human bronchial submucosal glands are innervated by both sympathetic and parasympathetic nerves. There are α and β receptors on tracheal submucosal glands. Stimulation of these receptors causes an increase in secretion of fluid and mucus. Epithelial cells on the airway lining do not have direct sympathetic innervation, but do possess β₂ receptors whose stimulation can also increase secretion of fluid. Mucociliary clearance is enhanced, removing trapped particulate matter.[14]

Parasympathetic Innervation and Effects

The lung is supplied by vagus nerves, with the recurrent laryngeal nerve (part of the thoracic vagus) innervating the trachea; other branches of the vagus enter the

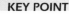

KEY POINT

In the human lung, glands and blood vessels are innervated by sympathetic nerve fibers, but airway smooth muscle has few if any such fibers, responding instead to circulating epinephrine by means of β receptors. Parasympathetic vagal nerves innervate the lung as well, supplying the airway smooth muscle and mucous glands.

lung at the hilum and innervate the intrapulmonary airways. In the trachea and remaining airways, parasympathetic nerves supply airway smooth muscle and glands. The vagus nerves in the lung release acetylcholine and are therefore termed *cholinergic*. Acetylcholine couples with muscarinic acetylcholine receptors on airway smooth muscle to cause bronchoconstriction and on submucosal glands to stimulate secretion. The action of acetylcholine is limited by the enzyme acetylcholinesterase, or cholinesterase, which breaks down acetylcholine.

Cholinergic nerve fibers in the lung are densest in the hilar region and decrease toward the airway periphery. Cholinergic muscarinic receptors also decrease in density in distal airways. Electrical stimulation of vagus nerves in dog studies causes more contraction in the intermediate bronchi than in the main bronchi or trachea.[15]

Muscarinic Receptors in the Airway

The genes for five subtypes of acetylcholine, or muscarinic, receptors have been identified, designated M₁ through M₅. Only four of these subtypes, M₁ to M₄, have been identified by chemical (ligand)-binding studies pharmacologically. Three of these muscarinic receptor subtypes have been identified in human lung: M₁, M₂, and M₃. Their location is illustrated in Figure 5-11, and the function of each is discussed.

M₁ Receptors. M₁ receptors are present at the parasympathetic ganglion, on the postjunctional membrane. Usually, acetylcholine ganglionic receptors are nicotinic, as described previously. However, the M₁ receptor may facilitate nicotinic receptor activity and nerve transmission, with an overall excitatory effect.

M₂ Receptors. M₂ receptors are localized to the presynaptic membrane of postganglionic parasympathetic nerve endings. These receptors are thought to be autoregulatory receptors whose stimulation by acetylcholine inhibits further acetylcholine release from the nerve ending, thereby limiting the cholinergic stimulation. This is analogous to the α₂ receptor inhibiting further release of norepinephrine from sympathetic nerve endings, identifying it as an autoreceptor as discussed previously (see

Cholinergic Neurotransmitter Function). Stimulation of prejunctional M_2 receptors in human airways *in vitro* results in strong inhibition of cholinergic parasympathetic-induced bronchoconstriction. Pilocarpine, a direct-acting cholinergic agonist (parasympathomimetic), is a selective stimulant of M_2 receptors.[16] Inhalation of pilocarpine blocks cholinergic reflex bronchoconstriction caused by sulfur dioxide in nonasthmatic human subjects, verifying that M_2 receptor stimulation can block cholinergic bronchoconstriction.[17]

In asthmatic subjects, pilocarpine does not inhibit bronchoconstriction. This suggests the possibility of M_2 receptor dysfunction in asthma, resulting in increased cholinergic bronchoconstriction. If M_2 receptors fail

to provide their normal inhibition of acetylcholine release and bronchial contraction, this may explain why blockade of β receptors can cause such severe bronchoconstriction in asthmatics. The normal balance of acetylcholine inhibition by M_2 receptors is lacking, and β blockade by drugs such as propranolol leaves acetylcholine stimulation of airway smooth muscle unchecked.

M_3 Receptors. M_3 receptors are present on submucosal glands and airway smooth muscle and possibly on surface goblet cells. Stimulation of M_3 receptors causes bronchoconstriction of smooth muscle and exocytosis and glandular secretion from submucosal mucous glands. M_3 receptors may also be present on airway epithelial cells, to increase ciliary beat. Antagonism

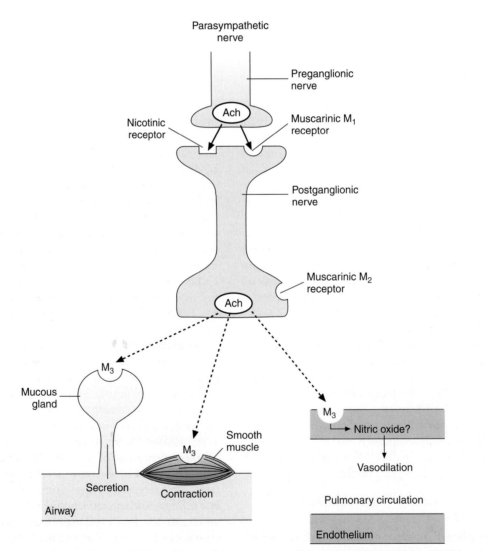

FIGURE 5-11 Location and effects of muscarinic receptor subtypes in the pulmonary system. *Ach,* Acetylcholine.

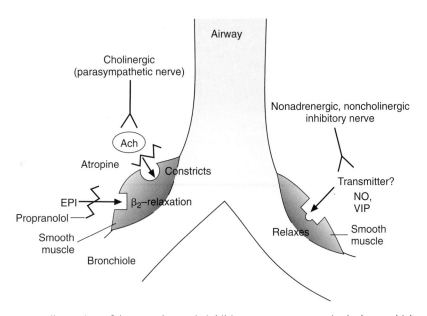

FIGURE 5-12 Illustration of the nonadrenergic inhibitory nervous system in the lung, which can cause relaxation of airway smooth muscle. Relaxation of smooth muscle occurs in the presence of cholinergic blockade by atropine and adrenergic blockade by propranolol. *Ach,* Acetylcholine; *EPI,* epinephrine; *NO,* nitric oxide; *VIP,* vasoactive intestinal peptide.

of M_3 receptors is the basis for a class of bronchodilator agents, the anticholinergic bronchodilators (see Chapter 7).

Muscarinic Receptors on Blood Vessels

Muscarinic M_3 receptors are located on endothelial cells of both the bronchial and pulmonary vasculature. Stimulation of M_3 receptors causes release of an endothelium-derived relaxant factor.[18] This relaxant factor, which produces vasodilation and is mediated by an increase in intracellular cyclic guanosine monophosphate (cGMP), has been identified as nitric oxide (NO) or a very similar nitrosocompound.[19]

Nonadrenergic, Noncholinergic Inhibitory Nerves

KEY POINT

In addition to sympathetic and parasympathetic nerves in the lung, there is evidence of a *nonadrenergic, noncholinergic (NANC)* system. This system has both inhibitory and excitatory branches.

There is evidence of a branch of nerves that are neither parasympathetic (cholinergic) nor sympathetic (adrenergic), which can cause relaxation of airway smooth muscle. These nerves have been termed *nonadrenergic, noncholinergic (NANC) inhibitory nerves.*[20] They are also referred to as simply *nonadrenergic inhibitory nerves* because adrenergic activity relaxes airway smooth muscle, and this is an additional but nonadrenergic neural method of relaxing such smooth muscle. Evidence of NANC inhibitory nerves is based on the following type of experimentation. When parasympathetic (cholinergic) receptors are blocked with an antagonist, such as atropine, and sympathetic (adrenergic) receptors are also blocked with a β blocker, such as propranolol, electrical field stimulation of the lung will produce relaxation of bronchial smooth muscle. A more detailed description of this methodology and evidence is given by Diamond and Altiere.[21] Figure 5-12 illustrates this inhibitory system that is neither adrenergic nor cholinergic and its possible neurotransmitter substances. A nonadrenergic inhibitory nervous system found in the gastrointestinal tract is primarily responsible for the relaxation of peristalsis and the internal anal sphincter. In the gastrointestinal tract, this system develops in conjunction with the parasympathetic branch. Embryologically, the gastrointestinal and respiratory tracts share a common origin, and the separation of the trachea and gut occurs around the fourth or fifth week of gestation. This adds plausibility to the presence of a nonadrenergic inhibitory system in the lungs similar to that in the gastrointestinal tract.

KEY POINT

Inhibitory effects on airway smooth muscle cause bronchodilation and may be mediated by the neurotransmitter vasoactive intestinal peptide (VIP) or even by nitric oxide (NO).

The exact neurotransmitter responsible for relaxation responses mediated by NANC inhibitory nerves is under investigation; however, the neurotransmitter vasoactive intestinal peptide (VIP) is the current front runner.[22] Vasoactive intestinal peptide can relax mammalian airway smooth muscle. Another possible neurotransmitter causing airway smooth muscle relaxation is nitric oxide (NO). The enzyme responsible for NO synthesis, nitric oxide synthase (NOS), has been found in nerve terminals around airway smooth muscle, and NO produces effects similar to those caused by NANC inhibitory nerve activation. In fact, Ricciardolo believes that NANC inhibition is mediated by NO, with the help of VIP.[23] Definitive identification of an NANC inhibitory neurotransmitter substance remains to be accomplished.

Nonadrenergic, Noncholinergic Excitatory Nerves

The existence of *nonadrenergic, noncholinergic excitatory nervous control* of airway smooth muscle has also been demonstrated using electrical field stimulation (EFS) techniques. This system is also referred to as simply *noncholinergic excitatory nervous control*, because cholinergic activity contracts airway smooth muscle, and this is an additional but noncholinergic neural method of exciting and constricting such smooth muscle. Stimulation of NANC excitatory nerves causes bronchial contraction. There are sensory *afferent* nerves termed *C-fibers* present in the airways, as well as around bronchial blood vessels and submucosal glands and within the airway epithelium,

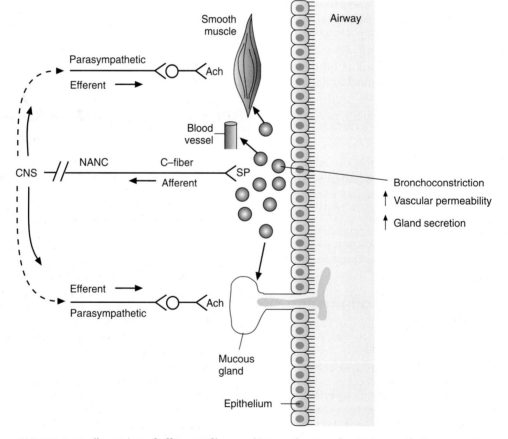

FIGURE 5-13 Illustration of afferent C-fibers making up the nonadrenergic, noncholinergic *(NANC)* excitatory nervous system in the lung. Activation of C-fibers causes both an afferent impulse with reflex parasympathetic activity and release of substance P, causing local effects in the airway. *Ach,* Acetylcholine; *CNS,* central nervous system; *SP,* substance P.

These afferent fibers follow vagal nerve tracts into the central nervous system, as shown in Figure 5-13.

KEY POINT

Excitatory effects such as bronchoconstriction are produced by afferent sensory fibers that have substance P as a neurotransmitter; these effects are caused by local release of substance P, as well as by afferent–efferent reflex arcs, involving efferent cholinergic transmission.

Sensory C-fiber nerves contain substance P, which is a tachykinin (a family of small peptide mediators). Substance P is also referred to as a *neuropeptide*. Sensory C-fibers can be stimulated by noxious substances such as capsaicin, found in chili peppers. When stimulated, C-fibers conduct impulses to the central nervous system that result in reflexes of cough and parasympathetically induced bronchoconstriction. Sensory C-fibers also release their neuropeptides, such as substance P, at the local site of the nerve fiber. Substance P and other tachykinins cause bronchoconstriction in the airways and vasodilation, increased vascular permeability, mucous gland secretion, and enhanced mucociliary activity. The NANC excitatory C-fiber system has been considered as a possible cause of the hyperreactive airway seen in asthma. The presence of C-fibers is less marked in human airways than in rodent species.

SELF-ASSESSMENT QUESTIONS

1. Which portion of the nervous system is under voluntary control: the autonomic or the skeletal muscle motor nerve portion?
2. What is the neurotransmitter at each of the following sites: neuromuscular junction, autonomic ganglia, most sympathetic end sites?
3. Where are muscarinic receptors found?
4. What is the effect of cholinergic stimulation on airway smooth muscle?
5. What is the effect of adrenergic stimulation on the heart?
6. Classify the drugs pilocarpine, physostigmine, propranolol, and epinephrine.
7. How do indirect-acting cholinergic agonists (parasympathomimetics) produce their action?
8. What effect would the drug atropine have on the eye and on airway smooth muscle?
9. What is the general difference between α and β receptors in the sympathetic nervous system?

SELF-ASSESSMENT QUESTIONS —cont'd

10. What is the primary mechanism for terminating the neurotransmitters acetylcholine and norepinephrine?
11. What is the predominant sympathetic receptor type found on airway smooth muscle?
12. Identify the adrenergic receptor preference for phenylephrine, norepinephrine, epinephrine, and isoproterenol.
13. What is the autoregulatory receptor on the sympathetic presynaptic neuron?
14. Classify the following drugs by autonomic class and receptor preference: dopamine, ephedrine, albuterol, phentolamine, propranolol, prazosin.
15. What is the autoregulatory receptor on the parasympathetic presynaptic neuron at the terminal nerve site?
16. Contrast α_1- and α_2-receptor effects, in general.
17. What substance may be the neurotransmitter in the NANC inhibitory nervous system in the lung?
18. What substance is the neurotransmitter in the NANC excitatory nervous system in the lung?

Answers to Self-Assessment Questions appear in Appendix A.

CLINICAL SCENARIO

A 42-year-old white female with a long-standing history of asthma presents to the emergency department (ED) of a local acute care hospital. She states that she has been feeling as if her "heart were racing" today. She currently uses a β-adrenergic bronchodilator (albuterol) as needed and inhales an anticholinergic bronchodilator (ipratropium bromide) before bedtime, both drugs administered by metered dose inhaler (MDI) inhalation.

On admission to the ED, she has the following vital signs: pulse (P), 155 beats/min and regular; blood pressure (BP), 146/90 mmHg; and respiratory rate (RR), 22 breaths/min, with mild distress.

Her breath sounds are clear to auscultation, and a chest radiograph (posteroanterior [PA]) shows no abnormalities. A lead II electrocardiogram (ECG) reveals supraventricular tachycardia (SVT). Oxygen saturation as revealed by pulse oximetry (SpO$_2$) is 90%. A resident orders oxygen at 2 L/min by nasal cannula, and intravenous propranolol for her SVT, which is given. Approximately 5 minutes later, her heart rate is reduced to 110 beats/min, but she begins to wheeze audibly and

Continued

complains of severe shortness of breath (SOB), and her respiratory pattern is labored at 26 breaths/min. She is anxious, and her pulse oximetry reading drops from 92% back to 72%.

What may have led to the wheezing and dyspnea of the patient?

What changes in the therapeutic approach would you suggest in a case such as this?

Answers to Clinical Scenario Questions appear in Appendix A.

References

1. Iversen LL: The uptake of catecholamines at high perfusion concentrations in the rat isolated heart: a novel catecholamine uptake process, *Br J Pharmacol* 25:18, 1965.
2. Iversen LL, Salt PJ: Inhibition of catecholamine uptake 2 by steroids in the isolated rat heart, *Br J Pharmacol* 40:528, 1970.
3. Ahlquist RP: A study of the adrenotropic receptors, *Am J Physiol* 153:586, 1948.
4. Lands AM, Arnold A, McAuliff JP, Luduena FP, Brown TG Jr: Differentiation of receptor systems activated by sympathomimetic amines, *Nature (London)* 214:597, 1967.
5. Langer SZ: Presynaptic regulation of the release of catecholamines, *Pharmacol Rev* 32:337, 1980.
6. Barnes PJ: Airway receptors, *Postgrad Med J* 65:532, 1989.
7. Partanen M, Laitinen A, Hervonen A, Toivanen M, Laitinen LA: Catecholamine- and acetylcholinesterase-containing nerves in human lower respiratory tract, *Histochemistry* 76:175, 1982.
8. Barnes PJ: Neural control of human airways in health and disease, *Am Rev Respir Dis* 134:1289, 1986.
9. Carstairs JR, Nimmo AJ, Barnes PJ: Autoradiographic visualization of beta-adrenoceptor subtypes in human lung, *Am Rev Respir Dis* 132:541, 1985.
10. Ariens EJ, Simonis AM: Physiological and pharmacological aspects of adrenergic receptor classification, *Biochem Pharmacol* 32:1539, 1983.
11. Emorine L, Blin N, Strosberg AD: The human 3-adrenoceptor: the search for a physiological function, *Trends Pharmacol Sci* 15:3, 1994.
12. Adolphson RL, Abern SB, Townley RG: Human and guinea pig respiratory smooth muscle: demonstration of alpha adrenergic receptors [abstract], *J Allergy* 47:110, 1971.
13. Falliers CJ, Tinkelman DG: Alternative drug therapy for asthma, *Clin Chest Med* 7:383, 1986.
14. Altiere RJ, Lindsay G: Sympathetic innervation. In Leff AR, editor: *Pulmonary and critical care pharmacology and therapeutics*, New York, 1996, McGraw-Hill.
15. Jacoby DB, Fryer AD: Parasympathetic innervation of the airways. In Leff AR, editor: *Pulmonary and critical care pharmacology and therapeutics*, New York, 1996, McGraw-Hill.
16. Barnes PJ: Muscarinic receptor subtypes in airways, *Life Sci* 52:521, 1993.
17. Minette PA, Lammers JW, Dixon CM, McCusker MT, Barnes PJ: A muscarinic agonist inhibits reflex bronchoconstriction in normal but not in asthmatic subjects, *J Appl Physiol* 67:2461, 1989.
18. Cuss FM, Barnes PJ: Epithelial mediators, *Am Rev Respir Dis* 136:S32, 1987.
19. Wylam ME: Pulmonary vascular pharmacology. In Leff AR, editor: *Pulmonary and critical care pharmacology and therapeutics*, New York, 1996, McGraw-Hill.
20. Richardson JB, Beland J: Nonadrenergic inhibitory nervous system in human airways, *J Appl Physiol* 41:764, 1976.
21. Diamond L, Altiere RJ: The airway nonadrenergic, noncholinergic inhibitory nervous system. In Leff AR, editor: *Pulmonary and critical care pharmacology and therapeutics*, New York, 1996, McGraw-Hill.
22. Stephens NL: Airway smooth muscle, Lung 179:333, 2002.
23. Ricciardolo FLM: Multiple roles of nitric oxide in the airways, *Thorax* 58:175, 2003.

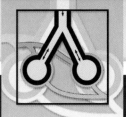

Chapter 6

Adrenergic (Sympathomimetic) Bronchodilators

DOUGLAS S. GARDENHIRE

CHAPTER OUTLINE

Clinical Indications for Adrenergic Bronchodilators
Indication for Short-Acting Agents
Indication for Long-Acting Agents
Indication for Racemic Epinephrine
Specific Adrenergic Agents and Formulations
Catecholamines
Resorcinol Agents
Saligenin Agents
Pirbuterol
A Prodrug: Bitolterol
Levalbuterol: The (R)-Isomer of Albuterol
Long-Acting β-Adrenergic Agents
Mode of Action
β-Receptor and α$_2$-Receptor Activation
α$_1$-Receptor Activation
Salmeterol, Formoterol, and Arformoterol:
Mechanism of Action

Routes of Administration
Inhalation Route
Oral Route
Parenteral Route
Adverse Side Effects
Tremor
Cardiac Effects
Tolerance to Bronchodilator Effect
Loss of Bronchoprotection
Central Nervous System Effects
Fall in Arterial Oxygen Pressure
Metabolic Disturbances
Propellant Toxicity and Paradoxical Bronchospasm
Sensitivity to Additives
The β-Agonist Controversy
Asthma Morbidity and Mortality
Respiratory Care Assessment of β-Agonist Therapy

CHAPTER OBJECTIVES

After reading this chapter, the reader will be able to:
1. Define *sympathomimetic*
2. Define *adrenergic*
3. List all currently available β-adrenergic agents used in respiratory therapy
4. Differentiate between the specific adrenergic agents and formulations

5. Describe the mode of action for each specific adrenergic agent and formulation
6. Describe the route of administration available for β agonists
7. Discuss adverse effects of β agonists
8. Clinically assess β-agonist therapy

KEY TERMS AND DEFINITIONS

Adrenergic bronchodilator — An agent that stimulates sympathetic nervous fibers, which allow relaxation of smooth muscle in the airway. Also known as a *sympathomimetic bronchodilator, or β_2 agonist*

Asthma paradox — Refers to the increasing incidence of asthma morbidity, and especially asthma mortality, despite advances in the understanding of asthma and availability of improved drugs to treat asthma

Bronchospasm — Narrowing of the bronchial airways, caused by contraction of smooth muscle

Catecholamines — A group of similar compounds having sympathomimetic action; they mimic the actions of epinephrine

Cyclic AMP (cAMP) — Nucleotide produced by β_2-receptor stimulation; it affects many cells, but causes relaxation of bronchial smooth muscle

Cyclic GMP (cGMP) — Nucleotide producing the opposite effect of cAMP, that is, it causes bronchoconstriction

Downregulation — Long-term desensitization of β receptors to β_2 agonists, caused by a reduction in the number of β receptors

Prodrug — A drug that exhibits its pharmacological activity once it is converted, inside the body, to its active form

α-Receptor stimulation — Causes vasoconstriction and a vasopressor effect; in the upper airway (nasal passages) this can provide decongestion

β_1-Receptor stimulation — Causes increased myocardial conductivity and increased heart rate, as well as increased contractile force

β_2-Receptor stimulation — Causes relaxation of bronchial smooth muscle, with some inhibition of inflammatory mediator release and stimulation of mucociliary clearance

Sympathomimetic — Producing effects similar to those of the sympathetic nervous system

---

Chapter 6 presents adrenergic drugs used as inhaled bronchodilators. The specific agents and the clinical indications for this class of drugs are summarized, along with their mechanism of action as mediated by β receptors. Structure–activity relations of available agents are presented as a basis for their difference in receptor selectivity and duration of action. Differences among routes of administration are discussed, and side effects are reviewed. A brief summary of the β-agonist debate over possible harmful effects with these agents is given.

CLINICAL INDICATIONS FOR ADRENERGIC BRONCHODILATORS

The general indication for use of an **adrenergic bronchodilator** is relaxation of airway smooth muscle in the presence of reversible airflow obstruction associated with acute and chronic asthma (including exercise-induced asthma), bronchitis, emphysema, bronchiectasis, and other obstructive airway diseases. Differences in the rate of onset, peak effect, and duration led to a distinction

in use between short-acting and long-acting agents. Appendix D outlines recommendations and guidelines for the use of β agonists in chronic obstructive pulmonary disease (COPD) and asthma.

Indication for Short-Acting Agents

Short-acting β_2 agonists such as albuterol, levalbuterol, or pirbuterol are indicated for relief of *acute* reversible airflow obstruction in asthma or other obstructive airway diseases.

Short-acting agents are termed "rescue" agents in the 1997 National Asthma Education and Prevention Program Expert Panel Report 2 (NAEPP EPR 2) guidelines.[1] Short- term acting agents may also be termed "relievers" as discussed in the Global Initiative for Asthma (GINA) guidelines.[2]

Indication for Long-Acting Agents

Long-acting agents, such as salmeterol, formoterol, and arformoterol are indicated for maintenance bronchodilation and control of **bronchospasm,** and for control of nocturnal symptoms in asthma or other obstructive diseases.

NAEPP EPR 2 guidelines and GINA consider salmeterol a "controller"; its slow time to peak effect makes it a poor rescue drug. In asthma, a long-acting bronchodilator is usually combined with antiinflammatory medication for control of airway inflammation and bronchospasm. Even though formoterol has a rapid onset of action, similar to that of albuterol, its slower

KEY POINT

The adrenergic bronchodilator group is indicated for the treatment of reversible airway obstruction in diseases such as asthma and COPD. These agents produce bronchodilation by stimulating β_2 receptors on airway smooth muscle.

peak effect and prolonged activity make it a better maintenance drug than an acute reliever or rescue agent.

Indication for Racemic Epinephrine

Racemic epinephrine is often used, either as an inhaled aerosol or by direct lung instillation, for its strong α-adrenergic vasoconstricting effect to reduce airway swelling after extubation or during epiglottitis, croup, or bronchiolitis, or to control airway bleeding during endoscopy.

SPECIFIC ADRENERGIC AGENTS AND FORMULATIONS

Table 6-1 lists the adrenergic bronchodilators currently approved for general clinical use in the United States as of the writing of this edition. Practitioners are urged to read package inserts on a drug before administration. Such inserts give details of dosage strengths and frequencies, adverse effects, shelf life, and storage requirements, all of which are needed for safe application. Table 6-1 is not intended to replace more detailed information supplied by the manufacturer on each of the bronchodilator agents. There are three subgroups of adrenergic bronchodilators based on distinct differences in duration of action:

Ultrashort-acting (duration, <3 hours): Epinephrine, isoproterenol, isoetharine

Short-acting (duration, 4–6 hours): Albuterol, levalbuterol, metaproterenol, pirbuterol, terbutaline

Long-acting (duration, 12 hours): Salmeterol, formoterol, arformeterol

Catecholamines

The sympathomimetic bronchodilators are all either catecholamines or derivatives of catecholamines. In Figure 6-1 the basic catecholamine structure is seen to be composed of a benzene ring with hydroxyl groups at the third and fourth carbon sites and an amine side chain attached at the first carbon position.

Catecholamine: One of a group of similar compounds having a sympathomimetic action, and a chemical structure consisting of an aromatic catechol nucleus and a dialiphatic amine side chain.

The terminal amine group (NH_2) and the benzene ring are connected by two carbon atoms, designated as α and β, a notation not to be confused with α and β receptors in the sympathetic nervous system. Examples of catecholamines are dopamine, epinephrine, norepinephrine, isoproterenol, and isoetharine. The first three occur naturally in the body. Catecholamines, or **sympathomimetic** amines, mimic the actions of epinephrine more or less precisely, causing tachycardia, elevated blood pressure, smooth muscle relaxation of bronchioles and skeletal muscle blood vessels, glycogenolysis, skeletal muscle tremor, and central nervous system stimulation.

Adrenergic Bronchodilators as Stereoisomers

Adrenergic bronchodilators can exist in two different spatial arrangements, producing isomers. Rotation about the β carbon on the ethylamine side chain of the basic molecular structure seen in Figure 6-1 produces two nonsuperimposable mirror images, termed *enantiomers* or simply *isomers*. Figure 6-2 illustrates epinephrine as a *stereoisomer*, showing the (R)- and (S)-isomers as the mirror image of each other. Enantiomers have similar physical and chemical properties, but not the same physiological effects. The (R)-isomer, or levo isomer, is active on airway β receptors, producing bronchodilation, and on extrapulmonary adrenergic receptors. The (S)-isomer, or dextro isomer, is not active on adrenergic receptors such as β receptors, and until recently the (S)-isomer was considered physiologically inert. The two mirror images of the isomers rotate light in opposite directions, and this is the basis for designating them as dextrorotatory (*d,* +) or levorotatory (*l,* -) Using their actual spatial configuration, the levo isomer and dextro isomer are referred to as the *(R)-isomer* (for *rectus,* right) and *(S)-isomer* (for *sinister,* left), respectively. Adrenergic bronchodilators such as epinephrine, albuterol, or salmeterol have been produced synthetically as racemic mixtures, or 50:50 equimolar mixes of the (R)-isomers and (S)-isomers. Natural epinephrine found in the adrenal gland occurs as the (R, or levo)-isomer only. Levalbuterol, released in 1999, represents the first *synthetic* inhaled solution available as the single (R)-isomer of racemic albuterol. The structures of the currently available inhaled β agonists to be discussed are shown in Figure 6-3. Only a single isomer form is shown, for simplification and clarity.

Epinephrine is a potent catecholamine bronchodilator that stimulates both α and β receptors. Because epinephrine lacks β_2-receptor specificity, there is a high prevalence of side effects such as tachycardia, blood pressure increase, tremor, headache, and insomnia. Epinephrine occurs naturally in the adrenal medulla and has a rapid onset, but a short duration, because of metabolism by catechol *O*-methyltransferase (COMT). It has been

TABLE 6-1

Inhaled Adrenergic Bronchodilator Agents Currently Available in the United States

Drug	Brand Name	Receptor Preference	Adult Dosage	Time Course (Onset, Peak, Duration)
Ultra Short-Acting Adrenergic Bronchodilator Agents *(< 3 hrs)*				
Epinephrine	Adrenalin Cl, Epinephrine Mist, Primatene Mist	α, β	SVN: 1% solution (1:100), 0.25-0.5 ml (2.5-5.0 mg) qid MDI: 0.22 mg/puff, puffs as ordered or needed	Onset: 3-5 min Peak: 5-20 min Duration: 1-3 hr
Racemic epinephrine	microNefrin, Nephron, S2	α, β	SVN: 2.25% solution, 0.25-0.5 ml (5.63-11.25 mg) qid	Onset: 3-5 min Peak: 5-20 min Duration: 0.5-2 hr
Isoetharine	Isoetharine HCl	β₂	SVN: 1% solution, 0.5 ml (5.0 mg) q4h	Onset: 1-6 min Peak: 15-60 min Duration: 1-3 hr
Short-Acting Adrenergic Bronchodilator Agents *(4 - 6 hrs)*				
Metaproterenol	Alupent	β₂	SVN: 0.4%, 0.6%, 5% solution, 0.3 ml (15 mg) tid, qid MDI: 650 µg/puff, 2 or 3 puffs tid, qid Tab: 10 mg and 20 mg, tid, qid Syrup: 10 mg per 5 ml	Onset: 1-5 min Peak: 60 min Duration: 2-6 hr
✓ Albuterol	Proventil, Proventil HFA, Ventolin, Ventolin HFA, ProAir, AccuNeb	β₂	SVN: 0.5% solution, 0.5 ml (2.5 mg), 0.63 mg, 1.25 mg and 2.5 mg unit dose, tid, qid MDI: 90 µg/puff, 2 puffs tid, qid Tab: 2 mg, 4 mg, and 8 mg, bid, tid, qid Syrup: 2 mg/5 ml, 1-2 tsp tid, qid	Onset: 15 min Peak: 30-60 min Duration: 5-8 hr
Pirbuterol	Maxair Autohaler	β₂	MDI: 200 µg/puff, 2 puffs q4-6h	Onset: 5 min Peak: 30 min Duration: 5 hr
✓ Levalbuterol	Xopenex, Xopenex HFA	β₂	SVN: 0.31 mg/3 ml tid, 0.63 mg/3 ml tid, or 1.25 mg/3 ml tid; Concentrate 1.25 mg/0.5 ml, tid MDI: 45 µg/puff, 2 puffs q4-6h	Onset: 15 min Peak: 30-60 min Duration: 5-8 hr
Long-Acting Adrenergic Bronchodilator Agents *(12 hrs)*				
Salmeterol	Serevent	β₂	DPI: 50 µg/blister bid	Onset: 20 min Peak: 3-5 hr Duration: 12 hr
Formoterol	Foradil	β₂	DPI: 12 µg/inhalation bid	Onset: 15 min Peak: 30-60 hr Duration: 12 hr
✓ Arformoterol	Brovana	β₂	SVN: 15 µg/2 ml unit dose, bid	Onset: 15 min Peak: 30-60 hr Duration: 12 hr

DPI, Dry powder inhaler; *MDI,* metered dose inhaler; *SVN,* small volume nebulizer.

administered both by inhalation and subcutaneous injection to treat patients with acute asthmatic episodes. It is also used as a cardiac stimulant, based on its strong β₁ effects. Self-administered, intramuscular injectable doses of 0.3 and 0.15 mg are marketed to control systemic hypersensitivity (anaphylactoid) reactions. This drug is more useful for the management of acute asthma rather than for daily maintenance therapy because of its pharmacokinetics and side effect profile. The parenteral form of epinephrine is a natural extract, consisting of only the (R, or levo)-isomer. The synthetic formulation of epinephrine for nebulization, microNefrin or Nephron, is a racemic mixture of the (R, or levo)- and (S, or dextro)-isomers. The mode of action of racemic epinephrine is the same as with natural epinephrine, giving both α and β stimulation. Because only the (R)-isomer is active on adrenergic receptors, a 1:100 strength formulation of natural epinephrine (injectable formulation) has been used for nebulization, whereas a 2.25% strength racemic mixture is used in nebulization. An epinephrine metered dose inhaler (MDI) can be found over-the-counter as Primatene Mist. The U.S. Food and Drug Administration (FDA) ruled in 2006 that Primatene Mist was not essential, which could lead to removal from market if the manufacturer does not convert to the hydrofluoroalkane (HFA) formulation by December 31, 2008.

Isoproterenol is a potent catecholamine bronchodilator that stimulates both β_1 (cardiac) and β_2 receptors. The drug was widely used for nebulization until the advent of the more β_2-specific agents such as isoetharine and later the resorcinols, saligenins, and others. Today, isoproterenol is no longer used or manufactured as a nebulizer solution. It is available parenterally, to treat bronchospasm during anesthesia and for use as a vasopressor in patients with shock.[3]

Isoetharine was one of the first β_2-specific adrenergic bronchodilators in the United States. As a catecholamine, it has a short duration of action, but a rapid onset. Cardiac (β_1) stimulation is minimal compared with isoproterenol or epinephrine.

Keyhole Theory of β_2 Specificity

The three catecholamine drugs described in the previous section differ in their receptor preference, ranging from α and β (epinephrine), to β nonspecific (isoproterenol), and finally to β_2 specific (isoetharine). The theory that explains the shift from α activity to β_2 specificity has been termed the *keyhole theory* of β sympathomimetic receptors: The larger the side-chain attachment to a catechol base, the greater the β_2 specificity. If the catecholamine structural pattern is seen as a keylike shape, then the larger the "key" (side chain), the more β_2 specific the drug. The increase in side chain substitutions can be seen in the drug structures presented in Figure 6-3, for the three catecholamines described and subsequent β_2-selective agents to be discussed.

Epinephrine has a methyl group attached to the terminal amine group and activates α and β receptors equally. *Isoproterenol* adds an additional methyl group with strong β stimulation and very little α stimulation. *Isoetharine* further increases the bulk of the amine side chain and adds an ethyl group, modifying the structure of isoproterenol and producing β_2-preferential activity. Actually, bronchodilator activity is reduced by an approximate factor of 10 compared with that of isoproterenol, but cardiovascular stimulation is less by a factor of 300.

Metabolism of Catecholamines

Despite the increase in β_2 specificity with increased side-chain bulk, all of the previously mentioned catecholamines are rapidly inactivated by the cytoplasmic

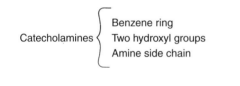

Catecholamines {
Benzene ring
Two hydroxyl groups
Amine side chain
}

Structure:

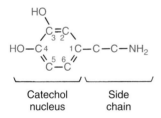

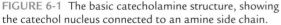

Catechol nucleus   Side chain

FIGURE 6-1 The basic catecholamine structure, showing the catechol nucleus connected to an amine side chain.

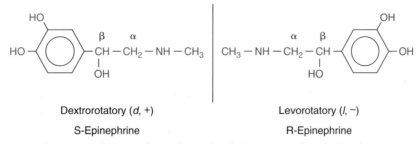

Dextrorotatory (*d*, +)   Levorotatory (*l*, −)

S-Epinephrine   R-Epinephrine

FIGURE 6-2 The structure of epinephrine, illustrating the (R)-isomer (levo, *l*, −) and (S)-isomer (dextro, *d*, +) as mirror images of each other, termed *enantiomers*. Natural epinephrine is (R)-epinephrine. Synthetic formulations for inhalation are racemic (50:50) mixtures of (R)- and (S)-isomers.

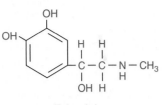

Epinephrine

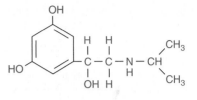

Metaproterenol

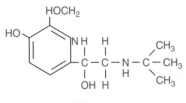

Pirbuterol

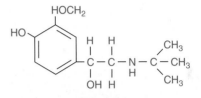

Albuterol
(R,S-isomer)

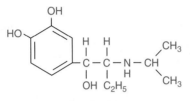

Isoetharine

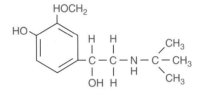

Levalbuterol
(R-isomer)

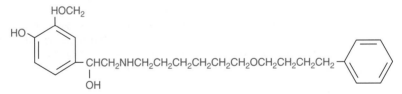

Salmeterol

FIGURE 6-3 Chemical structures of currently available inhaled adrenergic bronchodilators in the United States. With the exception of natural epinephrine and levalbuterol, all formulations are racemic mixtures and are shown in the same orientation for clarity. The isomers of racemic albuterol and levalbuterol are labeled to indicate the difference between these two drugs. Formoterol and arformoterol, not shown, are illustrated in Figure 6-8. (From Rau JL: Inhaled adrenergic bronchodilators: historical development and clinical application, *Respir Care* 45:854, 2000.)

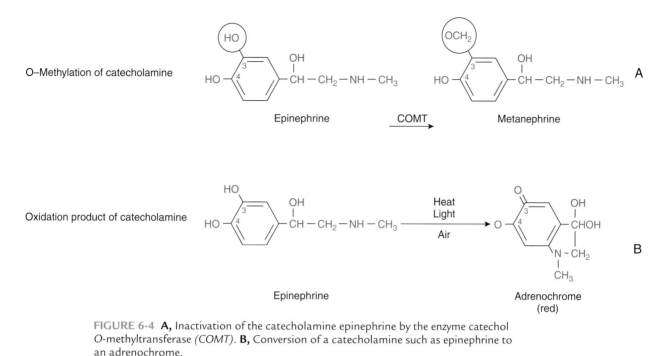

FIGURE 6-4 **A,** Inactivation of the catecholamine epinephrine by the enzyme catechol O-methyltransferase *(COMT)*. **B,** Conversion of a catecholamine such as epinephrine to an adrenochrome.

enzyme COMT. This enzyme is found in the liver and kidneys, as well as throughout the rest of the body. Figure 6-4, *A*, illustrates the action of COMT as it transfers a methyl group to the carbon-3 position on the catechol nucleus. The resulting compound, metanephrine, is inactive on adrenergic receptors. Because the action of COMT on circulating catecholamines is very efficient, the duration of action of these drugs is severely limited, with a range of 1.5 to at most 3 hours.

Catecholamines are also unsuitable for oral administration because they are inactivated in the gut and liver by conjugation with sulfate or glucuronide at the carbon-4 site. Because of this action, they have no effect when taken by mouth, limiting their route of administration to inhalation or injection. Catecholamines are also readily inactivated to inert adrenochromes by heat, light, or air (Figure 6-4, *B*). For this reason, racemic epinephrine, isoetharine, and isoproterenol are stored in amber-colored bottles. Nebulizer *rainout* (i.e., nebulized particles that condense and fall, under the influence of gravity) in the tubing may appear pinkish after treatment, and a patient's sputum may even appear pink-tinged after using aerosols of catecholamines.

Resorcinol Agents

Because the limited duration of action with catecholamines is hardly suitable for maintenance therapy of bronchospastic airways, drug researchers sought to

KEY POINT

The basic catecholamine structure, consisting of a catechol ring connected to an amine side chain, directly influences activity. β_2-Receptor specificity is considered to be due to side chain bulk *(keyhole theory)*. The short duration of action of catecholamines is due to metabolism by the enzyme COMT."

modify the catechol nucleus, which is so vulnerable to inactivation by COMT. As a result, the hydroxyl attachment at the carbon-4 site was shifted to the carbon-5 position, producing a resorcinol nucleus (see Figure 6-3). This change resulted in *metaproterenol* (named for the 3,5-attachments in the meta position) and *terbutaline* (for the tertiary butyl group). Because neither drug is acted on by COMT, both have a significantly longer duration of action of 4 to 6 hours compared with the short-acting catecholamine bronchodilators. Because of its bulky side chain, terbutaline is β_2-preferential, thus possessing minimal cardiac (β_1) effects. Both drugs can be taken orally because they resist inactivation by the sulfatase enzymes in the gastrointestinal tract and liver. For these reasons, the newer generation of resorcinols and other catecholamine derivatives was much better suited for maintenance therapy than the older catecholamine agents. Metaproterenol and terbutaline are slower to reach a peak effect

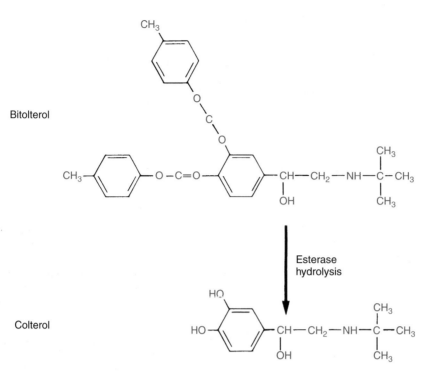

FIGURE 6-5 Illustration of the structure of bitolterol, showing conversion by esterase enzymes to its active catecholamine form, colterol, a β_2-preferential agonist.

(30 to 60 minutes) than epinephrine, isoproterenol, or isoetharine. Of these two agents only metaproterenol is available for inhalation, as a nebulizer solution or MDI. Terbutaline is available as a tablet to be taken by mouth or parenterally.

KEY POINT

Modification of the catecholamine structure produces *noncatecholamines* such as metaproterenol, albuterol, and terbutaline, which have a 4- to 6-hour duration and are β_2 preferential.

Saligenin Agents

A different modification of the catechol nucleus at the carbon-3 site resulted in the saligenin *albuterol*, referred to as *salbutamol* in Europe (see Figure 6-3). Albuterol is available in a variety of pharmaceutical vehicles in the United States. These include oral tablets, syrup, nebulizer solution, MDI, and extended release tablets. As with the resorcinol bronchodilators, this drug has a β_2-preferential effect, is effective by mouth, and has a duration of up to 6 hours, with a peak effect in 30 to 60 minutes.

Pirbuterol

Pirbuterol is another noncatecholamine adrenergic agent currently available as pirbuterol acetate (Maxair) in an MDI formulation with a breath-actuated inhaler delivery device (see Chapter 3). The strength is 0.2 mg per puff, and the usual dose is 2 puffs. Pirbuterol is structurally similar to albuterol except for a pyridine ring in place of the benzene ring (see Figure 6-3). The onset of activity by aerosol is 5 to 8 minutes, with a peak effect at 30 minutes and a duration of action of approximately 5 hours. Pirbuterol is said to be less potent on a weight basis than albuterol and similar in both efficacy and toxicity to metaproterenol.[4] The side effect profile is the same as with other β_2 agonists.

A Prodrug: Bitolterol

Bitolterol (Tornalate) differs from the previous agents discussed in that the administered form must be converted in the body to the active drug. Because of this, bitolterol is referred to as a **prodrug**. The sequence of activation is seen in Figure 6-5.

The bitolterol molecule consists of two toluate ester groups on the aromatic ring at the carbon-3 and

Albuterol Isomers

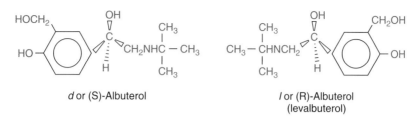

d or (S)-Albuterol   l or (R)-Albuterol
                                  (levalbuterol)

FIGURE 6-6 The (R)- and (S)-isomers of racemic albuterol. Levalbuterol is the single, (R)-isomer form of racemic albuterol and contains no (S)-isomer.

carbon-4 positions. These attachments protect the molecule from degradation by COMT. The large *N*-tertiary butyl substituent on the amine side chain prevents oxidation by monoamine oxidase (MAO). Bitolterol was administered as an inhalation solution, and once in the body the bitolterol molecule is hydrolyzed by esterase enzymes in the tissue and blood to the active bronchodilator colterol. The process of activation begins when the drug is administered and gradually continues over time. This results in a prolonged duration or sustained-release effect of up to 8 hours. Onset and peak effect are similar to those of the noncatecholamine agent metaproterenol, administered by inhalation. The active form, colterol, is a catecholamine and will be inactivated by COMT like any other catecholamine. The speed of this inactivation is offset by the gradual hydrolysis of bitolterol, to provide a prolonged duration of activity. The bulky side chain gives a preferential β_2 effect to the active form, colterol.[5]

In animal studies, bitolterol given orally or intravenously selectively distributed to the lungs. The inhalation route in humans seems preferable to treat the lungs locally, and the hydrolysis of bitolterol to colterol proceeds faster in the lungs than elsewhere, giving a selective effect and accumulation in the lungs. Colterol is excreted in urine and feces as free and conjugated colterol and as metabolites of colterol. Although interesting from a pharmacological viewpoint, bitolterol has been removed from market in the United States.

Levalbuterol: The (R)-Isomer of Albuterol (Xopenex)

Previous inhaled formulations of adrenergic bronchodilators were all synthetic racemic mixtures, containing both the (R)-isomer and the (S)-isomer in equal amounts. Levalbuterol is the pure (R)-isomer of racemic albuterol. Both stereoisomers of albuterol are shown in Figure 6-6. Although the (S)-isomer is physiologically

| Box 6-1 | Effects and Characteristics of the (S)-Isomer of Albuterol |

- Increases intracellular calcium concentration *in vitro*[8]
- Activity is blocked by the anticholinergic agent atropine[8]
- Does not produce pulmonary or extrapulmonary β_2-mediated effects[9]
- Enhances experimental airway responsiveness *in vitro*[10]
- Increases the contractile response of bronchial tissue to histamine or leukotriene C_4 (LTC_4) *in vitro*[11]
- Enhances eosinophil superoxide production with interleukin-5 (IL-5) stimulation[12]
- Is metabolized slower than (*R*)-albuterol *in vivo*[13]
- Preferentially retained in the lung when inhaled by MDI (*in vivo*)[14]

inactive on adrenergic receptors, there is accumulating evidence that the (S)-isomer is *not* completely inactive. Box 6-1 lists some of the physiological effects of (S)-albuterol noted in the literature.[6-12] The effects noted would antagonize the bronchodilating effects of the (R)-isomer of an adrenergic drug and promote bronchoconstriction. In addition, the (S)-isomer is more slowly metabolized than the (R)-isomer. Levalbuterol is the single (R)-isomer form of racemic albuterol, and is available in a HFA-propelled MDI, with nebulization solution in three strengths: a 0.31-mg, a 0.63-mg, and a 1.25-mg unit dose. Levalbuterol is also available as a concentrate, 1.25-mg in 0.5 mL. In a study by Nelson and associates,[13] the 0.63-mg dose was found comparable to the 2.5-mg racemic albuterol dose in onset and duration (Figure 6-7).

Side effects of tremor and heart rate changes were less with the single-isomer formulation. The 1.25-mg levalbuterol dose showed a higher peak effect on FEV_1 (forced expiratory volume in 1 second) with an 8-hour duration compared with racemic albuterol. Side effects with this dose were equivalent to those seen with racemic albuterol. It is significant that an equivalent

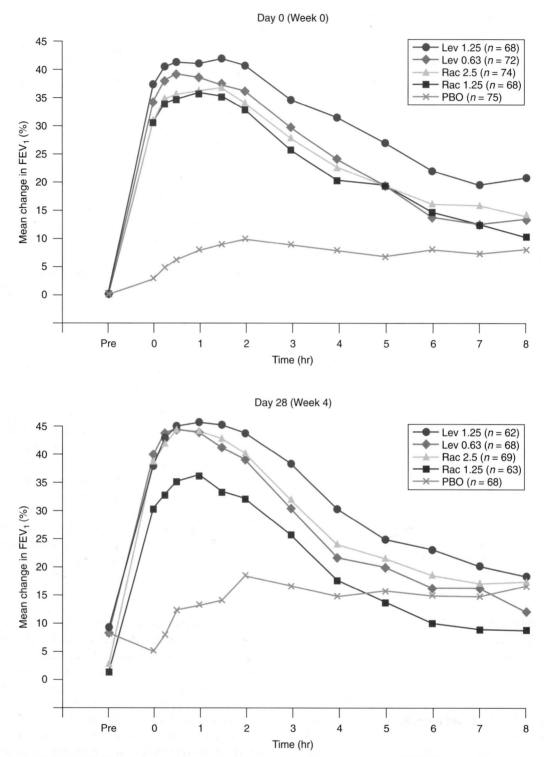

FIGURE 6-7 Mean percent change in forced expiratory volume in 1 second *(FEV₁)* from baseline (week 0) to the end of treatment (week 4) with various doses of levalbuterol, racemic albuterol, and placebo *(PLO)*. (From Nelson HS, Bensch G, Pleskow WW, DiSantostefano R, DeGraw S, Reasner DS, Rollins TE, Rubin PD: Improved bronchodilation with levalbuterol compared with racemic albuterol in patients with asthma, *J Allergy Clin Immunol* 102:943, 1998.)

clinical response was seen with one-fourth the racemic dose (0.63 mg) when using the pure isomer, although the racemic mixture contains 1.25 mg of the (R)-isomer (one-half of the total 2.5-mg dose). A detailed review of levalbuterol and of the physiological differences between the (R)-isomer and (S)-isomer of albuterol are available.[14]

Long-Acting β-Adrenergic Agents

The trend in adrenergic bronchodilators has been toward development from nonspecific, short-acting agents, such as epinephrine, to β_2-specific agents with action lasting 4 to 6 hours, such as albuterol and levalbuterol. A major limitation of β-adrenergic bronchodilators developed after isoproterenol and isoetharine was their 4- to 6-hour duration of action, which limited their usefulness in controlling nocturnal asthma symptoms and necessitated a less convenient, four-times-daily dosing schedule. Longer acting agents offer the advantages of less frequent dosing and protection through the night for asthmatic patients. These agents include extended release albuterol and newer drugs such as salmeterol (Serevent), formoterol (Foradil), and arformoterol (Brovana).

Long-acting bronchodilators are contrasted with short-acting agents. Short-acting agents include albuterol, levalbuterol, and pirbuterol, although these agents at one time were considered longer acting in comparison with the ultrashort-acting catecholamines such as isoetharine.

KEY-POINT

Salmeterol, formoterol, and *arformoterol* represent long-acting β_2 agonists with a 12-hour duration of action resulting from their unique pharmacodynamics (drug–receptor interaction).

Extended-Release Albuterol

An extended release form of albuterol is available as either Proventil Repetabs or Volmax. This is a 4- or 8-mg tablet taken orally with extended activity up to 12 hours. The extended activity of Repetabs is achieved with a tablet formulation that contains 2 mg of drug in the coating for immediate release and 2 mg in the core for release after several hours. The Volmax product uses an osmotic gradient to draw water into the tablet, dissolve the albuterol, and gradually release active drug through a pinhole in the tablet. Thus the 6-hour duration can be extended for 8 to 12 hours and mimics the effect of taking two doses.

Salmeterol (Serevent)

Salmeterol, a β_2-selective receptor agonist, is available in a dry powder formulation in the Diskus inhaler. Salmeterol xinafoate is a racemic mixture of two enantiomers, with the (R)-isomer containing the predominant β_2 activity.[15]

Bronchodilator Effect. Salmeterol represents a new generation of long-acting β_2-specific bronchodilating agents, whose bronchodilation profile differs from those of the agents previously discussed. The median time to reach a 15% increase in FEV_1 above baseline (considered the onset of bronchodilation) in asthmatic subjects is longer with salmeterol than albuterol; it has been reported as between 14 and 22 minutes[16,17] and generally is greater than 10 minutes.[18] The slower onset of action with salmeterol is significant for its clinical application (discussed subsequently). The time to peak bronchodilating effect is generally 3 to 5 hours, and its duration of action in maintaining an FEV_1 15% above pretreatment baseline is 12 hours or longer. At each point (onset, peak effect, and duration) salmeterol exhibits slower, longer times for effect compared with shorter acting bronchodilators such as albuterol.

With inhaled salmeterol xinafoate, an initial peak plasma concentration of 1 to 2 µg/L is seen 5 minutes after inhalation, with a second peak of 0.07 to 0.2 µg/L at 45 minutes; the second peak is probably due to absorption of swallowed dose. The drug is metabolized by hydroxylation, with elimination primarily in the feces.[19] The increased duration of action of salmeterol is due to its increased lipophilicity, conferred by the long side chain. The "tail" of the molecule anchors at an exosite in the cell membrane, allowing continual activation of the β receptor. The mode of action is discussed more fully below.

Formoterol (Foradil)

Formoterol is another β_2-selective agonist with a long-acting bronchodilatory effect of up to 12 hours in duration. A racemic mixture of (R,R)- and (S,S)-formoterol was approved by the FDA as Foradil for maintenance treatment of asthma in adults and children 5 years or older and for acute prevention of exercise-induced bronchospasm in adults and children 5 years or older. Formoterol is also indicated for the treatment of COPD and can be used in conjunction with other inhaled medications, such as inhaled corticosteroids, short-acting β agonist, and theophylline. Racemic formoterol is available as a dry powder aerosol for use with the Aerolizer dry powder inhaler (DPI). The current recommended

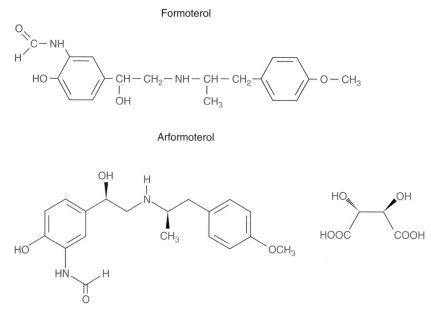

FIGURE 6-8 The chemical structure of formoterol and arformoterol, long-acting lipophilic β_2 agonists.

dose for adults and children 5 years or older is 12 µg twice daily by Aerolizer.

The chemical structure of formoterol is seen in Figure 6-8. As with salmeterol, the extensive side chain, or *tail,* makes formoterol more lipophilic than the shorter acting bronchodilators and is the basis for its longer duration of effect. The increased lipophilicity of both salmeterol and formoterol allows the drugs to remain in the lipid cell membrane. Even if a tissue preparation containing the drugs is perfused or washed, the drug activity persists. Salmeterol is more lipophilic than formoterol, and this along with its anchoring capability may explain why salmeterol is less prone to being "washed away" than formoterol.[18]

Bronchodilator Effect. Like salmeterol, formoterol has a prolonged duration of bronchodilating effect of up to 12 hours. Unlike salmeterol, the onset of action for formoterol is significantly faster. The time from inhalation to significant bronchodilation is similar to that of albuterol. It has been reported that 1 minute after inhalation of formoterol there is a significant increase in specific airway conductance (sGaw).[20] The onset of bronchodilation is generally considered to be 2 to 3 minutes with formoterol, compared with 10 minutes or longer with salmeterol. Figure 6-9 shows the dose-proportional response to inhaled (*R,R*)-formoterol, the single isomer isolated from the racemic mixture of (*R,R*)- and (*S,S*)-formoterol, compared with inhaled racemic albuterol.[21] In a study by van Noord and colleagues[22]

comparing racemic formoterol 24 µg, salmeterol 50 µg, and albuterol 200 µg, the increase in airway conductance after 1 minute was 44%, less than 16%, and 44%, respectively. The time to maximal increase in airway conductance was 2 hours, 2 to 4 hours, and 30 minutes, respectively, for the three drugs. The maximal increase was 135, 111, and 100%, respectively.[20,22]

The efficacy of formoterol in relaxing airway smooth muscle (its maximal effect) is higher than that of albuterol, which is higher than that of salmeterol. The lower intrinsic efficacy of salmeterol would make it a better agent than formoterol for patients with cardiovascular disease.[18]

Arformoterol (Brovana)

Arformoterol is the latest β_2-selective agonist with a long-acting bronchodilatory effect of up to 12 hours in duration. Arformoterol is the single, (R,R)-isomer form of racemic formoterol, which is approved by the FDA as Brovana for maintenance treatment of COPD. The current recommend adult dose is 15 µg, twice daily. Brovana is available in 2 mL unit-dose vials and is for nebulization only.

Antiinflammatory Effects

Both the short-acting and long-acting β agonists show antiinflammatory effects *in vitro.* Salmeterol, formoterol, and arformoterol inhibit human mast cell activation and degranulation *in vitro,* prevent an increase in

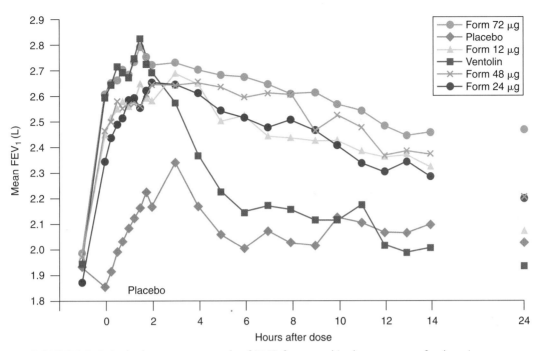

FIGURE 6-9 A single-dose crossover study of (R,R)-formoterol in the treatment of asthmatic adults. Shown are the dose-proportional FEV_1 responses and duration of action for the single isomer (R,R)-formoterol, a long-acting β_2 agonist.

vascular permeability with inflammatory mediators, and generally diminish the attraction and accumulation of airway inflammatory cells.[18] Despite these *in vitro* antiinflammatory effects, salmeterol and formoterol have not been shown to inhibit accumulation of inflammatory cells in the airway or the rise in inflammatory markers *in vivo*. Neither drug is considered to have a sufficient effect on airway inflammation in patients with asthma to replace antiinflammatory drugs such as corticosteroids.

Clinical Use

Long-acting β agonists are indicated for maintenance therapy of asthma that is not controlled by regular low-dose inhaled corticosteroids, and for chronic obstructive lung disease needing daily inhaled bronchodilator therapy for reversible airway obstruction. National guidelines recommend the introduction of a long-acting β agonist in step 3 care of asthma (asthma not controlled by lower doses of antiinflammatory medications).[23] Use of long-acting β agonists may prevent the need to increase the inhaled dose of corticosteroid. Several points should be noted in the clinical use of long-acting agents, because of their differences from shorter acting β agonists.

- Long-acting β_2 agonists are not recommended for rescue bronchodilation because repeated administration with their longer duration and increased lipophilic property risk accumulation and toxicity.[18]
- A shorter acting β_2 agonist, such as albuterol or other agents previously discussed, should be prescribed and available for asthmatics for treatment of breakthrough symptoms if additional bronchodilator therapy is needed between scheduled doses of a long-acting β_2 agonist; asthmatics must be well educated in the appropriate use of the two types of β agonists (shorter-acting versus long-acting).
- Although they have antiinflammatory effects, short-acting or long-acting β agonists are not a substitute for inhaled corticosteroids in asthma maintenance or for other antiinflammatory medications if such are required.
- The difference in rate of onset between salmeterol and formoterol may require classifying β_2 agonists as "fast" and "slow" in addition to "short" and "long" acting, with salmeterol being a slow and long-acting bronchodilator versus formoterol as a fast and long-acting bronchodilator.[24]

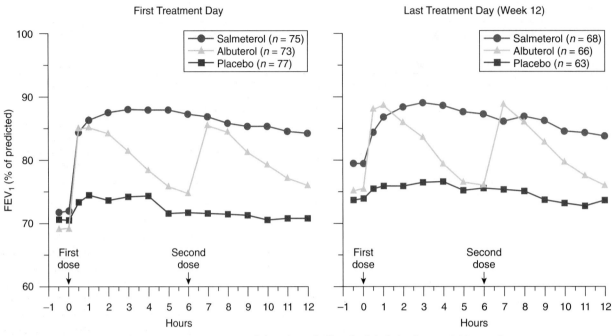

FIGURE 6-10 Mean FEV$_1$ response and duration of effect for inhaled salmeterol 42 µg twice daily, albuterol 180 µg four times daily, and placebo. (Modified from Pearlman DS, Chervinsky P, LaForce C, Seltzer JM, Southern DL, Kemp JP, Dockhorn RJ, Grossman J, Liddle RF, Yancey SW, *et al.*: A comparison of salmeterol with albuterol in the treatment of mild-to-moderate asthma, *N Engl J Med* 327:1420, 1992.)

The addition of a long-acting β$_2$ agonist to inhaled corticosteroids can lead to improved lung function and a decrease in symptoms.[25] A combination product of salmeterol and fluticasone in a Diskus inhaler (Advair Diskus) demonstrated superior asthma control and better lung function than either drug taken alone.[26-29] Because of their prolonged bronchodilation, long-acting β$_2$ agonists taken twice daily have a greater area under the FEV$_1$ curve compared with short-acting agents taken four times daily. This can be seen in Figure 6-10, which illustrates dose–response curves for albuterol and salmeterol. Unlike albuterol, which tends to return to baseline in 4 to 6 hours, salmeterol provides a more sustained level of bronchodilation, giving a higher baseline of lung function.[30] The same effect has been found in comparing twice-daily salmeterol with four-times-daily inhaled ipratropium bromide, a shorter acting anticholinergic bronchodilator discussed in Chapter 7.[31]

It is important to note that Salpeter and associates, in a meta-analysis, reported that long-acting β$_2$ agonists increased the risk of asthma hospitalizations and deaths compared with placebo.[32] In addition, Nelson and others also described an increase in death rate among patients using salmeterol; their findings reported the highest rate of death among African Americans.[33] Please note that neither of these studies took into account the severity of asthma, or whether the participants used other medications. This means that some participants' asthma may have been worse than others. Concerning cotreatments, the studies could not account for other medications participants may have been taking, or with what regularity they were taking them. The latter could have serious consequences if, for example, a participant stopped using inhaled corticosteroids that were prescribed to treat their asthma. Any of these variables—asthma severity, presence of cotreatments, and patient adherence—could affect data interpretation. Nevertheless, the labeling of these agents has been changed to warn that death can occur.

MODE OF ACTION

The bronchodilating action of the adrenergic drugs is due to stimulation of β$_2$ receptors located on bronchial smooth muscle. Distinctions among types of adrenergic receptors were identified in Chapter 5. In addition

TABLE 6-2

Adrenergic Receptor Types, With Their G Proteins, Effector Systems, Second Messengers, and Examples of Cell Responses

Receptor	G Protein	Effector	Second Messenger	Response
α_1	G_q	Phospholipase C (PLC)	Inositol trisphosphate (IP_3), diacylglycerol (DAG)	Vasoconstriction
α_2	G_i	Adenylyl cyclase (inhibits)	cAMP (inhibits)	Inhibition of neurotransmitter release
β (β_1, β_2, β_3)	G_s	Adenylyl cyclase (stimulates)	cAMP (increases)	Smooth muscle relaxation

cAMP, cyclic adenosine 3′,5′-monophosphate.

to β_2 receptors, some adrenergic bronchodilators can stimulate α and β_1 receptors, with the following clinical effects:

α-Receptor stimulation: Causes vasoconstriction (i.e., a *vasopressor* effect); in the upper airway (nasal passages) this can provide decongestion

β₁-Receptor stimulation: Causes increased myocardial conductivity and increased heart rate, as well as increased contractile force

β₂-Receptor stimulation: Causes relaxation of bronchial smooth muscle, with some inhibition of inflammatory mediator release and stimulation of mucociliary clearance

Both α and β receptors are examples of G protein–linked receptors. Table 6-2 lists each of the adrenergic receptor types, along with its particular type of G protein, effector system, and second messenger and an example of cell response in the lungs. As described in Chapter 2, the G protein is a heterotrimer whose α subunit differentiates the type of G protein. The G protein couples the adrenergic receptor to the effector enzyme, which in turn initiates the cell response by means of a particular intracellular second messenger. The mode of action with β-receptor, α_2-receptor, and α_1-receptor stimulation is described for each.

β-Receptor and α₂-Receptor Activation

The mode of action of β agonists and the β receptors has been well characterized, although the activity of α receptors is not as well understood. The mode of action for relaxation of airway smooth muscle when a β_2 receptor is stimulated is illustrated in Figure 6-11. Adrenergic agonists such as albuterol or epinephrine attach to β receptors, which are polypeptide chains that traverse the cell membrane seven times and have an extracellular NH_2 terminus and an intracellular carboxy (COOH)

terminus. This causes activation of the stimulatory G protein, designated G_s. The actual binding site of a β agonist is within the cell membrane, inside the "barrel" or circle formed by the transmembrane loops of the receptor chain. The β agonist forms bonds with elements of the third, fifth, and sixth transmembrane loops. When stimulated by a β agonist, the receptor undergoes a conformational change, which reduces the affinity of the α subunit of the G protein for guanosine diphosphate (GDP). The GDP is replaced by GTP, and the α subunit dissociates from the receptor and the β–γ portion of the G protein to link with the effector system. The effector system for the β receptor is adenylyl cyclase, a membrane-bound enzyme. Activation of adenylyl cyclase by the α subunit of the G_s protein causes increased synthesis of the second messenger, cyclic adenosine 3′,5′-monophosphate (cAMP). cAMP may cause smooth muscle relaxation by increasing the inactivation of myosin light chain kinase, an enzyme initiating myosin–actin interaction and subsequent smooth muscle contraction. An increase in cAMP also leads to a decrease in intracellular calcium.

A similar sequence of events is responsible for the action of α_2-receptor stimulation, which can inhibit further neurotransmitter release from the presynaptic neuron when stimulated by norepinephrine in a feedback, autoregulatory fashion (see Chapter 5). However, stimulation of α_2 receptors (not shown in Figure 6-11) results in activation of an inhibitory G protein, designated G_i, whose α subunit serves to inhibit the enzyme adenylyl cyclase, thereby lowering the rate of synthesis for intracellular cAMP.

α₁-Receptor Activation

Stimulation of an α_1 receptor by an agonist such as phenylephrine or epinephrine (which has affinity for both α and β receptors) results in vasoconstriction of

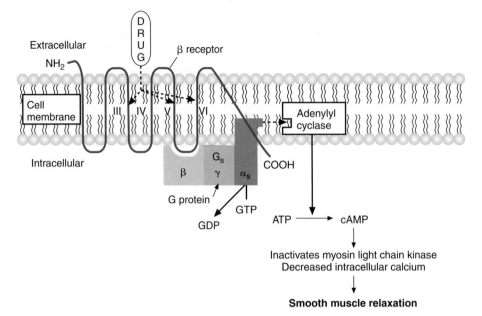

FIGURE 6-11 Diagram illustrating the mode of action by which stimulation of the G protein–linked β receptor by a β agonist causes smooth muscle relaxation.

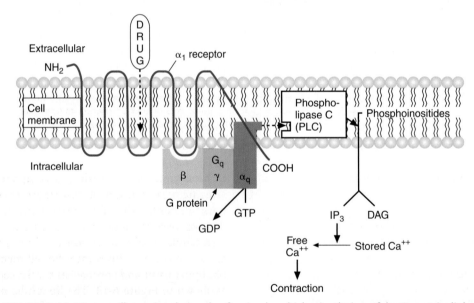

FIGURE 6-12 Diagram illustrating the mode of action by which stimulation of the G protein–linked α_1 receptor by an α agonist causes smooth muscle contraction, which can result in vasoconstriction of blood vessels.

peripheral blood vessels, including those in the airway. The mode of action for this effect as mediated by the G protein–linked α_1 receptor is illustrated in Figure 6-12. Stimulation of the α_1 receptor causes a conformational change in the receptor, which in turn activates the G protein designated G_q. With activation, GDP dissociates from the G protein, GTP binds to the α subunit

of the G protein, and the α subunit dissociates from the β–γ dimer, to activate the effector phospholipase C (PLC). Activation of the effector, PLC, leads to the conversion of membrane phosphoinositides into inositol 1,4,5-trisphosphate (IP_3) and diacylglycerol (DAG). IP_3 stimulates release of intracellular stores of calcium into the cytoplasm of the cell, and DAG activates protein

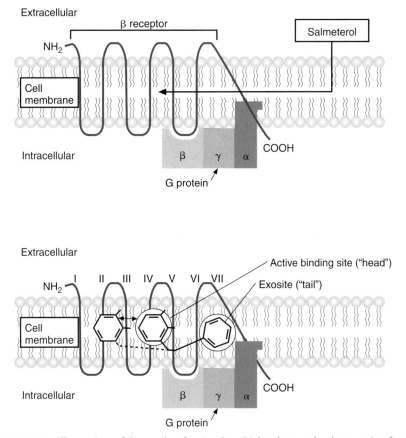

FIGURE 6-13 An illustration of the mode of action by which salmeterol, a long-acting β_2-specific bronchodilator, interacts with the β receptor by means of an exosite anchor, that is, its lipophilic side chain (the "tail"), allowing continual stimulation of the receptor via its active binding site (the "head").

kinase C. Contraction of vascular smooth muscle results.

Salmeterol, Formoterol, and Arformoterol: Mechanism of Action

The action of salmeterol in providing sustained protection from bronchoconstriction differs to a degree from that of the previously described adrenergic bronchodilators. The difference in salmeterol's pharmacodynamics is reflected in its pharmacokinetics with a slower onset and time to peak effect and a longer duration of action compared with previous adrenergic agents.

The structure of salmeterol is seen in Figure 6-3, along with that of other β agonists for comparison. The drug is a modification of the saligenin albuterol, with a long nonpolar (i.e., *lipophilic*) N-substituted side chain. Salmeterol thus consists of a polar, or *hydrophilic,* phenyl

ethanolamine "head," with a large lipophilic "tail" or side chain. As a result of this structure, salmeterol is lipophilic, unlike most β agonists, which are hydrophilic and approach the β receptor directly from the aqueous extracellular space. In contrast, salmeterol, as a lipophilic molecule, diffuses into the cell membrane phospholipid bilayer and approaches the β receptor laterally, as shown in Figure 6-13. The lipophilic nonpolar side chain then binds to an area of the β receptor referred to as the *exosite,* a hydrophobic region. With the side chain (tail) anchored in the exosite, the active saligenin head binds to and activates the β receptor at the same location as albuterol.

The binding properties of salmeterol, formoterol, and arformoterol differ from those of albuterol and other β agonists. Because the side chain of salmeterol is anchored at the exosite, the active head portion continually attaches to and detaches from the receptor site. This provides ongoing stimulation of the β receptor and is the basis for the persistent duration of action of salmeterol. This model of activity is supported by studies of the effect of β antagonists on the β-agonist action of salmeterol, as well as molecular binding studies. If albuterol is attached to the β receptor, the smooth muscle relaxation can be fully reversed by a β-blocking agent such as propranolol or sotalol, indicating a competitive blockade. When the β-blocking agent is removed, there is no further relaxation of smooth muscle. The albuterol has been displaced and the action of the drug is terminated. If salmeterol stimulates a receptor, a β antagonist such as propranolol will also reverse the effect of relaxation. However, when the propranolol is removed from the tissue, the relaxant effect of salmeterol is reestablished. This indicates that the salmeterol remains anchored in the receptor and is available to continually stimulate the β receptor once the blocking agent is removed.[15]

The prolonged activity of formoterol is also thought to be due to its lipophilicity, although formoterol is less lipophilic than salmeterol. Formoterol and arformoterol, which is moderately lipophilic, enters the bilipid cell membrane, where it is retained, with the lipid layer acting as a depot and giving a long-acting effect. At the same time, formoterol and arformoterol can approach the β receptor from the aqueous phase, giving it a rapid onset of action.[20]

ROUTES OF ADMINISTRATION

β-Adrenergic bronchodilators are currently available for inhalation (MDI, nebulizer solution, or DPI), oral administration (tablets or syrup), and parenteral administration (injection), although not all agents are found in each form. Regardless of the route of administration, there are three general patterns to the time course of bronchodilation with drugs in this group. The *catecholamines* show a rapid onset of 1 to 3 minutes, a peak effect at about 15 to 20 minutes, and a rapid decline in effect after 1 hour. The *noncatecholamines* (resorcinols and saligenins), with the exception of salmeterol, show an onset of 5 to 15 minutes, a peak effect at 30 to 60 minutes, and a duration of 4 to 6 hours. Salmeterol differs significantly, with a slower onset (>20 minutes) and peak effect (at about 3 hours), and a 12-hour duration. Formoterol and arformoterol is similar in duration to salmeterol but with an onset as rapid as that of albuterol. Aside from these general patterns, which depend on the type of drug used, the route of administration will further affect the time course of a drug. Inhaled and injected adrenergic bronchodilators have a quicker onset than orally administered agents.

KEY POINT

Routes of administration for β agonists can include inhalation (aerosol), oral, and parenteral, with minimal side effects seen with inhalation.

Inhalation Route

All of the β-adrenergic bronchodilators marketed in the United States are available for inhalational delivery, using an MDI, a nebulizer (including intermittent positive-pressure breathing nebulization), or a DPI. Catecholamines must be given by inhalation because they are ineffective orally. Inhalation is the preferred route for administering β-adrenergic drugs for all of the following reasons:

- Onset is rapid.
- Smaller doses are needed compared with those for oral use.
- Side effects such as tremor and tachycardia are reduced.
- Drug is delivered directly to the target organ (i.e., lung).
- Inhalation is painless and safe.

The use of aerosol delivery *during* an acute attack of airway obstruction has been questioned. However, several studies have failed to show substantial differences between inhaled and parenteral β-adrenergic agents in acute severe asthma.[34,35] There is no reason to avoid these bronchodilators as inhaled aerosols during acute episodes.[36] The inhalation route targets the lung directly. In fact, combining oral delivery with additional inhalation has been shown to produce good additive effects with albuterol.[37]

The major difficulties with aerosol administration are the time needed for nebulization (5 to 10 minutes), the possible embarrassment of using an MDI in public or at school, and inability to use an MDI correctly. Difficulty in correctly using an MDI can be remedied by using spacer devices or, alternatively, by using a gas-powered handheld nebulizer. A DPI can eliminate problems associated with both nebulizers and MDIs.

Continuous Nebulization

Administration of inhaled adrenergic agents by continuous nebulization has been used to manage severe asthma, in an effort to avoid respiratory failure, intubation, and mechanical ventilation. The *Guidelines for the Diagnosis and Management of Asthma* released by the 1997 National Asthma Education and Prevention Expert Panel Report 2 (NAEPP EPR 2) also recommend 2.5 to 5 mg of albuterol by nebulizer every 20 minutes for three doses, as well as 10 to 15 mg/hr by continuous nebulization.[1] Because a nebulizer treatment takes approximately 10 minutes, giving three treatments every 20 minutes requires repeated therapist attendance. Continuous administration by nebulizer may simplify such frequent treatments. The use of continuous nebulization of β-agonist bronchodilators was reviewed by Fink and Dhand,[38] who present a summary of studies, including dosages used. With continuous nebulization, there are no general standards for doses other than the recommendation from the NAEPP EPR 2; in the studies cited in Fink and Dhand,[38] dosages vary from 2.5 to 15 mg/hr and include schedules based on milligrams per kilogram per hour.

The impact and optimal use of continuous nebulization versus intermittent nebulization is not clear. In the five randomized controlled trials from 1993 to 1996 cited by Fink and Dhand,[38] there was similar improvement between continuous versus intermittent nebulization. One study by Lin and associates[39] showed faster improvement in patients with FEV_1 less than 50% of predicted, using continuous nebulization. A study by Shrestha and colleagues[40] compared a high dose (7.5 mg) and low dose (2.5 mg) of albuterol with both continuous and intermittent nebulization. FEV_1 improved more with continuous than intermittent nebulization, and the low dose of 2.5 mg was as effective as the higher dose of 7.5 mg with continuous administration. These and other results suggest that there is a benefit to continuous nebulization in severe airflow obstruction, but a dose less than 10 to 15 mg/hr may be effective, with less toxicity. Less clinician time is required for the administration of continuous nebulization. Fink and Dhand[38] suggest that for emergency department patients with severe airway obstruction, who do not respond sufficiently after 1 hour of intermittent nebulization of β agonists, continuous nebulization offers a practical approach to optimal dosing in a cost-effective manner.

Delivery Methods. Several delivery methods to accomplish continuous nebulization have been tried and reported. These include the following:
- Measured refilling of a small-volume nebulizer (SVN)
- Volumetric infusion pump with an SVN[41]
- Large-reservoir nebulizer such as the HEART or HOPE nebulizer

Toxicity and Monitoring. Continuous nebulization of $β_2$ agonists is not standard therapy, and patients receiving this treatment have serious airflow obstruction. Potential complications include cardiac arrhythmias, hypokalemia, and hyperglycemia. Unifocal premature ventricular contractions were reported in one patient by Portnoy and associates.[42] Significant tremor may also occur. Subsensitivity to continuous therapy was not observed by Portnoy and colleagues. Close monitoring of patients receiving continuous β agonists is necessary and includes observation, along with cardiac and electrolyte monitoring. Selective $β_2$ agonists, such as albuterol, should be used to reduce side effects.

Oral Route

The oral route has the advantages of ease, simplicity, short time required for administration, and exact reproducibility and control of dosage. However, in terms of clinical effects, this is not the preferred route. The time course of oral β agonists differs from that of inhaled β agonists. The onset of action begins in about 1.5 hours, with a peak effect reached after 1 to 2 hours and a duration of action between 3 and 6 hours.[43] Larger doses are required than with inhalation, and the frequency and degree of unwanted side effects increase substantially. The catecholamines are ineffective by mouth, as previously discussed. Noncatecholamine bronchodilators in the adrenergic group seem to lose their $β_2$ specificity with oral use, possibly because of the reduction of the side-chain bulk in a first pass through the liver.[44] Patient compliance on a three- or four-times-daily schedule may be better than with a nebulizer. If this is the case with an individual patient and the side effects are tolerable, then oral use may be indicated for bronchodilator therapy. The introduction of an oral tablet of albuterol with extended-action properties (Repetabs, Volmax) offers the possibility of protection from bronchoconstriction for longer than 8 hours. However, inhaled salmeterol and formoterol now offer a 12-hour duration. Either the extended release tablet or a long-acting β agonist is advantageous in preventing nocturnal asthma and deterioration of flow rates in the morning.

Parenteral Route

β-Adrenergic bronchodilators have been given subcutaneously as well as intravenously, usually in the emergency management of acute asthma. Subcutaneously, epinephrine 0.3 mg (0.3 ml of 1:1000 strength) every 15 to 20 minutes up to 1 mg in 2 hours and terbutaline 0.25 mg (0.25 ml of a 1-mg/ml solution) repeated in 15 to 30 minutes, not exceeding 0.5 mg in 4 hours, have been used. Shim[45] suggests that for practical purposes both aerosolized and subcutaneous routes should be used to manage acute obstruction, although there may be little difference in effect with the two routes. No difference in effect between epinephrine and terbutaline has been found when given subcutaneously.

The intravenous route has been used most commonly with isoproterenol and also with albuterol. Intravenous administration of these agents was thought useful during severe obstruction because these agents would be distributed throughout the lungs, whereas aerosol delivery would not allow them to penetrate the periphery. This assumption is questionable for both subcutaneous and intravenous bronchodilator therapy, because aerosols do exert an effect with obstruction. Intravenous isoproterenol is not clearly advantageous as a bronchodilator, although this route is used for cardiac stimulation in shock and bradycardia. The dose-limiting factor is tachycardia. Intravenous therapy is a last resort and requires an infusion pump, cardiac monitor, and close attention. Children's dosages range from 0.1 to 0.8 µg/kg/min, and adult dosages range from 0.03 to 0.2 µg/kg/min, until bronchial relaxation or side effects occur.[45] However, the combination of myocardial stimulation and hypoxia can cause serious arrhythmias, and intravenous isoproterenol should be avoided in acute asthma, in favor of β_2-specific agents. Albuterol has been given intravenously as a bolus between 100 to 500 µg or by infusion between 4 and 25 µg/min.[46] Although albuterol is more β_2 specific by aerosol than is isoproterenol, the usefulness of intravenous administration compared with oral, aerosol, or subcutaneous administration is not clearly established.

ADVERSE SIDE EFFECTS

Just as the adrenergic bronchodilators exert a therapeutic effect by stimulation of α-, β_1-, or β_2-adrenergic receptors, they can likewise cause unwanted effects as a result of stimulation of these receptors. In general, the term *side effect* indicates any effect other than the intended therapeutic effect. The most common clinically observed side effects of adrenergic bronchodilators are listed in Box 6-2 and are briefly discussed. It must be emphasized that the number and severity of these side effects vary from patient to patient; not every side effect is seen with each patient. It must be remembered that the later adrenergic agents (albuterol, bitolterol, pirbuterol, levalbuterol, and salmeterol) are much more β_2 specific than previous agents such as ephedrine, epinephrine, or isoproterenol. Because of this, there is a greater likelihood of cardiac stimulation causing tachycardia and blood pressure increases with the last three agents than with the newer drugs. The more recent agents are safe, and the side effects listed are more of a nuisance than a danger and are easily monitored by clinicians. The introduction of single-isomer β agonists

Box 6-2	Side Effects Seen With β-Agonist Use

- Tremor
- Palpitations and tachycardia
- Headache
- Insomnia
- Rise in blood pressure
- Nervousness
- Dizziness
- Nausea
- Tolerance to bronchodilator effect
- Loss of bronchoprotection
- Worsening ventilation–perfusion ratio (resulting in decreased arterial oxygen pressure, PaO_2)
- Hypokalemia
- Bronchoconstrictor reaction to solution additives (SVN) and propellants (MDI)

such as levalbuterol may show a further specificity and decrease in side effects, which are potentially caused by the detrimental effects of the (S)-isomer of β agonists.

KEY POINT

Adverse side effects can occur with β agonists and include tremor (very common), headache, insomnia, bronchospasm (with MDI use), palpitations, and some tolerance.

Tremor

The annoying effect of muscle tremor with β agonists is due to stimulation of β_2 receptors in skeletal muscle. It is dose related, and is the dose-limiting side effect of the β_2-specific agents, especially with oral administration. The adrenergic receptors mediating muscle tremor have been shown to be of the β_2 type.[47,48] As shown previously, this side effect is much more noticeable with oral delivery, which provides a rationale for aerosol administration of these agents. Tolerance to the side effect of tremor usually develops after a period of days to weeks with the oral route, and patients should be reassured of this when beginning to use these drugs.

Cardiac Effects

The older adrenergic agents with strong β_1- and α-stimulating effects were considered dangerous in the presence of congestive heart failure. The dose-limiting side effect with these agents is tachycardia. They increase cardiac output and oxygen consumption by stimulating β_1 receptors, leading to a decrease in cardiac efficiency, which is the work relative to oxygen consumption.

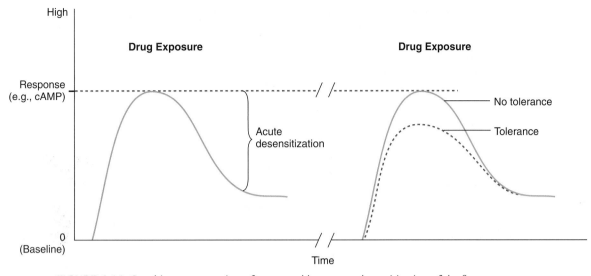

FIGURE 6-14 Graphic representation of acute and long-term desensitization of the β-receptor response to β agonists. Cell response during actual receptor stimulation by agonist immediately declines *(left side)*; subsequent exposure to drug will produce a lower peak initial response if tolerance or long-term desensitization occurs *(right side)*.

Newer agents have a preferential β_2 effect to minimize cardiac stimulation. However, tachycardia may also follow use of the newer agents, and there is evidence that this is due to the presence of β_2 receptors even in the heart.[49] β_2-Agonists cause vasodilation, and this can also cause a reflex tachycardia. Despite this effect, agents such as terbutaline or albuterol can actually improve cardiac performance. Albuterol and terbutaline can cause peripheral vasodilation and increase myocardial contractility without increasing oxygen demand by the heart.[34] The net effect is to reduce afterload and improve cardiac output with no oxygen cost. These agents are therefore attractive for use with airway obstruction combined with congestive heart failure. Seider and colleagues[50] reported that neither heart rate nor frequency of premature beats was significantly affected by inhaled terbutaline or ipratropium bromide (an anticholinergic bronchodilator) in 14 patients with chronic obstructive pulmonary disease (COPD) and ischemic heart disease. Although there are no written standards, most healthcare practitioners accept no more than a 20% change in pretreatment pulse after bronchodilator therapy has been initiated. This is why it is important to check the pulse rate before, during, and after bronchodilator therapy to evaluate cardiac response. If the pulse rate has increased more than 20% relative to the pretreatment pulse, stopping treatment with referral to the prescribing healthcare practitioner may be warranted to prevent unwanted cardiac effects.

Tolerance to Bronchodilator Effect

Adaptation to a drug with repeated use is a concern because use of the drug is actually reducing its effectiveness. With β agonists, there is *in vitro* evidence of an acute desensitization of the β receptor within minutes of exposure to a β agonist, as well as a longer term desensitization. This is illustrated in Figure 6-14, which shows both an acute decrease in response during sustained exposure of the receptor to the agonist and a long-term decrease in maximal response with subsequent drug exposure. This decrease in bronchodilator response has been observed with both short-acting and long-acting β agonists.

Exposure of cells with β receptors to isoproterenol causes a short-term, acute reduction in adenylyl cyclase activity and production of cAMP. The immediate desensitization is caused by an "uncoupling" of the receptor and the effector enzyme adenylyl cyclase.[51] A model for desensitization of the β receptor is diagrammed in Figure 6-15. When stimulated by a β agonist, the β receptor goes into a low-affinity binding state (i.e., has reduced affinity for binding with a β agonist). Simultaneously, the β agonist causes an increase in cAMP, which increases protein kinase A, also referred to as *β-adrenergic receptor kinase,* or *β-ARK*. β-ARK causes phosphorylation (transfer of phosphate groups, P) of the hydroxyl groups (OH) on the carboxy-terminal portion of the β receptor. This phosphorylation induces

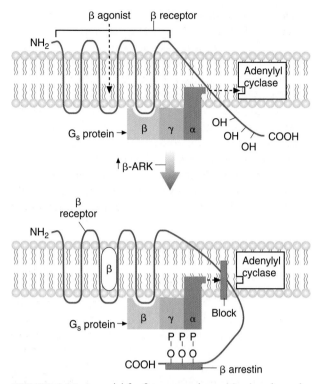

FIGURE 6-15 A model for β receptor desensitization through phosphorylation of the β receptor at the carboxy-terminal site by β-adrenergic receptor kinase *(β-ARK)*, blocking the action of the α_2 subunit on the effector enzyme adenylyl cyclase. *OH,* hydroxyl groups; *P,* phosphate groups.

binding of a protein named β-arrestin, which prevents the receptor from interacting with G_s and disrupts the coupling of G_s with the effector enzyme adenylyl cyclase. Removal of the β agonist allows the dissociation of both β-arrestin and the phosphate groups from the receptor, and the receptor returns to a fully active state.

Long-term desensitization is considered to be caused by a reduction in the number of β receptors. This is termed **downregulation**. Both norepinephrine and albuterol have caused a reduction of almost 50% *in vitro* in the number of β-adrenergic receptors in airway smooth muscle of guinea pigs.[51] Exposure of isolated human bronchus to isoproterenol or terbutaline produces similar desensitization.[52] Long-term desensitization is also illustrated in Figure 6-14, as indicated by the lower peak response to subsequent administration of an adrenergic agonist.

Although use of an inhaled β agonist does cause a reduction in peak effect, the bronchodilator response is still significant and stabilizes within several weeks with continued use.[18] Such tolerance is not generally considered clinically important and does not contraindicate

the use of these agents. The same phenomenon of tolerance is also responsible for diminished side effects, such as muscle tremor, among patients regularly using inhaled β-agonist bronchodilators.

In addition to loss of receptors (downregulation) by exposure to a β agonist, altered β-receptor function may be caused secondary to inflammation. Increased levels of phospholipase A_2 (PLA$_2$) may destabilize membrane support of the β receptor, changing its function. Cytokines such as interleukin-1β (IL-1β) may cause desensitization, and platelet-activating factor (PAF) inhibits the relaxing effect of isoproterenol on human tracheal tissue.

Corticosteroids can reverse the desensitization of β receptors and are said to be able to potentiate the response to β agonists.[53] Corticosteroids have the following effects, in relation to β-agonist and β-receptor function:

- Corticosteroids increase the proportion of β receptors expressed on the cell membrane *(upregulation)*
- Corticosteroids increase the proportion of β receptors in the high-affinity binding state
- Corticosteroids inhibit the release and action of inflammatory mediators such as PLA$_2$, cytokines, and PAF

β Agonists may in turn have a positive effect on corticosteroid function and activity. A review by Anderson explores possible mechanisms for the beneficial interaction of β agonists and corticosteroids.[25]

Loss of Bronchoprotection

A distinction was found by Ahrens and colleagues to exist between the *bronchodilating effect* and the *bronchoprotective effect* of β agonists.[54] The bronchodilating effect of a β agonist can be measured on the basis of airflow change, as indicated by, for example, a change in FEV$_1$ or peak expiratory flow rate (PEFR). The bronchoprotective effect refers to the reaction of the airways to challenge by provocative stimuli such as allergens or irritants and is measured with doses of histamine, methacholine, or cold air. Ahrens and colleagues[54] found that the protective effect with agonists such as metaproterenol or albuterol declines more rapidly than the bronchodilating effect. Not only is there a difference in time between these effects, but it was found that tolerance occurs with the bronchoprotective effect of a β agonist, just as with the bronchodilating effect. Results from a study by O'Connor and associates[55] are shown in Figure 6-16. The difference in dose of adenosine (AMP) and methacholine required to induce a 20% decline in FEV$_1$ (PC$_{20}$) after the inhalation of terbutaline

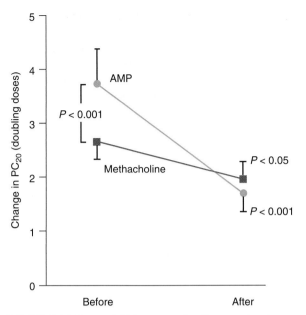

FIGURE 6-16 Data of O'Connor and colleagues showing a decrease in the provocational dose of adenosine (AMP) and methacholine after inhaling 500 µg of terbutaline compared with placebo, before and after a 7-day treatment period with terbutaline, indicating a loss of protection against airway stimuli with regular terbutaline use, especially with the inflammatory agent AMP. The higher the number of doubling doses needed for bronchoconstriction, the lower the airway responsiveness, that is, the greater the airway protection. (From O'Connor BJ, Aikman SL, Barnes PJ: Tolerance to the nonbronchodilator effects of inhaled β_2-agonists in asthma, *New Engl J Med* 327:1204, 1992.)

compared with placebo is seen before and after 7 days of steady treatment with terbutaline. Airway response to challenge is seen to occur with a significantly lower dose of either AMP or methacholine in subjects with mild asthma, *after* 7 days of β-agonist exposure, showing tolerance to the protective effect of terbutaline. The development of tolerance to the bronchoprotective effect of the long-acting β-agonist salmeterol was shown to occur both in the absence of corticosteroid therapy (by Bhagat and colleagues[56]) and with concomitant inhaled corticosteroid treatment (by Kalra and associates[57]). After the first 4 weeks of regular treatment with salmeterol, there was no increase in bronchial hyperresponsiveness or loss of bronchoprotection, in a study by Rosenthal and associates.[58] Sustained improvements were seen in pulmonary function and asthma symptom control.[58]

The mechanism underlying the increase in bronchial hyperresponsiveness with use of β agonists is not clear. Evidence accumulating on the effects of the (S)-isomer of β agonists suggests a possible cause.[59] The same

effects could conceivably be implicated in the reduction in maximal bronchodilator effect with repeated use.

Central Nervous System Effects

Commonly reported side effects of the adrenergic bronchodilators include headache, nervousness, irritability, anxiety, and insomnia, which are caused by central nervous system stimulation. Feelings of nervousness or anxiety may be due to the muscle tremor seen with these drugs, rather than to direct central nervous system stimulation. Excessive stimulation of the central nervous system, or at least symptoms of such, should be noted by clinicians and can warrant evaluation of the dosage used.

Fall in Arterial Oxygen Pressure

A fall in arterial oxygen pressure (Pa_{O_2}) has been noted with isoproterenol administration during asthmatic bronchospasm, as ventilation improves and the exacerbation is relieved. The same effect has subsequently been noted with newer β agonists such as albuterol and salmeterol.[60] The mechanism for this seems to be an increase in perfusion (i.e., blood flow) of poorly ventilated portions of the lung. It is known that regional alveolar hypoxia produces regional pulmonary vasoconstriction in an effort to shunt perfusion to lung areas of higher oxygen tension. This vasoconstriction is probably accomplished by α-sympathetic receptors.[61]

Administration of inhaled β agonists may reverse hypoxic pulmonary vasoconstriction by β_2 stimulation, increasing perfusion to underventilated lung regions.[62] Preferential delivery of the inhaled aerosol to better ventilated lung regions increases the ventilation–perfusion mismatch. It has been noted that such Pa_{O_2} drops are statistically significant but physiologically may be negligible.[60,63] Oxygen tension falls most in subjects with the highest initial Pa_{O_2}. Decreases in Pa_{O_2} rarely exceed 10 mmHg, and the Pa_{O_2} values tend to be on the flat portion of the oxyhemoglobin curve, so that drops in arterial oxygen saturation (Sa_{O_2}) are minimized. Oxygen tensions usually return to baseline within 30 minutes.

Metabolic Disturbances

Adrenergic bronchodilators can increase blood glucose and insulin levels, as well as decrease serum potassium levels. This is a normal effect of sympathomimetics. In diabetic patients, clinicians should be aware of a possible effect on glucose and insulin levels. Hypokalemia has also been reported after parenteral administration of albuterol and epinephrine.[64] The clinical importance of this is controversial and would be of concern mainly for patients with cardiac disease or in interpreting serum potassium levels obtained shortly after use of adrenergic bronchodilators. The mechanism of the effect on potassium is probably activation of the sodium–potassium pump by the β receptor, with enhanced transport of potassium from the extracellular to the intracellular compartment. Such metabolic effects are minimized with inhaled aerosols of β-adrenergic agents, because plasma levels of the drug remain low.

Propellant Toxicity and Paradoxical Bronchospasm

The use of chlorofluorocarbon (CFC; e.g., Freon)-powered MDIs can cause bronchospasm of hyperreactive airways. This reaction to the propellant was shown by Yarbrough and colleagues.[65] They found that 7% of 175 subjects who used an MDI with placebo and propellant experienced a decrease of 10% or more in their FEV_1. The incidence was about 4% when using an MDI with metaproterenol and propellant, probably because the bronchodilating effect overcame the propellant effect. In most cases, bronchospasm lasts less than 3 minutes. It appears there is no noticeable difference in adverse reactions among patients using a CFC MDI and those using a hydrofluoroalkane (HFA) MDI.[66] A dry powder formulation is an ideal alternative formulation to an MDI if sensitivity to propellants exists, assuming drug availability and adequate inspiratory flow rate. Use of a nebulizer instead of an MDI may also be considered if bronchospasm occurs in a patient. Finally, the oral route offers an alternative to the inhalation route of administration. Cocchetto and associates[67] reviewed the literature on paradoxical bronchospasm with use of inhalation aerosols.

Sensitivity to Additives

An increasingly publicized problem for those with hyperreactive airways is sensitivity to sulfite preservatives, with resulting bronchospasm. Sulfiting agents are used as preservatives for food and are also used as antioxidants for bronchodilator solutions to prevent degradation and inactivation. Sulfites include sodium or potassium sulfite, bisulfite, and metabisulfite. When a sulfite is placed in solution, at warm temperature in an acid pH such as saliva, it converts to sulfurous acid and sulfur dioxide. Sulfur dioxide is known to cause bronchoconstriction in asthmatic patients. Solutions of isoetharine, isoproterenol (Isuprel), and racemic epinephrine (Nephron and microNefrin) all contain sulfites as preservatives. There have been reports of coughing and wheezing, as well as pruritus, after use of sulfite-containing bronchodilators. Other additives and preservatives that can potentially have an effect on airway smooth muscle include benzalkonium chloride (BAC), ethylenediamine tetraacetic acid (EDTA), and hydrochloric or sulfuric acid to adjust pH of the solution. Asmus and colleagues[68] recommend that only additive-free, sterile-filled unit-dose bronchodilator solutions be used for nebulizer treatment of acute airflow obstruction, especially if doses are given hourly or continuously. Clinicians should check aerosol formulations for BAC or EDTA, and if symptoms of bronchoconstriction occur, consider these as a possible cause.

THE β-AGONIST CONTROVERSY

The **asthma paradox** is a descriptive phrase for the increasing incidence of asthma morbidity, and especially asthma mortality, despite advances in the understanding of asthma and availability of improved drugs to treat asthma. Many studies have implicated the use of short-acting β agonists in asthma near-death emergencies and deaths,[69,70] worsening clinical outcomes,[71,72] and increased hyperreactivity.[73,74] The events described in these studies may have been related to lack of corticosteroid use, thus leaving uncontrolled asthma symptoms to be treated only with short-acting β agonists.

Short-acting drugs, such as albuterol, and long-acting agents, such as salmeterol, have not in general been associated with a significant worsening of asthma.[75] However, more recent evidence has indicated that long-acting β agonists may have a potential to increase asthma hospitalization or cause death.[32,33] It has been noted that regular use of fenoterol and isoproterenol, but not other β agonists, may lead to worsening asthma control.[59] Tolerance to the bronchodilator effect does occur with the use of β agonists, although this stabilizes and does not progress. There is an increase in bronchial hyperreactivity after institution of regular β-agonist therapy, which is not well explained. There is currently evidence to suggest that this effect may be caused or enhanced by the (S)-enantiomer of β agonists, which has a range of proinflammatory effects.

Asthma Morbidity and Mortality

A complete analysis of the relation between β agonists and worsening asthma based on the literature seems to indicate that there is *not* a class effect of these drugs

KEY POINT

The β agonists have been questioned as a possible factor in the increase in asthma mortality, leading to the "β-agonist controversy."

causing deterioration of asthma.[59] Although it is not clear that β-agonist use increases risk of morbidity or death from asthma, asthma mortality is reported to be rising in the United States and worldwide, despite more available treatment options, including β_2-specific and longer acting adrenergic broncho dilators.[76] There are several causes, not all involving β-agonist therapy, that may potentially lead to worsening asthma severity.

- Use of β agonists may allow allergic individuals to expose themselves to allergens and stimuli, with no immediate symptoms to warn them, but with development of progressive airway inflammation and increasing bronchial hyperresponsiveness.
- Repeated self-administration of β agonists gives temporary relief of asthma symptoms through bronchodilation, which may cause underestimation of severity and delay in seeking medical help. The β agonists do not block progressive airway inflammation, which can lead to death from lethal airway obstruction and hypoxia.
- Use of β agonists to alleviate symptoms of wheezing and resistance may lead to insufficient use, through poor patient education, poor patient compliance, or both, of antiinflammatory therapy to control the basic inflammatory nature of asthma.
- Accumulation of the (S)-isomer with racemic β agonists could exert a detrimental effect on asthma control.
- There is increased airway irritation with environmental pollution and lifestyle changes.[77]

Discussion of the relation of β-agonist use to asthma morbidity and mortality should review the use of β agonists in the context of the National Asthma Education and Prevention Program (NAEPP) guidelines. The 1991, 1997, and 2002 documents all stress that asthma is a disease of chronic airway inflammation. Treatment with regular β-agonist therapy in severe asthma (asthma requiring step 2 care or greater) does not address the underlying inflammatory process. In evaluating β-agonist therapy in asthma, one must evaluate concomitant antiinflammatory therapy (or the lack of it), as well as environmental management of the asthma.

RESPIRATORY CARE ASSESSMENT OF β-AGONIST THERAPY

- Assess the effectiveness of drug therapy on the basis of indication(s) for the aerosol agent: Presence of reversible airflow resulting from primary bronchospasm or obstruction secondary to an inflammatory response or secretions, either acute or chronic.
- Monitor flow rates with bedside peak flow meters, by portable spirometry, or on the basis of laboratory reports of pulmonary function before and after bronchodilator studies, to assess reversibility of airflow obstruction.
- Perform respiratory assessment: Breathing rate and pattern, and breath sounds by auscultation, before and after treatment.
- Assess pulse before, during, and after treatment; a 20% increase from baseline may constitute changing medication or discontinuing therapy.
- Assess the patient's subjective reaction to treatment, for any change in breathing effort or pattern.
- Assess arterial blood gases or pulse oximeter saturation, as needed, for acute states with asthma or COPD, to monitor changes in ventilation and gas exchange (oxygenation).
- Note the effect of β agonists on blood glucose (increase) and K^+ (decrease) laboratory values, if high doses, such as with continuous nebulization or emergency department treatment, are used.
- Long term: Monitor pulmonary function studies of lung volumes, capacities, and flows.
- Instruct asthmatic patients in the use and interpretation of disposable peak flow meters to assess the severity of asthmatic episodes and to ensure there is an action plan for treatment modification.
- Patient education should emphasize that β agonists do not treat underlying inflammation or prevent progression of asthma, and additional antiinflammatory treatment or more aggressive medical therapy may be needed if there is a poor response to the rescue β agonist.
- Instruct and then verify correct use of the aerosol delivery device (SVN, MDI, reservoir, DPI).
- Instruct patients in the use, assembly, and especially cleaning of aerosol inhalation devices.

For long-acting β agonists:

- Assess ongoing lung function, including predose FEV_1 over time and variability in peak expiratory flows.
- Assess amount of rescue β-agonist use and nocturnal symptoms.

- Assess number of exacerbations, unscheduled clinic visits, and hospitalizations.
- Assess days of absence resulting from symptoms.
- Assess ability to reduce the dose of concomitant inhaled corticosteroids.

SELF-ASSESSMENT QUESTIONS

1. Identify three adrenergic bronchodilators used clinically that are catecholamines.
2. Which of the catecholamine bronchodilators given by aerosol is β_2 specific?
3. What is the duration of action of the catecholamine bronchodilators?
4. Identify two advantages introduced with the modifications of the catecholamine structure in adrenergic bronchodilators.
5. Identify the usual dose by aerosol for an SVN for levalbuterol and albuterol.
6. What is an extremely common side effect with β_2-adrenergic bronchodilators?
7. Identify the approximate duration of action for isoetharine, pirbuterol, and salmeterol.
8. Identify the generic drug for each of the following brand names: Alupent, Tornalate, Maxair, Serevent, Ventolin.
9. Which route of administration is more likely to have greater severity of side effects with a β agonist, oral or inhaled aerosol?
10. You notice a pinkish tinge to aerosol rainout in the large-bore tubing connecting a patient's mouthpiece to a nebulizer after a treatment with racemic epinephrine; what has caused this?
11. A patient exhibits paradoxical bronchoconstriction from the Freon propellant when using his albuterol by MDI. Suggest an alternative for the patient.
12. If you are working with an asthmatic with occasional symptoms of wheezing and chest tightness, which respond well to an inhaled β agonist, would you suggest using salmeterol?
13. Suggest a β agonist that would be appropriate for he patient in question 12.

Answers to Self-Assessment Questions are found in Appendix A.

CLINICAL SCENARIO

A 24-year-old white male moved to the metropolitan Atlanta area in the fall of the previous year. He presents to your outpatient clinic with a complaint of difficulty in breathing. He has no history of asthma or other previous pulmonary disease. He is an accountant with a medium-size firm. He noticed a few "chest colds" from October through January, but these resolved with over-the-counter cold medications such as decongestants and cough suppressants. It is now late May, and during a golf game he had difficulty breathing. He described a tightness in his chest and the sound of wheezing on interview. The course had recently been mown. The pollen count was quite high at the time, and there was an increased ozone concentration, leading to a smog alert on the day of his game. He also complained of waking up several times during the night with mild shortness of breath.

His respiratory rate (RR) is 14 breaths/min, with no obvious distress at rest; blood pressure (BP) is 128/74 mmHg; heart rate (HR) is 76 beats/min; and temperature (T) is within normal limits. His oxygen saturation by pulse oximetry (Spo_2) is 93% on room air. On auscultation you detect mild expiratory wheezing bilaterally.

How could you assess the presence of airflow obstruction in this patient?

Given his symptoms, your physical findings, and a reduced peak flow, would you recommend a β agonist?

If you recommend a bronchodilator, suggest an appropriate agent.

How could you assess his response to a β-agonist bronchodilator?

At this point, suggest a β agonist to prescribe for his use at home or work when he leaves the clinic.

What type of instructions and follow-up would you suggest for this patient?

Answers to Clinical Scenario Questions are found in Appendix A.

References

1. National Asthma Education and Prevention Program, National Heart, Lung, and Blood Institute, National Institutes of Health: Expert Panel Report 2: *Guidelines for the diagnosis and management of asthma*, NIH Publication 97–4051. Bethesda, Md, 1997, National Institutes of Health. (Available at http://www.nhlbi.nih.gov/guidelines/asthma/asthgdln.pdf; accessed February 2007.)

2. Global Initiative for Asthma (GINA), National Heart, Lung, and Blood Institute, National Institutes of Health: *GINA Report, Global Strategy for Asthma Management and Prevention,* November, 2006. Bethesda, MD, 2006, National Institutes of Health (Available at: http://www.ginasthma.com/Guidelineitem.asp??l1=2&l2=1&intId=60, Accessed March 2007.), 2005, National Institutes of Health. (Available at http://www.ginasthma.com/Guidelineitem.asp?l1=2&l2=1&intId=1169&archived=1;accessed March 2007).

3. *Drug Facts and Comparisons*, St. Louis, Mo, 2006, Facts and Comparisons, Wolters Kluwer Health.

4. Richards DM, Brogden RN: Pirbuterol: a preliminary review of its pharmacological properties and therapeutic efficacy in reversible bronchospastic disease, *Drugs* 30:7, 1985.

5. Orgel HA, Kemp JP, Tinkelman DG, Webb DR Jr: Bitolterol and albuterol metered-dose aerosols: comparison of two long-acting beta-2 adrenergic bronchodilators for treatment of asthma, *J Allergy Clin Immunol* 75:55, 1985.

6. Mitra S, Ugur M, Ugur O, Goodman HM, McCullough JR, Yamaguchi H: (S)-Albuterol increases intracellular free calcium by muscarinic receptor activation and a phospholipase C–dependent mechanism in airway smooth muscle, *Mol Pharmacol* 53:347, 1998.

7. Lipworth BJ, Clark DJ, Koch P, Arbeeny C: Pharmacokinetics and extrapulmonary β_2 adrenoceptor activity of nebulised racemic salbutamol and its R and S isomers in healthy volunteers, *Thorax* 52:849, 1997.

8. Johansson FJ, Rydberg I, Aberg G, Andersson RG: Effects of albuterol enantiomers on *in vitro* bronchial reactivity, *Clin Rev Allergy Immunol* 14:57, 1996.

9. Templeton AG, Chapman ID, Chilvers ER, Morley J, Handley DA: Effects of S-salbutamol on human isolated bronchus, *Pulm Pharmacol Ther* 11:1, 1998.

10. Volcheck GW, Gleich GJ, Kita H: Pro- and anti-inflammatory effects of beta adrenergic agonists on eosinophil response to IL-5, *J Allergy Clin Immunol* 101:S35, 1998.

11. Schmekel B, Rydberg I, Norlander B, Sjosward KN, Ahlner J, Andersson RG: Stereoselective pharmacokinetics of S-salbutamol after administration of the racemate in healthy volunteers, *Eur Respir J* 13:1230, 1999.

12. Dhand R, Goode M, Reid R, Fink JB, Fahey PJ, Tobin MJ: Preferential pulmonary retention of (S)-albuterol after inhalation of racemic albuterol, *Am J Respir Crit Care Med* 160:1136, 1999.

13. Nelson HS, Bensch G, Pleskow WW, DiSantostefano R, DeGraw S, Reasner DS, Rollins TE, Rubin PD: Improved bronchodilation with levalbuterol compared with racemic albuterol in patients with asthma, *J Allergy Clin Immunol* 102:943, 1998.

14. Rau JL: Introduction of a single isomer beta agonist, *Respir Care* 45:962, 2000.

15. Johnson M, Butchers PR, Coleman RA, Nials AT, Strong P, Sumner MJ, Vardey CJ, Whelan CJ: The pharmacology of salmeterol, *Life Sci* 52:2131, 1993.

16. Kemp JP, Bierman CW, Cocchetto DM: Dose–response study of inhaled salmeterol in asthmatic patients with 24-hour spirometry and Holter monitoring, *Ann Allergy* 70:316, 1993.

17. Boyd G, Anderson K, Carter R: Placebo controlled comparison of the bronchodilator performance of salmeterol and salbutamol over 12 hours, *Thorax* 45:340P, 1990.

18. Moore RH, Khan A, Dickey BF: Long-acting inhaled β_2-agonists in asthma therapy, *Chest* 113:1095, 1998.

19. Brogden RN, Faulds D: Salmeterol xinafoate: a review of its pharmacological properties and therapeutic potential in reversible obstructive airways disease, *Drug Eval* 42:895, 1991.

20. Bartow RA, Brogden RN: Formoterol: an update of its pharmacological properties and therapeutic efficacy in the management of asthma, *Drugs* 56:303, 1998.

21. Vaickus L, Claus R: (R,R)-Formoterol: rapid onset and 24 hour duration of response after a single dose [abstract], *Am J Respir Crit Care Med* 161:A191, 2000.

22. van Noord JA, Smeets JJ, Raaijmakers JA, Bommer AM, Maesen FP: Salmeterol versus formoterol in patients with moderately severe asthma: dose and duration of action, *Eur Respir J* 9:1684, 1996.

23. National Asthma Education and Prevention Program, National Heart, Lung, and Blood Institute, National Institutes of Health: Expert Panel Report: *Guidelines for the diagnosis and management of asthma—update on selected topics 2002*, NIH Publication 02–5074. Bethesda, Md, 2002, National Institutes of Health. (Available at http://www.nhlbi.nih.gov/guidelines/asthma/asthmafullrpt.pdf; accessed March 2007.)

24. Politiek MJ, Boorsma M, Aalbers R: Comparison of formoterol, salbutamol and salmeterol in methacholine-induced severe bronchoconstriction, *Eur Respir J* 13:988, 1999.

25. Anderson GP: Interactions between corticosteroids and β-adrenergic agonists in asthma disease induction, progression, and exacerbation, *Am J Respir Crit Care Med* 161:S188, 2000.

26. Walters JA, Wood-Baker R, Walters EH: Long-acting β_2-agonists in asthma: an overview of Cochrane systematic reviews, *Respir Med* 99:384, 2005.

27. Castle W, Fuller R, Hall J, Palmer J: Serevent nationwide surveillance study: comparison of salmeterol with salbutamol in asthmatic patients who require regular bronchodilator treatment, *BMJ* 306:1034, 1993.

28. Bateman ED, Boushey HA, Bousquet J, Busse WW, Clark TJ, Pauwels RA, Pedersen SE, GOAL Investigators Group: Can guideline-defined asthma control be achieved? The Gaining Optimal Asthma ControL study, *Am J Respir Crit Care Med* 170:836, 2004.

29. Shapiro G, Lumry W, Wolfe J, Given J, White MV, Woodring A, Baitinger L, House K, Prillaman B, Shah T: Combined salmeterol 50 mcg and fluticasone propionate 250 mcg in the Diskus device for the treatment of asthma, *Am J Respir Crit Care Med* 161:527, 2000.

30. Pearlman DS, Chervinsky P, LaForce C, Seltzer JM, Southern DL, Kemp JP, Dockhorn RJ, Grossman J, Liddle RF, Yancey SW: *et al*.: A comparison of salmeterol with albuterol in the treatment of mild-to-moderate asthma, *N Engl J Med* 327:1420, 1992.

31. Mahler DA, Donohue JF, Barbee RA, Goldman MD, Gross NJ, Wisniewski ME, Yancey SW, Zakes BA, Rickard KA, Anderson WH: Efficacy of salmeterol xinafoate in the treatment of COPD, *Chest* 115:957, 1999.

32. Salpeter SR, Buckley NS, Ormiston TM, Salpeter EE: Meta-analysis: effect of long-acting β-agonists on severe asthma exacerbations and asthma-related deaths, *Ann Intern Med* 144:904, 2006.

33. Nelson HS, Weiss ST, Bleecker ER, Yancey SW, Dorinsky PM, SMART Study Group: The Salmeterol Multicenter Asthma Research Trial: a comparison of usual pharmacotherapy for asthma or usual pharmacotherapy plus salmeterol, *Chest* 129:15, 2006.

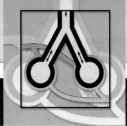

Chapter 7

Anticholinergic (Parasympatholytic) Bronchodilators

DOUGLAS S. GARDENHIRE

CHAPTER OBJECTIVES

After reading this chapter, the reader will be able to:

1. Differentiate between *parasympathomimetic* and *parasympatholytic*
2. Differentiate between *cholinergic* and *anticholinergic*
3. Differentiate between *muscarinic* and *antimuscarinic*
4. List all available anticholinergic agents used in respiratory therapy
5. Discuss the indication for anticholinergic agents
6. Explain the mode of action for anticholinergic agents
7. Describe the route of administration available for anticholinergic agents
8. Discuss adverse effects for anticholinergic agents
9. Discuss the clinical application for anticholinergic agents

KEY TERMS AND DEFINITIONS

Anticholinergic bronchodilator — An agent that blocks parasympathetic nervous fibers, which allow relaxation of smooth muscle in the airway

Antimuscarinic bronchodilator — Same as anticholinergic bronchodilator: an agent that blocks the effect of acetylcholine at the cholinergic site

Cholinergic — An agent that produces the effect of acetylcholine.

Muscarinic — Same as cholinergic: an agent that produces the effect of acetylcholine or an agent that mimicks acetylcholine

Parasympatholytic — Blocking parasympathetic nervous fibers

Parasympathomimetic — Producing effects similar to the parasympathetic nervous system

C hapter 7 discusses a second class of bronchodilators: the anticholinergic agents. Anticholinergic drugs given by inhaled aerosol can block cholinergic-induced airway constriction. Their mode of action is reviewed along with their pharmacologic effects, based on their structural differences. Specific agents are profiled and their clinical effect in chronic obstructive pulmonary disease (COPD) and asthma is discussed.

CLINICAL INDICATION FOR USE

A summary of recommendations and guidelines for use of anticholinergic (**antimuscarinic**) bronchodilators in the treatment of COPD and asthma can be found in Appendix D.

KEY POINT

Anticholinergic agents given by inhalation offer a second class of *bronchodilating agents.*

Indication for Anticholinergic Bronchodilator

Ipratropium and tiotropium are indicated as bronchodilators for maintenance treatment in COPD, including chronic bronchitis and emphysema.

Indication for Combined Anticholinergic and β-Agonist Bronchodilators

A combination anticholinergic and β agonist, such as ipratropium and albuterol (Combivent), is indicated for use in patients receiving regular treatment for COPD and who require additional bronchodilation for relief of airflow obstruction.

Ipratropium is also commonly used in severe asthma in addition to β agonists, especially bronchoconstriction that does not respond well to β-agonist therapy.

Anticholinergic Nasal Spray

A nasal spray formulation is indicated for symptomatic relief of allergic and nonallergic perennial rhinitis and the common cold.

SPECIFIC ANTICHOLINERGIC (PARASYMPATHOLYTIC) AGENTS

Parasympatholytic (anticholinergic, or antimuscarinic) agents that are given by aerosol include ipratropium, a combination of ipratropium and albuterol, and tiotropium. Dose and administration for each agent are given in Table 7-1.

Atropine sulfate had been administered as a nebulized solution, using either the injectable solution or, preferably, solutions marketed for aerosolization, however, this agent is no longer aerosolized. Both duration of bronchodilation and the incidence of side effects are dose dependent. Dosages for children based on dose-response curves had been given as 0.05 mg/kg three or four times daily.[1] Dosages for adults are based on a schedule of 0.025 mg/kg three or four times daily.[2] Although greater bronchodilation and duration were seen with dosage schedules of 0.05 or 0.1 mg/kg for adults, the side effects of dry mouth, blurred vision, and tachycardia became unacceptable. Because it is a tertiary ammonium compound and not fully ionized, atropine is readily absorbed from the gastrointestinal tract and respiratory mucosa. Systemic side effects (which are discussed subsequently) were seen in doses required for effective bronchodilation when given as an inhaled aerosol. The drug is not recommended for inhalation as a bronchodilator because of its widespread distribution

TABLE 7-1

Inhaled Anticholinergic Bronchodilator Agents*

Drug	Brand Name	Adult Dosage	Time Course (Onset, Peak, Duration)
Ipratropium bromide	Atrovent	MDI: 18 µg/puff, 2 puffs qid	*Onset:* 15 min *Peak:* 1-2 hr *Duration:* 4-6 hr
	Atrovent HFA	HFA MDI: 17 µg/puff. 2 puffs qid SVN: 0.02% solution (0.2 mg/ml), 500 µg tid, qid Nasal spray: 0.03%, 0.06%; 2 sprays per nostril 2 to 4 times daily (dosage varies)	
Ipratropium bromide and albuterol	Combivent	MDI: ipratropium 18 µg/puff and albuterol 90 µg/puff, 2 puffs qid	*Onset:* 15 min *Peak:* 1-2 hr *Duration:* 4-6 hr
	DuoNeb	SVN: ipratropium 0.5 mg and albuterol 2.5 mg	
Tiotropium bromide	Spiriva	DPI: 18 µg/inhalation, 1 inhalation daily (one capsule)	*Onset:* 30 min *Peak:* 3 hr *Duration:* 24 hr

DPI, Dry powder inhaler; *MDI,* metered dose inhaler; *SVN,* small volume nebulizer; *HFA,* hydrofluoroalkane.
*A holding chamber is recommended with MDI administration to prevent accidental eye exposure.

in the body and the availability of the approved agents ipratropium and tiotropium.

Ipratropium bromide (Atrovent) is a nonselective antagonist of M_1, M_2, and M_3 receptors (for a discussion of muscarinic receptors, see Chapter 5). Ipratropium is currently available in three formulations for bronchodilator use: as a chlorofluorocarbon-propelled metered dose inhaler (CFC MDI) with 18 µg/puff, a hydrofluoroalkane-propelled MDI (HFA MDI) with 17 µg/puff, and a nebulizer solution of 0.02% concentration in a 2.5-ml vial, giving a 500-µg dose per treatment. This agent is an *N*-isopropyl derivative of atropine. As a quaternary ammonium derivative of atropine, ipratropium is fully ionized and does not distribute well across lipid membranes, limiting its distribution more to the lung when inhaled. Ipratropium is approved specifically for the maintenance treatment of airflow obstruction in COPD.

Ipratropium is poorly absorbed into the circulation from either the nasal mucosa, when given by nasal spray, or from the airway, when inhaled orally by aerosol. Approximately 20% of the nasal dose and the MDI dose is absorbed, with only 2% of the larger nebulizer solution absorbed into the bloodstream. Ipratropium is partially metabolized by ester hydrolysis to inactive products. It is minimally bound to plasma proteins such as albumin (<9%), and the elimination half-life is about 1.6 hours.

The profile of clinical effect for ipratropium differs from that of inhaled β-adrenergic agonists. The onset of bronchodilation begins within minutes but proceeds more slowly to a peak effect 1 to 2 hours after inhalation. The β agonists can peak between 20 and 30 minutes depending on the agent. In asthma, the duration of bronchodilator effect is about the same for ipratropium as for β agonists. However, in COPD the duration is longer by 1 to 2 hours.[3]

Ipratropium bromide (Atrovent nasal spray) is also available for treatment of rhinopathies and rhinorrhea, including nonallergic perennial rhinitis, viral infectious rhinitis (colds), and allergic rhinitis, if intranasal corticosteroids fail to control symptoms.[4] The nasal spray is available in two strengths, with a 0.03% solution delivering 21 µg/spray and the 0.06% solution delivering 42 µg/spray. The 0.03% strength is given as two sprays per nostril two or three times daily, and the 0.06% strength is given as two sprays per nostril three or four times daily. Optimal dosage varies. Intranasal ipratropium has been shown to significantly reduce the volume of nasal secretions and symptoms in patients with allergic rhinitis and in those with nonallergic rhinitis.[4] Side effects with the nasal spray are largely local and have included nasal dryness, itching, and epistaxis in a few patients. Dry mouth and dry throat have also occurred. Systemic symptoms such as blurred vision or urinary hesitancy are rare.

Ipratropium and albuterol (Combivent) is a combination MDI product, with the usual doses of each agent (18 μg/puff of ipratropium, 90 μg/puff of albuterol). The combination therapy has been shown to be more effective in stable COPD than either agent alone.[5] Another agent, DuoNeb, is available as a combination of ipratropium (0.5 mg) and albuterol base (2.5 mg).

Glycopyrrolate is a quaternary ammonium derivative of atropine that, like ipratropium, does not distribute well across lipid membranes in the body. It is usually administered parenterally as an antimuscarinic agent during reversal of neuromuscular blockade, as an alternative to atropine, with fewer ocular or central nervous system side effects. The injectable solution has been nebulized in a 1-mg dose for bronchodilation. Gal and colleagues[6] reported a comparison of glycopyrrolate with atropine and established dose–response curves. Glycopyrrolate has an onset of action of approximately 15 to 30 minutes, a peak effect at 0.5 to 1 hour, and a duration of approximately 6 hours. Although the injectable formulation of glycopyrrolate is used as a less expensive alternative to the Atrovent brand of ipratropium, it is not approved for inhalation.

Tiotropium bromide (Spiriva), a **muscarinic** receptor antagonist, is a long-acting bronchodilator. It is a quaternary ammonium compound structurally related to ipratropium. Like ipratropium, tiotropium is poorly absorbed after inhalation. Inhalation of a single dose gives a peak plasma level within 5 minutes, with a rapid decline to very low levels within 1 hour.[7,8] Tiotropium exhibits receptor subtype selectivity for M_1 and M_3 receptors. The drug binds to all three muscarinic receptors (M_1, M_2, and M_3) but dissociates much more slowly than ipratropium from the M_1 and M_3 receptors. This results in a selectivity of action on M_1 and M_3 receptors. Atropine and ipratropium both block all three types of muscarinic receptor. The M_2 receptor is an autoreceptor inhibiting further release of acetylcholine, so that blockade can increase acetylcholine release and may offset the bronchodilating effect of atropine or ipratropium.[8] In patients with COPD, tiotropium gives a bronchodilating effect for up to 24 hours, with adequate dose. The drug also gives a prolonged, dose-dependent protection against inhaled methacholine challenge.[9]

Several studies have examined the bronchodilating effect of various doses of tiotropium, in comparison with both placebo and ipratropium.[9-11] A single dose of 18 μg inhaled once daily from a dry powder inhaler (DPI), the HandiHaler,[12] provided significant bronchodilation for up to 24 hours, with a low side effect profile. An increase of 15% from baseline FEV_1 (forced expiratory volume in 1 second) occurred 30 minutes after inhalation, with a peak effect at about 3 hours. Three hours after inhalation, improvement in FEV_1 was greater for tiotropium than for ipratropium. After a dose of tiotropium, the trough, or lowest, value for FEV_1 remained above that of ipratropium, because of the prolonged action of tiotropium. Ipratropium had a more rapid onset of action than tiotropium, but after the initial dosing this difference loses relevance because tiotropium maintains a higher level of baseline bronchodilation. In a meta-analysis, Barr and associates found that tiotropium reduces COPD exacerbations and hospitalizations, improves quality-of-life symptoms, and may slow the decline in a patient's FEV_1.[13]

> **KEY POINT**
>
> The anticholinergic bronchodilators are specifically *parasympatholytic*, that is, *antimuscarinic* agents, blocking the effect of acetylcholine at the cholinergic (muscarinic) receptors on bronchial smooth muscle.

> **KEY POINT**
>
> The only approved anticholinergic agents for inhalation as an aerosol at this time are *ipratropium* (Atrovent), which is available as an MDI, an SVN solution, and an intranasal spray; and *tiotropium* (Spiriva), available only as a DPI.

CLINICAL PHARMACOLOGY

Structure–Activity Relations

Chemical structures of the two naturally occurring belladonna alkaloids, atropine and scopolamine (also called hyoscine), are illustrated in Figure 7-1. Atropine, including its sulfate (atropine sulfate), and scopolamine are both tertiary ammonium compounds that differ from each other only by an oxygen bridging the carbon-6 and carbon-7 positions. Quaternary ammonium derivatives of atropine include atropine, ipratropium, and tiotropium. Another quaternary atropine derivative, which has been administered experimentally as a bronchodilator by aerosol, is glycopyrrolate (Robinul) (not shown in Figure 7-1).

Tertiary ammonium forms such as atropine sulfate or scopolamine are easily absorbed into the bloodstream, distribute throughout the body, and in particular cross the blood–brain barrier to cause central nervous system changes. Quaternary ammonium forms (such as ipratropium, tiotropium, and glycopyrrolate) are fully ionized and poorly absorbed into the bloodstream or central

Anticholinergic (Parasympatholytic) Agents
TERTIARY AMMONIUM COMPOUNDS

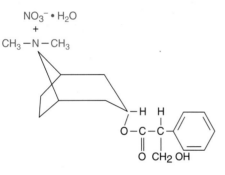

Atropine

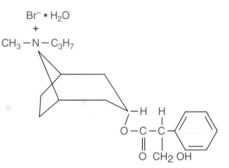

Scopalamine
(Hyoscine)

QUATERNARY AMMONIUM COMPOUNDS

Atropine
methylnitrate

Ipratropium
bromide

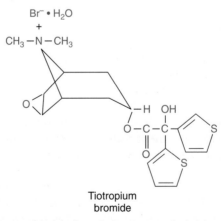

Tiotropium
bromide

FIGURE 7-1 Chemical structures of anticholinergic (parasympatholytic) agents: tertiary compounds, such as atropine and scopolamine, and quaternary compounds such as ipratropium and tiotropium.

TABLE 7-2

Comparison of Cholinergic Antagonism (Antimuscarinic Effects) With Cholinergic Effects (Muscarinic Effects)

Cholinergic Effect	Anticholinergic Effect
Decreased heart rate	Increased heart rate
Miosis (contraction of iris, eye)	Mydriasis (pupil dilation)
Contraction (thickening) of lens, eye	Cycloplegia (lens flattened)
Salivation	Drying of upper airway
Lacrimation	Inhibition of tear formation
Urination	Urinary retention
Defecation	Antidiarrheal or constipation
Secretion of mucus	Mucociliary slowing
Bronchoconstriction	Inhibition of constriction

TABLE 7-3

Pharmacological Effects of Tertiary Versus Quaternary Anticholinergic Agents Given by Inhaled Aerosol

	Tertiary (e.g., Atropine)	Quaternary (e.g., Ipratropium and Tiotropium)
Respiratory tract	Bronchodilation	Bronchodilation
	Decreased mucociliary clearance	Little or no change in mucociliary clearance
	Blockage of hypersecretion	Blockage of nasal hypersecretion
Central nervous system	Altered CNS function (dose related)	No effect
Eye	Mydriasis	Usually no effect*
	Cycloplegia	
	Increased intraocular pressure	
Cardiac	Minor slowing of heart rate (small dose); increased heart rate (larger dose)	No effect
Gastrointestinal	Dry mouth, dysphagia; slows motility	Dry mouth
Genitourinary	Urinary retention	Usually no effect†

CNS, Central nervous system.
*Assumes aerosol is not sprayed into eye; use with caution in glaucoma.
†Use with caution in prostatic enlargement or urinary retention.

nervous system. As a result, the systemic side effects seen with aerosol administration of the tertiary ammonium atropine sulfate do not occur or are minimal with a quaternary ammonium such as ipratropium. In general, quaternary ammonium agents given by inhalation are poorly absorbed from the lung. They are not rapidly removed from the aerosol deposition site and do not cross the blood–brain barrier as atropine sulfate does, giving them a wider therapeutic margin in relation to side effects.

Pharmacological Effects of Anticholinergic (Antimuscarinic) Agents

The general effects of **cholinergic** (muscarinic) stimulation and the corresponding effects produced by anticholinergic (antimuscarinic) action are listed in Table 7-2. Specific effects differ for tertiary and quaternary ammonium compounds because of their absorption differences as previously outlined for their structure–activity

relations. These effects and their differences are summarized in Table 7-3 and discussed subsequently.

Tertiary Ammonium Compounds

Tertiary compounds include *atropine sulfate, scopolamine,* and *L-Hyoscyamine sulfate.* They are well absorbed across mucosal surfaces and their effects increase with dose. Effects are summarized for these agents for the organ systems.

Respiratory Tract Effects. Atropine sulfate, a prototype tertiary compound, inhibits and reduces mucociliary clearance, as demonstrated by Groth and associates.[14] Atropine seems to block hypersecretion stimulated by cholinergic agonists in both the lower airway and the nose (upper airway) more than basal secretion.[15] Atropine relaxes airway smooth muscle, the basis for its use in asthma.

Central Nervous System Effects. Tertiary compounds cross the blood–brain barrier and produce dose-related effects. Small doses of 0.5 of 1.0 mg can cause effects that include restlessness, irritability, drowsiness, fatigue, or, alternatively, mild excitement. Increased doses can cause disorientation, hallucinations, or coma. Inhaled atropine has been reported to cause an acute psychotic reaction.[16,17]

Eye Effects. Tertiary anticholinergic compounds given by inhalation will distribute through the bloodstream and can affect vision. They block contraction of the iris to cause pupil dilation and paralyze the ciliary muscle of the lens to prevent thickening of the lens for near accommodation, causing blurred vision. These effects can raise intraocular pressure in glaucoma. Atropine-like agents are contraindicated in narrow-angle glaucoma.

Cardiac Effects. Atropine in small doses causes minor slowing of the heart rate; larger doses increase heart rate through vagal blockade.

Gastrointestinal Effects. Anticholinergic agents generally cause dryness of the mouth as a result of inhibition of salivary gland secretions, and atropine is used for this effect to reduce upper airway secretions before surgery and anesthesia or when reversing neuromuscular blockade (see Chapter 18). Larger doses can cause dysphagia. Gastrointestinal motility is slowed, an effect that is the basis for the inclusion of atropine in the brand Lomotil, an antidiarrheal. Inhibition of gastrointestinal motility and emptying has been noted with normal doses of atropine given by aerosol to asthmatics.[18]

Genitourinary Effects. Atropine-like agents can inhibit parasympathetic-controlled relaxation of the urinary sphincter. With prostate gland enlargement this can produce acute urinary retention. Atropine-like drugs can predispose to male impotency, because penile erection is also under parasympathetic control. Ejaculation is a sympathetic function.

Quaternary Ammonium Compounds

Quaternary compounds include the approved aerosol agent ipratropium, as well as tiotropium and glycopyrrolate. The following effects are discussed primarily for ipratropium, which is well known as an inhaled bronchodilator. In general, quaternary ammonium compounds will not cross lipid membranes easily and therefore do not distribute throughout the body when inhaled. Agents such as ipratropium will produce an anticholinergic effect at the site of delivery. With inhalation this will be the nose or mouth and the upper and lower airway.

Respiratory Tract Effects. Ipratropium has minimal or no effect on mucociliary clearance or mucus

viscosity, despite the fact that the aerosol is delivered topically to the airways. The drug does cause bronchodilation by blocking cholinergic contractile action. In the nasal passages, however, ipratropium does reduce hypersecretion, the basis for its use in rhinitis.

Central Nervous System Effects. Because quaternary compounds do not cross the blood–brain barrier, they do not cause CNS effects as the tertiary agents do.

Eye Effects. As long as ipratropium and other quaternary agents are not sprayed directly in the eye, there are no effects on intraocular pressure, pupil size, or lens accommodation when inhaled as an aerosol. Topical delivery to the eye can cause pupillary dilation (mydriasis) and lens paralysis (cycloplegia). Subjects using quaternary ammonium antimuscarinic bronchodilators must be cautioned to protect the eyes from aerosol drug.

Cardiac Effects. Ipratropium has minimal effects on heart rate or blood pressure when given by inhaled aerosol.

Gastrointestinal Effects. There is little effect on gastrointestinal motility with inhaled ipratropium in most patients. However, a portion of the aerosol dose is swallowed, thereby allowing exposure of the gastrointestinal tract to the drug. There has been a report of meconium ileus in an adult cystic fibrosis patient receiving nebulized ipratropium.[19] Use of a reservoir device with MDI administration can reduce oropharyngeal impaction and the amount of swallowed drug.

Genitourinary Effects. Ipratropium has no effect on urinary ability when tested in males 50 to 70 years of age.[20]

KEY POINT

Quaternary compounds, such as ipratropium, are fully ionized and less absorbed in body tissues than *tertiary compounds,* such as atropine sulfate. Consequently, side effects with quaternary compounds are localized to the site of drug exposure.

MODE OF ACTION

In Chapter 5 the autonomic innervation of the airway is outlined. This consists of the traditional sympathetic and parasympathetic branches, as well as nonadrenergic, noncholinergic (NANC) inhibitory and excitatory branches.

The sympathetic branch does not actually extend its fibers beyond the peribronchial ganglia or plexa

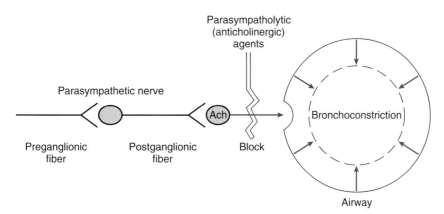

FIGURE 7-2 Conceptual overview of the action of anticholinergic (parasympatholytic) bronchodilating agents in preventing cholinergic-induced bronchoconstriction. *Ach,* Acetylcholine.

to the airway, although adrenergic receptors are present throughout the airway, especially in the periphery. Parasympathetic nerves do enter the lung at the hila, deriving from the vagus, and travel along the airways. Parasympathetic postganglionic fibers terminate on or near the airway epithelium, submucosal mucous glands, smooth muscle, and probably mast cells. Parasympathetic innervation and muscarinic receptors are concentrated in the larger airways, although present from the trachea to the respiratory bronchioles.

In the normal airway a basal level of bronchomotor tone is caused by parasympathetic activity. This basal level of tone can be abolished by anticholinergic agents such as atropine, indicating it is mediated by acetylcholine. Administration of **parasympathomimetic** (cholinergic) agents such as methacholine (e.g., in bronchial provocation testing) can intensify the level of bronchial tone to the point of constriction in healthy subjects and more so in asthmatic patients.

Cholinergic stimulation of muscarinic receptors on airway smooth muscle and submucosal glands causes contraction and release of mucus. Anticholinergic agents such as atropine or ipratropium are antimuscarinic; they competitively block the action of acetylcholine at parasympathetic postganglionic effector cell receptors. Because of this action, anticholinergic agents block cholinergic-induced bronchoconstriction, as seen in Figure 7-2.

An important point to realize with use of a blocking agent, such as an **anticholinergic bronchodilator**, is that the effect seen will depend on the degree of tone present that can be blocked. In healthy subjects, there will be minimal airway dilation with an anticholinergic agent because there is only a basal or resting level of tone to be blocked. Variation in the clinical effect of such

drugs will be partially due to variation in the degree of parasympathetic activity. One particular mechanism for parasympathetic activity in the lung is vagally mediated reflex bronchoconstriction, which is discussed in the next section.

KEY POINT

The anticholinergic agents ipratropium and tiotropium are indicated for the treatment of airflow obstruction in COPD.

Vagally Mediated Reflex Bronchoconstriction

A portion of the bronchoconstriction seen in COPD may be due to a mechanism of vagally mediated reflex innervation of airway smooth muscle (Figure 7-3).

Sensory C-fiber nerves respond to a variety of stimuli, such as irritant aerosols (hypotonic or hypertonic), cold air and high airflow rates, cigarette smoke, noxious fumes, and mediators of inflammation such as histamine. When activated, they produce an afferent nerve impulse to the central nervous system, which results in a reflex cholinergic efferent impulse, to cause constriction of airway smooth muscle and release of secretion from mucous glands, as well as cough.

Because atropine and its derivatives are competitive inhibitors of acetylcholine at the neuroeffector junction, such antagonists should block parasympathetic reflex bronchoconstriction. Atropine has been shown to inhibit exercise-induced asthma and psychogenic bronchospasm, as well as bronchoconstriction caused by β-blockade or cholinergic agents. Application of a topical anesthetic such as 4% lidocaine by aerosol to the large

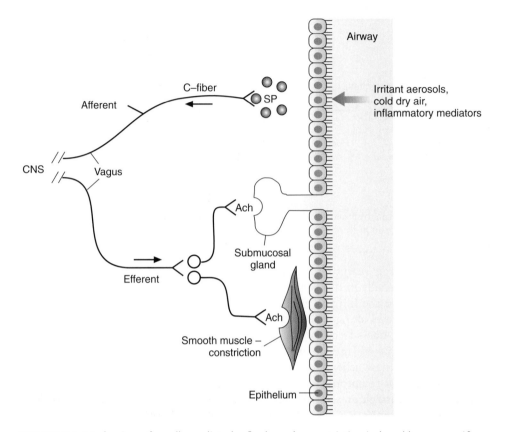

FIGURE 7-3 Mechanism of vagally mediated reflex bronchoconstriction induced by nonspecific stimuli on sensory C-fibers. *Ach,* Acetylcholine; *CNS,* central nervous system; *SP,* substance P.

airways has also inhibited reflex bronchoconstriction, by blocking the sensory irritant receptors in the epithelial lining.

Changes in the airway may also sensitize the subepithelial cough receptors, making them more responsive to lower thresholds of stimulation. This is often seen during colds that involve lung congestion. Lung inflation during a deep breath stimulates the cough receptors, resulting not only in coughing but also increased bronchomotor tone. It has been suggested that greater bronchial reactivity in asthmatic patients or patients with COPD may be caused by mucosal edema and deformation of airway tissue, which increases the sensitivity of

> **KEY POINT**
>
> At least a portion of the airflow obstruction in COPD may be due to *vagally mediated reflex bronchoconstriction* caused by stimulation of afferent sensory C-fibers, which trigger reflex, efferent vagal nerve activity, and constriction.

these receptors in response to irritants. Several reviews of cholinergic mechanisms of airway obstruction have been published.[21-25]

Muscarinic Receptor Subtypes

Anticholinergic agents cause bronchodilation by blocking muscarinic receptor subtypes: M_1 receptors at the parasympathetic ganglia, which facilitate cholinergic neurotransmission and bronchoconstriction, and M_3 receptors on airway smooth muscle, which cause bronchoconstriction. Muscarinic receptor subtypes are reviewed in Chapter 5 and are illustrated for the lung in Figure 7-4. M_1 receptors on the postganglionic parasympathetic neuron facilitate cholinergic nerve transmission, leading to release of acetylcholine. Acetylcholine stimulates M_3 receptor subtypes on airway smooth muscle and submucosal glands, causing contraction of smooth muscle and exocytosis of secretion from the mucous gland. The M_2 receptor subtype at cholinergic nerve endings inhibits further acetylcholine release from the postganglionic neuron.

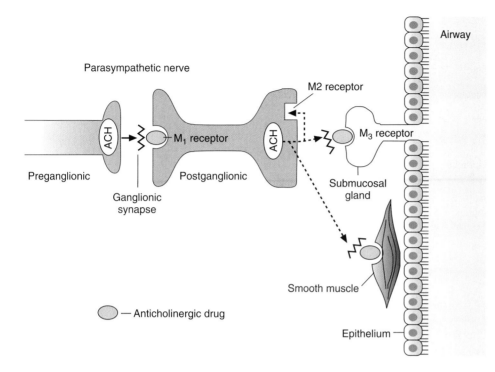

FIGURE 7-4 Identification and location of muscarinic receptor subtypes M_1, M_2, and M_3 in the vagal nerve, submucosal gland, and bronchial smooth muscle in the airway, showing nonspecific blockade by anticholinergic drugs such as ipratropium. *ACH*, Acetylcholine.

TABLE 7-4		

Muscarinic Receptor Subtypes: Their G Proteins and Effector Systems

Receptor	G Protein	Effector
M_1	G_q	Phospholipase C
M_2	G_i	Adenylyl cyclase (decreases)
M_3	G_q	Phospholipase C
M_4	G_i	Adenylyl cyclase (decreases)
M_5	G_q	Phospholipase C leads to an increase

M_3 receptors are G protein–linked receptors, as introduced in Chapter 2 and again in Chapter 5. Table 7-4 lists the various muscarinic receptor subtypes and their G proteins, along with their effector enzymes. Stimulation of the M_3 receptor subtype activates a G_q protein that in turn activates phospholipase C (PLC). Phospholipase C causes the breakdown of phosphoinositides into inositol trisphosphate (IP_3) and diacylglycerol (DAG). This ultimately leads to an increase in the cytoplasmic concentration of free calcium and smooth muscle contraction or gland exocytosis. As

shown in Figure 7-5, the competitive blockade of M_3 receptors by anticholinergic agents prevents this sequence. The blockade of M_1 receptor subtypes by anticholinergic agents also inhibits nerve transmission by acetylcholine at the ganglionic synapse. Both ipratropium and tiotropium also block the M_2 receptor. This receptor inhibits continued release of acetylcholine. As a result, blockade of the M_2 receptor can enhance acetylcholine release, possibly counteracting the bronchodilator effect of M_3 receptor blockade. As noted in the discussion of ipratropium and tiotropium, tiotropium has selective affinity for M_1 and M_3 receptors because it dissociates much more rapidly from the M_2 receptor and remains bound to the M_1 and M_3 subtypes.

The use of agents such as ipratropium for allergic and nonallergic rhinitis is based on the parasympathetic control of submucosal glands in the nasal mucosa. Acetylcholine stimulates muscarinic receptors in the nose, where approximately 55% are M_3 and the rest are M_1.[26] M_2 receptors were not identified in human nasal mucosa in an autoradiographic study by Okayama and associates.[27] Blockade of muscarinic M_1 and M_3 receptors on submucosal nasal glands by ipratropium given as a nasal spray prevents gland secretion and rhinitis.

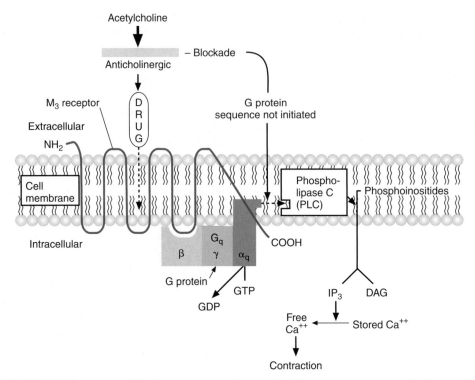

FIGURE 7-5 Illustration of the M_3 receptor as a G protein–linked receptor, showing the G_q protein; its effector system, phospholipase C; and the mechanism of smooth muscle constriction, which is blocked by an anticholinergic agent preventing stimulation of the M_3 receptor. *DAG,* Diacylglycerol; *IP₃,* inositol trisphosphate; *GDP,* guanosine diphosphate; *GTP,* guanosine triphosphate.

KEY POINT

The anticholinergic bronchodilators are *nonspecific blockers of muscarinic receptor subtypes* (M_1, M_2, and M_3) in the airway. Blockade of the M_3 receptor subtype on bronchial smooth muscle prevents activation of the linking G_q protein, its effector system phospholipase C (PLC), and subsequent increase in free calcium with bronchoconstriction or gland exocytosis.

KEY POINT

Blockade of M_1 and M_3 receptors in the nasal passages prevents gland secretion and rhinitis.

ADVERSE EFFECTS

It has been stated that the safety profile of quaternary ammonium antimuscarinic bronchodilators (e.g., ipratropium or tiotropium) is superior to that of β agonists, particularly with regard to cardiovascular effects.[9]

Changes in electrocardiogram, blood pressure, or heart rate are not usually seen. There is no worsening of ventilation–perfusion abnormalities in COPD, which would otherwise cause an increase in hypoxemia. A tolerance to bronchodilation and loss of bronchoprotection have not been observed. The lack of these effects is due to the poor absorption and systemic distribution of quaternary compounds such as ipratropium. A detailed review of the clinical pharmacology and toxicology of ipratropium is provided by Cugell.[28]

The side effects seen with the MDI and small volume nebulizer (SVN) formulations of ipratropium, the agent with the most clinical experience, are primarily related to the local, topical delivery to the upper and lower airway with inhalation. Similar side effects would be expected with other antimuscarinic agents such as tiotropium. The most common side effect seen with this class of bronchodilator is dry mouth. Possible side effects are listed in Box 7-1. The SVN solution has also been associated with additional side effects in a few patients: pharyngitis, dyspnea, flulike symptoms, bronchitis, and upper respiratory infection. It should be noted that

Box 7-1	Side Effects Seen With Anticholinergic Aerosol Ipratropium*

MDI AND SVN (COMMON)
- Dry mouth
- Cough

MDI (OCCASIONAL)
- Nervousness
- Irritation
- Dizziness
- Headache
- Palpitation
- Rash

SVN
- Pharyngitis
- Dyspnea
- Flulike symptoms
- Bronchitis
- Upper respiratory infections
- Nausea
- Occasional bronchoconstriction
- Eye pain
- Urinary retention (<3%)

MDI, Metered dose inhaler; SVN, small volume nebulizer.
*Side effects were reported in a small percentage (<3 to 5%) of patients.
Precautions: Use with caution in patients with narrow-angle glaucoma, prostatic hypertrophy, bladder neck obstruction, constipation, bowel obstruction, or tachycardia.

the amount of drug in the nebulizer dose is more than 10 times greater than in the MDI dose (500 µg versus 40 µg). If the patient receives approximately 10% of an inhaled aerosol to the lung, a much larger dose is given with an SVN. The orally swallowed portion will be proportionally higher also. Systemic side effects such as tachycardia, palpitations, urinary hesitancy, constipation, blurred vision, or increased ocular pressure are less likely with quaternary agents such as ipratropium or tiotropium than with tertiary agents such as atropine. Although ipratropium is not contraindicated in subjects with prostatic hypertrophy, urinary retention, or glaucoma, the drug should be used with caution and adequate evaluation for possible systemic side effects in these subjects.

The eye must be protected from drug exposure with aerosol use resulting from accidental spraying or with nebulizer delivery. Blockade of muscarinic receptors causes mydriasis by blocking the sphincter muscle of the iris and inhibits the ciliary muscle of the lens, preventing

lens thickening (accommodation). As the iris dilates outward and the lens remains flattened, drainage of intraocular aqueous humor is reduced. In patients with narrow-angle glaucoma, intraocular pressure can rise. Because many COPD patients are older, the presence of narrow-angle glaucoma may be more common. Subjects using quaternary ammonium antimuscarinic bronchodilators must be informed of this hazard and should use proper aerosol inhalation technique. A holding chamber should be used with MDI administration. With nebulizer delivery, the mouthpiece should be kept in the mouth and a reservoir tube attached to the expiratory side of the T mouthpiece to vent aerosol away from the face. The ideal nebulizer would be a dosimetric device with no ambient exposure from the device on exhalation. If the nebulizer solution is delivered by facemask (which is not recommended), the eyes should be closed or covered to prevent drug exposure. Because of the greater risk of eye exposure with a nebulizer, especially disposable, constant-output devices, an MDI with holding chamber is recommended for delivery of this class of bronchodilator.

KEY POINT

The most common side effects with quaternary ammonium antimuscarinic bronchodilators are dry mouth and perhaps a cough caused by the aerosol particles.

KEY POINT

Direct spraying in the eye must be avoided to prevent ocular effects. Subjects with COPD can show a greater response in reversibility of airflow obstruction with an anticholinergic agent than a β agonist.

CLINICAL APPLICATION

Anticholinergic (antimuscarinic) aerosols have been investigated for use with asthma and with COPD. Table 7-5 compares the general effects seen with anticholinergic bronchodilators and β-adrenergic bronchodilators.

Use in Chronic Obstructive Pulmonary Disease

Antimuscarinic agents were found to be more potent bronchodilators than β-adrenergic agents in bronchitis–emphysema, and this is likely to be their primary clinical application. This difference is illustrated in Figure 7-6 with data from Tashkin and colleagues.[29] In that 90-day, multicenter study, the investigation compared 40 µg of ipratropium with 1.5 mg of metaproterenol, both given by MDI, in a population of patients with COPD. Explanations for the superiority of anticholinergic action in COPD are debated but may relate to the complicated, inflammatory, noncholinergic pathways seen in asthma, especially due to stimuli mentioned previously in the section on vagally mediated reflex bronchoconstriction. Conversely, the pathology of COPD may reveal the reason for the superior effect of anticholinergic over β-adrenergic drugs. Ipratropium has been approved by the U.S. Food and Drug Administration (FDA) specifically for use in the treatment of COPD, although the drug is also prescribed for treatment of asthma.

An analysis of data from the clinical trials of ipratropium compared with a β agonist for FDA approval was conducted by Rennard and associates.[30] Their analysis showed that use of ipratropium over the 90-day interval tested was associated with improved baseline lung function and response to acute bronchodilator use. Subjects using β agonists over the same period had little change in baseline lung function and a small decrease in airway response to acute bronchodilator treatment.

Tiotropium, an antimuscarinic bronchodilator, offers a prolonged duration of action of up to 24 hours with a single daily inhalation. In dose-ranging trials an inhaled dose of 18 µg once per day has been found to give significant bronchodilation in patients with COPD with few side effects.[9,11] Figure 7-7 illustrates the effect on FEV_1 with single inhaled doses of tiotropium of various strengths in comparison with placebo.[9] There is also prolonged dose-dependent protection against inhaled methacholine challenge. Both the bronchodilating and the bronchoprotective effect can be compared with the 6-hour effect of ipratropium. Perhaps one of the more important effects of a long-acting drug such as tiotropium is the elevation in baseline, predose FEV_1. Unlike ipratropium, lung function is maintained more consistently at a higher level throughout the day with tiotropium. This may have a significant effect on quality of life and reduction of breathlessness in patients with COPD. Beeh and colleagues report that an inhaled dose of 18 µg once per day improved lung function as

TABLE 7-5

Comparison of Effects for Anticholinergic and β-Adrenergic Bronchodilators

	Anticholinergic	β Agonist
Onset	Slightly slower	Faster
Time to peak effect	Slower	Faster
Duration	Longer	Shorter
Tremor	None	Yes
Fall in Pao_2	None	Yes
Tolerance	None	Yes
Site of action	Larger, central airways	Central and peripheral airways

Pao_2, Arterial oxygen pressure.

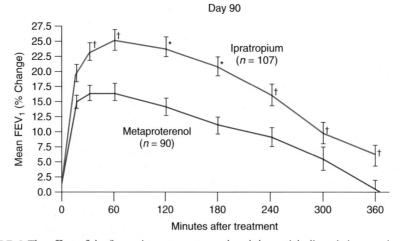

Day 90

FIGURE 7-6 The effect of the β agonist metaproterenol and the anticholinergic ipratropium on FEV_1 in patients with COPD after 90 days of treatment ($^*P < 0.01$; $^†P < 0.05$). [From Tashkin DP, Ashutosh K, Bleecker ER, Britt EJ, Cugell DW, Cummiskey JM, DeLorenzo L, Gilman MJ, Gross GN, Gross NJ, et al.: Comparison of the anticholinergic bronchodilator ipratropium bromide with metaproterenol in chronic obstructive pulmonary disease: a 90-day multi-center study, *Am J Med* 81(suppl 5A):59, 1986. From Excerpta Medica, Inc.]

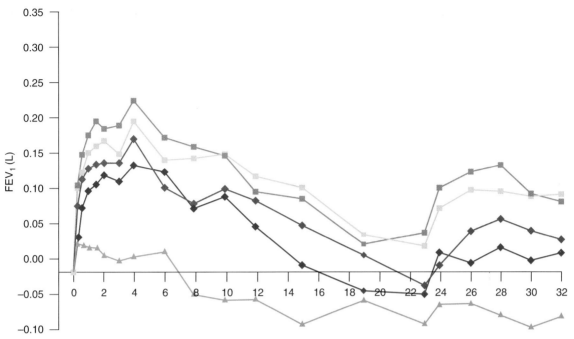

FIGURE 7-7 Bronchodilator responses measured on the basis of FEV_1 in patients with COPD given single doses of tiotropium, a long-acting antimuscarinic bronchodilator. Symbols: solid squares, 80 µg; open squares, 40 µg; solid diamonds, 20 µg; open diamonds, 10 µg; solid triangles, placebo. (Data from Maesen FP, Smeets JJ, Sledsens TJ, Wald FD, Cornelissen PJ: Tiotropium bromide, a new long-acting antimuscarinic bronchodilator: a pharmacodynamic study in patients with chronic obstructive pulmonary disease (COPD), *Eur Respir J* 8:1506, 1995.)

well as reduced exacerbations in patients with COPD of different severities.[31] Adams and associates also found improvement in lung function and dyspnea in COPD patients.[32] The prolonged effect may also be useful in controlling nocturnal asthma symptoms, where cholinergic mechanisms appear to increase airway tone.[33]

Current COPD guidelines do not dictate the use of any one specific bronchodilator.[34,35] However, it is noted that the use of a short-term β_2 agonist and an anticholinergic, such as ipratropium, improves the forced expiratory volume in 1 second (FEV_1) in patients with COPD.[35] The use of a long-term anticholinergic, such as tiotropium, improves the health of patients with COPD.[35] The use of a single agent or combination will be dictated by the patient's response.

Use in Asthma

Anticholinergic (antimuscarinic) agents such as ipratropium do not have a labeled indication for asthma in the United States. Current asthma guidelines state that ipratropium may have some additive benefit when given with inhaled β agonists[36,37] Antimuscarinic

bronchodilators are not clearly superior to β-adrenergic agents in treating asthma. Antimuscarinic and β-adrenergic agents have an approximately equal effect on flow rates in many patients. These agents may be especially useful in the following applications when prescribed for asthmatic patients[38]:

- Nocturnal asthma, in which the slightly longer duration of action may protect against nocturnal deterioration of flow rates[39]
- Psychogenic asthma, which may be mediated through vagal parasympathetic fibers
- Asthmatic patients with glaucoma, angina, or hypertension who require treatment with β-blocking agents
- As an alternative to theophylline in patients with notable side effects from that drug
- Acute, severe episodes of asthma not responding well to β agonists

A large, randomized controlled study by Qureshi and colleagues[40] in 434 children 2 to 8 years of age with acute moderate to severe asthma found that the overall rate of hospitalization was lowered with addition of inhaled ipratropium to nebulized albuterol.[40] However, the most striking effect on admission was seen in children with severe asthma (peak expiratory flow, <50% predicted). A meta-analysis of the addition of anticholinergic bronchodilators to β agonists in children and adolescents, conducted by Plotnick and Ducharme,[41] concluded that adding multiple doses of anticholinergic (antimuscarinic) bronchodilators to β_2 agonists was safe, improved lung function, and may avoid hospital admission in 1 of 11 treated patients. Multiple doses should be preferred to single doses of antimuscarinic agents.

Combination Therapy: β-Adrenergic and Anticholinergic Agents in Chronic Obstructive Pulmonary Disease

Theoretically, a combination of β-adrenergic and anticholinergic agents should offer advantages in the treatment of COPD (and asthma as well), based on the following considerations:

- Complementarity of sites of action exists, with anticholinergic effect seen in the more central airways and β-agonist effect in the smaller, more peripheral airways.
- Mechanisms of action from anticholinergic and β-adrenergic agents are separate and complementary.

Pharmacokinetics of shorter acting agents (albuterol or ipratropium) in the two classes of bronchodilator are somewhat complementary, with β agonists peaking sooner but also terminating sooner, while anticholinergics tend to peak more slowly and last longer. However, this consideration is not relevant with longer acting agents in both classes, such as salmeterol, formoterol, arformoterol, and tiotropium.

Additive Effect of β Agonists and Anticholinergic Agents

Conflicting results have been found on the question of whether the bronchodilator effect of β agonists is increased by adding an anticholinergic agent, in either COPD or asthma.[42-46] Many of the studies performed with combined anticholinergic and β-agonist bronchodilator therapy suffer from small sample sizes and poor statistical power. Before the approval of combined albuterol and ipratropium (Combivent), a large, well-controlled study was conducted over 85 days with 462 patients at 24 centers.[5] Patients represented stable COPD. The study showed superior efficacy of the combination therapy of ipratropium and albuterol compared with either agent alone. Figure 7-8 shows a comparison

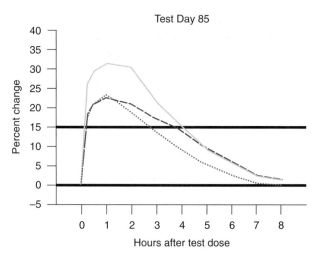

FIGURE 7-8 Percentage change in FEV_1 on test day 85, for combined ipratropium and albuterol compared with either drug alone, in patients with COPD. Dotted line, albuterol; dashed line, ipratropium; solid line, ipratropium plus albuterol. (From COMBIVENT Inhalation Aerosol Study Group: In chronic obstructive pulmonary disease, a combination of ipratropium and albuterol is more effective than either agent alone: an 85-day multicenter trial, *Chest* 105:1411, 1994.)

of ipratropium plus albuterol with albuterol or ipratropium alone on the percentage change in FEV_1, from this study. The mean *peak* increases in FEV_1 were 31 to 33% for combined drug therapy, compared with 24 to 25% for ipratropium alone and 24 to 27% for albuterol alone. Flow rates were significantly better on all test days. Symptom scores did not differ among the three groups, however. As a large, well-designed study, these results support combination anticholinergic and β-agonist therapy in COPD.

KEY POINT

Combined anticholinergic and β-agonist therapy may give additive bronchodilating results in COPD and in severe, acute asthma.

Sequence of Administration

The order in which an MDI of β_2 agonist and an anticholinergic are administered has been debated. Because an anticholinergic bronchodilator acts in the central, larger airways, some practitioners argue that it should be given *before* the β_2 agonist. No data have been given to support this sequence, however. The β_2 agonist is often given first, and this can be rationalized for two reasons: (1) β_2 agonists have a more rapid onset of action than does an anticholinergic bronchodilator; and (2) β_2 receptors are distributed in large and small airways. The order of administration is probably not important. Combination products such as Combivent and DuoNeb (ipratropium and albuterol) make order of administration a moot point.

RESPIRATORY CARE ASSESSMENT OF ANTICHOLINERGIC BRONCHODILATOR THERAPY

- Assess effectiveness of drug therapy based on the indication(s) for the aerosol agent: Presence of reversible airflow resulting from primary bronchospasm or obstruction secondary to an inflammatory response or secretions, either acute or chronic.
- Monitor flow rates using bedside peak flow meters, portable spirometry, or laboratory reports of pulmonary function. Before-and-after bronchodilator studies performed with a β agonist may not reliably predict response to an anticholinergic (antimuscarinic) agent such as ipratropium.
- Perform respiratory assessment: Breathing rate and pattern, and breath sounds by auscultation, before and after treatment.
- Assess pulse before, during, and after treatment.
- Assess patient's subjective reaction to treatment, for any change (positive or negative) in breathing effort or pattern.
- Assess arterial blood gases, or pulse oximeter saturation, as needed, for acute states with COPD or asthma, to monitor changes in ventilation and gas exchange (oxygenation).
- Long term: Monitor pulmonary function studies of lung volumes, capacities, and flows.
- Instruct and then verify correct use of aerosol delivery device (SVN, MDI, reservoir, DPI). Emphasize that the eye must be protected from aerosol sprays. Instruct patients in use, assembly, and especially cleaning of aerosol inhalation devices.

   For long-acting antimuscarinic bronchodilators:
- Assess ongoing lung function, including predose FEV_1 over time.
- Assess amount of concomitant β-agonist use and nocturnal symptoms.
- Assess number of exacerbations, unscheduled clinic visits, and hospitalizations.
- Assess days of absence because of symptoms.

SELF-ASSESSMENT QUESTIONS

1. What was the first FDA-approved anticholinergic bronchodilator for aerosol inhalation?
2. What is the usual recommended dose of ipratropium by MDI and by SVN?
3. Identify a long-acting anticholinergic bronchodilator and give its duration of action.
4. What is the usual clinical indication for use of an anticholinergic bronchodilator such as ipratropium?
5. Which disease state, asthma or COPD, may show greater response to an anticholinergic bronchodilator rather than a β agonist?
6. With which type of anticholinergic agent are you more likely to observe systemic side effects: the tertiary ammonium or quaternary ammonium compounds?
7. What are the most common side effects seen with inhaled ipratropium and tiotropium?
8. Can ipratropium be used with subjects who have glaucoma?
9. Can ipratropium be alternated with or combined with a β agonist in the treatment of COPD and asthma?
10. What precautions should you observe if administering ipratropium by SVN?
11. What is the clinical indication for the use of an anticholinergic intranasal spray?

Answers to Self-Assessment Questions are found in Appendix A.

CLINICAL SCENARIO

Mr. James C. is a 66-year-old retired, well-educated middle level manager for a major film company. He is referred to a pulmonologist for his complaint of shortness of breath. On interview he states that he has increasingly noticed exertional dyspnea with mild physical activity over the past few months. With questioning, he admits to occasional social alcohol intake of either 1 or 2 beers or a couple of mixed drinks several times a week. He has been happily married to the same woman since he was 24. He also admits to regular cigarette smoking of about 1 pack/day since he was 20 years old. He leads a sedentary life with no physical exercise. He states that he does have a chronic cough, which is worse in the morning, although he denies

Continued

much productivity. He appears to be well nourished, is articulate, and his color is good. No cyanosis or use of accessory muscles is noted at rest.

Physical examination reveals very mild digital clubbing, a slightly increased anteroposterior (AP) diameter, diminished and distant breath sounds bilaterally with some rhonchi, mildly hyperresonant percussion notes, no jugular venous distention upright or supine, and no peripheral edema. His vital signs are as follows: blood pressure (BP), 146/90; temperature (T), 37.2° C; pulse (P), 88 beats/min; respiratory rate (RR), 16 breaths/min with no laboring. His arterial blood gas (room air) results are as follows: pH, 7.40; arterial carbon dioxide pressure (Pa_{CO_2}), 42.5 mmHg; arterial oxygen pressure (Pa_{O_2}), 62 mmHg; base excess, 1.9 mEq/L; and hemoglobin (Hgb), 14.5 g/dl.

His pulmonary function results are as follows:

Observed	% Predicted
Forced vital capacity (FVC), 2.98 L	74
Forced expiratory volume in 1 second (FEV_1), 1.94 L	60
FEV_1/FVC, 65%	83
Residual volume/total lung capacity (RV/TLC), 42%	124
Diffusing capacity of the lung for carbon monoxide (DL_{CO}), 18.4 (ml/min/mmHg)	70

Mr. C's chest radiograph (PA, lateral) shows some loss of lung markings, mild flattening of the hemidiaphragms, and increased AP diameter. His electrolytes and white cell count are normal.

His chief complaint, smoking history, physical findings, and laboratory results all indicate early manifestations of COPD. He is mildly hypoxemic at rest (Pa_{O_2}, 62 mmHg), but his acid–base status is normal. Moderate airflow obstruction is present as evidenced by the FEV_1 of 1.94 L, an FEV_1/FVC of 65%, and an increased RV/TLC ratio. Gas exchange is impaired, as seen in the below-normal DL_{CO}. There is no evidence of cardiac failure or acute exacerbation at this time. His diagnosis is COPD with mixed bronchitis and emphysema.

Would you recommend a bronchodilator for Mr. C.?

What type of bronchodilator would you think best to start for Mr. C.?

If Mr. C. has trouble with MDI use, what actions could you take?

What lifestyle change(s) would you emphasize to Mr. C.?

Answers to Clinical Scenario Questions are found in Appendix A.

References

1. Cavanaugh MJ, Cooper DM: Inhaled atropine sulfate: dose response characteristics, *Am Rev Respir Dis* 114:517, 1976.
2. Pak CC, Kradjan WA, Lakshminarayan S, Marini JJ: Inhaled atropine sulfate: dose–response characteristics in adult patients with chronic airflow obstruction, *Am Rev Respir Dis* 125:331, 1982.
3. Gross NJ: Anticholinergic agents: clinical application. In Leff AR, editor: *Pulmonary and critical care pharmacology and therapeutics,* New York, 1996, McGraw-Hill.
4. Meltzer EO: Intranasal anticholinergic therapy of rhinorrhea, *J Allergy Clin Immunol* 90:1055, 1992.
5. COMBIVENT Inhalation Aerosol Study Group: In chronic obstructive pulmonary disease, a combination of ipratropium and albuterol is more effective than either agent alone: an 85-day multicenter trial, *Chest* 105:1411, 1994.
6. Gal TJ, Suratt PM, Lu J: Glycopyrrolate and atropine inhalation: comparative effects on normal airway function, *Am Rev Respir Dis* 129:871, 1984.
7. Witek TJ Jr: Anticholinergic bronchodilators, *Respir Care Clin N Am* 5:521, 1999.
8. Barnes PJ: The pharmacological properties of tiotropium, *Chest* 117:63S, 2000.
9. Maesen FP, Smeets JJ, Sledsens TJ, Wald FD, Cornelissen PJ: Tiotropium bromide, a new long-acting antimuscarinic bronchodilator: a pharmacodynamic study in patients with chronic obstructive pulmonary disease (COPD), *Eur Respir J* 8:1506, 1995.
10. Van Noord JA, Bantje TA, Eland ME, Korducki L, Cornelissen PJ; on behalf of the Dutch Tiotropium Study Group: A randomised controlled comparison of tiotropium and ipratropium in the treatment of chronic obstructive pulmonary disease, *Thorax* 55:289, 2000.
11. Littner MR, Ilowite JS, Tashkin DP, Friedman M, Serby CW, Menjoge SS, Witek TJ Jr: Long-acting bronchodilation with once-daily dosing of tiotropium (Spiriva) in stable chronic obstructive pulmonary disease, *Am J Respir Crit Care Med* 161:1136, 2000.
12. Chodosh S, Flanders J, Serby CW, Hochrainer D, Witek TJ: Effective use of HandiHaler dry powder inhalation system over a broad range of COPD disease severity [abstract], *Am J Respir Crit Care Med* 159:A524, 1999.
13. Barr RG, Bourbeau J, Camargo CA Jr, Ram FS. Tiotropium for stable chronic obstructive pulmonary disease: a meta-analysis. *Thorax* 61:854, 2006.
14. Groth ML, Langenback EG, Foster WM: Influence of inhaled atropine on lung mucociliary function in humans, *Am Rev Respir Dis* 144:1042, 1991.
15. Wanner A: Effect of ipratropium bromide on airway mucociliary function, *Am J Med* 81(suppl 5A):32, 1986.
16. Bergman KR, Pearson C, Waltz GW, Evans R III: Atropine-induced psychosis, an unusual complication of therapy with inhaled atropine sulfate, *Chest* 78:891, 1980.

17. Herschman ZL, Silverstein J, Blumberg G, Lehrfield A: Central nervous system toxicity from nebulized atropine sulfate, *J Toxicol Clin Toxicol* 29:273, 1991.

18. Botts LD, Pingleton SK, Schroeder CE, Robinson RG, Hurwitz A: Prolongation of gastric emptying by aerosolized atropine, *Am Rev Respir Dis* 131:725, 1985.

19. Mulherin D, Fitzgerald MX: Meconium ileus equivalent in association with nebulized ipratropium bromide in cystic fibrosis, *Lancet* 335:552, 1990.

20. Molkenboer JFWM, Lardenoye JG: The effect of Atrovent on micturition function, double-blind crossover study, *Scand J Respir Dis* 103(suppl):154, 1979.

21. Barnes PJ: Autonomic control of airway function in asthma, *Chest* 91(suppl):45S, 1987.

22. Bleecker ER: Cholinergic and neurogenic mechanisms in obstructive airways disease, *Am J Med* 81(suppl 5A):2, 1986.

23. Hogg JC: The pathophysiology of asthma, *Chest* 82(suppl):8S, 1982.

24. Leff A: Pathophysiology of asthmatic bronchoconstriction, *Chest* 82(suppl):13S, 1982.

25. Simonsson BG, Jacobs FM, Nadel JA: Role of autonomic nervous system and the cough reflex in the increased responsiveness of airways in patients with obstructive airway disease, *J Clin Invest* 46:1812, 1967.

26. Baraniuk JN: Muscarinic receptors. In Leff AR, editor: *Pulmonary and critical care pharmacology and therapeutics*, New York, 1996, McGraw-Hill.

27. Okayama M, Baraniuk JN, Hausfeld JN, Merida M, Kaliner MA: Autoradiographic localization of muscarinic receptor subtypes in human nasal mucosa, *J Allergy Clin Immunol* 89:1144, 1992.

28. Cugell DW: Clinical pharmacology and toxicology of ipratropium bromide, *Am J Med* 81(suppl 5A):18, 1986.

29. Tashkin DP, Ashutosh K, Bleecker ER, Britt EJ, Cugell DW, Cummiskey JM, DeLorenzo L, Gilman MJ, Gross GN, Gross NJ, et al.: Comparison of the anticholinergic bronchodilator ipratropium bromide with metaproterenol in chronic obstructive pulmonary disease: a 90-day multi-center study, *Am J Med* 81(suppl 5A):59, 1986.

30. Rennard SI, Serby CW, Ghafouri M, Johnson PA, Friedman M: Extended therapy with ipratropium is associated with improved lung function in patients with COPD: a retrospective analysis of data from seven clinical trials, *Chest* 110:62, 1996.

31. Beeh KM, Beier J, Buhl R, Stark-Lorenzen P, Gerken F, Metzdorf N; ATEM-Studiengruppe: Efficacy of tiotropium bromide in patients with COPD of different severities. *Pneumologie* 60:341, 2006.

32. Adams SG, Anzueto A, Briggs DD, Menjoge SS, Kesten S: Tiotropium in COPD patients not previously receiving maintenance respiratory medication. *Respir Med* 100:1495, 2006.

33. Morrison JFJ, Pearson SB, Dean HG: Parasympathetic nervous system in nocturnal asthma, *Br Med J* 296:1427, 1988.

34. Celli BR, MacNee W; ATS/ERS Task Force: Standards for the diagnosis and treatment of patients with COPD: a summary of the ATS/ERS position paper. *Eur Respir J* 23:932, 2004. (Available at http://www.thoracic.org/sections/publications/statements/pages/respiratory-disease-adults/copdexecsum.html; accessed March 2007.)

35. Global Initiative for Chronic Obstructive Lung Disease: Executive Summary: December 2006, *Global strategy for the diagnosis, management, and prevention of COPD*. National Heart, Lung, and Blood Institute (Bethesda, Md) and World Health Organization (Geneva, Switzerland), 2006. (Available at http://www.goldcopd.org/Guidelineitem.asp?l1=2&l2=1&intId=996; accessed March 2007.)

36. National Asthma Education and Prevention Program, National Heart, Lung, and Blood Institute, National Institutes of Health: Expert Panel Report 2: *Guidelines for the diagnosis and management of asthma*, NIH Publication 97–4051. Bethesda, Md, 1997, National Institutes of Health. (Available at http://www.nhlbi.nih.gov/guidelines/asthma/asthgdln.pdf; accessed February 2007.)

37. Global Initiative for Asthma (GINA), National Heart, Lung, and Blood Institute, National Institutes of Health: *GINA Report, Global Strategy for Asthma Management and Prevention*, November, 2006. Bethesda, MD, 2006, National Institutes of Health (Available at: http://www.ginasthma.com/Guidelineitem.asp??l1=2&l2=1&intId=60, Accessed March 2007.)

38. Weber RW: Role of anticholinergics in asthma [editorial], *Ann Allergy* 65:348, 1990.

39. Cox ID, Hughes DTD, McDonnell KA: Ipratropium bromide in patients with nocturnal asthma, *Postgrad Med J* 60:526, 1984.

40. Qureshi F, Pestian J, Davis P, Zaritsky A: Effect of nebulized ipratropium on the hospitalization rates of children with asthma, *N Engl J Med* 339:1030, 1998.

41. Plotnick LH, Ducharme FM: Should inhaled anticholinergics be added to β₂ agonists for treating acute childhood and adolescent asthma? A systematic review, *Br Med J* 317:971, 1998.

42. Rebuck AS, Chapman KR, Abboud R, Pare PD, Kreisman H, Wolkove N, Vickerson F: Nebulized anticholinergic and sympathomimetic treatment of asthma and chronic obstructive airways disease in the emergency room, *Am J Med* 82:59, 1987.

43. Owens MW, George RB: Nebulized atropine sulfate in the treatment of acute asthma, *Chest* 99:1084, 1991.

44. Karpel JP: Bronchodilator responses to anticholinergic and β-adrenergic agents in acute and stable asthma, *Chest* 99:871, 1991.

45. Lightbody IM, Ingram CG, Legge JS, Johnston RN: Ipratropium bromide, salbutamol and prednisolone in bronchial asthma and chronic bronchitis, *Br J Dis Chest* 72:181, 1978.

46. Petrie GR, Palmer KNV: Comparison of aerosol ipratropium bromide and salbutamol in chronic bronchitis and asthma, *Br Med J* 1:430, 1975.

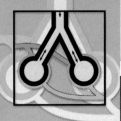

Chapter 8

Xanthines

DOUGLAS S. GARDENHIRE

CHAPTER OUTLINE

Clinical Indications for the Use of Xanthines
Use in Asthma
Use in Chronic Obstructive Pulmonary Disease
Use in Apnea of Prematurity
Specific Xanthine Agents
General Pharmacological Properties
Structure–Activity Relations
Proposed Theories of Activity
Titrating Theophylline Doses
Equivalent Doses of Theophylline Salts
Serum Levels of Theophylline
Dosage Schedules

Theophylline Toxicity and Side Effects
Factors Affecting Theophylline Activity
Clinical Uses
Use in Asthma
Use in Chronic Obstructive Pulmonary Disease
Nonbronchodilating Effects of Theophylline
Use in Apnea of Prematurity

CHAPTER OBJECTIVES

After reading this chapter, the reader will be able to:
1. Define *xanthine*
2. List all available xanthines used in respiratory therapy
3. Differentiate between the clinical indications and uses of xanthines

4. Discuss the proposed theories of activity for xanthines
5. Discuss adverse effects and toxicity of xanthines
6. Be able to clinically assess xanthine therapy

KEY TERMS AND DEFINITIONS

Alkaloids — A group of alkaline substances taken from plants, which react with acids to form salts, (e.g., theophylline).

Methylxanthines — A chemical group of drugs derived form xanthines. There are three methylated (CH₃) xanthines: caffeine, theophylline, and theobromine

Phosphodiesterase (PDE) — A group of enzymes that change intracellular signaling.

Xanthine — A nitrogenous compound found in many organs and in the blood and urine.

Chapter 8 reviews the pharmacology of the **xanthine** drugs, such as theophylline. Theophylline has been traditionally used to treat patients with asthma and chronic obstructive pulmonary disease (COPD) in both stable and acute phases. The mechanism of action of xanthines is unclear, and their clinical use in asthma and COPD has been relegated to that of second- or third-line agents, although this remains an issue of some debate.

KEY POINT

Theophylline, and its salt, *aminophylline,* are members of the *methylxanthine* group of drugs, which also includes *dyphylline.*

CLINICAL INDICATIONS FOR THE USE OF XANTHINES

KEY POINT

Clinical uses of theophylline include the management of asthma, COPD, and apnea of prematurity in neonates.

Theophylline has traditionally been used in the management of asthma and COPD. Theophylline and caffeine have been used to treat apnea of prematurity. A now-obsolete use of theophylline was as a diuretic. Although theophylline is usually classified as a bronchodilator, it actually has a relatively weak bronchodilating effect compared with β_2 agonists. Its therapeutic action in asthma and COPD may occur by other means, such as stimulation of the ventilatory drive or direct strengthening of the diaphragm. Any of these actions could result in the clinical outcome of improved ventilatory flow rates. This is further discussed subsequently in the section Clinical Uses.

Use in Asthma

Sustained-release theophylline is indicated as an alternative for maintenance (step 2) therapy of mild, persistent asthma or greater in patients older than 5 years of age, and is listed as an alternative in step 3 for patients younger than 5 years of age. Sustained-release theophylline is considered a less preferred alternative to low-dose inhaled corticosteroids or cromolyn-like agents as second-line maintenance drug therapy in stable asthma. The 1997 National Institutes of Health (NIH) guidelines on asthma do not clearly give a preference between theophylline and the antileukotriene agents (zafirlukast and montelukast), which were newly released at the time of the Expert Panel 2 recommendations.[1] Many clinicians believe that the antileukotrienes are preferable to theophylline in terms of side effects and therapeutic margin. Theophylline remains an alternative in the 2002 update on selected topics from the National Asthma Education and Prevention Program (NAEPP) Expert Panel.[2]

Methylxanthines are not generally recommended for acute exacerbations of asthma in the 1997 Expert Panel 2 report giving guidelines for managing asthma. Guidelines on drug therapy of asthma including the role of theophylline can be found in Appendix D.

Use in Chronic Obstructive Pulmonary Disease

Current guidelines for the treatment of stable COPD state that bronchodilators are central to symptom management. The Global Initiative for Chronic Obstructive Lung Disease (GOLD) states that inhaled bronchodilators are preferred when available. Theophylline is considered effective in COPD but, because of potential toxicity, is recommended as an alternative to the inhaled bronchodilators such as β_2 agonists or anticholinergic agents.[3] Barr and associates conducted a meta-analysis on the use of xanthines for the treatment of COPD exacerbations. There findings suggest that xanthines should not be used in the treatment of COPD exacerbations.[4] Guidelines on drug management of COPD from the National Heart,

Lung, and Blood Institute (NHLBI) and the World Health Organization (WHO) are given in Appendix D.

Use in Apnea of Prematurity

If pharmacological therapy is needed to stimulate breathing in apnea of prematurity (AOP), methylxanthines are considered the first-line agents of choice. Theophylline has been most extensively used, but Bhatia[5] suggests that caffeine citrate may be the agent of choice. Caffeine citrate better penetrates the cerebrospinal fluid and has a higher therapeutic index with fewer side effects compared with theophylline. Caffeine citrate (Cafcit) has been approved for administration either intravenously or orally.

SPECIFIC XANTHINE AGENTS

Theophylline is related chemically to the natural metabolite xanthine, which is a precursor of uric acid. Figure 8-1 gives the general xanthine structure, along with that of theophylline (1,3-dimethylxanthine) and caffeine (1,3,7-trimethylxanthine). Because of their methyl attachments, these agents are often referred to as **methylxanthines**. Another xanthine is theobromine. All three agents are found as **alkaloids** in plant species. Caffeine is found in coffee beans and kola nuts. Caffeine and theophylline are contained in tea leaves, and caffeine and theobromine are in cocoa seeds or beans. Historically, these natural plant substances have all been used as brews for their stimulant effect.

There are several synthetic modifications to the naturally occurring methylxanthines. These include dyphylline [7-(2,3-dihydroxypropyl)theophylline], proxyphylline [7-(2-hydroxypropyl)theophylline], and enprofylline (3-propylxanthine). Table 8-1 lists xanthine derivatives, along with selected brand names and available formulations.

Theophylline is available in a variety of formulations, including sustained-release oral forms, as aminophylline for oral or intravenous administration, and in rectal suppository forms. Aminophylline has been tried unsuccessfully by aerosol with asthmatic subjects.[6] The aerosol is irritating to the pharynx, has a bitter taste, and can cause coughing and wheezing.

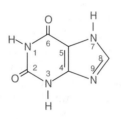

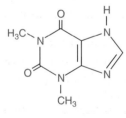

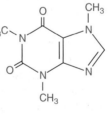

Xanthine

Theophylline   Caffeine

FIGURE 8-1 Chemical structure of xanthine and its methylated derivatives theophylline and caffeine.

GENERAL PHARMACOLOGICAL PROPERTIES

KEY POINT

Xanthines generally have *stimulant* properties, exemplified by the xanthine caffeine. Other effects of this class of drug include diuresis and smooth muscle relaxation (e.g., bronchodilation).

The xanthine group has the following general physiological effects in humans:
- Central nervous system stimulation
- Cardiac muscle stimulation

TABLE 8-1

Xanthine Derivatives Used as Bronchodilators in Obstructive Airways Diseases, With Selected Brand Names and Available Formulations

Xanthine Derivative	Selected Brand Names	Formulations
Theophylline	Slo-Phyllin, Theolair, Quibron-T/SR Dividose, Bronkodyl, Elixophyllin, Theo-Dur, Uni-Dur, Uniphyl	Tablets, capsules, syrup, elixir, extended-release tablets, capsules, injection
Oxtriphylline	Choledyl SA	Tablets, syrup, elixir, sustained-release tablets
Aminophylline	Aminophylline	Tablets, oral liquid, injection, suppositories
Dyphylline	Dylix, Lufyllin	Tablets, elixir

- Diuresis
- Bronchial, uterine, and vascular smooth muscle relaxation
- Peripheral and coronary vasodilation
- Cerebral vasoconstriction

Some of the effects seen with xanthines are well known to those who drink caffeinated beverages (e.g., coffee, colas, and tea). Coffee in particular can be used for the central nervous system stimulatory effect to remain awake. The diuretic effect after drinking coffee or cola is also well known. Caffeine or theophylline can also cause tachycardia, and the cerebral vasoconstricting effect has been used to treat migraine headaches. A special agent intended for this use is Cafergot, each tablet of which contains 100 mg of caffeine and 1 mg of ergotamine tartrate.

Caffeine and theophylline differ in the intensity of the effects listed previously. These differences are summarized in Table 8-2. Caffeine has more central nervous system–stimulating effect than theophylline, and this includes ventilatory stimulation. In clinical use, theophylline is generally classified as a bronchodilator, because of the relaxing effect on bronchial smooth muscle.

Structure–Activity Relations

Figure 8-2 illustrates the general xanthine structure and the effect of attachments at various sites on the molecule. Also, the chemical structure of theophylline is shown in comparison with that of the theophylline derivatives dyphylline and enprofylline. The methyl attachments at the nitrogen-1 and nitrogen-3 positions for theophylline enhance its bronchodilating effect, as well as its toxic side effects, which are discussed later in this chapter. In contrast, the structure of caffeine (see Figure 8-1) has an additional methyl group at the nitrogen-7 position, thereby decreasing its bronchodilator effect in relation to theophylline. Dyphylline has the same methyl attachments at the nitrogen-1 and nitrogen-3 positions as theophylline but also has a large attachment at the nitrogen-7 position that decreases its bronchodilator potential. Enprofylline, which is not clinically available in the United States at this time, has potent bronchodilating effects, probably because of the large substitution at the nitrogen-3 position.

KEY POINT

The exact *mode of action* of xanthines is unclear; antagonism of adenosine receptors may occur, perhaps as a partial mechanism for the effects of drugs such as theophylline.

TABLE 8-2

Differences in Intensity of Effects for Caffeine and Theophylline

Effect	Caffeine	Theophylline
Central nervous system stimulation	+++	++
Cardiac stimulation	+	+++
Smooth muscle relaxation	+	+++
Skeletal muscle stimulation	+++	++
Diuresis	+	+++

Proposed Theories of Activity

The exact mechanism of action of xanthines, and theophylline in particular, is not known.[7] It was originally thought that xanthines caused smooth muscle relaxation by inhibition of phosphodiesterase, leading to an increase in intracellular cyclic adenosine 3′,5′-monophosphate (cyclic AMP, or cAMP). An increase in cAMP causes relaxation of bronchial smooth muscle. The effect of increased cAMP is described in Chapter 6 in the discussion of β-adrenergic agents. However, this explanation to account for therapeutic xanthine actions has been questioned. Several alternative theories concerning the action of xanthines have been proposed in addition to phosphodiesterase inhibition. Each of the proposed theories of activity for xanthines is briefly described and commented on in the following sections.

Inhibition of Phosphodiesterase

Theophylline is a weak and nonselective inhibitor of cAMP-specific **phosphodiesterase (PDE)**. The pathway by which this inhibition can lead to an increase in intracellular cAMP, with consequent bronchial relaxation or antiinflammatory effects, is illustrated in Figure 8-3, *A*. However, at the dosage levels used clinically in humans, theophylline is a poor inhibitor of the enzyme.[8] As a result, this may not be the best theory on how xanthines exert a therapeutic effect. *PDE* is a generic term referring to at least 11 distinct families that have been identified as hydrolyzing cAMP or cyclic guanosine 3′,5′-monophosphate (cyclic GMP, or cGMP) and that have unique tissue and subcellular distributions. The various PDE families differ in substrate specificity, inhibitor sensitivity, and cofactor requirements.[7] There are two cAMP-hydrolyzing PDEs, referred to as *PDE3* and *PDE4*, that may play a role in asthma. PDE4 is expressed in airway smooth muscle, pulmonary nerves, and many

General Xanthine Structure

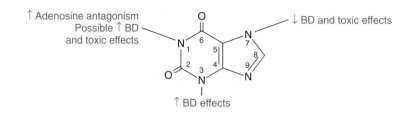

Xanthine Agents

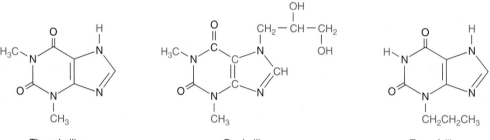

Theophylline

Dyphylline

Enprofylline

FIGURE 8-2 Effect of attachments at various sites on the xanthine molecule and comparative illustration of the structures of theophylline, dyphylline, and enprofylline. *BD,* Bronchodilation.

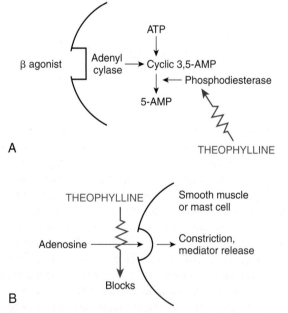

FIGURE 8-3 Two proposed mechanisms of action by which theophylline and xanthines reverse airway obstruction.
A, Inhibition of phosphodiesterase. **B,** Blockade of adenosine receptors. *AMP,* Adenosine monophosphate; *ATP,* adenosine triphosphate.

proinflammatory and immune cells. PDE4 inhibitors suppress processes thought to contribute to asthma inflammation by blocking the degradation of cAMP in target cells and tissue. The antiinflammatory effect of theophylline and xanthines is reviewed in the discussion of the clinical application of these drugs in COPD and asthma.

Antagonism of Adenosine

An alternative explanation of bronchodilation is that theophylline acts by blocking the action of adenosine. This mechanism is illustrated in Figure 8-3, *B.* Adenosine is a purine nucleoside that can stimulate A_1 and A_2 receptors. A_1-Receptor stimulation inhibits cAMP, whereas A_2-receptor stimulation increases cAMP. Inhaled adenosine has produced bronchoconstriction in asthmatic patients. Theophylline is a potent inhibitor of both A_1 and A_2 receptors and could block smooth muscle contraction mediated by A_1 receptors.

This explanation is contradicted by the action of enprofylline, which is about five times more potent than theophylline for relaxing smooth muscle, yet lacks a sufficient attachment at the nitrogen-1 position to provide adenosine antagonism.[9] This can be seen in Figure 8-2 by comparing the structures of theophylline and enprofylline. In addition, A_1 receptors are sparse in smooth muscle, and isolated animal tissue preparations have actually shown smooth muscle relaxation through adenosine stimulation of the A_2 receptors.

Catecholamine Release

A third explanation of xanthine action is that these agents cause the production and release of endogenous catecholamines, which in turn could cause muscle tremor, tachycardia, and bronchial relaxation. Studies on plasma levels of catecholamines such as epinephrine have reported conflicting results, with both an increase and no change reported.[10]

TITRATING THEOPHYLLINE DOSES

In the past, clinical use of the xanthine theophylline, in its many forms, was questioned because of wide variability in its therapeutic effect. It was subsequently found that individuals metabolize theophylline at differing rates, which makes it difficult to determine therapeutic doses. This is complicated further by the fact that different forms of the drug are not always equivalent.

Equivalent Doses of Theophylline Salts

The standard with which salts of theophylline are compared is anhydrous theophylline. Anhydrous theophylline is 100% theophylline. By contrast, salts of theophylline such as oxtriphylline (Choledyl SA) are not pure theophylline by weight. A 200-mg dose of Choledyl contains approximately 130 mg of theophylline, whereas Theo-Dur (a brand of theophylline) is 100% anhydrous theophylline. A 200-mg dose of Choledyl SA will not give the same amount of theophylline as a 200-mg dose of Theo-Dur. Table 8-3 lists the equivalent dose of pure theophylline provided by the salts, such as oxtriphylline and aminophylline.

Because oxtriphylline is 64% theophylline, a dose equivalent to 100 mg of theophylline anhydrous would be 156 mg of oxtriphylline (100 mg/0.64 = 156 mg). Similarly, 127 mg of aminophylline dihydrate (theophylline ethylenediamine) would be required for equivalency to 100 mg of theophylline anhydrous. It should be noted that dyphylline is not a theophylline but a derivative of theophylline. It does not form theophylline in the body and is about one-tenth as potent as theophylline. This is consistent with its structure–activity relation, described previously.

TABLE 8-3		
Theophylline Content of Salts of Theophylline, With Amount Needed for Equivalence to 100% Anhydrous Theophylline		
Theophylline Salt	**Theophylline (%)**	**Equivalent Dose**
Theophylline anhydrous	100	100 mg
Theophylline monohydrate	91	110 mg
Aminophylline anhydrous	86	116 mg
Aminophylline dihydrate	79	127 mg
Oxtriphylline	64	156 mg

Serum Levels of Theophylline

In 1972, Jenne and colleagues indicated that the optimal serum theophylline level for maximal bronchodilation in adults was between 10 and 20 µg/ml.[11] The effects associated with a range of serum levels are as follows:

<5 µg/ml: No effects seen

10 to 20 µg/ml: Therapeutic range

>20 µg/ml: Nausea

>30 µg/ml: Cardiac arrhythmias

40 to 45 µg/ml: Seizures

> **KEY POINT**
>
> Because individuals vary in the rate at which theophylline is metabolized, dosage must be titrated to clinical effectiveness, avoidance of side effects, and, most precisely, a *therapeutic serum level* of 10 to 12 µg/ml in COPD and between 5 and 15 µg/ml in asthma management.

Since the originally proposed serum levels of 10 to 20 µg/ml, the recommended range has been changed to a somewhat more conservative 5 to 15 µg/ml for the management of asthma.[12] American Thoracic Society (ATS) recommendations for the use of theophylline in COPD suggest a target serum level of 10 to 12 µg/ml.[3] Both of these ranges seek maximal therapeutic effect with minimal toxicity and side effects. It is stressed that the ranges listed for toxic effects are general. It is possible for an individual to bypass the nauseous phase of toxicity and immediately enter the seizure phase.

Although there is a dose-related response to higher serum levels of theophylline, there is evidence that the response does not continue at the same rate of increase as levels rise. This is illustrated in Figure 8-4. The improvement in forced expiratory volume in 1 second

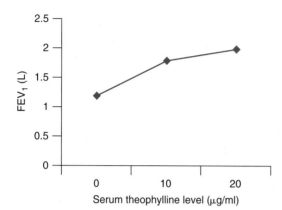

FIGURE 8-4 Conceptual illustration of the decreasing rate of improvement with theophylline levels above 10 µg/ml, even though levels may be in the therapeutic range of 10 to 20 µg/ml. (For illustrative purposes only; not to be used to predict clinical response to serum levels.) *FEV$_1$*, Forced expiratory volume in 1 second. (Data from Tashkin DP: Measurement and significance of the bronchodilator response. In Jenne JW, Murphy S, editors: *Drug therapy for asthma: research and clinical practice,* New York, 1987, Marcel Dekker.)

(FEV$_1$) tends to flatten above a serum level of 10 to 12 µg/ml, whereas the toxic effects of theophylline (discussed subsequently) tend to increase even within the therapeutic range of 10 to 20 µg/ml.[13]

Dosage Schedules

Because of the variability in the rate at which individuals metabolize theophylline and the other factors that affect theophylline metabolism and clearance rates, dosage schedules are used to titrate the drug. These schedules are found in the product literature, references such as *Drug Facts and Comparisons* and *Physicians' Desk Reference,* and general pharmacology texts.

For rapid theophyllinization, the patient may be given an oral loading dose of 5 mg/kg, *provided the patient was not previously receiving theophylline.* This dose is based on anhydrous theophylline. Lean body weight should be used in calculating theophylline doses, because theophylline does not distribute into fatty tissue. In titrating the dose, each 0.5-mg/kg dose of theophylline given as a loading dose will result in a serum level of approximately 1 µg/ml. If theophylline was taken previously by the patient, a serum theophylline level should be measured if at all possible.

For chronic therapy, a slow titration is helpful, with an initial dose of 16 mg/kg/24 hr or 400 mg/24 hr, whichever is less. These dosages may need to be modified in the presence of factors such as age (younger children versus the elderly), congestive heart disease, or liver

disease. The effects of these factors on serum theophylline levels and on dosage are discussed subsequently. The dosage guidelines given have been obtained from theophylline product information.

Dosage of theophylline can be guided by the clinical reaction of the patient or, better, by measurement of serum drug levels. Without a serum drug level, the dose of theophylline should be based on the benefit provided and should be reduced if the patient experiences toxic side effects. When monitoring serum theophylline levels, take the sample at the time of peak absorption of the drug, that is, 1 to 2 hours after administration for immediate-release forms and 5 to 9 hours after the morning dose for sustained-release forms.

The previous examples of dosage schedules are by no means complete for all situations; they are intended only as an example of such schedules and of the complexity involved in treating patients with theophylline. Complete tables for different ages and clinical applications should be consulted when administering theophylline.

THEOPHYLLINE TOXICITY AND SIDE EFFECTS

> **KEY POINT**
>
> Theophylline has a *narrow therapeutic margin,* and side effects such as gastric upset, headache, insomnia, nervousness, palpitations, and diuresis occur frequently, even within the therapeutic range of dosing. Blood levels of theophylline are affected by many factors, which can either increase or decrease the amount of drug in the body.

An unfortunate and important problem with the use of theophylline is its narrow therapeutic margin. This refers to the fact that there is very little difference between the dose and serum level that give therapeutic benefit and those that cause toxic side effects. In fact, even within the therapeutic serum levels of 10 to 20 µg/ml, distressing side effects can be experienced. The most common adverse reactions usually seen with theophylline are listed in Box 8-1.

Gastric upset, headache, anxiety, and nervousness are not unusual as less toxic side effects of theophylline and can result in loss of school time or workdays. The diuretic effect should be noted in patients with excess airway secretions (e.g., patients with bronchitis or cystic fibrosis), with adequate fluid replacement done when necessary to prevent dehydration and thickening of secretions.

Box 8-1	Adverse Reactions Seen With Theophylline Treatment, Organized by Organ System*

CENTRAL NERVOUS SYSTEM
- Headache
- Anxiety
- Restlessness
- Insomnia
- Tremor
- Convulsions

GASTROINTESTINAL
- Nausea
- Vomiting
- Anorexia
- Abdominal pain
- Diarrhea
- Hematemesis
- Gastroesophageal reflux

RESPIRATORY
- Tachypnea

CARDIOVASCULAR
- Palpitations
- Supraventricular tachycardia
- Ventricular arrhythmias
- Hypotension

RENAL
- Diuresis

*Effects are not listed in order of severity or progression.

Box 8-2	Factors That Can Increase or Decrease Blood Levels of Theophylline and Affect Dosage Requirements

Increase	Decrease
Alcohol (0.9 g/kg)	β Agonists
β-Blocking agents	Aminoglutethimide
Calcium channel blockers	Barbiturates
Cimetidine, ranitidine	Carbamazepine
Corticosteroids	Cigarette smoking
Disulfiram	Isoniazid (+ or −)*
Influenza virus vaccine	Isoproterenol (IV)
Interferon	Ketoconazole
Ephedrine	Loop diuretics (+ or −)
Estrogen	Moricizine
Macrolide antibiotics	Phenytoin
(e.g., clarithromycin)	Rifampin
Mexiletine	Sulfinpyrazone
Methotrexate	
Pentoxifylline	
Quinolones, oral	
contraceptives	
Tacrine	
Ticlopidine	
Troleandomycin	
Zileuton	
Cirrhosis	
Congestive heart failure	
Hepatitis	
Pneumonia	
Renal failure	

IV, Intravenous.
*+, Increase in theophylline level; −, decrease in theophylline level. Data from Weinberger M, Hendeles L: Theophylline in asthma, *N Engl J Med* 334:1380, 1996; American Thoracic Society: Standards for the diagnosis and care of patients with chronic obstructive pulmonary disease, *Am J Respir Crit Care Med* 152:S77, 1995.

Reactions to levels of theophylline also can be unpredictable from patient to patient. Studies are cited in which reported serum levels of 78.5 and 104.8 µg/ml caused only gastrointestinal symptoms, whereas mean levels of 35 µg/ml caused cardiac arrhythmias or seizures.[13] Also, minor side effects may provide little warning before serious toxic effects such as arrhythmias or seizures occur.

FACTORS AFFECTING THEOPHYLLINE ACTIVITY

Theophylline is metabolized in the liver and eliminated by the kidneys. Any condition that affects these organs can affect theophylline levels in the body. Interactions between other drugs and theophylline can affect serum levels of the drug. Some of the common drugs and conditions that increase or decrease theophylline levels are listed in Box 8-2.

Viral hepatitis or left ventricular failure can cause elevated serum levels of theophylline for a given dose because of decreased liver metabolism of the drug. An opposite effect, that is, decreased serum levels, is caused by cigarette smoking, which stimulates the production of liver enzymes that inactivate methylxanthines.[14] This necessitates higher theophylline doses. Some drugs used for the treatment of tuberculosis, such as isoniazid, and the loop diuretics, such as furosemide (Lasix) or bumetanide (Bumex), are unpredictable in their effect and may either increase or decrease theophylline levels. Measurement of serum levels is extremely important when using these agents with theophylline.

The β agonists and theophylline have an additive effect and are often combined when treating patients with asthma or COPD. Theophylline may antagonize the sedative effect of the benzodiazepines (e.g., Valium). Theophylline can also reverse the paralyzing effect of nondepolarizing neuromuscular blocking agents (pancuronium and atracurium) in a dose-dependent manner. This is important to realize when paralyzing patients with severe asthma to facilitate ventilatory support and when intravenous administration of aminophylline is used.

CLINICAL USES

Recent guidelines for the pharmacological management of asthma and COPD do not indicate theophylline as first-line therapy (see Appendix D). The disadvantages of theophylline are its narrow therapeutic margin, toxic effects, unpredictable blood levels and need for individual dosing, and numerous drug–drug and drug–condition interactions. The use of theophylline in asthma and COPD is described in the following sections.

Use in Asthma

KEY POINT

Theophylline has been relegated to the level of a second- or third-line drug in treating *asthma*, and is considered if β agonists and antiinflammatory therapy fail to control symptoms.

The role of theophylline preparations in the management of acute and stable asthma and COPD has been debated.[15,16] In the treatment of asthma, theophylline is suggested for use after reliever agents, such as a β_2 agonist, and other controller agents, such as inhaled steroids, or mediator antagonists (cromolyn-like drugs) targeting the underlying inflammation.[1,2]

Use in Chronic Obstructive Pulmonary Disease

KEY POINT

In COPD the *nonbronchodilating effects* of theophylline, such as ventilatory drive stimulation, and enhanced respiratory muscle function are of value, although its use is debated.

Use as a maintenance agent in COPD is indicated if anticholinergics and a β_2 agonist fail to provide adequate control. Development of long-acting β_2 agonists, such as salmeterol, formoterol, and arformoterol, offers an additional drug choice to preserve lung function in COPD before using theophylline, especially if theophylline was used to prevent nocturnal symptoms. The increased FEV_1 with salmeterol gives more consistent improvement in lung function on a 12-hour basis and maintains a higher baseline of lung function.[17]

Theophylline, and its salt aminophylline, are listed as one of several bronchoactive agents for managing an acute exacerbation of COPD, in the GOLD guidelines; however, use of other bronchodilators is preferred.[3]

KEY POINT

COPD guidelines suggest the use of inhaled β agonists (e.g., albuterol) and anticholinergics (e.g., ipratropium) over the use of theophylline because of its side effects.

Because of side effects in the gastrointestinal system, xanthines are contraindicated in subjects with active peptic ulcer or acute gastritis. Suppositories should not be used if the rectum or lower colon is irritated. If stomach upset occurs with theophylline, the drug may be taken with food. Ingestion of large amounts of caffeine from other sources such as tea or coffee may precipitate side effects when taking theophylline.

Nonbronchodilating Effects of Theophylline

Although theophylline is classified as a bronchodilator, it actually has a relatively weak bronchodilating action. The efficacy of theophylline in obstructive lung disease may be due to its nonbronchodilating effects on ventilation. This concept of the effectiveness of theophylline is consistent with the finding of significant clinical improvement despite little increase in expiratory flow rates in asthmatic patients.[18] Mahler and colleagues[19] documented the effect of theophylline in reducing dyspnea in COPD subjects when there was no reversibility of obstruction and no objective improvement in lung function, gas exchange, or exercise performance capability. The nonbronchodilating effects of theophylline are listed with a brief commentary.

Respiratory Muscle Strength

Theophylline can increase the force of respiratory muscle contractility, and this effect is thought to inhibit or even reverse muscle fatigue and subsequent ventilatory failure. Theophylline can have the same effect on skeletal limb muscle. Aubier and associates[18] demonstrated increased diaphragmatic strength and transdiaphragmatic pressure generation by using electromyographic stimuli before and after theophylline administration.

Respiratory Muscle Endurance

Methylxanthines also show evidence of increasing respiratory muscle endurance, as well as strength. This can prevent fatigue of the respiratory muscles, especially with increased resistance. Xanthines have been shown to increase the time that an external inspiratory load could be sustained.[19]

Central Ventilatory Drive

The methylxanthines have also been shown to increase ventilatory drive at the level of the central nervous system. In particular, theophylline can increase phrenic nerve activity for a given level of chemical stimulus.[20] This effect on ventilatory drive seems to occur at the level of the midbrain and may involve the neurotransmitter dopamine.

Cardiovascular Effects

Theophylline use may have nonbronchodilating advantages in subjects with COPD who also have cardiac disease or cor pulmonale. Theophylline can increase cardiac output, decrease pulmonary vascular resistance, and improve myocardial muscle perfusion in ischemic regions.[21]

Antiinflammatory Effects

Theophylline also has some antiinflammatory effects, which may also explain its efficacy despite the fact that the drug is a relatively weak bronchodilator.[15,22] Evidence indicates that theophylline can produce some degree of immunomodulation, and an antiinflammatory and bronchoprotective effect through inhibition of cAMP-specific phosphodiesterase enzymes, particularly PDE3 and PDE4, in proinflammatory cells and tissues. Theophylline has been shown to cause the following (see references for detailed antiinflammatory effects of theophylline[15,22-24]):

- Decreased migration of activated eosinophils into bronchial mucosa with allergen stimuli and reduced eosinophil survival
- Reduced T-cell proliferation and accumulation in atopic asthma with corresponding improvement in pulmonary function
- Inhibition of proinflammatory cytokines, such as interleukin (IL)-1β, tumor necrosis factor-α, and interferon-γ, and increased production of the antiinflammatory cytokine IL-10
- Attenuation of the late-phase response to histamine in patients with allergic asthma
- Reduced airway responsiveness to stimuli such as histamine, methacholine, allergen, sulfur dioxide, distilled water, cyanates, and adenosine

The antiinflammatory and immunomodulating effects of theophylline occur at lower plasma concentrations such as 9 to 10 µg/ml, in contrast with those usually recommended for bronchodilation, and may result in a steroid-sparing effect.[23] Inhibitors of PDE4, with more selectivity than theophylline and reduced toxic effect profile, may offer a new class of antiinflammatory agents.[7]

Use in Apnea of Prematurity

When nonpharmacological methods are not successful in AOP, xanthines such as theophylline and caffeine are still considered a first-line choice of drug therapy, as stated in the indications for this class of drug. Theophylline is biotransformed to caffeine in neonates.[25] However, caffeine is preferable to theophylline for a variety of pharmacological reasons, as follows[5]:

- Caffeine penetrates more readily than theophylline into cerebrospinal fluid and can be effective in infants refractory to theophylline therapy.
- Caffeine is a more potent stimulant of the central nervous system and the respiratory system than theophylline.
- Dosing regimens are simpler and give more predictable results with caffeine than with theophylline, most likely because of smaller plasma fluctuations with caffeine.
- Caffeine has a wider therapeutic margin, with fewer side effects than theophylline.

A standard preparation of caffeine, caffeine citrate (Cafcit), is available, which can be administered either orally or intravenously. The recommended loading dose is 20 mg/kg of caffeine citrate (equivalent to 10 mg/kg of caffeine). This is followed 24 to 48 hours later by a single daily maintenance dose of 5 mg/kg of caffeine citrate (2.5 mg/kg of caffeine). Serum concentrations of 5 to 20 mg/L of caffeine have been found effective.[6]

SELF-ASSESSMENT QUESTIONS

1. What drug in the xanthine group is used most often therapeutically?
2. What is the difference between aminophylline and theophylline?
3. What is the recommended therapeutic plasma level for theophylline in asthma?
4. How do you know whether a given dose of theophylline will produce a satisfactory treatment effect in an asthmatic?
5. Identify at least three adverse side effects seen with theophylline.
6. What is meant by a "narrow therapeutic margin"?
7. Although theophylline is a weak bronchodilator, what other effects make it useful in treating chronic airflow obstruction?
8. True or False: theophylline causes bronchodilation and improved airflow solely by inhibiting phosphodiesterase, which breaks down cAMP.

Answers to Self-Assessment Questions are found in Appendix A.

CLINICAL SCENARIO

A 70-year-old white male arrived to the hospital emergency department. He was severely short of breath (SOB) and could take only a few steps before complaining of dyspnea. He reported coughing up thick, greenish sputum, with some tinges of blood in the last few days. He appeared oriented, coherent, and somewhat malnourished, with thin arms. On interview he admitted to smoking two packs of cigarettes a day since age 18, stopping about 2 years ago. He has had six hospitalizations within the last 2 years. Current medications include ipratropium bromide by MDI, 2 puffs four times daily, with a β_2 agonist by MDI as needed, 1 to 3 puffs. He has been using the β_2 MDI regularly during the last month, at least four times daily.

On physical examination, he was very SOB, even at rest, and used accessory muscles with a respiratory rate (RR) of 22 breaths/min. There was little discernible chest expansion. His breath sounds were distant in all areas, with expiratory wheezes, and air movement appeared poor. He was afebrile; pulse (P), 120 beats/min; blood pressure (BP), 170/112 mmHg. He was admitted with a diagnosis of acute exacerbation of COPD.

Laboratory values on admission showed normal electrolytes, but his white blood cell (WBC) count was 15.2×10^3/cc and his hemoglobin was 10.6 g/dl. Arterial blood gas values on room air were as follows: pH, 7.40; arterial carbon dioxide pressure ($Paco_2$), 42.4 mmHg; arterial oxygen pressure (Pao_2), 64 mmHg; base excess, +1.9 mEq/L; and arterial oxygen saturation (Sao_2), 90%.

A chest radiograph (posteroanterior, PA) shows hyperinflation of the lung fields, with flattened diaphragms.

What is the first drug that is indicated by this individual's blood sample values?

Would you continue use of ipratropium bromide; if so, what dose would you suggest?

What additional bronchodilator therapy could you recommend?

What is the rationale for use of theophylline in this patient?

What would you check before initiating therapy with theophylline?

What serum theophylline level would you target, if the patient is started on theophylline?

What agent could be recommended before theophylline is started?

Answers to Clinical Scenario Questions are found in Appendix A.

References

1. National Asthma Education and Prevention Program, National Heart, Lung, and Blood Institute, National Institutes of Health: Expert Panel Report 2: *Guidelines for the diagnosis and management of asthma,* NIH Publication 97-4051. Bethesda, Md, 1997, National Institutes of Health. (Available at http://www.nhlbi.nih.gov/guidelines/asthma/asthgdln.pdf; accessed February 2007.)
2. National Asthma Education and Prevention Program, National Heart, Lung, and Blood Institute, National Institutes of Health: Expert Panel Report: *Guidelines for the diagnosis and management of asthma—update on selected topics 2002,* NIH Publication 02-5074. Bethesda, Md, 2002, National Institutes of Health. (Available at http://www.nhlbi.nih.gov/guidelines/asthma/asthmafullrpt.pdf; accessed March 2007.)
3. Global Initiative for Chronic Obstructive Lung Disease: Executive Summary: December 2006, *Global strategy for the diagnosis, management, and prevention of COPD.* National Heart, Lung, and Blood Institute (Bethesda, Md) and World Health Organization (Geneva, Switzerland), 2006. (Available at http://www.goldcopd.org/Guidelineitem.asp?l1=2&l2=1&intId=996; accessed March 2007.)
4. Barr RG, Rowe BH, Camargo CA: Methylxanthines for exacerbations of chronic obstructive pulmonary disease, *Cochrane Database Syst Rev* 2:CD002168, 2003.
5. Bhatia J: Current options in the management of apnea of prematurity, *Clin Pediatr* 39:327, 2000.
6. Stewart BN, Block AJ: A trial of aerosolized theophylline in relieving bronchospasm, *Chest* 69:718, 1976.
7. Giembycz MA: Phosphodiesterase 4 inhibitors and the treatment of asthma, *Drugs* 59:193, 2000.
8. Jenne JW: Physiology and pharmacodynamics of the xanthines, In Jenne JW, Murphy S, editors: *Drug therapy for asthma: research and clinical practice,* New York, 1987, Marcel Dekker.
9. Persson CGA, Karlsson J: *In vitro* responses to bronchodilator drugs, In Jenne JW, Murphy S, editors: *Drug therapy for asthma: research and clinical practice,* New York, 1987, Marcel Dekker.
10. Svedmyr N: Theophylline, *Am Rev Respir Dis* 136(suppl):568, 1987.
11. Jenne JW, Wyze MS, Rood FS, MacDonald FM: Pharmacokinetics of theophylline: application to adjustment of the clinical dose of aminophylline, *Clin Pharmacol Ther* 13:349, 1972.
12. Kaliner M: Goals of asthma therapy, *Ann Allergy Asthma Immunol* 75:169, 1995.
13. Kelly HW: Theophylline toxicity, In Jenne JW, Murphy S, editors: *Drug therapy for asthma: research and clinical practice,* New York, 1987, Marcel Dekker.
14. Powell JR, Vozeh S, Hopewell P, Costello J, Sheiner LB, Riegelman S: Theophylline disposition in acutely ill hospitalized patients: the effect of smoking, heart failure, severe airway obstruction and pneumonia, *Am Rev Respir Dis* 118:229, 1978.
15. Weinberger M, Hendeles L: Theophylline in asthma, *N Engl J Med* 334:1380, 1996.

16. Lam A, Newhouse MT: Management of asthma and chronic airflow limitation: are methylxanthines obsolete? *Chest* 98:44, 1990.

17. Mahler DA, Donohue JF, Barbee RA, Goldman MD, Gross NJ, Wisniewski ME, Yancey SW, Zakes BA, Rickard KA, Anderson WH: Efficacy of salmeterol xinafoate in the treatment of COPD, *Chest* 115:957, 1999.

18. Aubier M, De Troyer A, Sampson M, Macklem PT, Roussos C: Aminophylline improves diaphragmatic contractility, *N Engl J Med* 305:249, 1981.

19. Supinski GS: Effects of methylxanthines on respiratory skeletal muscle and neural drive. In Jenne JW, Murphy S, editors: *Drug therapy for asthma: research and clinical practice*, New York, 1987, Marcel Dekker.

20. Mahler DA, Matthay RA, Snyder PE, Wells CK, Loke J: Sustained-release theophylline reduces dyspnea in nonreversible obstructive airway disease, *Am Rev Respir Dis* 131:22, 1985.

21. Ziment I: Pharmacologic therapy of obstructive airway disease, *Clin Chest Med* 11:461, 1990.

22. Sullivan P, Bekir S, Jaffar Z, Page C, Jeffery P, Costello J: Antiinflammatory effects of low-dose oral theophylline in atopic asthma, *Lancet* 343:1006, 1994.

23. Page CP: Recent advances in our understanding of the use of theophylline in the treatment of asthma, *J Clin Pharmacol* 39:237, 1999.

24. Markham A, Faulds D: Theophylline: a review of its potential steroid sparing effects in asthma, *Drugs* 56:1081, 1998.

25. Yeh TF: *Drug therapy in the neonate and small infant*, St. Louis, Mo, 1985, Mosby.

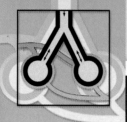

Chapter 9

Mucus-Controlling Drug Therapy

BRUCE K. RUBIN, JAMES B. FINK, MARKUS O. HENKE

CHAPTER OUTLINE

CHAPTER OBJECTIVES

After reading this chapter, the reader will be able to:

1. Interpret the physiology and mechanisms of mucus secretion and clearance
2. Name the types of mucoactive medications and their presumed modes of action
3. Describe the medications approved for the therapy of mucus clearance disorders and their approved indications
4. Identify the contraindications to the use of mucoactive medications
5. Explain the interaction between airway clearance devices or physical therapy and mucoactive medications

KEY TERMS AND DEFINITIONS

Abhesives — A coating of film that prevents or reduces adhesion

Elasticity — A rheologic property characteristic of solids; it is represented by the storage modulus G'

Expectorant — A medication meant to increase the volume or hydration of airway secretions

Gel — A macromolecular description of pseudo-plastic material having both viscosity and elasticity

Glycoprotein — A protein with covalently attached oligosaccharide units. The principle constituent of mucus and a high-molecular-weight glycoprotein, it gives mucus its physical/chemical properties such as viscoelasticity.

Mucin — The principal airway gel-forming mucins MUC2, MUC5AC, and MUC5B are proteins with attached oligosaccharide (sugar) side chains. Mucin is the principal constituent of mucus

Mucoactive agent — A term connoting any medication or drug that has an effect on mucus secretion; may include *mucolytic, expectorant, mucospissic, mucoregulatory,* or *mucokinetic agents*

Mucokinetic agent — A medication that increases ciliary clearance of respiratory mucus secretions

Mucolytic agent — A medication that degrades polymers in secretions. *Classic mucolytics* have free thiol groups to degrade mucin and *peptide mucolytics* break pathologic filaments of neutrophil-derived DNA or actin in sputum. Classic mucolytics are ineffective for the therapy of airway disease and are not recommended, whereas dornase alfa appears to be effective for the therapy of cystic fibrosis (CF) and perhaps bronchiectasis

Mucoregulatory agent — A drug that reduces the volume of airway mucus secretion and appears to be especially effective in hypersecretory states such as bronchorrhea, diffuse panbronchiolitis (DPB), CF, and some forms of asthma

Mucospissic agent — A medication that increases the viscosity of secretions and may be effective in the therapy of bronchorrhea

Mucus — Secretion, from surface goblet cells and submucosal glands, composed of water, proteins, and glycosylated mucins. The glycoprotein portion of the secretion is termed *mucin*. Mucus (noun) is the secretion; *mucous* (adjective) is the cell or gland type

Oligosaccharide — A sugar that is the individual carbohydrate unit of glycoproteins.

Rheology — Study of the deformation and flow (strain) of matter

Sol — A macromolecular description of the respiratory secretion in true solution, with the physical property of viscosity (usually referred to as the *periciliary layer*)

Sputum — Expectorated secretions that contain respiratory tract, oropharyngeal, and nasopharyngeal secretions as well as bacteria and products of inflammation including polymeric DNA and actin. Purulent sputum contains very little mucin and is similar in composition to pus

Viscosity — A rheologic property characteristic of liquids and represented by the loss modulus G

Chapter 9 presents an in-depth review of the mucociliary system and the nature of mucus, as a basis for discussing pharmacologic agents used in the treatment of respiratory secretions. The two drugs currently used in North America by aerosol administration, N-acetylcysteine or NAC (Mucomyst) and dornase alfa (Pulmozyme), are discussed, along with a number of investigational agents and future directions for mucoactive drug therapy are outlined.

DRUG CONTROL OF MUCUS: A PERSPECTIVE

KEY POINT

Mucoactive therapy should be considered after therapy to decrease infection and inflammation.

One of the major defense mechanisms of the lung is the self-renewing, self-cleansing mucociliary escalator. Failure of this system results in mechanical obstruction of the airway, often with thickened, adhesive secretions. In many diseases associated with abnormal mucociliary function a slowing of mucus transport is reported.[1,2] Whether such slowing is due to changes in the physical properties of mucus or to decreased ciliary activity, or both, is not always clear. Mucus is found in several areas of the body, including the airways, gastrointestinal tract, and genital tract. Regardless of its location, mucus is protective, lubricating, and waterproofing, and protects against osmotic or inflammatory changes. The mucus barrier can also entrap microorganisms, preventing chronic bacterial infection and biofilm formation.

Historically in respiratory care, drug therapy for secretions has been aimed at liquefying thick mucus to a watery state. Because mucus is a **gel** with physical properties of viscosity *and* elasticity, drug therapy for mucus clearance disorders should optimize the physical state of the mucus gel for efficient clearance. As a result, the term **mucolytic,** indicating breakdown of mucus, is better replaced with **mucoactive agent.** A review of mucus physiology presents the concepts necessary for discussing the current and future pharmacologic management of secretions. The amount of this chapter devoted to understanding the production, nature, and regulation of respiratory mucus reflects the current situation in which the knowledge of airway mucus has outstripped the development of therapies.

CLINICAL INDICATION FOR USE

> **KEY POINT**
>
> Mucus is protective, lubricating, waterproofing, and protecting against osmotic or inflammatory changes. The normal mucus barrier can entrap microorganisms preventing chronic bacterial infection and biofilm formation.

The general indication for mucoactive therapy is to reduce the accumulation of airway secretions, with concomitant improvement in pulmonary function and gas exchange, and the prevention of repeated infection and airway damage. Diseases in which mucoactive therapy is indicated are those with hypersecretion or poor clearance of airway secretions. These include cystic fibrosis (CF), acute and chronic bronchitis, pneumonia, diffuse panbronchiolitis (DPB), primary ciliary dyskinesia,

asthma, and bronchiectasis. Not all patients with mucus retention benefit from mucoactive drug therapy; those with adequately preserved expiratory airflow and cough have greater response.

Use of mucoactive therapy to promote secretion clearance should be considered after therapy to decrease infection and inflammation, and after minimizing or removing irritants to the airway, including tobacco smoke.[3]

IDENTIFICATION OF AGENTS

Table 9-1 lists general information on **mucoactive agents** that are approved, available, or commonly administered as inhaled aerosols in the United States. Table 9-2 lists similar information for other countries.[4] Greater detail is given on indications, dosage and administration, hazards and side effects, and assessment of drug therapy when presenting each agent.

Mucoactive agents differ in their mechanism of action. Secretion properties that impair airway clearance also differ between different diseases, and at different times in the course of a disease. The source and properties of airway secretions, as well as the mechanisms of action for the mucoactive agents, are the basis for clinical use of this class of drugs.

PHYSIOLOGY OF THE MUCOCILIARY SYSTEM

Source of Airway Secretions

The conducting airways in the lung and the nasal cavity to the oropharynx are lined by a mucociliary system, illustrated diagrammatically in Figure 9-1. The secretion lining the surface of the airway is called **mucus,** and has been described as having two phases: a gel layer (0.5-20 μm) that is propelled toward the larynx by the cilia, and floats on top of a watery periciliary layer (7 μm, the height of a fully extended cilium).[3] Cells responsible for secretion in the airway and the source of components found in respiratory mucus have been summarized by Basbaum and associates (1988).[5] Although there are many cell types in the mammalian airway, the essential secretory structures of the mucociliary system are the following:
- Surface epithelial cells
  - Pseudo-stratified, columnar, ciliated epithelial cells
  - Surface goblet (or surface mucous) cells
  - Clara cells in the distal airway
- Submucosal glands, with serous and mucous cells

Submucosal glands are found in cartilaginous airways. Beyond the distal airways, these mucus-producing

TABLE 9-1

Mucoactive Agents Available for Aerosol Administration

Drug	Brand Name	Adult Dosage	Use
N-Acetylcysteine (NAC)	10% Mucomyst 20% Mucomyst	SVN: 3-5 ml	Bronchitis, efficacy not proven for any dose of NAC for any lung disease
Dornase alfa	Pulmozyme	SVN: 2.5 mg/ampoule, one ampoule daily*	Cystic fibrosis
Aqueous aerosols: water, saline	N/A	SVN: 3-5 ml, as ordered USN: 3-5 ml, as ordered	Sputum induction, secretion, mobilization

*Use recommended nebulizer system—see package insert.
N/A, Not applicable; SVN, small volume nebulizer; USN, ultrasonic nebulizer.

TABLE 9-2

International Pharmacopoeia Listing of Mucolytic Drugs

Country	AGENT															Total
	NAC	Amb	Brom	Carbo	Dornase	Epraz	Erdos	Eth-cys	Guaif	Letos	MESNA	Meth-cys	Sob	Stepro	Thiop	
Argentina	+	+	+	–	–	–	–	–	–	–	–	–	–	–	–	3
Australia	+	–	+	–	+	–	–	–	–	–	–	–	–	–	–	3
Belgium	+	+	+	+	+	+	+	–	+	–	+	–	–	–	–	9
Brazil	+	+	+	+	+	–	–	–	–	–	–	–	+	–	–	6
Finland	+	–	+	+	–	–	+	–	+	–	–	–	–	–	–	5
France	+	+	+	+	–	–	+	–	–	+	–	–	–	–	–	6
Germany	+	+	–	+	–	–	–	–	–	–	–	–	–	–	–	3
Ireland	+	–	+	+	+	–	–	–	+	–	–	+	–	–	–	6
Italy	+	+	+	+	+	–	–	–	+	+	–	–	+	+	+	10
Japan	+	+	+	+	–	+	–	+	+	–	–	+	–	–	–	8
Netherlands	+	–	+	+	+	–	–	–	–	–	+	–	–	–	–	5
New Zealand	+	–	+	–	+	–	–	–	–	–	–	–	–	–	–	3
Russia	+	+	+	+	+	–	–	–	–	–	+	–	–	–	–	6
South Africa	+	–	+	+	–	–	–	–	+	–	+	–	–	–	–	5
Sweden	+	–	+	–	+	–	–	–	–	–	–	–	–	–	–	3
Switzerland	+	+	+	+	+	–	–	–	–	–	+	–	–	–	–	6
Taiwan	+	+	+	+	–	–	–	–	+	–	–	+	–	–	–	6
UK	–	–	–	+	+	–	–	–	–	–	–	+	–	–	–	3
USA	–	–	–	–	+	–	–	–	+	–	–	–	–	–	–	2
Total	17	10	16	14	12	2	3	1	8	2	5	4	2	1	1	–

+, In pharmacopoeias (see reference); –, not in pharmacopoeias.
NAC, N-Acetylcysteine; Amb, ambroxol; Brom, bromhexine; Carbo, carbocysteine (S-carboxymethylcysteine); Dornase, dornase alfa; Epraz, eprazinone hydrochloride; Erdos, erdosteine; Eth-cys, L-ethylcysteine; Guaif, guaifenesin; Letos, letosteine; MESNA, sodium 2-mercaptoethane sulfonate; Meth-cys, methyl cysteine (mecysteine) hydrochloride; Sob, sobrerol; Stepro, stepronin; Thiop, thiopronine.
Reprinted with permission from Rogers DF: Mucoactive drugs for asthma and COPD: any place in therapy? *Expert Opin Investig Drugs* 11:15, 2002.

cells are not found. Mucus secreted by surface epithelial cells and glands in the airway provide for basic protection of the respiratory tract, including humidification and warming of inspired gas, mucociliary transport of debris, waterproofing and insulation, and antibacterial activity.[3]

Terminology

There has been confusion regarding the nomenclature used to classify mucoactive medications. Although some authors have used "mucolytic" as a generic term for these agents, it is clear that most of these medications are thought to mobilize secretions by mechanisms other

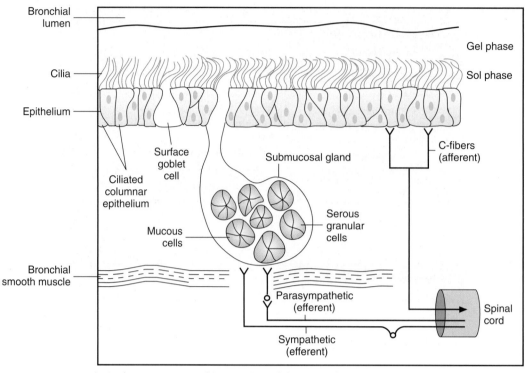

FIGURE 9-1 Principal components and innervation of the mucociliary system in the respiratory tract.

than by the direct "thinning" of mucus. For example, whereas the mucociliary transportability of sputum may be improved by reducing sputum viscosity while preserving elasticity, the cough clearability of secretions appears to be greater with increased viscosity and decreased adhesivity. Knowledge of mucus properties has given us tools to better understand the mechanisms of airway disease and mucoactive therapy. The currently accepted terminology is defined at the start of this chapter. For more details on current terminology, and its evolution, see References 6-8.

Surface Epithelial Cells

The surface of the trachea and bronchi includes primarily ciliated cells and goblet cells, at a ratio of approximately 5:1. There are more than 6000 goblet cells per square millimeter of normal airway mucosa. Goblet cells do not seem to be directly innervated in human lung, although they respond to irritants by increasing the production of mucus. Figures 9-2 and 9-3 show scanning electron micrographs of the mucus lining (Figure 9-2) and of the bronchiolar surface with the mucus stripped away (Figure 9-3). In addition to ciliated and goblet cells, microvilli, which may have a reabsorptive function, can be seen in Figure 9-3.

Submucosal Mucous Glands

Submucosal glands below the epithelial surface are thought to provide much of the airway surface mucin. The submucosal gland is under parasympathetic (vagal) control and responds to cholinergic stimulation by increasing the amount of mucus secreted. There is also evidence suggesting that submucosal glands in the respiratory tract are innervated by sympathetic axons and the peptidergic nerve system.

Two types of cells, mucous and serous, are found in the glands. Figure 9-4 shows a section of the ferret airway stained for mucin, with the surface mucous (goblet) cells and the submucosal gland serous and mucous cells identified.

Secretions from the serous and mucous cells mix in the submucosal gland and are transported through a ciliated duct onto the airway lumen.

Ciliary System

KEY POINT

The airway secretion consists of the *mucous layer,* where *mucus glycoprotein* is located, and a watery, *periciliary layer.*

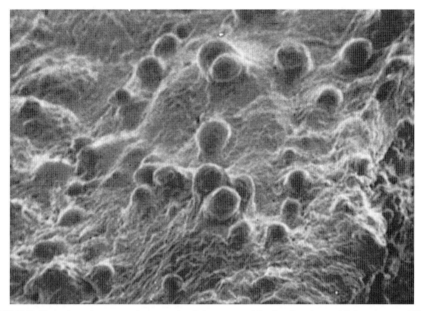

FIGURE 9-2 Scanning electron micrograph of the mucus blanket in a bronchiole, prepared from hamster lung. (From Nowell JA, Tyler WS: Scanning electron microscopy of the surface morphology of mammalian lungs, *Am Rev Respir Dis* 103:313, 1971.)

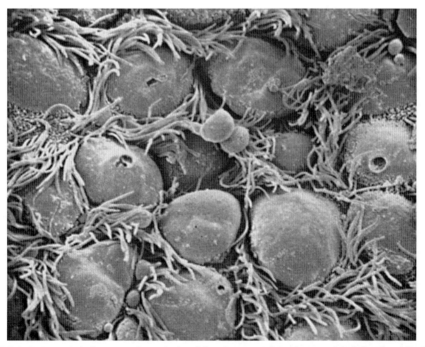

FIGURE 9-3 Scanning electron micrograph of the airway surface shows epithelial cells with cilia, possible surface goblet cells dehiscing, and some microvilli. (From Nowell JA, Tyler WS: Scanning electron microscopy of the surface morphology of mammalian lungs, *Am Rev Respir Dis* 103:313, 1971.)

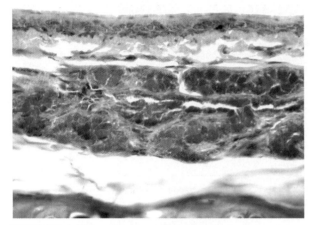

FIGURE 9-4 Light microscopy demonstrating immunohistochemical staining of the ferret airway, using horseradish peroxidase–conjugated *Dolichos biflorus* agglutinin *(DBA)*. The tracheal section shows the mucociliary apparatus including surface mucous (goblet) cells, ciliated epithelial cells, and serous and mucous glands.

Droplets of mucus from the secretory cells form plaques in the distal, nonciliated airway, and these coalesce into a continuous layer in the more proximal ciliated airway. Mucociliary transport results from the movement of the mucus gel by the beating cilia. There are approximately 200 cilia on each cell. Cilia are about 7 μm in length in larger airways, and shorten to 5 μm or slightly less in smaller bronchioles. Luk and Dulfano examined the ciliary beat frequency on biopsy samples from various tracheobronchial regions, and found rates of 8-18 Hz (Hz = 1 cycle/s) at 37° C.[9] A ciliary beat is made up of an *effective* (power) stroke and a *recovery* stroke with about a 1:2 ratio. In the effective stroke, the cilium moves in an upright position through a full forward arc, to contact the underside of the mucus layer and propel it forward. In the recovery stroke, the cilium swings back around to the starting point near the cell surface, to avoid pulling secretions back. Cilia beat in a coordinated or metachronal wave of motion to propel airway secretions. A functional surfactant layer lies at the tips of the cilia and separates the periciliary fluid from the mucus gel. This layer allows the cilia to effectively transmit kinetic energy to the mucus without becoming entangled. This layer also facilitates mucus spreading as a continuous layer and prevents water loss from the periciliary fluid. The properties of cilia are described in detail in an earlier review.[10]

Factors Affecting Mucociliary Transport

Mucociliary transport velocity varies in the normal lung and has been estimated at about 1.5 mm/min in peripheral airways and 20 mm/min in the trachea. Transport rates are slower in the presence of the following conditions or substances, many of which are associated with airway damage:

- Chronic obstructive pulmonary disease (COPD), cystic fibrosis (CF)
- Airway drying (such as with the use of dry gas for mechanical ventilation)
- Narcotics
- Endotracheal suctioning, airway trauma, and tracheostomy
- Cigarette smoke
- Atmospheric pollutants (SO_2, NO_2, ozone) may transiently increase transport, especially at low concentration. At higher, toxic concentrations or with prolonged exposure these decrease transport rates
- Hyperoxia and hypoxia

Table 9-3 summarizes the effects of drug groups, commonly used in respiratory care, on ciliary beat, mucus output, and overall transport.

Food Intake and Mucus Production

A common belief is that drinking dairy milk increases the production of mucus, or *phlegm,* and congestion in the respiratory tract. Respiratory care personnel may be asked for advice on withholding milk from children with colds, respiratory infections, or chronic respiratory conditions such as CF. Pinnock et al.[11] inoculated 60 healthy subjects with rhinovirus-2 in a study designed to answer the question, Does milk make mucus? Milk intake ranged from 0 to 11 glasses a day. They reported no association between milk and dairy product intake and upper or lower respiratory tract symptoms of congestion or nasal secretion weight. There was a trend for cough to be "loose" with increasing intake of milk, although this was not significant. None of the subjects were allergic to cow's milk. The authors concluded that the data do not support the withholding of milk or the belief that milk increases respiratory tract congestion.

NATURE OF MUCUS SECRETION

A healthy person is thought to produce about 100 ml of mucus per 24 hours, and the secretion is clear, viscoelastic, and sticky. Apparently most of this secretion is reabsorbed

TABLE 9-3

Effects of Various Drug Groups on Mucociliary Clearance

Drug Group	Ciliary Beat	Mucus Production	Transport
β-Adrenergic agents	Increase	Increase*	±
Cholinergic agents	Increase	Increase†	Increase
Methylxanthines	Increase	Increase†	±
Corticosteroids	None	Decrease†	None

*Data from Wanner A: Clinical aspects of mucociliary transport, *Am J Respir Dis* 116:73, 1977.
†Data from Iravani J, Melville GN: Mucociliary activity in the respiratory tract as influenced by prostaglandin E, *Respiration* 32:305, 1975.

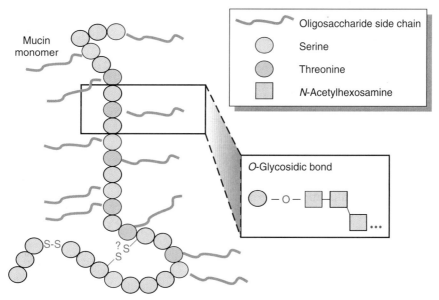

FIGURE 9-5 Basic structure and constituents of the mucus macromolecule.

in the bronchial mucosa, with only 10 ml or so reaching the glottis. This amount is rarely noticed by the individual. During disease, the volume of secretions can increase dramatically, and the secretions are expectorated or swallowed. One of the primary functions of respiratory tract mucus is thought to be transporting and removing trapped inhaled particles, cellular debris, or dead and aging cells.

KEY POINT

Mucociliary clearance is affected by numerous drug groups, including surfactants and anticholinergic agents.

Structure and Composition of Mucus

The structure and major constituents of the mucus secreted by submucosal glands and surface goblet cells are pictured in Figure 9-5 and have been reviewed.[5,7,12-14]

Airway mucus forms a protective barrier between the respiratory tract epithelium and the environment. Mucus is composed mainly of water and ions, with approximately 5% of the content due to proteins secreted by airway cells and lipids.[15-17] In health, the **mucin** glycoproteins are the major macromolecular component of the mucus gel. Mucins are responsible for the protective and clearance properties of mucus.[18-20]

There are two major classes of mucins: the secreted and the membrane-tethered mucins.[21,22] Several secreted mucins (MUC2, MUC5AC, MUC5B, and MUC6) have genes that are clustered on chromosome 11p15 and contain domains with significant homology to the von Willebrand factor D domains that are sites for oligomerization.[23] In sputum, MUC5AC and MUC5B are the major oligomeric mucins.[24] MUC5AC appears to be produced primarily by the goblet cells in the tracheobronchial surface epithelium, whereas MUC5B is secreted primarily by the submucosal glands.[25] The membrane-tethered mucins, MUC1, MUC3, MUC4, MUC12, and MUC13, contain a transmembrane domain and a short cytoplasmic domain.[23] At least 12 mucin genes (*MUC1, MUC2, MUC4, MUC5AC, MUC5B, MUC7, MUC8, MUC11, MUC13, MUC15, MUC19,* and *MUC20*) have been observed at the mRNA level in tissues of the lower respiratory tract from healthy individuals.[21,23,26-32]

Mucus is a complex, high molecular weight macromolecule consisting of a mucin protein backbone to which carbohydrate *(oligosaccharide)* side chains are attached. At the time of writing, 21 distinct mucin proteins have been identified but airway mucus is almost entirely composed of the MUC5AC and MUC5B secreted gel-forming mucins. The carbohydrate content is 80% or more of the total weight of the macromolecule. This structure has been likened to a bottlebrush in appearance. This general structure of protein and attached oligosaccharide side chains is termed a *glycoprotein*. Mucin forms a flexible, threadlike strand from 200 nm up to 6 μm in length[33] that is linearly cross-linked with disulfide bonds from adjacent cysteine residues. Strands may perhaps be further cross-linked with each other by hydrogen bonding and van der Waals forces. The result is a gel that consists of a high water content (90 to 95%) organized around the structural elements and that is intensely hydrophilic and spongelike.[34,35]

Under normal circumstances, bonding within mucus produces low viscosity but moderate elasticity. Although mucus incorporates water during its formation, a gel is both a liquid and a solid. An analogy is gelatin, which is mostly water but organizes into a semisolid by its chemical structure as the liquid gels. It is important clinically that sufficient water must be available to form mucus with normal physical properties, but once formed, mucus does not readily incorporate topically applied water.[36]

Phospholipids are also present in the serous cell granules of the submucosal glands. When released onto the airway surface, they may serve as lubricants affecting the surface-active and adhesive properties of mucus, both of which can affect mucociliary transport function.[3]

In addition to the mucus gel secreted in the airway, bronchial secretions contain serum and secreted proteins, lipids, and electrolytes. Antibacterial defense in the airway is provided by mucin, secretory IgA, IgG, lysozyme, lactoferrin, defensins, and peroxidase and serine proteases. Bronchial secretions control the potentially destructive action of protease enzymes with two major antiproteases: α_1-protease inhibitor and secretory leukoprotease inhibitor (sLPI), a cationic protein found in serous secretory glandular cells.[3] In healthy airways, the antiproteases are present in higher quantities than the protease enzymes and provide a protease screen.[37]

Epithelial Ion Transport

KEY POINT

Epithelial ion exchange in the airway surface liquid maintains normal periciliary fluid depth.

The composition and volume of the periciliary fluid layer is regulated in part by ion transport across the epithelial cells lining the airway lumen. If the periciliary layer is not approximately the height of an extended cilium, effective mucus movement cannot occur.[38] Defective ion transport contributes to the cycle of retained secretions and infection seen in CF.[39,40] Normal airway epithelial ion transport is illustrated in Figure 9-6.

In the basal, unstimulated state, sodium (Na^+) absorption into the epithelial cell is the dominant ion exchange that absorbs liquid from the airway periciliary layer. Sodium absorption occurs as an active transport process through sodium channels (epithelial sodium channel or ENaC) on the apical (airway) side of the cell. Sodium in the epithelial cell is then pumped from the cell, driven by a sodium/potassium-ATPase pump on the basolateral membrane of the epithelial cell shown in Figure 9-6. When sodium is absorbed from the airway

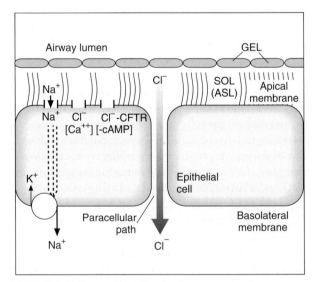

FIGURE 9-6 Illustration of ion-exchange mechanisms across the normal airway epithelium controlling absorption/secretion for the periciliary airway surface liquid *(ASL),* or sol. Under basal conditions, sodium (Na^+) is absorbed along with liquid, with no net chloride (Cl^-) secretion from the cell into the liquid layer. *cAMP,* Cyclic adenosine 3′,5′-monophosphate; *CFTR,* cystic fibrosis transmembrane ion conductance regulator.

surface liquid, there is an accompanying absorption of chloride ions and water.[41] Chloride secretion can occur through at least two different types of chloride channel in the cell apex. One channel is dependent on cyclic adenosine 3′,5′-monophosphate (cAMP), the cystic fibrosis transmembrane ion conductance regulator (CFTR) channel; the other channel is calcium activated.

To summarize, under normal conditions, healthy airway epithelia can absorb salt and water driven by an active sodium transport and normal epithelia can also secrete liquid into the periciliary fluid driven by active chloride transport through ion channels and passively through aquaporins or water channels.

Mucus in Disease States

KEY POINT

Mucus or mucociliary clearance can be abnormal in pulmonary diseases such as chronic bronchitis, asthma, or cystic fibrosis.

The normal clearance of airway mucus can be altered by changes in the volume, hydration, or composition of the secretion. Mucus is produced and secreted by surface goblet cells and submucosal gland cells. Water content is a function of transepithelial chloride secretion, active sodium absorption, and water transport. The composition of respiratory mucus is undergoing investigation based on structural analysis techniques.[42,43]

Knowledge of these features of respiratory mucus may lead to a better understanding of diseases characterized by an abnormal production of mucus such as chronic bronchitis and asthma, where there is mucus hypersecretion, and CF, where there is decreased mucus secretion. Although it had been hypothesized that patients with CF hypersecrete viscous mucus leading to airway obstruction, it has now been shown that these patients possibly secrete far less mucin than either healthy people or persons with chronic bronchitis and that the adhesive (but not viscous) secretions that characterize CF airway disease are composed almost entirely of DNA-rich pus.[44] Airway damage may predispose to bacterial infections in chronic bronchitis because of impaired clearance of mucus, while failure of CF cells to secrete mucus may not only cause epithelial cell dysfunction but may lay the airway epithelium bare and vulnerable to chronic bacterial infection.

Sputum is expectorated mucus mixed with inflammatory cells, cellular debris, polymers of DNA and filamentous (F)-actin, as well as bacteria. Mucus is usually cleared by airflow and ciliary movement, and sputum is cleared by cough.[45] Purulent, green sputum is caused by the neutrophil-derived enzyme myeloperoxidase, indicating neutrophil activation; this sputum contains very little mucin and can be considered pus.[46] Bronchial obstruction by secretions, either mucus or pus, can increase airflow resistance and lead to complete airway obstruction and atelectasis.[12] Thus, regardless of whether the airway is full of mucus or pus, effective airway clearance is vital to airway hygiene.

Chronic Bronchitis

Chronic bronchitis (CB) is defined clinically as daily sputum expectoration for 3 months of the year for at least 2 consecutive years, usually in a tobacco smoker or ex-smoker. In the CB airway there is hyperplasia of submucosal glands and goblet cells. The number of goblet cells increases, and there is hypertrophy of the submucosal glands, as measured by the Reid index of gland-to-airway wall thickness ratio.[47] When studied *in vitro*, it was found that submucosal glands from subjects with CB produce excessive amounts of mucus.[48] Tobacco smoke is considered the most important predisposing factor to airway irritation and mucus hypersecretion, but other factors can include viral infections, pollutants, and genetic predisposition.[12,49]

It has been reported that chronic sputum expectoration is associated with a more rapid decline in lung function and, for persons with COPD, more frequent admissions to hospital.[50]

Asthma

Mucus hypersecretion can occur during an acute asthmatic episode or can be a chronic feature of asthma accompanying airway inflammation. Turner-Warwick and Openshaw reported that as many as 80% of patients with asthma report increased sputum expectoration.[51]

In acute severe and fatal asthma there is profound hypersecretion of highly viscous and rigid mucus leading to complete airway obstruction.[52] Because most of these patients have received large amounts of β-agonist bronchodilators, sometimes even by the intravenous route or by continuous nebulization, it is likely that β receptors are fully saturated. β Agonists induce the secretion of viscous mucus, so it is possible that under these circumstances the aggressive use of β agonists may contribute to fatal airway obstruction.[53]

Bronchorrhea

Bronchorrhea is defined as the production of watery sputum of 100 ml or more per day. This occurs in about 9% of patients with chronic asthma.[54] Some of these patients respond well to antiinflammatory therapy such as corticosteroids,[55] indomethacin by aerosol,[56] or macrolide antibiotics.[57] These are all considered **muco-regulatory** medications and are most effective when bronchorrhea is associated with airway inflammation. Patients with congenital fucosidosis also have a form of bronchorrhea due to the inability of mucins to polymerize. This form of bronchorrhea does not respond to mucoregulatory therapy.[58]

Plastic Bronchitis

Plastic bronchitis is a rare disease characterized by the formation of large gelatinous or rigid branching airway casts.[59] These casts are large and more cohesive than those seen in ordinary mucus plugging. The casts can be spontaneously expectorated and occasionally patients will cough up large impressions of their tracheobronchial tree. Casts are often described as "pudding like" or "toothpaste." Many are too thick to be easily suctioned through a bronchoscope and too friable to be grasped and removed with forceps. However, some patients are able to spontaneously expectorate even large casts. Not all patients expectorate casts and this may delay the diagnosis or lead to underdiagnosis.

The prevalence of plastic bronchitis is unknown. This disease may also overlap with diseases such as asthma, and with the severe mucus plugging sometimes seen in bronchopulmonary *aspergillosis* or middle lobe syndrome. Differentiating between severe asthma with mucus plugging and plastic bronchitis can be difficult.

The mortality rate among patients with plastic bronchitis has been estimated as 6%-50% for those with "inflammatory" casts, as 28%-60% for those with "noninflammatory" casts, and as low as 0% for those producing casts associated with acute chest syndrome in sickle cell disease. Patients who die usually succumb to respiratory failure related to central airway obstruction.

There is only anecdotal evidence that any specific therapy is beneficial and this evidence has, in general, been provided only by single case reports. If chylous casts are present, dietary modification or thoracic duct ligation when appropriate may help. In patients with asthma or atopy and cellular casts, therapy should be directed toward treating underlying inflammation. Oral or inhaled corticosteroids and culture-directed therapy of infection have been reported to help. The 14- and 15-member macrolide antibiotics are known to be both immunomodulatory and mucoregulatory drugs. Rubin, BK and Henke, MO have had success using macrolides as immunomodulating agents in two patients

with eosinophilic plastic bronchitis (unpublished data). Macrolides have been successfully used in other disorders, primarily in DPB and CF. There is clear evidence that these effects are not related to the antimicrobial activity of the macrolide.[59,60]

Cystic Fibrosis

CF is a chronic hereditary disease characterized by impaired function of the CFTR protein. There is chronic airway infection, often with *Pseudomonas* and other gram-negative organisms. There is also chronic airway inflammation and, together, infection and inflammation lead to bronchiectasis, progressive pulmonary function decline, and eventually death. Although it was once thought that there was mucus hypersecretion and airway mucus obstruction in CF, it is now known that the CF airway secretions contain very little mucin. The airways in CF are almost entirely filled with pus derived from neutrophil degradation.

It is not yet clear how abnormal CFTR function leads to chronic infection and inflammation. Airway epithelia in CF show excessive absorption of sodium (Na^+) compared with normal epithelia. There is a limited ability for the epithelial cells to secrete chloride (Cl^-) through the chloride CFTR channels (see Figure 9-6) stimulated by cAMP. The result of excessive Na^+ absorption and limited Cl^- secretion may lead to decreased water and increased reabsorption of the periciliary fluid.[41] Abnormal phospholipid balance in CF secretions may also increase sputum adhesion and stickiness by altering surface properties of the secretion.[3] It has been shown that although CF sputum is not particularly viscous, it is biophysically similar to bronchiectasis sputum.[61]

PHYSICAL PROPERTIES OF MUCUS

As previously stated, the biochemical characteristics of mucus determine its physical properties, which influence the efficiency of mucus transport.

> **KEY POINT**
>
> *Physical properties* of mucus include *viscosity, elasticity, cohesivity,* and *adhesivity;* normal ranges of these properties are needed for adequate mucus transport to occur.

Adhesive Forces

Adhesion refers to forces between unlike molecules. In the airway, adhesive forces refer to the attractive forces between the mucus and airway surface. Adhesion

VISCOSITY AND ELASTICITY

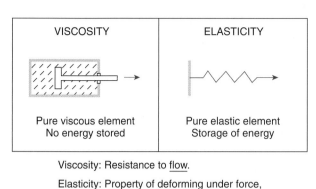

Viscosity: Resistance to flow.

Elasticity: Property of deforming under force,
resuming shape.

FIGURE 9-7 Illustration of concepts of viscosity and elasticity.

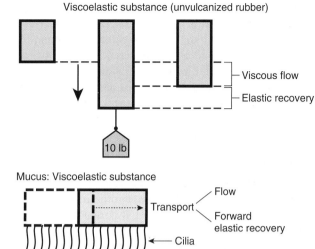

FIGURE 9-8 Illustration of the viscous and elastic properties affecting the movement of viscoelastic substances such as unvulcanized rubber and mucus.

severely reduces the ability to clear secretions by airflow (cough).[62] Mucokinetic agents are either **abhesives** like surfactant, which reduces the adhesivity of secretions, or agents that increase the power of expiratory airflow and cough. Mucolytics may work, in part, by severing the bonding of mucus to the epithelium, thus reducing inertial (frictional) adhesion.

Cohesive Forces

Cohesion refers to forces between like molecules. Cohesive forces result from the elongation of the mucus macromolecule. A property of spinnability has been described as a surrogate measure of cohesivity.

Rheology is the study of the deformation and flow (strain) of matter. The rheologic behavior of mucus describes the way it responds to forces (stress). **Viscosity**, or loss modulus, is the resistance of a fluid to flow. More specifically, viscosity is the proportionality constant (ratio) of applied force to rate of flow. The properties of an ideal or Newtonian liquid can be described by the loss modulus. **Elasticity**, or storage modulus, is the ability of a deformed material to return to its original shape. Ideal solids store energy during deformation, and this energy is available when the force is removed. The properties of an ideal or Hookean solid can be described by the storage modulus. The complex modulus (G^*) is the vectorial sum of viscosity and elasticity and is useful for describing the deformation of a pseudo-plastic gellike mucus. Figure 9-7 illustrates the concept of viscosity and of elasticity.[63-65]

Mucus as a Viscoelastic Material

The mucus gel is a viscoelastic material and therefore responds to an applied stress both as a fluid and as a solid. As a solid, a gel has elastic deformation, storing

energy with applied force, and as a liquid, a gel flows under applied force, losing *(dissipating)* energy. As the tips of the cilia contact the gel during the forward power stroke, the gel is stretched and its elastic recovery causes it to snap forward. At the same time, the mucus gel flows forward as a liquid under the forward beat of the cilia.

This model of gel transport is seen in Figure 9-8, using unvulcanized rubber as an example of a viscoelastic substance.

If such a rubber strip is loaded on one end with a weight and allowed to hang, it would initially stretch as an elastic solid. If the applied force remains, the strip will slowly elongate because of its viscosity (i.e., the rubber would "flow"). After removing the weight, the rubber recovers most of the elastic elongation because of stored energy, but will not recover the entire length because of flow. Mucus behaves similarly. Mucociliary transport results from both flow and forward elastic recovery. For this reason, the physical properties of viscosity and elasticity are important for efficient transport of respiratory secretions. In general, normal mucus has a relatively low viscosity, and its elasticity is high enough to provide forward propulsive energy.

Spinnability (Cohesivity) of Mucus

The ability of mucus to be drawn out into threads was initially identified for cervical mucus; it was termed "spinnability" and described in the German literature as "Spinnbarkeit." It was noted that this property was essential for the motility of sperm and female reproduction. The property of spinnability was subsequently studied by Puchelle and colleagues for respiratory mucus.[66] They used a device to stretch mucus vertically at a constant rate, and measured the spinnability of a mucus thread as the maximal length to which the thread could be drawn before breaking. In general, there was a significant and positive correlation between spinnability of mucus and its mucociliary transport rate. Spinnability was found to increase with increasing elasticity. Spinnability varied widely, however, with low viscosities, and mucus with high spinnability showed normal ciliary transport even though viscosity and elasticity were abnormally low. Spinnability, and therefore mucus transport, was also found to decrease as the purulence of sputum from CB patients increased. Spinnability gives information about internal cohesion forces in mucus. *Cohesivity* is defined as interfacial tension multiplied by the new area created after a test substance is pulled apart and cohesivity can be approximated by measuring spinnability. *Tenacity* is defined as the product of cohesivity and adhesive work—tenacity is one of the strongest determinants of the ability of sputum to be cleared by cough and the greater the tenacity of sputum, the worse the cough clearability.

Non-Newtonian Nature of Mucus

Evaluation of mucus properties is complicated by the fact that mucus exhibits non-Newtonian rheology. In an ideal Newtonian liquid, the applied force to rate of flow remains constant with changing force. A non-Newtonian substance, such as mucus, has changing viscosity (defined as the proportionality constant of force to flow) with varying applied force (shear rate). As the shear rate increases, the apparent viscosity of mucus decreases. Some mucus also exhibits a shear-thinning phenomenon: viscosity decreases at a low shear rate *after* the mucus is subjected to a high shear rate.[67] Such changes in viscosity are consistent with rupture or change of the macromolecular chains and cross-linking network of the gel. Mucus is usually *thixotropic*—stable at rest but becoming more fluid with applied force. Under forces exceeding the apparent yield stress mucus can undergo a sudden, catastrophic drop in viscosity caused by the dynamic and permanent rearrangement or rupture of polymer structure.

Because of its non-Newtonian behavior, evaluation of the properties of mucus and of the effect of drugs on those properties is complicated and must be performed under standardized conditions of dynamic shear rate and across the linear portion of the stress–strain curve. Otherwise, as noted by Shah and colleagues,[43]

interpretation of research findings on mucus viscosity is inaccurate.[68]

There are a number of review articles and compendia devoted to the physiology of mucus secretion in the lung and the nature of mucus.[7,9,12,16,45,69-72]

MUCOACTIVE AGENTS

> **KEY POINT**
>
> There are currently two agents administered by aerosol to modify airway secretions: *acetylcysteine* and *dornase alfa*.

At the time of this edition, there are two agents that have been used for administration as an aerosol, to treat abnormal pulmonary secretions: these are *N*-acetylcysteine (NAC) and dornase alfa. Both agents are mucolytic in their action, disrupting disulfide bonds in mucus, or enzymatically breaking down DNA in airway secretions, respectively. Although not an approved agent, bicarbonate solutions of 2% concentration have been instilled in 2- to 5-ml amounts into the airway, to raise the pH and alter mucus bonding. Table 9-4 summarizes the spectrum of agents, both in current use and with the potential to improve mucus clearance.

TABLE 9-4

Drugs Currently Used or Under Investigation as Mucus- and Secretion-Controlling Agents in the Respiratory Tract for Aerosolization

Drug	Description
NAL, nacystelyn	Classic mucolytic
Dornase alfa	Peptide mucolytic
P2Y$_2$ agent (denufosol)	Increases epithelial mucus and chloride secretion
Hyperosmolar saline	Expectorant
Dry powder mannitol	Expectorant
Thymosin β$_4$	Peptide mucolytic
Surfactants	Abhesive phospholipid, mucokinetic
β Agonists	Secretagogues and potentially mucokinetic if airflow increases
Macrolide antibiotics	Mucoregulatory
Anticholinergic agents	Mucoregulatory
Corticosteroids	Mucoregulatory
Gene therapy	Normalizes secretory cell function and mucociliary clearance

NAL, *N*-Acetylcysteine lysinate.

Mucolysis and Mucociliary Clearance

Mucolytic agents decrease the elasticity and viscosity of mucus because the gel structure is broken down. Because elasticity is crucial for mucociliary transport, mucolytics have the potential for a negative effect on normal physiological mucus clearance. Reduction of mucus gel to a more liquid state *may* facilitate aspiration of secretions with the use of suction catheters.[73] Ideally, the goal should be to facilitate physiological clearance by optimizing the viscoelasticity of mucus. The status of mucolytic agents in pulmonary disease was well reviewed at several conferences on the scientific basis of respiratory care.[74-76]

The therapeutic options for controlling mucus hypersecretion are outlined as follows:

1. **Remove causative factors where possible.**
   a. Treat infections
   b. Stop smoking!
   c. Avoid pollution and allergens
2. **Optimize tracheobronchial clearance.**
   a. Use bronchodilators—only if there is an increase in expiratory airflow
   b. Administer bronchial hygiene measures
      (1) Cough, deep breathing
      (2) Postural drainage
      (3) Other airway clearance devices and maneuvers
   c. Improve airflow by exercise and nutrition rehabilitation
3. **Use mucoactive agents when indicated.**

Mucolytics and Expectorants

Classic mucolytics reduce mucins by severing disulfide bonds or charge shielding.

N-ACETYL-L-CYSTEINE (NAC)

Indications for Use

KEY POINT

Acetylcysteine does *not* improve mucus clearance when given as an aerosol and therefore should never be used as a mucoactive medication.

As a mucolytic, NAC has been used in the treatment of conditions associated with viscous mucus secretions, although this is not an approved use of the drug. A second use of NAC is as an antioxidant antidote to reduce hepatic injury with acetaminophen overdose.[77] The drug is given orally for this use. Despite *in vitro* mucolytic activity and a long history of use, there are no data that demonstrate that oral or aerosolized NAC is effective therapy for any lung disease[78] and, in fact, its use may be harmful. This may be due, in part, to NAC selectively depolymerizing the essential mucin polymer structure and leaving the pathologic polymers of DNA and F-actin intact. Because there are no data that show NAC to be effective for lung disease and because of the high risk of side effects we do not recommend its use.

Other mucoactive agents under development include mucolytics such as *N*-acetylcysteine lysinate, or nacystelyn,[79] and low molecular weight dextran.[80]

Mode of Action

NAC disrupts the structure of the mucus polymer by substituting free thiol (sulfhydryl) groups for the disulfide bonds connecting mucin proteins.

The substituted sulfhydryl group in mucus does not provide a bond or cross-linking between strands, and as a result both the viscosity and the elasticity of the mucus are lowered. When in physical contact with mucus (but not sputum), NAC begins to reduce viscosity immediately. Its mucolytic activity increases with higher pH and is optimal at a local pH of 7.0 to 9.0. The solution of NAC contains a chelating agent, ethylenediaminetetraacetic acid. A light-purple solution indicates metal ion removal and does not change the safety or efficacy of the drug. It is suggested that opened vials of the drug be stored in a refrigerator and discarded after 96 hours to prevent contamination. Additional details in the manufacturer's package insert should be reviewed.

Hazards

The most serious potential complication with NAC is bronchospasm due to its acidity (pH 2.2). This is more likely in asthmatic patients and is less common when using the 10%, rather than the 20%, solution. The risk can be ameliorated by pretreatment with a bronchodilator. If this is done, a bronchodilator with rapid onset should be used. Other complications can include stomatitis, nausea, and rhinorrhea. Mechanical obstruction of the airway can occur and suction should be available with artificial airways. The disagreeable odor of NAC is due to the release of hydrogen sulfide, and this may provoke nausea or vomiting. In prolonged nebulization, the manufacturer suggests that after three-fourths of the solution is nebulized, the remaining one-fourth should be diluted with an equal volume of sterile water to prevent the formation of a highly concentrated residue, which could irritate the airway. An aerosol of NAC may leave a sticky film on hands or face.

Incompatibility With Antibiotics in Mixture

NAC is incompatible in mixture with the following antibiotics and should not be combined in physical solution.

- Sodium ampicillin
- Amphotericin B
- Erythromycin lactobionate
- Tetracyclines (tetracycline, oxytetracycline)
- Aminoglycosides

Incompatibility is taken to mean the formation of a precipitate; a change in color, clarity, or odor; or other physical or chemical change. NAC is reactive with a number of substances including rubber, copper, iron, and cork. Most conventional nebulizers made of plastic or glass are suitable for administering the drug. Aluminum, chromed metal, tantalum, sterling silver, and stainless steel are also safe to use, although silver may tarnish. A complete list of incompatibilities for NAC can be found in the manufacturer's literature.

DORNASE ALFA (PULMOZYME)

KEY POINT

Dornase alfa is indicated for clearance of purulent secretions in *cystic fibrosis*.

Peptide mucolytics, such as dornase alfa, reduce extracellular DNA and F-actin polymers. Dornase alfa (Pulmozyme) is a recombinant form of the human DNase I enzyme, which digests extracellular DNA material. Dornase alfa is occasionally referred to as rhDNase, for "recombinant human DNase." In February 1994 the U.S. Food and Drug Administration (FDA) approved dornase alfa for general use in treating the abnormally tenacious DNA-containing sputum seen in CF.

Dornase alfa was the first approved mucoactive agent for the treatment of CF. Dornase alfa is safe and effective, even in patients with more severe pulmonary disease defined as a forced vital capacity (FVC) less than 40% of the predicted value.[81] Efficacy has not yet been demonstrated for therapy of acute exacerbations of CF lung disease or for the treatment of other chronic airway diseases.[82] A small phase 1 study demonstrated no efficacy in non-CF bronchiectasis and there was a

suggestion that the use of dornase worsened disease in this adult population.[83] This may be due to the fact that secretions in bronchiectasis and COPD are composed primarily of mucin and related proteins,[84] whereas CF airway secretions include significantly less mucin and mucus, being composed almost entirely of neutrophil-derived pus.[44]

Indication and Use in Cystic Fibrosis

Dornase alfa is indicated for the management of CF, to reduce the frequency of respiratory infections requiring parenteral antibiotics, and to improve or preserve pulmonary function in these subjects.

The bulk and surface properties of respiratory secretions in CF are due to the presence of DNA from necrosing neutrophils present during chronic respiratory infections and to surfactant phospholipid hydrolysis by products of inflammation. In the presence of infection, neutrophils are attracted to the airways, degenerate, and release DNA, which further increases the viscosity of secretions. DNA is an extremely viscous polyanion.[85,86] DNA in secretions may also contribute to reduced effectiveness of aminoglycoside antibiotics such as gentamicin. This could be caused by binding of the antibiotic to the polyvalent anions of DNA.

Mode of Action

The peptide mucolytic agent dornase alfa is similar in action to the proteolytic enzyme pancreatic dornase, which was approved for human use by inhalation in 1958 but is no longer available.[86] Dornase alfa reduces the viscosity and adhesivity of infected respiratory secretions when given by aerosol. This is illustrated in Figure 9-9.

When mixed with purulent sputum from subjects with CF, dornase alfa lowered the viscosity and adhesivity of the sputum.[86] This was associated with a decrease in the size of the DNA in the sputum. The change in sputum viscosity with the addition of dornase alfa is dose dependent, with greater reduction occurring at higher concentrations of the drug.

Pancreatic dornase, termed *Dornavac* by the manufacturer, the product previously removed from the market, was a bovine pancreatic DNase. This product could cause serious bronchospasm when inhaled.[87] In addition, the foreign protein might generate anti-DNase antibodies and cause allergic reactions. Differences between the human and bovine pancreatic DNase I molecules in an immunogenic region imply that some of the adverse reactions to pancreatic dornase could have been caused by an immune response. Serum antibodies to

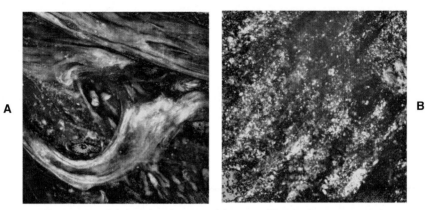

FIGURE 9-9 Illustration of the mode of action of dornase alfa in reducing DNA polymers in cystic fibrosis sputum. Shown is a confocal micrograph of cystic fibrosis sputum stained (with YOYO-1) for DNA before **(A)** and after **(B)** treatment with dornase alfa *in vitro*. The long DNA polymers are degraded into short units after dornase treatment.

DNase were found in some patients who had been given multiple doses of bovine pancreatic DNase. Adverse effects with bovine DNase may also have been caused by the presence of contaminating proteinases, trypsin and chymotrypsin, in the drug.[86] On the other hand, studies revealed no allergic response or serum anti-DNase antibodies with inhaled dornase alfa in healthy subjects or in those with CF.[85]

Dose and Administration

The aerosol product, dornase alfa, is available as single-use ampoule, with 2.5 mg of drug in 2.5 ml of clear, colorless solution. The solution should be refrigerated and protected from light. The usual dose is 2.5 mg daily, delivered by one of the following tested and approved nebulizers: Hudson RCI UP-DRAFT II OPTI-NEB nebulizer with tee (Teleflex Medical, Research Triangle Park, NC) or the Acorn II nebulizer (Vital Signs, Totowa, NJ) with a DeVilbiss Pulmo-Aide compressor (Sunrise Medical, Carlsbad, CA), or the PARI LC PLUS nebulizer (PARI Respiratory Equipment, Midlothian, VA) with PARI Inhaler Boy compressor.[88] Although other nebulizer systems may perform suitably in nebulizing dornase alfa, this should not be assumed without testing. Optimal delivery of the enzyme requires a nebulizer system capable of suitable aerosol generation (i.e., particle size and quantity). This is especially important when administering very expensive drugs or aerosol medications with a narrow therapeutic index.

Adverse Effects

Side effects with dornase alfa differed little from those of placebo in clinical trials, and the discontinuation rate was similar for dornase alfa (3%) and placebo (2%).

Anti-DNase antibody production was not found with inhaled dornase alfa. Common side effects with use of the drug have included voice alteration, pharyngitis, laryngitis, rash, chest pain, and conjunctivitis. Other, less common side effects reported include respiratory symptoms (cough increase, dyspnea, pneumothorax, hemoptysis, rhinitis, and sinusitis), flu syndrome and malaise, gastrointestinal obstruction, hypoxia, and weight loss. Contraindications include hypersensitivity to the medication.

Clinical Application and Evaluation

The intent of treatment with dornase alfa is to preserve or improve lung function in CF, while reducing the frequency and severity of respiratory infections by improving secretion clearance. A reduction in use of intravenous antibiotic therapy and the need for hospitalizations has also been reported. Evaluation of drug treatment is based not only on lung function but also on a reduction in the number and severity of infectious exacerbations and thus the need for antibiotics and hospitalization.[89]

F-ACTIN–DEPOLYMERIZING DRUGS: GELSOLIN AND THYMOSIN β₄

Chronic inflammation is characterized by inflammatory cell necrosis and release of undegraded DNA, filamentous actin (F-actin), and intracellular enzymes from neutrophils. These inflammatory products are present in the sputum from patients with CF. DNA and F-actin in the sputum copolymerize to form a rigid network that is entangled in the mucin gel. Peptide mucolytics degrade these filaments while leaving the glycoprotein network relatively intact. Gelsolin, an 85-kDa actin-severing peptide, has been shown to reduce the viscosity of CF sputum in a dose-dependent manner. Similarly, thymosin β_4 decreases sputum cohesivity in a dose-dependent and time-dependent manner.[90-92] Thymosin β_4 sequesters actin in cystic fibrosis sputum and decreases sputum cohesivity in vitro.[92] In vitro studies have shown that administration of F-actin–depolymerizing agents along with dornase alfa results in greater reduction in sputum cohesivity and viscoelasticity than either agent alone.[93,94] Actin-depolymerizing agents both destabilize the actin–DNA filament network and increase the depolymerizing activity of dornase alfa on the DNA filaments.

EXPECTORANTS

KEY POINT

Potassium iodide and glyceryl guaiacolate are considered *expectorants* or *mukokinetic agents,* rather than mucolytics, but these drugs have not been shown to have therapeutic efficacy and they should not be used. Future mucus-controlling agents may be able to normalize and optimize physical properties of mucus to improve clearance.

Iodide-Containing Agents

Iodide-containing agents (e.g., supersaturated potassium iodide, or SSKI) are generally considered to be **expectorants**. They are thought to stimulate the secretion of airway fluid. Iodopropylideneglycerol (IPG) may acutely increase tracheobronchial clearance as measured by radiolabeled aerosol in patients with chronic bronchitis.[95] However, in a double-blinded cross-over study in subjects with stable CB, therapy with IPG failed to demonstrate any changes in pulmonary function, gas trapping, or sputum properties.[96]

Sodium Bicarbonate

Sodium bicarbonate (2%) is a base that has occasionally been used for direct tracheal irrigation or as an aerosol. By increasing the local bronchial pH, sodium bicarbonate weakens the bonds between the side chains of the mucus molecule, resulting in lowering of the mucus viscosity and elasticity. Local bronchial irritation may occur with a bronchial pH of greater than 8.0. Sodium bicarbonate has not been clinically demonstrated to improved airway mucus clearance. There is little to recommend its use.

Guaifenesin

Guaifenesin is usually considered an expectorant rather than a mucolytic. It can be ciliotoxic when applied directly to the respiratory epithelium.[97] It may stimulate the cholinergic pathway and induce increased mucus secretion from the airway submucosal glands, but neither guaifenesin nor glycerol guaiacolate has been demonstrated to be clinically effective in randomized controlled trials.

Dissociating Solvents

Urea is a dissociating agent that can break ionic and hydrogen bonds. In mucin gels, urea disrupts the hydrogen bonds between the oligosaccharide side chains of the neighboring mucus molecules, with subsequent decrease in the physical entanglements between the molecules and decreased viscosity of the mucus. Urea may also decrease the interaction between DNA molecules. Because the mucolytic action of urea occurs only at very high concentrations of urea (3-8 mol/L),[98,99] it is not appropriate for human use.

Oligosaccharides

The oligosaccharide side chains make up about 80% of the mucin structure. These hydrogen bonds are weak and can be disrupted by agents such as dextran, mannitol, and lactose. The lower molecular weight fractions of dextran are primarily responsible for the mucoactive effects of dextran. Furthermore, an osmotic effect of dextran with increased hydration of the mucus could also result in improved clearance of secretions. Dextran administration via aerosol has been shown to improve tracheal mucus velocity in dogs.[80]

The charged oligosaccharide heparin has a greater mucolytic and mucokinetic capacity compared with the neutral oligosaccharide dextran. Heparin may cause both hydrogen bond disruption and improved ionic interactions. Aerosolized low molecular weight heparin shows promise in the treatment of asthma, presumably by interfering with antigen–receptor binding.[100]

P2Y$_2$ Agonists

Chloride conductance through the Ca^{2+}-dependent chloride channels is preserved in the CF airway. The tricyclic nucleotides UTP and ATP regulate ion transport through P2Y$_2$ purinergic receptors, which increase intracellular calcium. UTP aerosol, alone or in combination with amiloride, increases the transepithelial potential difference and the clearance of inhaled radioaerosol.[101] There is active development of novel P2Y$_2$ purinergic receptor agonists for clinical use.[102,103]

MUCOKINETIC AGENTS

KEY POINT

Other agents modifying airway secretions include inhaled anticholinergics such as atropine, tricyclic nucleotides, phospholipids, antiproteases, and gene therapy.

Mucokinetic agents increase cough clearance by increasing expiratory airflow or by reducing sputum adhesivity and tenacity.

Bronchodilators

β Agonists increase ciliary beat frequency, but this has little effect on mucus clearance. Of greater importance is that these medications can increase expiratory airflow in persons with an asthmatic component of airway disease.[104] However, airway muscle relaxation can also decrease expiratory airflow by producing dynamic airway collapse in persons with "floppy airways," such as those with airway malacia or bronchiectasis. β Agonists are also mucus secretagogues and therefore can potentially increase mucus plugging if they increase dynamic collapse and decrease expiratory airflow.

SURFACE-ACTIVE PHOSPHOLIPIDS

Surfactant is produced in the conducting airways as well as in the alveoli and is essential for mucociliary and cough clearance. A thin surfactant layer between the periciliary fluid and the mucus gel prevents airway dehydration, permits mucus spreading on extrusion from glands, and allows efficient ciliary coupling with mucus and, more importantly, ciliary release from mucus once kinetic energy is transmitted. With airway inflammation, surface-active phospholipids such as surfactant are often degraded by secretory phospholipases and inflammatory peptides can further inhibit surfactant function. In the absence of surfactant, mucus sticks to the epithelium, rendering cough less effective. There is severe loss of surfactant in the inflamed airway of patients with chronic bronchitis or CF.[105,106]

It has been reported in randomized, double-blind, placebo-controlled, multicenter studies that surfactant aerosol improves pulmonary function and sputum transportability in patients with chronic bronchitis or with CF, and that this effect is dose dependent. There were no significant side effects attributable to the surfactant therapy.[107] As a wetting and spreading agent, surfactant also has the ability to increase the lower airway deposition of other aerosol medications, such as dornase alfa or gene therapy vectors, and may increase small particle translocation through the mucus layer.[108]

MUCOREGULATORY MEDICATIONS

Another approach to reducing the burden of airway secretions is to decrease hypersecretion by goblet cells and submucosal glands. Medications that decrease mucus hypersecretion are referred to as **mucoregulatory medications**. These medications include antiinflammatory drugs such as corticosteroids, which are effective at decreasing the inflammatory stimulus that leads to mucus hypersecretion. Aerosolized indomethacin has also been used in Japan to treat patients with diffuse panbronchiolitis who have impairment due to mucus hypersecretion.[109]

Anticholinergic medications are also extensively used as mucoregulatory medications. Atropine is routinely given perioperatively to prevent laryngospasm and to decrease mucus secretion associated with endotracheal intubation. Atropine and its derivatives are mucoregulatory medications in that they do not "dry" secretions but will decrease hypersecretion that is mediated through M_3 cholinergic mechanisms. The quaternary ammonium derivatives of atropine, including ipratropium bromide and tiotropium, do not significantly cross the blood–airway barrier and, as such, their use is not associated with typical systemic effects of anticholinergic medications such as flushing or tachycardia. Ipratropium bromide is widely used as a bronchodilator medication in patients with chronic bronchitis. Studies have also shown that the long-term use of ipratropium is associated with a reduction in the volume of mucus secretion in patients with chronic bronchitis.[110] More specific M_3 antagonists hold the promise of improved mucoregulatory efficacy of this class of medications with less risk of adverse effects.

Some of the more interesting of the mucoregulatory medications are the macrolide antibiotics. These antibiotics were discovered about 50 years ago and derivatives of erythromycin A have been widely used for the treatment of bacterial infection. Since the mid-1960s data have been accumulating demonstrating that these medications also have immunomodulatory properties. This means that they decrease hyperimmunity or inflammation to more normal and beneficial levels. The mechanism for these properties appears to be different from that of the corticosteroids. These immunomodulatory and mucoregulatory properties of macrolide antibiotics have been exploited for the treatment of diffuse panbronchiolitis (DBP), a chronic inflammatory airway disease with great morbidity and mortality when untreated. DPB is seen primarily in Japan and Korea. Its etiology is unknown but the disease results in chronic sinobronchitis with mucus hypersecretion and debilitation. Antibiotics and corticosteroids are ineffective for the treatment of DPB. By virtue of their immunomodulatory and mucoregulatory properties, the macrolide antibiotics have been demonstrated to be the most effective agents for the treatment of DPB.[111] Accumulating evidence suggests that the 14- and 15-membered macrolides, but not the 16-member macrolides, may also be highly effective for the therapy of CF airway disease.[112,113] The mechanism of action of the macrolides as mucoregulatory agents is under intensive study.[114] It is anticipated that the development of macrolide medications without antibiotic properties will significantly extend the spectrum of use of these medications.

OTHER MUCOACTIVE AGENTS

Antiproteases

Persons with CF have increased activity of serine proteases on the respiratory epithelial surface. Neutrophils, when activated or degenerating, release proteases such as elastase that can directly damage epithelial cells and impair airway clearance. It has been shown that neutrophil proteases cause a secretory response from submucosal glands with an increase in mucus production.[115]

Intravenous administration or inhalation of α_1-antitrypsin suppresses the activity of neutrophil elastase and restores the bacteria-killing capacity of neutrophils. Recombinant secretory leukocyte protease inhibitor (rsLPI), when given to a small number of CF patients at a dose of 100 mg bid for 2 weeks, decreased neutrophil elastase and interleukin-8 in airway fluid but was ineffective at a dose of 50 mg bid. No significant side effects were reported.[116] Although promising, a number of issues need to be resolved before these or similar agents can be used to prevent damage due to unchecked protease activity in patients with CF.

Hyperosmolar Saline

For many years, sputum induction produced by hyperosmolar saline inhalation has been used to obtain specimens for the diagnosis of pneumonia. In a pilot study, 58 CF subjects were randomly assigned to receive 10 ml of either 0.9% normal saline or 6% hypertonic saline twice daily by ultrasonic nebulization.[117] Spirometry was performed before treatment, at the end of 2 weeks of treatment, and 2 weeks posttherapy. At the end of treatment there was a significant increase in FEV_1 (forced expiratory volume in 1 second) in the hypertonic saline group, with a return to baseline by 28 days. Despite pretreatment with 600 µg of inhaled albuterol, several patients had an acute decrease in FEV_1 after inhaling hypertonic saline. Similarly, hyperosmolar dry powder mannitol improves quality of life and pulmonary function in adult subjects with non-CF bronchiectasis and significantly improves the surface adhesivity and cough clearability of expectorated sputum.[118]

Subsequent studies, summarized in the Cochrane Database of Systematic Reviews, confirm that the long term use of inhaled hyperosmolar saline improves pulmonary function in patients with CF[119-121] and inhaled hyperosmolar saline or mannitol is beneficial in non-CF bronchiectasis.[122] Although this therapy is readily available and inexpensive, it has been reported that hypertonic saline aerosol is not as effective as dornase alfa in the therapy of CF lung disease.[123] Furthermore, hypertonic saline has an unpleasant taste and induces coughing; these features may limit its acceptance and hence its efficacy as a long-term therapy.

GENE THERAPY

Gene transfer therapy represents a novel use for aerosols. Efforts in this arena have centered largely on complementary DNA transfer of the normal CFTR gene in CF patients. Gene transfer was first attempted by inserting the normal CFTR gene into a replication-defective *Adenovirus* vector by bolus bronchoscopic delivery of the vector. An unanticipated host immune response to the vector led to reevaluation of this strategy.[124]

For gene transfer to be effective, the vector and its package must be nonimmunogenic, stable to shear forces during aerosolization, and safe to transfected cells. The vector should not increase cell turnover. It should either stably integrate into the progenitor (basal) cell genome or be safe and effective with repeated administration and should be able to reach the cellular target of relevance. Part of the difficulty with CF is that this cellular target has not been clearly identified as epithelial cell, goblet cell, submucous gland, or all of these. The amount of gene and vector and persistence in the airway must also be determined for each vector and delivery system.[125,126]

Viral vectors that have been studied include adenoviruses, adeno-associated virus, and lentivirus. *Adenoviruses* naturally target the airway epithelium. *Adeno-associated viruses (AAVs)* are very small organisms that require a "helper" virus to replicate. These viruses are capable of site-directed insertion into DNA, reducing the risk of insertional mutagenesis (initiating cancer by activation of an oncogene or inactivation of an oncogene suppressor). Gene therapy with the AAV appears to be especially promising.[127] *Lentiviruses* are retroviruses such as human immunodeficiency virus (HIV). They are able to transfect cells that are not terminally differentiated, such as the basal or airway progenitor cell, but insertional mutagenesis is a substantial risk.[128]

The primary nonviral vectors studied to date have been cationic *liposomes.* These lipid capsules are able to form complexes with DNA and then enter cells. With the first generation of liposome vectors, the efficiency of gene transfer was poor; however, this has improved dramatically with newer systems.[129,130]

USING MUCOACTIVE THERAPY WITH PHYSIOTHERAPY AND AIRWAY CLEARANCE DEVICES

A number of physical factors affect secretion clearance. Cephalad airflow bias is responsible for the movement of mucus in airways during normal ventilation.[131-133] The narrowing of airways on exhalation increases the velocity and shearing forces in the airway, creating a cephalad airflow bias with tidal breathing. This bias is amplified during coughing, when increased transmural pressure causes the airways to fold and constrict, increasing airflow velocity even further.[134]

In acute airway diseases leading to ciliary dysfunction and/or mucus hypersecretion, cough is the primary mechanism for secretion clearance from the central airways, and cephalad airflow contributes increasingly to peripheral airway clearance. Cough is one of the most common respiratory complaints of patients seeking medical attention.[135] During a normal cough, the expiratory airflow rises to a maximum along with narrowing of the intrathoracic airways. The narrowing of the airways is a product of high airflows and pressure differentials across the lung. Airflow velocity varies inversely with the cross-sectional area of the airways, creating high linear velocity, increased turbulence, high shearing forces within the airway, and high kinetic energy. These forces shear secretions and debris from the airway walls, propelling them toward the central and upper airway, where they are expectorated or swallowed. In chronic obstructive pulmonary disease, narrowing airways may close prematurely, trapping gas, reducing expiratory flow rates, and limiting the effectiveness of the cough.

Gravity

Gravity is not a primary mechanism for normal mucociliary transport. In health, the viscosity of the normal mucus blanket is sufficient to resist the flow of mucus into gravity-dependent terminal bronchioles. Conventional chest physiotherapy (CPT) incorporating postural drainage results in significantly greater expectoration than no treatment in patients with cystic fibrosis (CF).[136] Conventional CPT has become the "gold standard" with which all other bronchial hygiene techniques are compared. However, there is no proven benefit to adding postural drainage to less conventional CPT, such as those described below, and postural drainage carries a risk for patients with gastroesophageal reflux or muscle weakness.

Insufflation–Exsufflation

An insufflation–exsufflation device inflates the lungs with positive pressure followed by a negative pressure to simulate a cough.[137] The cycle begins with an inspiratory pressure of 25 to 35 cmH$_2$O for 1 to 2 seconds, followed by an expiratory pressure of 30 to 40 cmH$_2$O for 1 to 2 seconds. It can be used with an oronasal mask or attached to an artificial airway.

Active Cycle of Breathing and Forced Expiratory Technique Maneuver

The active cycle of breathing (ACB) technique involves a combination of breathing control (relaxed diaphragmatic breathing), thoracic expansion control (deep breaths), and forced expiration from progressively increasing lung volumes. Although often used by patients with CF, there are no controlled studies documenting benefit from this mode of airway clearance.

The forced expiratory technique (FET) consists of a breath taken in to mid-lung volume and air squeezed out by contracting the chest wall and abdominal muscles with the mouth and glottis kept open. The huff should not be a violent or explosive exhalation.[138,139] Exercise should be encouraged with patients, who often find that it is associated with requirements for shorter ACB sessions.

Autogenic Drainage

Autogenic drainage (AD) aims to "optimize" airflow in the various generations of bronchi to move secretions without forced expirations.[140,141] It has not been demonstrated to be as effective as CPT in mobilizing secretions. This technique incorporates staged breathing starting with small tidal breaths from expiratory reserve volume (ERV), repeated until secretions "collect" in the central airways. Patients are instructed to suppress cough, and a larger volume is taken for a series of 10-20 breaths, followed by a series of even larger (approaching vital capacity [VC]) breaths, in turn followed by several huff coughs. This technique requires a great deal of patient cooperation, and is recommended only for patients >8 years of age and for those who have a good sense of their own breathing. Some uncontrolled studies have reported similar secretion clearance with AD and postural drainage (PD).[142,143]

Exercise

Exercise causes increased sputum production compared with rest.[144,145] Exercise appears to augment bronchial hygiene, and should be encouraged, as tolerated; however, it should not substitute for other bronchial hygiene regimens.

Positive Airway Pressure

Positive airway pressure (PAP) techniques can be effective alternatives to chest physical therapy in expanding the lungs and mobilizing secretions. Evidence suggests that PAP therapy is more effective than incentive spirometry and intermittent positive pressure breathing (IPPB) in the management of postoperative atelectasis[146,147] and as an adjunct to enhance the benefits of aerosol bronchodilator delivery.[148,149] Cough, FET, and other airway clearance techniques are components of PAP therapy.

Pursed-lip breathing is a procedure that many patients with chronic obstructive lung disease have taught themselves to relieve air trapping caused by collapse of unstable airways during expiration. The resistance at the mouth during a pursed-lip exhalation transmits back pressure to splint the airways open, preventing compression and premature closure (much like a fixed orifice resistor). Pursed-lip breathing represents a functional predecessor to modern strategies of applying positive expiratory pressure to the airway. By preventing expiratory airway collapse, PAP may improve the distribution of ventilation throughout the lungs, via collateral intrabronchiolar channels.[150,151]

High-Frequency Techniques

High-frequency oscillation (HFO) of the air column in the conducting airways has been shown to enhance clearance of secretions. HFO can be generated by devices providing the oscillations at the airway opening or on the chest wall. The oscillations can be mechanically generated and administered to the patient, or self-generated by expiration through an oscillatory device. High-frequency oscillations can influence mucus clearance through a variety of mechanisms, including alteration of mucus rheology, enhanced mucus–airflow interaction, and reflex mechanisms.

Shearing at the air–mucus interface could be a significant factor in the enhanced tracheal mucus clearance during HFO.[152] Although the mechanism for the reduction in viscoelasticity is unknown, likely possibilities involve cooperative unfolding of the physical entanglements between the primary network of mucus glycoproteins and other structural macromolecules, the rupture of cross-linking bonds such as disulfide bridges, or the fragmentation of larger molecules such as DNA or F-actin, which are present as a by-product of infection and can increase mucus viscoelasticity due to their interactions with glycoproteins. Pilot studies suggest that dornase alfa is most effective for CF when given during HFO therapy as opposed to before or after therapy.

High-frequency chest wall compression (HFCWC) increases tracheal mucus clearance rates and correlates with improved ventilation. HFCWC may reduce the viscoelastic and cohesive properties of mucus,[42,153] thus making it more easily clearable. In addition, the high-frequency oscillations may reinforce the interaction with cilia or the natural harmonics of the chest wall. The oscillations may stimulate release of fresh secretions by a vagal reflex mechanism.

Oscillation of the Airway

The Flutter mucus clearance device combines the techniques of positive expiratory pressure (PEP) with high-frequency oscillations at the airway opening. The weight of the ball serves as a PEP device (approximately 10 cmH$_2$O), and the internal shape of the bowl allows the ball to flutter, generating oscillations of about 15 Hz (2-32 Hz), varying with position of the device. The proposed mechanism of effect includes shearing of mucus from the airway wall by oscillatory action; stabilization of airways, preventing early airway closure; facilitation of cephalad flow of mucus; and changes in mucus rheology.

Although the Flutter has been available since about 1994, little has been published on its efficacy. In one study[154] the amount of sputum expectorated by subjects with CF was more than three times the amount expectorated with either voluntary cough or postural drainage. Another study reported that Flutter valve therapy was an acceptable alternative to conventional CPT in hospitalized patients with CF.[155] However, these results have not been confirmed by other studies, the relevance of expectorated sputum volume to clinical effectiveness is unproven, and most of the more recent studies of the Flutter have not shown it to be effective for airway clearance.[156-160] We generally do not recommend the use of this device.

Intrapulmonary percussive ventilation (IPV) of the lungs involves the use of a pneumatic device called a Percussionator to treat atelectasis, enhance the mobilization and clearance of retained secretions, and deliver nebulized medications to the distal airways.[161] With IPV, the patient breathes through a mouthpiece that delivers high-flow minibursts at rates exceeding 200 cycles/min. During these percussive bursts of gas into the airway, continuous airway pressure is maintained while the pulsatile percussive intraairway pressure rises progressively. Each percussive cycle is programmed by holding a thumb button for 5 to 10 seconds for the percussive inspiratory cycle, and releasing the button for exhalation. Treatments of approximately 20 minutes are recommended by the manufacturer. Impaction pressures of 25 to 40 psig (pounds-force per square inch gauge) are delivered at a frequency ranging from <100 to 225 percussive cycles/min at 40 psig. Some small studies have reported comparable results with IPV and standard chest physical therapy.[162-164]

Chest Wall Oscillation

The vest consists of a large-volume variable-frequency air pulse delivery system attached to a nonstretchable inflatable vest that is worn by the patient so that it extends over the entire torso down to the iliac crest. Pressure pulses that fill the vest and vibrate the chest wall are controlled by the patient (with a foot pedal) and applied during expiration or the entire respiratory cycle. Pulse frequency is adjustable from 5 to 25 Hz, with pressure in the vest varying from 28 mmHg at 5 Hz to 39 mmHg at 25 Hz. However, it is generally recommended that the oscillatory frequency be held at a single frequency between 10 and 15 Hz for the duration of therapy. In theory, vibrations to the chest wall cause transient increases in airflow in the lungs, to improve gas–liquid interactions and the movement of mucus. The frequency of oscillations (cycles per second) and flow bias (inspiratory vs. expiratory) are important in determining effectiveness.[165,166] The Vest has been reported to be effective for secretion clearance in patients with CF.[167-169] Conjecture that this device has a role in lung expansion for patients other than those with cystic fibrosis in the acute care setting has not been empirically established.

FUTURE MUCUS-CONTROLLING AGENTS

To improve mucus transport, both elasticity and viscosity must be considered. Mucolytics have been targeted only at lowering the viscosity of mucus. In the context of the normal physiology of ciliary movement, logic dictates that thicker and denser strands of mucus would be moved more efficiently by ciliary contact and elastic recovery than would thin, low-viscosity solutions. The conceptual analogy is that of raking water—little transport will occur. This assumes mucus clearance is being optimized *physiologically*. Endotracheal aspiration of secretions by suction would be easier with low-viscosity mucus. Research supports the theory that elasticity is important for mucus transport.[68,170]

It has been suggested that the treatment of bronchial hypersecretion would be better aimed at *normalizing* the rheological properties of mucus to optimize transport, rather than at simply lysing or liquefying bronchial secretions as traditionally done. Indeed, cough clearance is enhanced by a highly cohesive and viscous secretion that is not sticking to the airway wall. In this sense it can be considered easier to expel a solid pea from a pea shooter than it would be to "shoot" out pea soup.

Purulent sputum has high elasticity *and* viscosity, and mucolytic agents such as dornase alfa might restore normal transport properties by lowering tenacity, viscosity, and elasticity. With low viscoelasticity (e.g., bronchorrhea), restructuring or cross-linking agents would increase both viscosity and elasticity to improve transport. Such agents have been termed **mucospissic**.[171,172] Agents with mucospissic activity include sodium tetraborate, Congo red, and tetracycline.[170] The thickening effect of tetracycline can occur with oral and aerosol administration, although more so with direct aerosol. Tetracycline may bind to mucus proteins to increase viscosity and elasticity, although exact binding sites remain unclear.

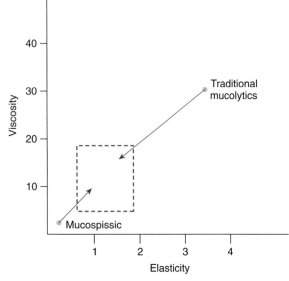

FIGURE 9-10 Conceptual representation of an optimal range of viscosity and elasticity of mucus for mucociliary transport.

With very adhesive sputum (CF, asthma, chronic bronchitis) mucokinetic agents that decrease tenacity while preserving viscoelasticity might be useful. At present there are no drugs available as mucus-controlling agents in the United States that will selectively modify viscosity or elasticity.

Further investigation may produce clinically useful agents tailored to specific secretion problems, as illustrated in Figure 9-10. The first step has been to recognize the complex rheologic and tenacious nature of mucus and the necessity for cross-linking to provide adequate elasticity for efficient ciliary transport. The second step has been to increase our understanding of the structure of mucus and regulation of its production. Finally, a better understanding of adhesivity and cohesivity, the components of tenacity, has focused attention on control of the abnormal surface properties of mucus and sputum and their role in cough clearance.

RESPIRATORY CARE ASSESSMENT OF MUCOACTIVE DRUG THERAPY

Assessment of drug therapy for respiratory secretions is difficult: FEV_1 is relatively insensitive to changes in mucociliary clearance. The rate of change in lung function over time is a better marker. In addition, during maintenance therapy, the volume of sputum expectorated is variable from day to day and does not reflect effective therapy. Therefore, the following assessments should be performed.

Before Treatment

• Assess patient's adequacy of cough and level of consciousness to determine need for mechanical suctioning or need for adjunct bronchial hygiene (postural drainage or percussion, PEP therapy) to clear airway with treatment, or whether treatment is contraindicated.

During Treatment and Short Term

• Instruct and then verify correct use of aerosol nebulization system, including cleaning.
• Assess therapy based on indication for drug: mucolysis and improved clearance of secretions.
  • Monitor airflow changes for adverse effects such as a fall in FEV_1.
• Assess breathing pattern and rate.
• Assess patient's subjective reaction to treatment, that is, changes in breathing effort or pattern.
• Discontinue therapy if patient experiences adverse reactions.

Long Term

• Monitor number and severity of respiratory tract infections, need for antibiotic therapy, emergency visits, and hospitalizations.
• Monitor pulmonary function for improvement or slowing of the rate of deterioration.

General Contraindications

• In general, if the FEV_1 is less than 25% of predicted, it becomes difficult to mobilize and expectorate secretions. Theoretically, with profound airflow compromise, secretion clearance could decline.
• Use mucoactive therapy with caution in patients with severely compromised vital capacity and expiratory flow, such as in the presence of end-stage pulmonary disease or neuromuscular disorders.
• Gastroesophageal reflux and/or inability of the patient to protect the airway are risk factors for postural drainage, if that is necessary with mucoactive therapy. Mucoactive agents should be discontinued if there is evidence of clinical deterioration.
• Patients with acute bronchitis or exacerbation of chronic disease (CF and COPD) may be less responsive to mucoactive therapy, possibly because of infection and muscular weakness, which can further reduce airflow dependent mechanisms.

SELF-ASSESSMENT QUESTIONS

1. Identify the two mucolytic agents approved for inhalation as an aerosol in the United States—give the generic and brand names.
2. What is the mode of action for dornase alfa?
3. What is the clinical indication for use of dornase alfa?
4. What are contraindications to the use of mucolytic medications?
5. How do macrolide antibiotics affect mucus and what are their indications for use?
6. How should dornase alfa be administered when high-frequency oscillation is used?
7. What is a common side effect seen with NAC by aerosol?
8. What are the indications for the use of acetylcysteine?
9. How and when should bicarbonate aerosol or instillation be used?

Answers to Self-Assessment Questions appear in Appendix A.

CLINICAL SCENARIO

A 17-year-old woman with CF was admitted to your hospital with an acute respiratory infection (pulmonary exacerbation). She is pleasant, mature, and well informed concerning her disease. She complains of an increased cough, increased sputum production, with some hemoptysis, and weight loss over the past 2 weeks.

History: She was diagnosed with CF at the age of 2 years because of failure to thrive, and did well clinically until age 12. She has had a nasal polypectomy, and a G-tube placed for night feeding several years ago, which resulted in a weight gain of 30 pounds (13.6 kg). She is chronically infected with resistant *Pseudomonas* and *Stenotrophomonas* and she has grown atypical *Mycobacterium* in the past. She has been admitted with exacerbations of CF twice in the past year. She has been taking 300 mg of tobramycin (TOBI) bid by aerosol at home regularly this year, with courses of oral ciprofloxacin when symptoms of respiratory infection surfaced.

Physical examination: Vital signs are as follows: temperature (T), 37.5° C; pulse (P), 110 and regular; respiratory rate (RR), 26 breaths/min; blood pressure (BP), 110/50. Oxygen saturation by pulse oximetry (SpO_2) is 0.92 in ambient air. She has mild dyspnea while walking. Auscultation of the chest revealed crackles in all fields, with more in the right upper lobe. Extremities showed clubbing with no cyanosis. She has a cough productive of greenish, thick sputum. No nasal polyps are visible to examination.

Laboratory: Electrolytes were normal; hemoglobin, 14.3 g/dl; hematocrit, 44%; white blood cell count (WBC), 13.4×10^3 cells/mm^3. Chest radiograph (posteroanterior [PA] and lateral) shows diffuse chronic changes with thick interstitial markings consistent with bronchiectasis, and a normal cardiac silhouette. There is an infiltrate in the right upper lobe. Her pulmonary function test results show the following:

Observed	% Predicted
Forced vital capacity (FVC)	72
Forced expiratory volume in 1 second (FEV$_1$)	55
Functional residual capacity	121

Hospital course: After her admission, she was treated for the next 21 days with a course of IV antibiotics in addition to her usual medications of pancreatic enzymes and vitamin supplements, albuterol by aerosol before chest physical therapy, nocturnal tube feedings, and oxygen 1 LPM (liter per minute) at night. Her symptoms of dyspnea and her weight improved. She continues to have a productive cough with thick sputum, although the hemoptysis has disappeared. She is clinically stable, and is ready to be discharged.

What aerosol medications would be indicated for her?

What outcomes would you assess to determine the effectiveness of dornase alfa in her case?

Answers to Clinical Scenario Questions appear in Appendix A.

References

1. Denton R, Forsman W, Hwang SH, Litt M, Miller CE: Viscoelasticity of mucus: its role in ciliary transport of pulmonary secretions, *Am Rev Respir Dis* 98:380, 1968.
2. Sackner MA: Effect of respiratory drugs on mucociliary clearance, *Chest* 73(6 Suppl):958, 1978.
3. Puchelle E, de Bentzmann S, Zahm JM: Physical and functional properties of airway secretions in cystic fibrosis: therapeutic approaches, *Respiration* 62(suppl 1):2, 1995.
4. Rogers DF: Mucoactive drugs for asthma and COPD: any place in therapy?, *Expert Opin Investig Drugs* 11:15, 2002.
5. Basbaum C, Carlson D, Davidson E, Verdugo P, Gail DB: NHLBI workshop summary: cellular mechanisms of airway secretion, *Am Rev Respir Dis* 137:479, 1988.
6. Reid L, Clamp JR: The biochemical and histochemical nomenclature of mucus, *Br Med Bull* 34:5, 1978.

7. Basbaum CB: Airway mucin: chairman's summary, *Am Rev Respir Dis* 144:S2, 1991.

8. King M, Rubin BK: Mucus-controlling agents: past and present, *Respir Care Clin N Am* 5:575, 1999.

9. Luk CK, Dulfano MJ: Effect of pH, viscosity and ionic-strength changes on ciliary beating frequency of human bronchial explants, *Clin Sci (Lond)* 64:449, 1983.

10. Sleigh MA, Blake JR, Liron N: The propulsion of mucus by cilia, *Am Rev Respir Dis* 137:726, 1988.

11. Pinnock CB, Graham NM, Mylvaganam A, Douglas RM: Relationship between milk intake and mucus production in adult volunteers challenged with rhinovirus-2, *Am Rev Respir Dis* 141:352, 1990.

12. Lundgren JD, Shelhamer JH: Pathogenesis of airway mucus hypersecretion, *J Allergy Clin Immunol* 85:399, 1990.

13. Rose MC, Voynow JA: Respiratory tract mucin genes and mucin glycoproteins in health and disease, *Physiol Rev* 86:245, 2006.

14. Perez-Vilar J, Boucher RC: Reevaluating gel-forming mucins' roles in cystic fibrosis lung disease, *Free Radic Biol Med* 37:1564, 2004.

15. Boat TF, Cheng PW: Biochemistry of airway mucus secretions, *Fed Proc* 39:3067, 1980.

16. Kaliner M, Marom Z, Patow C, Shelhamer J: Human respiratory mucus, *J Allergy Clin Immunol* 73:318, 1984.

17. Kaliner M, Shelhamer JH, Borson B, Nadel J, Patow C, Marom Z: Human respiratory mucus, *Am Rev Respir Dis* 134:612, 1986.

18. Thornton DJ, Sheehan JK, Lindgren H, Carlstedt I: Mucus glycoproteins from cystic fibrotic sputum: macromolecular properties and structural "architecture," *Biochem J* 276:667, 1991.

19. Sheehan JK, Richardson PS, Fung DC, Howard M, Thornton DJ: Analysis of respiratory mucus glycoproteins in asthma: a detailed study from a patient who died in status asthmaticus, *Am J Respir Cell Mol Biol* 13:748, 1995.

20. Davies JR, Hovenberg HW, Linden CJ, Howard R, Richardson PS, Sheehan JK, Carlstedt I: Mucins in airway secretions from healthy and chronic bronchitic subjects, *Biochem J* 313:431, 1996.

21. Reid CJ, Gould S, Harris A: Developmental expression of mucin genes in the human respiratory tract, *Am J Respir Cell Mol Biol* 17:592, 1997.

22. Davies JR, Herrmann A, Russell W, Svitacheva N, Wickstrom C, Carlstedt I: Respiratory tract mucins: structure and expression patterns, *Novartis Found Symp* 248:76, 2002.

23. Rose MC, Nickola TJ, Voynow JA: Airway mucus obstruction: mucin glycoproteins, *MUC* gene regulation and goblet cell hyperplasia, *Am J Respir Cell Mol Biol* 25:533, 2001.

24. Kirkham S, Sheehan JK, Knight D, Richardson PS, Thornton DJ: Heterogeneity of airways mucus: variations in the amounts and glycoforms of the major oligomeric mucins MUC5AC and MUC5B, *Biochem J* 361:537, 2002.

25. Wickstrom C, Davies JR, Eriksen GV, Veerman EC, Carlstedt I: MUC5B is a major gel-forming, oligomeric mucin from human salivary gland, respiratory tract and endocervix: identification of glycoforms and C-terminal cleavage, *Biochem J* 334:685, 1998.

26. Thornton DJ, Carlstedt I, Howard M, Devine PL, Price MR, Sheehan JK: Respiratory mucins: identification of core proteins and glycoforms, *Biochem J* 316:967, 1996.

27. Rose MC, Gendler SJ: Airway mucin genes and gene products, In: Rogers DF, Lethem MI, editors: *Airway mucus basic mechanisms and clinical perspectives*, Basel, Switzerland, 1997, Birkhauser.

28. Leikauf GD, Borchers MT, Prows DR, Simpson LG: Mucin apoprotein expression in COPD, *Chest* 121(5 suppl):166S, 2002.

29. Williams SJ, Wreschner DH, Tran M, Eyre HJ, Sutherland GR, McGuckin MA: Muc13, a novel human cell surface mucin expressed by epithelial and hemopoietic cells, *J Biol Chem* 276:18327, 2001.

30. Pallesen LT, Berglund L, Rasmussen LK, Petersen TE, Rasmussen JT: Isolation and characterization of MUC15, a novel cell membrane-associated mucin, *Eur J Biochem* 269:2755, 2002.

31. Chen Y, Zhao YH, Kalaslavadi TB, Hamati E, Nehrke K, Le AD, Ann DK, Wu R: Genome-wide search and identification of a novel gel-forming mucin MUC19/Muc19 in glandular tissues, *Am J Respir Cell Mol Biol* 30:155, 2004.

32. Higuchi T, Orita T, Nakanishi S, Katsuya K, Watanabe H, Yamasaki Y, Waga I, Nanayama T, Yamamoto Y, Munger W, *et al*: Molecular cloning, genomic structure, and expression analysis of MUC20, a novel mucin protein, up-regulated in injured kidney, *J Biol Chem* 279:1968, 2004.

33. Rogers DF: Airway submucosal gland and goblet cell secretion, In: Chung KF, Barnes PJ, editors: *Pharmacology of the respiratory tract*, New York, 1993, Marcel Dekker.

34. Lopez-Vidriero MT: Airway mucus: production and composition, *Chest* 80(6 suppl):799, 1981.

35. Matthews LW, Spector S, Lemm J, Potter JL: Studies on pulmonary secretions. I. The overall chemical composition of pulmonary secretions from patients with cystic fibrosis, bronchiectasis, and laryngectomy, *Am Rev Respir Dis* 88:199, 1963.

36. Dulfano MJ, Adler K, Wooten O: Physical properties of sputum. IV. Effects of 100 per cent humidity and water mist, *Am Rev Respir Dis* 107:130, 1973.

37. Birrer P: Proteases and antiproteases in cystic fibrosis: pathogenetic considerations and therapeutic strategies, *Respiration* 62(suppl 1):25, 1995.

38. Clarke LL, Boucher R: Ion and water transport across airway epithelia, In: Chung KF, Barnes PJ, editors: *Pharmacology of the respiratory tract: experimental and clinical research*, New York, 1993, Marcel Dekker.

39. Boucher RC: Human airway ion transport: part one, *Am J Respir Crit Care Med* 150:271, 1994.

40. Boucher RC: Human airway ion transport: part two, *Am J Respir Crit Care Med* 150:581, 1994.

41. Knowles MR, Olivier KN, Hohneker KW, Robinson J, Bennett WD, Boucher RC: Pharmacological treatment of abnormal ion transport in the airway epithelium in cystic fibrosis, *Chest* 107:71S, 1995.

42. Tomkiewicz RP, Biviji A, King M: Effects of oscillating air flow on the rheological properties and clearability of mucous gel simulants, *Biorheology* 31:511, 1994.

43. Shah SA, Santago P, Rubin BK: Quantification of biopolymer filament structure, *Ultramicroscopy* 104:244, 2005.

44. Henke MO, Renner A, Huber RM, Seeds MC, Rubin BK: MUC5AC and MUC5B mucins are decreased in cystic fibrosis airway secretions, *Am J Respir Cell Mol Biol* 31:86, 2004.

45. Rubin BK, van der Schans CP: Therapy for mucus clearance disorders, In: Lenfant C, editor: *Biology of the lung series*, New York, 2004, Marcel Dekker.

46. Hodgkin JE: *Chronic obstructive pulmonary disease: current concepts in diagnosis and comprehensive care*, Park Ridge, Ill, 1979, American College of Chest Physicians.

47. Reid L: Measurement of the bronchial mucous gland layer: a diagnostic yardstick in chronic bronchitis, *Thorax* 15:132, 1960.

48. Sturgess J, Reid L: An organ culture study of the effect of drugs on the secretory activity of the human bronchial submucosal gland, *Clin Sci* 43:533, 1972.

49. Rubin BK, Kishioka C, van der Schans CP, Dowell A, Fiel S: Mucus and mucoactive therapy in chronic bronchitis, *Clin Pulm Med* 5:1, 1998.

50. Vestbo J, Prescott E, Lange P, Copenhagen City Heart Study Group: Association of chronic mucus hypersecretion with FEV$_1$ decline and chronic obstructive pulmonary disease morbidity, *Am J Respir Crit Care Med* 153:1530, 1996.

51. Turner-Warwick M, Openshaw P: Sputum in asthma, *Postgrad Med J* 63(suppl 1):79, 1987.

52. Rubin BK, Tomkiewicz R, Fahy JV, Green FH: Histopathology of fatal asthma: drowning in mucus, *Pediatr Pulmonol Suppl* 23:88, 2001.

53. Webber SE, Widdicombe JG: The actions of methacholine, phenylephrine, salbutamol and histamine on mucus secretion from the ferret *in vitro* trachea, *Agents Actions* 22:82, 1987.

54. Shimura S, Sasaki T, Sasaki H, Takishima T: Chemical properties of bronchorrhea sputum in bronchial asthma, *Chest* 94:1211, 1988.

55. Marom Z, Shelhamer J, Alling D, Kaliner M: The effects of corticosteroids on mucous glycoprotein secretion from human airways *in vitro*, *Am Rev Respir Dis* 129:62, 1984.

56. Tamaoki J, Chiyotani A, Kobayashi K, Sakai N, Kanemura T, Takizawa T: Effect of indomethacin on bronchorrhea in patients with chronic bronchitis, diffuse panbronchiolitis, or bronchiectasis, *Am Rev Respir Dis* 145:548, 1992.

57. Marom ZM, Goswami SK: Respiratory mucus hypersecretion (bronchorrhea): a case discussion—possible mechanisms(s) and treatment, *J Allergy Clin Immunol* 87:1050, 1991.

58. Rubin BK, MacLeod PM, Sturgess J, King M: Recurrent respiratory infections in a child with fucosidosis: is the mucus too thin for effective transport?, *Pediatr Pulmonol* 10:304, 1991.

59. Madsen P, Shah SA, Rubin BK: Plastic bronchitis: new insights and a classification scheme, *Paediatr Respir Rev* 6:292, 2005.

60. Rubin BK, Henke MO: Immunomodulatory activity and effectiveness of macrolides in chronic airway disease, *Chest* 125(2 suppl):70S, 2004.

61. Bush A, Payne D, Pike S, Jenkins G, Henke MO, Rubin BK: Mucus properties in children with primary ciliary dyskinesia: comparison with cystic fibrosis, *Chest* 129:118, 2006.

62. Albers GM, Tomkiewicz RP, May MK, Ramirez OE, Rubin BK: Ring distraction technique for measuring surface tension of sputum: relationship to sputum clearability, *J Appl Physiol* 81:2690, 1996.

63. King M, Rubin BK: Rheology of airway mucus: Relationship with transport, In: Takishima T, Shimura S, editors: *Airway secretion: physiological bases for the control of mucous hypersecretion*, New York, 1994, Marcel Dekker.

64. Rubin BK, King M: Mucus physiology and pathophysiology: therapeutic aspects, In: Derenne JP, Similowski T, Whitelaw WA, editors: *Acute respiratory failure in chronic obstructive lung disease*, New York, 1996, Marcel Dekker.

65. Rubin BK: Frontiers in mucus clearance, In: Goldstein AL, editor: *Frontiers in biomedicine*, New York, 2000, Kluwer Academic/Plenum Publishers.

66. Puchelle E, Zahm JM, Duvivier C: Spinability of bronchial mucus: relationship with viscoelasticity and mucous transport properties, *Biorheology* 20:239, 1983.

67. Lourenco RV: Bronchial mucous secretions: introduction, *Chest* 63(suppl):56S, 1973.

68. Dulfano MJ, Adler KB: Physical properties of sputum. VII. Rheologic properties and mucociliary transport, *Am Rev Respir Dis* 112:341, 1975.

69. Hirsch SR: Airway mucus and the mucociliary system, In: Middleton E Jr, Reed CE, Ellis EF, editors: *Allergy: principles and practice*, St. Louis, Mo, 1983, Mosby.

70. Kilburn KH: A hypothesis for pulmonary clearance and its implications, *Am Rev Respir Dis* 98:449, 1968.

71. King M, Gilboa A, Meyer FA, Silberberg A: On the transport of mucus and its rheologic simulants in ciliated systems, *Am Rev Respir Dis* 110:740, 1974.

72. Marin MG: Pharmacology of airway secretion, *Pharmacol Rev* 38:273, 1986.

73. Shah S, Fung K, Brim S, Rubin BK: An *in vitro* evaluation of the effectiveness of endotracheal suction catheters, *Chest* 128:3699, 2005.

74. Rogers DF: Mucus hypersecretion in chronic obstructive pulmonary disease, *Novartis Found Symp* 234:65, 2001.

75. Barton AD: Aerosolized detergents and mucolytic agents in the treatment of stable chronic obstructive pulmonary disease, *Am Rev Respir Dis* 110:104, 1974.

76. Wanner A, Rao A: Clinical indications for and effects of bland, mucolytic, and antimicrobial aerosols, *Am Rev Respir Dis* 122:79, 1980.

77. Macy AM: Preventing hepatotoxicity in acetaminophen overdose, *Am J Nurs* 79:301, 1979.

78. Decramer M, Rutten-van Molken M, Dekhuijzen PN, Troosters T, van Herwaarden C, Pellegrino R, van Schayck CP, Olivieri D, Del Donno M, De Backer W, *et al*: Effects of N-acetylcysteine on outcomes in chronic obstructive pulmonary disease (Bronchitis Randomized on NAC Cost-Utility Study, BRONCUS): a randomised placebo-controlled trial, *Lancet* 365:1552, 2005.

79. App EM, Baran D, Dab I, Malfroot A, Coffiner M, Vanderbist F, King M: Dose-finding and 24-h monitoring for efficacy and safety of aerosolized Nacystelyn in cystic fibrosis, *Eur Respir J* 19:294, 2002.

80. Feng W, Garrett H, Speert DP, King M: Improved clearability of cystic fibrosis sputum with dextran treatment *in vitro*, *Am J Respir Crit Care Med* 157:710, 1998.

81. McCoy K, Hamilton S, Johnson C, Pulmozyme Study Group: Effects of 12-week administration of dornase alfa in patients with advanced cystic fibrosis lung disease, *Chest* 110:889, 1996.

82. Wilmott RW, Amin RS, Colin AA, DeVault A, Dozor AJ, Eigen H, Johnson C, Lester LA, McCoy K, McKean LP, *et al*: Aerosolized recombinant human DNase in hospitalized cystic fibrosis patients with acute pulmonary exacerbations, *Am J Respir Crit Care Med* 153:1914, 1996.

83. O'Donnell AE, Barker AF, Ilowite JS, Fick RB, rhDNase Study Group: Treatment of idiopathic bronchiectasis with aerosolized recombinant human DNase I, *Chest* 113:1329, 1998.

84. Henke MO, Saha AS, Rubin BK: The role of airway secretions in COPD: clinical applications, *COPD* 3:377, 2005.

85. Aitken ML, Burke W, McDonald G, Shak S, Montgomery AB, Smith A: Recombinant human DNase inhalation in normal subjects and patients with cystic fibrosis: a phase 1 study, *JAMA* 267:1947, 1992.

86. Shak S, Capon DJ, Hellmiss R, Marsters SA, Baker CL: Recombinant human DNase I reduces the viscosity of cystic fibrosis sputum, *Proc Natl Acad Sci USA* 87:9188, 1990.

87. Raskin P: Bronchospasm after inhalation of pancreatic dornase, *Am Rev Respir Dis* 98:697, 1968.

88. Fiel SB, Fuchs HJ, Johnson C, Gonda I, Clark AR, Pulmozyme rhDNase Study Group: Comparison of three jet nebulizer aerosol delivery systems used to administer recombinant human DNase I to patients with cystic fibrosis, *Chest* 108:153, 1995.

89. Ramsey BW, Dorkin HL: Consensus conference: practical applications of Pulmozyme. September 22, 1993, *Pediatr Pulmonol* 17:404, 1994.

90. Rubin BK, Kater AP, Goldstein AL: Thymosin β_4 sequesters actin in cystic fibrosis sputum and decreases sputum cohesivity, *Chest* 130:1433, 2006.

91. Pollard TD, Blanchoin L, Mullins RD: Molecular mechanisms controlling actin filament dynamics in nonmuscle cells, *Annu Rev Biophys Biomol Struct* 29:545, 2000.

92. Rubin BK, Kater AP, Goldstein AL: Thymosin β4 sequesters actin in cystic fibrosis sputum and decreases sputum cohesivity *in vitro*, *Chest* 130:1433, 2006.

93. Vasconcellos CA, Allen PG, Wohl ME, Drazen JM, Janmey PA, Stossel TP: Reduction in viscosity of cystic fibrosis sputum *in vitro* by gelsolin, *Science* 263:969, 1994.

94. Dasgupta B: Rheological properties in cystic fibrosis and airway secretions with combined rhDNase and gelsolin treatment, In: Singh M, Savena VP, editors: *Advances in physiological fluid dynamics*, New Delhi, India, 1996, Narosa.

95. Pavia D, Agnew JE, Glassman JM, Sutton PP, Lopez-Vidriero MT, Soyka JP, Clarke SW: Effects of iodopropylidene glycerol on tracheobronchial clearance in stable, chronic bronchitic patients, *Eur J Respir Dis* 67:177, 1985.

96. Rubin BK, Ramirez O, Ohar JA: Iodinated glycerol has no effect on pulmonary function, symptom score, or sputum properties in patients with stable chronic bronchitis, *Chest* 109:348, 1996.

97. Rubin BK: An *in vitro* comparison of the mucoactive properties of guaifenesin, iodinated glycerol, surfactant, and albuterol, *Chest* 116:195, 1999.

98. Waldron-Edward D, Skoryna SC: The mucolytic activity of amides: a new approach to mucus dispersion, *Can Med Assoc J* 94:1249, 1966.

99. Marriott C, Richards JH: The effects of storage and of potassium iodide, urea, *N*-acetyl-cysteine and Triton X-100 on the viscosity of bronchial mucus, *Br J Dis Chest* 68:171, 1974.

100. Ahmed T, Garrigo J, Danta I: Preventing bronchoconstriction in exercise-induced asthma with inhaled heparin, *N Engl J Med* 329:90, 1993.

101. Stutts MJ, Fitz JG, Paradiso AM, Boucher RC: Multiple modes of regulation of airway epithelial chloride secretion by extracellular ATP, *Am J Physiol* 267:C1442, 1994.

102. Noone PG, Hamblett N, Accurso F, Aitken ML, Boyle M, Dovey M, Gibson R, Johnson C, Kellerman D, Konstan MW, *et al*: Cystic Fibrosis Therapeutics Development Research Group: Safety of aerosolized INS 365 in patients with mild to moderate cystic fibrosis: results of a phase I multi-center study, *Pediatr Pulmonol* 32:122, 2001.

103. Deterding R, Retsch-Bogart G, Milgram L, Gibson R, Daines C, Zeitlin PL, Milla C, Marshall B, Lavange L, Engels J, *et al*: Cystic Fibrosis Foundation Therapeutics Development Network: Safety and tolerability of denufosol tetrasodium inhalation solution, a novel P2Y$_2$ receptor agonist: results of a phase 1/phase 2 multicenter study in mild to moderate cystic fibrosis, *Pediatr Pulmonol* 39:339, 2005.

104. Newhouse MT: Primary ciliary dyskinesia: what has it taught us about pulmonary disease? *Eur J Respir Dis Suppl* 127:151, 1983.

105. Girod S, Galabert C, Lecuire A, Zahm JM, Puchelle E: Phospholipid composition and surface-active properties of tracheobronchial secretions from patients with cystic fibrosis and chronic obstructive pulmonary diseases, *Pediatr Pulmonol* 13:22, 1992.

106. Griese M, Essl R, Schmidt R, Ballmann M, Paul K, Rietschel E, Ratjen F: BEAT Study Group: Sequential analysis of surfactant, lung function and inflammation in cystic fibrosis patients, *Respir Res* 6:133, 2005.

107. Anzueto A, Jubran A, Ohar JA, Piquette CA, Rennard SI, Colice G, Pattishall EN, Barrett J, Engle M, Perret KA, *et al*: Effects of aerosolized surfactant in patients with stable chronic bronchitis: a prospective randomized controlled trial, *JAMA* 278:1426, 1997.

108. Schurch S, Gehr P, Im HV, Geiser M, Green F: Surfactant displaces particles toward the epithelium in airways and alveoli, *Respir Physiol* 80:17, 1990.

109. Tamaoki J, Chiyotani A, Kobayashi K, Sakai N, Kanemura T, Takizawa T: Effect of indomethacin on bronchorrhea in patients with chronic bronchitis, diffuse panbronchiolitis, or bronchiectasis, *Am Rev Respir Dis* 145:548, 1992.

110. Tamaoki J, Chiyotani A, Tagaya E, Sakai N, Konno K: Effect of long term treatment with oxitropium bromide on airway secretion in chronic bronchitis and diffuse panbronchiolitis, *Thorax* 49:545, 1994.

111. Shinkai M, Rubin BK: A global perspective on macrolide use, *Jpn J Antibiotics* 58:129, 2005.

112. Shinkai M, Park CS, Rubin BK: Immunomodulatory effects of macrolide antibiotics, *Clin Pulm Med* 12:341, 2005.

113. Jaffé A, Bush A: Anti-inflammatory effects of macrolides in lung disease, *Pediatric Pulmonol* 31:464, 2001.

114. Rubin BK, Tamaoki J, editors: *Antibiotics as anti-inflammatory and immunomodulatory agents,* Basel, Switzerland, Birkhäuser, 2004.

115. Kishioka C, Okamoto K, Kim J, Rubin BK: Regulation of secretion from mucous and serous cells in the excised ferret trachea, *Respir Physiol* 126:163, 2001.

116. McElvaney NG, Nakamura H, Birrer P, Hebert CA, Wong WL, Alphonso M, Baker JB, Catalano MA, Crystal RG: Modulation of airway inflammation in cystic fibrosis: *in vivo* suppression of interleukin-8 levels on the respiratory epithelial surface by aerosolization of recombinant secretory leukoprotease inhibitor, *J Clin Invest* 90:1296, 1992.

117. Eng PA, Morton J, Douglass JA, Riedler J, Wilson J, Robertson CF: Short-term efficacy of ultrasonically nebulized hypertonic saline in cystic fibrosis, *Pediatr Pulmonol* 21:77, 1996.

118. Daviskas E, Anderson SD, Gomes K, Briffa P, Cochrane B, Chan HK, Young IH, Rubin BK: Inhaled mannitol for the treatment of mucociliary dysfunction in patients with bronchiectasis: effect on lung function, health status and sputum, *Respirology* 10:46, 2005.

119. Donaldson SH, Bennett WD, Zeman KL, Knowles MR, Tarran R, Boucher RC: Mucus clearance and lung function in cystic fibrosis with hypertonic saline, *N Engl J Med* 354:241, 2006.

120. Elkins MR, Robinson M, Rose BR, Harbour C, Moriarty CP, Marks GB, Belousova EG, Xuan W, Bye PT; National Hypertonic Saline in Cystic Fibrosis (NHSCF) Study Group: A controlled trial of long-term inhaled hypertonic saline in patients with cystic fibrosis, *N Engl J Med* 354:229, 2006.

121. Wark PA, McDonald V, Jones AP: Nebulised hypertonic saline for cystic fibrosis, *Cochrane Database Syst Rev* 3:CD001506, 2005.

122. Wills P, Greenstone M: Inhaled hyperosmolar agents for bronchiectasis, *Cochrane Database Syst Rev* 1:CD002996, 2002.

123. Suri R, Metcalfe C, Lees B, Grieve R, Flather M, Normand C, Thompson S, Bush A, Wallis C: Comparison of hypertonic saline and alternate-day or daily recombinant human deoxyribonuclease in children with cystic fibrosis: a randomised trial, *Lancet* 358:1316, 2001.

124. Knowles MR, Hohneker KW, Zhou Z, Olsen JC, Noah TL, Hu PC, Leigh MW, Engelhardt JF, Edwards LJ, Jones KR, *et al*: A controlled study of adenoviral-vector-mediated gene transfer in the nasal epithelium of patients with cystic fibrosis, *N Engl J Med* 333:823, 1995.

125. Rochat T, Morris MA: Gene therapy for cystic fibrosis by means of aerosol, *J Aerosol Med* 15:229, 2002.

126. Flotte TR, Laube BL: Gene therapy in cystic fibrosis, *Chest* 120(3 suppl):124S, 2001.

127. Moss RB, Rodman D, Spencer LT, Aitken ML, Zeitlin PL, Waltz D, Milla C, Brody AS, Clancy JP, Ramsey B, *et al*: Repeated adeno-associated virus serotype 2 aerosol-mediated cystic fibrosis transmembrane regulator gene transfer to the lungs of patients with cystic fibrosis: a multicenter, double-blind, placebo-controlled trial, *Chest* 125:509, 2004.

128. Copreni E, Penzo M, Carrabino S, Conese M: Lentivirus-mediated gene transfer to the respiratory epithelium: a promising approach to gene therapy of cystic fibrosis, *Gene Ther* 11(suppl 1):S67, 2004.

129. Eastman SJ, Scheule RK: Cationic lipid:pDNA complexes for the treatment of cystic fibrosis, *Curr Opin Mol Ther* 1:186, 1999.

130. Montier T, Delepine P, Pichon C, Ferec C, Porteous DJ, Midoux P: Non-viral vectors in cystic fibrosis gene therapy: progress and challenges, *Trends Biotechnol* 22:586, 2004.

131. King M, Kelly S, Cosio M: Alteration of airway reactivity by mucus, *Respir Physiol* 62:47, 1985.

132. Gross D, Zidulka A, O'Brien C, Wight D, Fraser R, Rosenthal L, King M: Peripheral mucociliary clearance with high-frequency chest wall compression, *J Appl Physiol* 58:1157, 1985.

133. Warwick WJ: Mechanisms of mucous transport, *Eur J Respir Dis Suppl* 127:162, 1983.

134. Camner P: Studies on the removal of inhaled particles from the lungs by voluntary coughing, *Chest* 80(6 suppl):824, 1981.

135. Irwin RS, Madison JM: The diagnosis and treatment of cough, *N Engl J Med* 343:171, 2000.

136. Thomas J, Cook DJ, Brooks D: Chest physical therapy management of patients with cystic fibrosis: a meta-analysis, *Am J Respir Crit Care Med* 151:846, 1995.

137. Bach JR: Update and perspective on noninvasive respiratory muscle aids. 2. The expiratory aids, *Chest* 105:1538, 1994.

138. Hasani A, Pavia D, Agnew JE, Clarke SW: Regional lung clearance during cough and forced expiration technique (FET): effects of flow and viscoelasticity, *Thorax* 49:557, 1994.

139. Hasani A, Pavia D, Agnew JE, Clarke SW: Regional mucus transport following unproductive cough and forced expiration technique in patients with airway obstruction, *Chest* 105:1420, 1994.

140. Chevaillier J: Autogenic drainage (AD), In: Lawson D, editor: *Cystic fibrosis: horizons*, Chichester, 1984, John Wiley & Sons.

141. Shom MH: Autogenic drainage: a modern approach to physiotherapy in cystic fibrosis, *J R Soc Med* 82(suppl 16):32, 1989.

142. Giles DR, Wagener JS, Accurso FJ, Butler-Simon N: Short-term effects of postural drainage with clapping vs autogenic drainage on oxygen saturation and sputum recovery in patients with cystic fibrosis, *Chest* 108:952, 1995.

143. Salh W, Bilton D, Dodd M, Webb AK: Effect of exercise and physiotherapy in aiding sputum expectoration in adults with cystic fibrosis, *Thorax* 44:1006, 1989.

144. Zach MS, Purrer B, Oberwaldner B: Effect of swimming on forced expiration and sputum clearance in cystic fibrosis, *Lancet* 2:1201, 1981.

145. Bilton D, Dodd M, Webb AK: Evaluation of exercise as an adjunct to physiotherapy in the treatment of cystic fibrosis, *Thorax* 44:859, 1989.

146. Ricksten SE, Bengtsson A, Soderberg C, Thorden M, Kvist H: Effects of periodic positive airway pressure by mask on postoperative pulmonary function, *Chest* 89:774, 1986.

147. Paul WL, Downs JB: Postoperative atelectasis: intermittent positive pressure breathing, incentive spirometry, and face-mask positive end-expiratory pressure, *Arch Surg* 116:861, 1981.

148. Andersen JB, Klausen NO: A new mode of administration of nebulized bronchodilator in severe bronchospasm, *Eur J Respir Dis Suppl* 119:97, 1982.

149. Frischknecht-Christensen E, Norregaard O, Dahl R: Treatment of bronchial asthma with terbutaline inhaled by conespacer combined with positive expiratory pressure mask, *Chest* 100:317, 1991.

150. Andersen JB, Qvist J, Kann T: Recruiting collapsed lung through collateral channels with positive end-expiratory pressure, *Scand J Respir Dis* 60:260, 1979.

151. Andersen JB, Jespersen W: Demonstration of intersegmental respiratory bronchioles in normal human lungs, *Eur J Respir Dis* 61:337, 1980.

152. Dasgupta B, Tomkiewicz RP, Boyd WA, Brown NE, King M: Effects of combined treatment with rhDNase and airflow oscillations on spinnability of cystic fibrosis sputum *in vitro*, *Pediatr Pulmonol* 20:78, 1995.

153. van Hengstum M, Festen J, Beurskens C, Hankel M, van den Broeke W, Corstens F: No effect of oral high frequency oscillation combined with forced expiration manoeuvres on tracheobronchial clearance in chronic bronchitis, *Eur Respir J* 3:14, 1990.

154. Konstan MW, Stern RC, Doershuk CF: Efficacy of the Flutter device for airway mucus clearance in patients with cystic fibrosis, *J Pediatr* 124:689, 1994.

155. Gondor M, Nixon PA, Mutich R, Rebovich P, Orenstein DM: Comparison of Flutter device and chest physical therapy in the treatment of cystic fibrosis pulmonary exacerbation, *Pediatr Pulmonol* 28:255, 1999.

156. Mahesh VK, McDougal JA, Haluszka L: Efficacy of the Flutter device for airway mucus clearance in patients with cystic fibrosis, *J Pediatr* 128:165, 1996.

157. Pryor JA, Webber BA, Hodson ME, Warner JO: The Flutter VRP1 as an adjunct to chest physiotherapy in cystic fibrosis, *Respir Med* 88:677, 1994.

158. Homnick DN, Anderson K, Marks JH: Comparison of the Flutter device to standard chest physiotherapy in hospitalized patients with cystic fibrosis: a pilot study, *Chest* 114:993, 1998.

159. App EM, Kieselmann R, Reinhardt D, Lindemann H, Dasgupta B, King M, Brand P: Sputum rheology changes in cystic fibrosis lung disease following two different types of physiotherapy: Flutter vs autogenic drainage, *Chest* 114:171, 1998.

160. Girard JP, Terki N: The Flutter VRP1: a new personal pocket therapeutic device used as an adjunct to drug therapy in the management of bronchial asthma, *J Investig Allergol Clin Immunol* 4:23, 1994.

161. McInturff SL, Shaw LI: Intrapulmonary percussive ventilation, *Respir Care* 30:884, 1985.

162. Natale JE, Pfeifle J, Homnick DN: Comparison of intrapulmonary percussive ventilation and chest physiotherapy: a pilot study in patients with cystic fibrosis, *Chest* 105:1789, 1994.

163. Homnick DN, White F, de Castro C: Comparison of effects of an intrapulmonary percussive ventilator to standard aerosol and chest physiotherapy in treatment of cystic fibrosis, *Pediatr Pulmonol* 20:50, 1995.

164. Newhouse PA, White F, Marks JH, Homnick DN: The intrapulmonary percussive ventilator and Flutter device compared to standard chest physiotherapy in patients with cystic fibrosis, *Clin Pediatr (Phila)* 37:427, 1998.

165. King M, Zidulka A, Phillips DM, Wight D, Gross D, Chang HK: Tracheal mucus clearance in high-frequency oscillation: effect of peak flow rate bias, *Eur Respir J* 3:6, 1990.

166. King M, Phillips DM, Gross D, Vartian V, Chang HK, Zidulka A: Enhanced tracheal mucus clearance with high frequency chest wall compression, *Am Rev Respir Dis* 128:511, 1983.

167. Hansen LG, Warwick WJ: High-frequency chest compression system to aid in clearance of mucus from the lung, *Biomed Instrum Technol* 24:289, 1990.

168. Arens R, Gozal D, Omlin KJ, Vega J, Boyd KP, Keens TG, Woo MS: Comparison of high frequency chest compression and conventional chest physiotherapy in hospitalized patients with cystic fibrosis, *Am J Respir Crit Care Med* 150:1154, 1994.

169. Kluft J, Beker L, Castagnino M, Gaiser J, Chaney H, Fink RJ: A comparison of bronchial drainage treatments in cystic fibrosis, *Pediatr Pulmonol* 22:271, 1996.

170. Gelman RA, Meyer FA: Mucociliary transference rate and mucus viscoelasticity dependence on dynamic storage and loss modulus, *Am Rev Respir Dis* 120:553, 1979.

171. Davis SS, Deverell LC: Rheological factors in mucociliary clearance: the assessment of mucotropic agents using an *in vitro* model, *Mod Probl Paediatr* 19:207, 1976.

172. Braga PC, Ziment I, Allegra L: Classification of agents that act on bronchial mucus, In: Braga PC, Allegra L, editors: *Drugs in bronchial mucology*, New York, 1989, Raven Press.

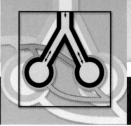

Chapter 10

Surfactant Agents

DOUGLAS S. GARDENHIRE

CHAPTER OUTLINE

Perspective
   Physical Principles
   Application to the Lung
Clinical Indications for Exogenous Surfactants
Identification of Surfactant Preparations
Exogenous Surfactants
   Composition of Pulmonary Surfactant
   Production and Regulation of Surfactant Secretion
   Types of Exogenous Surfactant Preparations
Specific Exogenous Surfactant Preparations
   Beractant (Survanta)
   Calfactant (Infasurf)
   Poractant Alfa (Curosurf)

Mode of Action
Clinical Outcome
Hazards and Complications of Surfactant Therapy
   Airway Occlusion, Desaturation, and Bradycardia
   High Arterial Oxygen (Pao_2) Values
   Overventilation and Hypocarbia
   Apnea
   Pulmonary Hemorrhage
Future Directions in Surfactant Therapy
Respiratory Care Assessment of Surfactant Therapy

CHAPTER OBJECTIVES

After reading this chapter, the reader will be able to:

1. Define *surfactant*
2. List all available exogenous surfactant agents used in respiratory therapy
3. Describe the mode of action for exogenous surfactant agents
4. Discuss the route of administration for exogenous surfactant agents
5. Recognize hazards and complications of exogenous surfactant therapy
6. Assess the use of surfactant therapy

KEY TERMS AND DEFINITIONS

LaPlace's Law — Physical principle describing and quantifying the relation between the internal pressure of a drop or bubble, the amount of surface tension, and the radius of the drop or bubble

Prophylactic treatment — Prevention of respiratory distress syndrome (RDS) in very low birth weight infants, and in infants with higher birth weight but with evidence of immature lungs, who are at risk for developing RDS

Rescue treatment — Retroactive, or "rescue," treatment of infants who have developed RDS

Surface tension — The attraction of molecules in a liquid–air interface, such as the liquid lining in lung tissue and the air, pulling the surface molecules inward

Surfactant — An agent that lowers surface tension

Chapter 10 reviews pharmacological agents termed **surfactants**, which are intended to alter the surface tension of alveoli and the resulting pressures needed for alveolar inflation. The physical principles of surfactants and surface tension forces are reviewed as a basis for introducing agents that have been used or are currently used in respiratory care. The use of current exogenous surfactant agents in the treatment of respiratory distress syndrome of the newborn is presented.

PERSPECTIVE

Physical Principles

> **KEY POINT**
>
> Surfactant agents regulate surface tension in films at gas–liquid interfaces. The interrelation of surface tension, drop or bubble size, and pressure is described by LaPlace's Law.

Exogenous surfactants are administered to replace missing pulmonary surfactant in respiratory distress syndrome (RDS) of the newborn. Surface-active agents act on liquids to affect surface tension. The following terms and concepts form the basis for an understanding of the application of surfactant preparations and their effects in the airway. (2n – 28 weeks neonate)

Surfactant: Surface-active agent that lowers surface tension. Examples include soap and various forms of detergent. Surfactants, or surface-active agents, have also been termed *detergents* for this reason.

Surface tension: Force caused by attraction between like molecules that occurs at liquid–gas interfaces and holds the liquid surface intact. The units of measure for surface tension are usually dynes per centimeter (dyn/cm), indicating the force required to cause a 1-cm rupture in the surface film. Because a liquid's molecules are more attracted to each other than to the surrounding gas, a droplet or spherical shape usually results (Figure 10-1, A).

LaPlace's Law: Physical principle describing and quantifying the relation between the internal pressure of a drop or bubble, the amount of surface tension, and the radius of the drop or bubble (Figure 10-1, B). For a bubble, which is a liquid film with gas inside and out, LaPlace's Law is as follows:

$$Pressure = (4 \times surface\ tension)/radius$$

In alveoli there is only a single air–liquid interface, and LaPlace's Law is as follows:

$$Pressure = (2 \times surface\ tension)/radius$$

Application to the Lung

Because an alveolus has a liquid lining, surface tension forces apply. The higher the surface tension of the liquid, the greater is the compressing force inside the alveolus, which can cause collapse or difficulty in opening the alveolus. In foamy, bubbly pulmonary edema, the surface tension of the liquid allows the formation of the bubbly froth. In both cases, low compliance or pulmonary edema, lowering the surface tension will ease alveolar opening or cause the foam bubbles to collapse and liquefy.

CLINICAL INDICATIONS FOR EXOGENOUS SURFACTANTS

Exogenous surfactants are clinically indicated for the treatment or prevention of RDS in the newborn.

Prophylactic treatment: Prevention of RDS in very low birth weight infants, and in infants with higher birth weight but with evidence of immature lungs, who are at risk for developing RDS.

Rescue treatment: Retroactive, or "rescue," treatment of infants who have developed RDS.

The basic problem in RDS is lack of pulmonary surfactant as a result of lung immaturity. This results in high

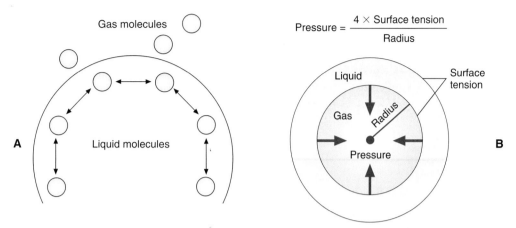

FIGURE 10-1 **A,** The concept of like liquid molecules producing the attractive force resulting in surface tension. **B,** LaPlace's Law illustrated for a bubble with two air–liquid interfaces. For alveoli (with only one air–liquid interface), the relation is as follows: Pressure = (2 × surface tension)/radius.

surface tensions in the liquid-lined, gas-filled alveoli. Increased ventilating pressure is required to expand the alveoli during inspiration, which will lead to ventilatory and respiratory failure in the infant without ventilatory support. This concept, and the effect of exogenous surfactant, is shown in Figure 10-2. Exogenous surfactants are also being investigated for efficacy in the treatment of acute respiratory distress syndrome (ARDS), acute lung injury (ALI), and meconium aspiration syndrome (MAS), although this is not an approved clinical application at this time.[1]

IDENTIFICATION OF SURFACTANT PREPARATIONS

Table 10-1 lists surfactant formulations that currently have U.S. Food and Drug Administration (FDA) approval for general clinical use in the United States. Detailed differences between these formulations and details of their dosing and administration are given subsequently for each agent in separate sections.

EXOGENOUS SURFACTANTS

KEY POINT

Three surfactant agents are currently used for treatment of *neonatal respiratory distress syndrome* (RDS). Beractant (Survanta), calfactant (Infasurf), and poractant alfa (Curosurf) are *modified natural* agents.

The term *exogenous,* used to describe this class of drugs, refers to the fact that these are surfactant preparations from outside the patient's own body. These preparations may be obtained from other humans, from animals, or by laboratory synthesis. The clinical use of exogenous surfactants has been to replace the missing pulmonary surfactant of the premature or immature lung in RDS of the newborn. These agents have also been investigated for use in ARDS, and may prove to be beneficial, although results have not been entirely consistent.[2,3]

Composition of Pulmonary Surfactant

Pulmonary surfactant is a complex mixture of lipids and proteins (Box 10-1). The surfactant mixture is produced by alveolar type II cells. Their primary function, although not necessarily their only function, is to regulate the surface tension forces of the liquid alveolar lining. Surfactant regulates surface tension by forming a film at the air–liquid interface. Surfactant lowers surface tension as it is compressed during expiration, thus reducing the amount of pressure and inspiratory effort required to reexpand the alveoli during a succeeding inspiration. The amount of extracellular (i.e., outside the type II cell) surfactant in animals is 10 to 15 mg/kg body weight in adults and 5 to 10 times that in mature newborns.[4] Figure 10-3 illustrates the source, basic composition, and regulation of pulmonary surfactant in the alveolus. Each of the major components is described in the following sections.

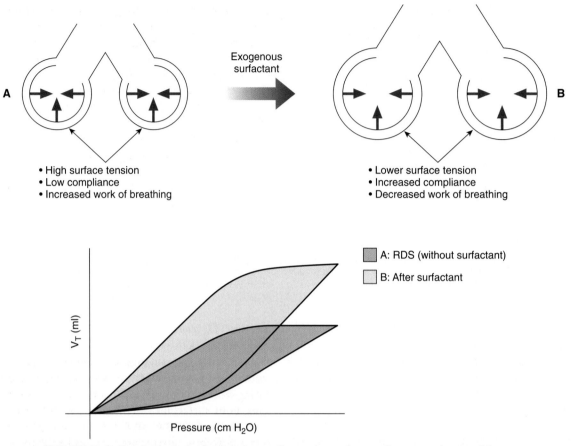

FIGURE 10-2 *Top:* **A,** The lack of pulmonary surfactant in respiratory distress syndrome of the newborn results in high surface tension of the alveolar liquid lining and the need for high inspiratory pressures to expand alveoli. **B,** Exogenous surfactants reduce the high surface tension to reduce the pressures needed for alveolar expansion. *Bottom:* A graph illustrating the change in the pressure-volume relation without pulmonary surfactant *(A)* and after exogenous surfactant therapy *(B).* V_T, Tidal volume.

TABLE 10-1		
Exogenous Surfactant Preparations Currently Approved for Use in the United States*		
Drug	**Brand Name**	**Formulation and Initial Dose**
Beractant	Survanta	8-ml vial, 25 mg phospholipids/ml with 0.5-1.75 mg/ml triglycerides, 1.4-3.5 mg/ml free fatty acids, and <1 mg/ml protein *Dose:* 100 mg phospholipids/kg (4 ml/kg) in four divided doses by tracheal instillation
Calfactant	Infasurf	6-ml vial of 35 mg phospholipids/ml, 0.65 mg proteins *Dose:* 3 ml/kg in two divided doses of 1.5 ml/kg
Poractant alfa	Curosurf	1.5-ml vial (80 mg phospholipids) with 1 mg of proteins or 3-ml vial (160 mg phospholipids) with 2 mg of proteins *Dose:* 2.5 ml/kg (200 mg/kg) in two divided doses by tracheal instillation

subsequent doses: of 1.25 ml/kg × 12 hrs at need

*Individual agents are discussed subsequently in a separate section. Detailed information on each should be obtained from the manufacturer's drug insert.

KEY POINT

Endogenous *pulmonary surfactant* is 90% lipids and 10% protein. The major phospholipid is *dipalmitoylphosphatidylcholine (DPPC)*.

Lipids

Lipids make up about 85 to 90% of surfactant by weight. The lipid component of surfactant is approximately 90% phospholipids, such as phosphatidylcholine,

Box 10-1	Composition of Whole Surfactant From Bronchoalveolar Lavage Fluid (% by Weight)

LIPIDS (85–90%)
- Phospholipids (~90%)
  - Phosphatidylcholine
    - Half is dipalmitoylphosphatidylcholine, DPPC
  - Phosphatidylglycerol
  - Phosphatidylethanolamine
  - Phosphatidylserine
  - Phosphatidylinositol
  - Sphingomyelin
- Neutral lipids (10%)
  - Cholesterol and others

PROTEINS (10%)
- Surfactant protein A (SP-A)
- Surfactant protein B (SP-B)
- Surfactant protein C (SP-C)
- Surfactant protein D (SP-D)

phosphatidylglycerol, sphingomyelin, and others, and 10% other lipids, most of which is cholesterol.[5] Phospholipids have both lipophilic and hydrophilic properties and are able to achieve low surface tensions at air–liquid interfaces. Phosphatidylcholine makes up about 75 to 80% of the phospholipids in surfactant, and about half of this is dipalmitoylphosphatidylcholine, or DPPC, which is also known as *lecithin*. DPPC is the surfactant component predominantly responsible for the reduction of alveolar surface tension. The hydrophilic choline residue of DPPC associates with the liquid phase in alveoli, while the hydrophobic palmitic acid residue projects into the air phase.[6]

Proteins

KEY POINT

Surfactant-associated proteins, such as SP-A, SP-B, and SP-C, regulate the function of endogenous pulmonary surfactant.

The total protein portion of surfactant is about 10% by weight. Approximately 80% of this portion is contaminating serum proteins and 20% is surfactant-specific proteins. Four surfactant-specific proteins (SPs) have been identified so far: SP-A, SP-B, SP-C, and SP-D.[4] Proteins of the surfactant mixture are reviewed by Johansson and associates.[7]

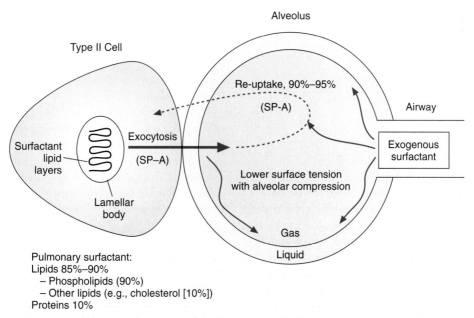

FIGURE 10-3 The production and reuptake of surfactant by type II cells. Exogenous surfactant is also taken up, to become part of the surfactant pool for alveoli.

All of the components of surfactant are synthesized by the alveolar type II cell. The type I cell, which is the basic alveolar epithelial cell on 95% of the alveolar surface, has no known role in surfactant synthesis or metabolism. The type II cell also secretes other proteins, such as cytokines, growth factors, and antibacterial proteins, into the alveolar space. The role of the surfactant-associated proteins is well reviewed by Hawgood and Poulain[8] and Possmayer.[9]

Surfactant Protein A (SP-A). SP-A is a high molecular weight, water-soluble glycoprotein. This protein is specific to surfactant and has also been denoted as SP-35, apoprotein A, and SAP-35.[4] SP-A seems to regulate both secretion and exocytosis of surfactant from the type II cell, as well as the reuptake of surfactant for recycling and reuse.

Surfactant Proteins B and C (SP-B and SP-C). SP-B and SP-C are low molecular weight, hydrophobic proteins that improve the adsorption and spreading of the phospholipid throughout the air–liquid interface in the alveolus.

Surfactant Protein D (SP-D). SP-D is a fourth protein identified in natural endogenous surfactant. SP-D has similarities to SP-A as a large, water-soluble protein, although differences exist in their molecular configuration.[8] There is no clear role for SP-D in surfactant function at this time, calling into question whether SP-D is correctly designated as a surfactant-associated protein.

Production and Regulation of Surfactant Secretion

KEY POINT

Exogenous surfactant agents enter into the alveolar pool and replace deficient natural surfactant.

The surfactant lipids are synthesized in the alveolar type II cells and stored in vesicles termed *lamellar bodies* (see Figure 10-3). Surfactant in the lamellar bodies is then secreted by exocytosis out of the type II cell and into the alveolus. The major stimulus for secretion of lamellar bodies into the alveolar space appears to be inflation of the lung, with a chemically coupled stretch response.[10] SP-A and SP-B facilitate the formation of an intermediate lattice form of surfactant, termed *tubular myelin*, before it reaches the air–liquid interface. SP-C also helps to "break" the lipid layers of surfactant, so that adsorption and spreading of the compound as a monolayer will proceed quickly through the air–liquid interface. Surfactant is converted to small vesicles, which can be taken back into the type II cell or taken in alveolar macrophages. The two major alveolar forms of surfactant are large surfactant aggregates (lamellar bodies and tubular myelin–like structures) and small vesicles or aggregates.[11] The secretion of surfactant material from the type II cell is estimated as 10% of the intracellular pool every hour,[12] with an alveolar half-life between 15 and 30 hours.[5] The constant secretion of surfactant is balanced by two clearance mechanisms: endocytosis back into the type II cells, and clearance/degradation by alveolar macrophages.[8] In addition, clearance can occur by degradation within the alveoli, and by mucociliary removal and transport.[5]

A key feature of surfactant production, which is the basis for the success of replacement therapy with exogenous compounds, is the recycling activity in surfactant production. Most surfactant (90 to 95%) is taken back into the alveolar type II cell, reprocessed, and resecreted. It is for this reason that exogenously administered surfactant is successful in replacing missing surfactant, with one or two doses. The exogenous surfactant is taken into the type II cells and becomes the surfactant pool, through the reuptake and recycling mechanism. The reuptake is regulated, at least partly, by SP-A. It is clear that surfactant-specific proteins, or apoproteins, are critical for both the surface-active functioning of surfactant and the metabolic regulation of the surfactant pool. This process is well described by Wright and Clements[6] and Morton.[2] The normal function of endogenous surfactant also depends on the structural organization of the compound. Smaller surfactant aggregates have less SP-A and are less surface active than larger aggregates.[4]

Pulmonary surfactant has also been found to contribute to host defense by increasing bacterial killing, modifying macrophage function, and downregulating the inflammatory response through decreased mediator release from inflammatory cells.[13] Surfactant also enhances ciliary beat frequency and maintains patency of conducting airways.[11]

Types of Exogenous Surfactant Preparations

Exogenous surfactant preparations can be placed into three categories. These categories and examples of each are given in Table 10-2, and described in the following sections. A more complete technical description is given by Jobe and Ikegami.[4]

TABLE 10-2		
Types of Surfactant Preparations and Examples		
Category	**Description**	**Examples**
Natural	Surfactant from natural sources (human or animal) with addition or removal of substances	Survanta (bovine) Curosurf (porcine) Infasurf (bovine)
Synthetic	Surfactant that is prepared by mixing *in vitro*–synthesized substances that may or may not be in natural surfactant	None at present
Synthetic natural	Surfactant prepared *in vitro* by genetic engineering	None at present

Natural/Modified Natural Surfactant

Natural surfactant is an apt descriptive term for the category of surfactants obtained from animals or humans by alveolar wash or from amniotic fluid. The large surface-active aggregates of natural surfactant are recovered from the fluid by centrifugation or simple filtration. Because these are natural surfactants, the ingredients necessary for effective function to regulate surface tension are present. Specifically, this includes the surface proteins needed for adsorption and spreading. Depending on the source, natural surfactants can be expensive and time consuming to obtain and prepare. In addition, there is concern over contamination with viral infectious agents or immunological stimulation and antibody production in response to foreign proteins. Natural surfactant preparations are usually modified by the addition or removal of certain components. Examples of natural surfactants are given in Table 10-2. The natural surfactant Survanta, as an example, is obtained as an extract of minced cow lung, supplemented with other ingredients such as DPPC, palmitic acid, and tripalmitin. Usually, the modifications to the natural surfactant material are designed to improve functioning in the lung and to reduce protein contamination and provide sterility. Although Survanta contains the hydrophobic proteins SP-B and SP-C, the protein SP-A is missing, and this may shorten the duration of effect.

Other examples of a modified natural surfactant include *surfactant TA (Surfacten),* prepared by Mitsubishi Pharma in Japan and used by Fujiwara and colleagues

in their work.[14] Surfactant TA is a reconstituted chloroform–methanol extract from minced cow lungs, with DPPC and other lipids added. *Curosurf* is another modified natural surfactant, obtained as a pig lung extract. *Infasurf* is a chloroform–methanol extract of fluid lavaged from calf lung and, like Survanta, contains only the surfactant proteins SP-B and SP-C, but not SP-A.[15] *Alveofact* is an organic solvent extract of cow lung lavage containing 99% phospholipids and neutral lipids and 1% surfactant proteins B and C (SP-B and SP-C).[16]

Synthetic Surfactant

Synthetic surfactants are mixtures of synthetic components. The characteristic feature of artificial surfactants is that none of the ingredients are obtained from natural sources, such as human, cow, or pig lung. Synthetic surfactants do not contain any of the surfactant proteins, including SP-B or SP-C, that are found in the natural preparations. A major advantage of this class of surfactant is its freedom from contaminating infectious agents and additional foreign proteins that may be antigenic to the recipient. A possible disadvantage is the lack of equivalent performance between the organic chemicals substituted for the naturally occurring surfactant proteins, such as SP-A, -B, or -C. At present, no synthetic surfactant is available. Exosurf (colfosceril palmitate), which was the only synthetic surfactant on the market, has been removed.[1] However, a new synthetic surfactant, Surfaxin (lucinactant) is currently being considered by the FDA. In a study conducted by Moya and colleagues[17] found that Surfaxin was better at reducing RDS and bronchopulmonary dysplasia than Exosurf, but not less than those administered Survanta. Another study by Sinha and others[18] found no difference between Surfaxin and Curosurf.

Synthetic Natural Surfactant

An ideal solution to the problems of concern in both natural and artificial surfactants would be genetically engineered surfactant produced by recombinant DNA technology. In such a preparation the phospholipid, lipid, and protein ingredients of the natural surfactant aggregate would be produced by characterizing, by *in vitro* cloning, the gene or genes responsible for human surfactant. There are no products available for general use at this time, but work progresses on their development. The genes and amino acid sequence for each of the surfactant proteins have been characterized.[19-21] A genetically engineered surfactant that closely resembles the structure and effect of natural human surfactant would be the ideal preparation.

SPECIFIC EXOGENOUS SURFACTANT PREPARATIONS

KEY POINT

Exogenous surfactants are given either *prophylactically* in RDS or as *rescue* treatment.

Three exogenous surfactant preparations have been approved for general clinical use in the United States at the time of this edition. Each of these preparations is described in greater detail.

Beractant (Survanta)

Beractant (Survanta) is considered a modified natural surfactant. It is a natural bovine lung extract mixed with colfosceril palmitate (DPPC), palmitic acid, and tripalmitin. These last three ingredients are used to standardize the composition of the drug preparation, as well as to reproduce the surface tension–lowering properties of natural surfactant. The ingredients are suspended in 0.9% saline. The composition of beractant, given in the product literature, is described in Table 10-1. The extract from minced bovine lung contains natural phospholipids; neutral lipids; fatty acids; and the low molecular weight, hydrophobic surfactant proteins SP-B and SP-C. The hydrophilic, high molecular weight protein SP-A is not contained in beractant. SP-A helps regulate surfactant reuptake and secretion by the alveolar type II cells. However, the addition of SP-A to beractant by Yamada and colleagues[22] did not improve the biophysical activity (spreading and absorption) or the physiological activity (lung compliance change) of the mixture.

Beractant is available as Survanta from Ross Products Division of Abbott Laboratories (Columbus, OH) in a vial containing 8 ml of suspension, with a concentration of 25 mg/ml, in a 0.9% sodium chloride solution. The suspension does not require reconstitution. This gives a maximal total dose of 200 mg of phospholipids in a single vial of 8 ml of suspension.

Indications for Use

Specific guidelines for use of beractant are as follows:
- Prophylactic therapy of premature infants less than 1250 g birth weight or with evidence of surfactant deficiency and risk of RDS; the agent should be given within 15 minutes of birth or as soon as possible.
- Rescue treatment of infants with evidence of RDS; the agent should be given within 8 hours of age.

Dosage

The recommended dose of beractant is 100 mg of phospholipids per kilogram of birth weight. Because there are 25 mg of phospholipids per milliliter in the beractant suspension, this is equivalent to a dose of 4 ml/kg of birth weight. For example, a 2000-g (2-kg) infant would require 8 ml, or the entire vial of suspension.

Repeat doses of beractant are given no sooner than 6 hours later if there is evidence of continuing respiratory distress. The manufacturer's literature recommends that manual hand-bag ventilation *not* be used for the repeat dose in place of mechanical ventilation. Ventilator adjustment may be necessary, however.

Administration

Beractant suspension is off-white to light brown in color. If settling has occurred in the suspension, the vial can be swirled gently but should not be shaken. The suspension is kept refrigerated and must be warmed by allowing it to stand at room temperature for at least 20 minutes. Artificial warming methods should not be used.

The calculated dose is given in quarters from a syringe and instilled into the trachea through a 5-French catheter placed into the endotracheal tube (ETT). The catheter is removed and the infant is manually ventilated for at least 30 seconds, or until stable, between doses. The remaining doses are given in similar fashion. During each quarter dose the infant is placed in a different position.

Unopened vials that have been warmed to room temperature may be returned for refrigerated storage within 8 hours. This should be done no more than once. Used vials should be discarded with residual drug. The preceding general description of beractant (Survanta) is intended to be instructional.

Calfactant (Infasurf)

Calfactant is another modified natural surfactant preparation from calf lung (bovine). It is an organic solvent extract of calf lung surfactant obtained by cell-free bronchoalveolar lavage. The extract contains phospholipids, neutral lipids, and hydrophobic proteins SP-B and SP-C. The preparation is a suspension, which does not require reconstitution. Its composition is given in Table 10-1. Each milliliter contains 35 mg of total phospholipids, including 26 mg of phosphatidylcholine, of which 16 mg is disaturated phosphatidylcholine, and

0.65 mg of proteins, which includes 0.26 mg of SP-B. The protein SP-A is not contained in the preparation. The formulation is heat sterilized and contains no preservatives.

Indications for Use

Specific guidelines for use of calfactant (Infasurf) are as follows:
- The prevention (prophylaxis) of RDS in premature infants less than 29 weeks of gestational age and at high risk for RDS
- The treatment (rescue) of premature infants less than or equal to 72 hours of age who develop RDS and require endotracheal intubation

Dosage

The recommended dose of calfactant is 3 ml/kg body weight at birth. The dose should be delivered as two divided doses of 1.5 ml/kg. Each 6 ml of suspension contains enough preparation (210 mg of phospholipids) to treat a 2-kg infant. It is noted in the drug insert that calfactant prophylaxis should be administered as soon as possible, preferably no more than 30 minutes after birth.

Repeat doses, up to a total of three doses, can be given 12 hours apart. Repeat doses as early as 6 hours after the previous dose can be given if the infant is still intubated and requires 30% or greater oxygen for an arterial oxygen pressure (Pao_2) of 80 mmHg or less (manufacturer's literature).

Administration

Calfactant can be administered to an intubated infant either by side-port delivery or with a catheter. The preparation does not require reconstitution. Calfactant is an off-white suspension that requires gentle swirling or agitation, but not shaking, in the vial to ensure dispersion. Flecks may be visible in the suspension and foaming at the surface.

Side-port Adaptor. The dose is given in two aliquots of 1.5 ml/kg each. Position the infant with either the right or left side dependent for each aliquot. The suspension is instilled in small bursts timed to coincide with the inspiratory cycle, over 20 to 30 breaths. It is recommended that the infant be evaluated between repositioning for the second aliquot.

Catheter Administration. The dose is divided into four equal aliquots, with the catheter removed between each instillation, and mechanical ventilatory support for 0.5 to 2 minutes. Each aliquot is given with the infant in a different position (prone, supine, right lateral, and left lateral).

Poractant Alfa (Curosurf)

Poractant alfa is a natural surfactant obtained as an extract of porcine lung. It is a suspension consisting of approximately 99% phospholipids (80 mg of phospholipids in the 1.5-ml vial and 160 mg of phospholipids in the 3-ml vial) and about 1% surfactant-associated proteins, including SP-B.

Indications for Use

Specific guidelines for use of poractant alfa (Curosurf) are as follows:
- For the treatment (rescue) of premature infants with RDS, reducing mortality and pneumothoraces
- Unlabeled uses: severe meconium aspiration syndrome in term infants; respiratory failure caused by group B streptococcal infection in neonates

Dosage

The initial dose of poractant alfa is 2.5 ml/kg birth weight. Subsequent doses of 1.25 ml/kg birth weight can be given twice at 12-hour intervals if needed. The maximum recommended total dose (initial plus repeat doses) is 5 ml/kg.

Administration

Before use, the vial should be slowly warmed to room temperature. The vial should be turned upside-down to uniformly disperse the suspension without shaking. Poractant alfa does not need to be reconstituted. The dose is administered through a 5-French catheter positioned in the ETT, with the tip in the distal end of the ETT but not extended beyond the end of the ETT.

The dose is given in two divided aliquots. The infant is positioned with either the right or left side down for the first aliquot. The catheter is then removed and the infant is manually ventilated with 100% oxygen for 1 minute. When the infant is stable, the second aliquot is instilled with the alternate side down, after which the catheter is removed. The airway should not be suctioned for 1 hour unless significant airway obstruction is evident.

MODE OF ACTION

The mode of action of exogenous surfactants is to replace and replenish a deficient endogenous surfactant pool in neonatal RDS. As previously described, endogenous surfactant normally secreted by alveolar type II cells leaves the alveolar space and reenters the type II cells in the form of small vesicles. In the intracellular space, surfactant components are recycled. Exogenously administered surfactant that reaches the alveolar space can be recycled into the type II cells and form a surfactant pool to regulate surface tension.

CLINICAL OUTCOME

There can be a dramatic improvement in oxygenation after surfactant administration, but Davis and associates[23] did not report a corresponding increase in compliance. Although exogenous surfactant should lower surface tension and thereby increase lung compliance, there is disagreement in the literature over whether the primary clinical effect of exogenous surfactant is one of increasing lung compliance.[24] Fujiwara and colleagues[14] noted that there was clearing of the chest radiograph associated with a good clinical response to surfactant, suggesting that surfactant treatment increased the functional residual capacity (FRC). A study by Goldsmith and associates[25] measured an increase in the FRC within 15 minutes of treatment with natural surfactant, correlating with the time of blood gas improvements. The surfactant stabilizes alveoli on expiration and prevents collapse, increasing residual volume and FRC. An increase in oxygenation would be seen with this effect.[24] An increase in lung volume resulting from improved residual volume and FRC shifts the tidal ventilation to a new pressure–volume curve. At higher lung volumes, chest wall elastic recoil is higher. A shift to the flatter part of the pressure–volume curve could give the same tidal volume for a given pressure change, masking the actual increase in static compliance.[21]

HAZARDS AND COMPLICATIONS OF SURFACTANT THERAPY

KEY POINT

There are possible *hazards* to the use of exogenous surfactants, including airway occlusion, desaturation, bradycardia, overoxygenation and overventilation, apnea, and pulmonary hemorrhage.

Some of the complications in exogenous surfactant therapy are due to the dosing procedure, and others can be caused by the therapeutic effect of the drug itself. In the dosing procedure, relatively large volumes of suspension are instilled into neonatal-size airways, and this can block gas exchange, causing desaturation and bradycardia.

The effect of the drug in improving pulmonary compliance can lead to overventilation, excessive volume delivery from pressure-limited ventilation, and overoxygenation with dangerously high Pa_{O_2} levels. As a result, the following complications or hazards can occur with surfactant therapy. In general, complications of prematurity may affect the response to exogenous surfactant.

Airway Occlusion, Desaturation, and Bradycardia

Because the current method of administration is by direct tracheal instillation, a large volume of surfactant suspension may cause an acute obstruction of infant airways, with subsequent hypoxemia and bradycardia.[26] Repetitive small additions of the dose and a transient increase in ventilating pressure may help distribute the surfactant to the periphery.

High Arterial Oxygen (Pa_{O_2}) Values

A good response to exogenous surfactant will result in better (higher) lung compliance, increased FRC, and concomitant improvement in oxygenation. Fractional inspired oxygen ($F_{I_{O_2}}$) settings must be lowered if Pa_{O_2} improves, to prevent overoxygenation and the possibility of retinopathy of prematurity.

Overventilation and Hypocarbia

As lung compliance improves, peak ventilating pressure, expiratory baseline pressures, and ventilatory rate must be adjusted, or overventilation, leading to *hypocapnia* (low blood CO_2), and pneumothorax may occur.

Apnea

Apnea has been noted to occur with the intratracheal administration of surfactant.

Pulmonary Hemorrhage

In a study of infants weighing less than 700 g at birth, the incidence of pulmonary hemorrhage was 10% with Exosurf compared with 2% in the control group. This increase was not seen in infants greater than 700 g at birth. Pulmonary hemorrhage was more frequent in infants who were younger, smaller, male, and with a patent ductus arteriosus.

FUTURE DIRECTIONS IN SURFACTANT THERAPY

KEY POINT

Exogenous surfactants are being investigated for clinical use in disease states such as *ARDS, MAS,* and *pneumonia*.

In addition to RDS of the newborn, surfactant replacement therapy has been considered in meconium aspiration syndrome. In a meta-analysis, Soll and Dargaville report that surfactant therapy may be beneficial in reducing respiratory illness severity and reducing infants' need for extracorporeal membrane oxygenation (ECMO).[27] Surfactant therapy had been studied for a variety of adult respiratory disorders. This topic is comprehensively reviewed by Hamm and colleagues.[5] Acute respiratory distress syndrome (ARDS) in the adult is a potential target for surfactant therapy. In RDS of the newborn, the primary abnormality of lung function is related to surfactant deficiency. In ARDS with adults, the surfactant deficiency is secondary to lung injury with complex inflammatory responses.[5] This would suggest a difference in clinical response to surfactant therapy between premature infants and adults with ARDS. In addition, dose amount and administration techniques may need to be modified for therapy in adults, who have large lung volumes compared with infants. If lung injury in ARDS is non-uniform in distribution, exogenous surfactant, especially if aerosolized, may distribute unevenly to more compliant lung areas instead of to areas needing surfactant the most.[11]

The availability of newer surfactant preparations, specifically human recombinant surfactants, may offer better results to improve outcomes in adults with ARDS.[21]

Other adult respiratory disorders in which either surfactant replacement therapy or abnormal surfactant regulation may occur include pneumonia, lung transplants, sarcoidosis, hypersensitivity pneumonitis, idiopathic pulmonary fibrosis, alveolar proteinosis, obstructive lung disease including asthma, radiation pneumonitis, and drug-induced pulmonary disease.[28]

RESPIRATORY CARE ASSESSMENT OF SURFACTANT THERAPY

- Monitor pulse and cardiac rhythm during and after administration.
- Monitor the infant for signs of airway occlusion (desaturation and bradycardia) during and after administration; if obstruction is evident, remove the infant from the ventilator and manually ventilate; in addition, saline lavage may be needed as well as aggressive suctioning to clear the airway.
- Monitor color and activity level of the infant.
- Monitor chest rise for level of ventilation, or use electronic monitor if available.
- Monitor arterial oxygen saturation and adjust F_{IO_2} accordingly to prevent hyperoxia or hypoxia.

- Monitor transcutaneous P_{CO_2} if possible, and be prepared to adjust level of ventilation as needed to prevent hypercarbia or hypocarbia.
- Assess lung mechanics (exhaled volumes or peak inspiratory pressures) during mechanical ventilation to determine effectiveness of the exogenous agent in normalizing lung compliance. The instilled drug may cause changes within minutes in some cases.
- Consider possible adverse effects if pulse, cardiac rhythm, or arterial/transcutaneous blood gas values deteriorate.

SELF-ASSESSMENT QUESTIONS

1. What is the definition of a *surface-active substance?*
2. In general, what is the clinical indication for use of exogenous surfactants?
3. What type (category) of exogenous surfactant is each of the following: beractant, calfactant, and poractant alfa?
4. What are the major ingredients of natural pulmonary surfactant?
5. Give the dosage schedule of each of the current exogenous surfactants.
6. What is the difference between "rescue" and "prophylaxis" treatment with these agents?
7. Identify at least three possible adverse effects with the use of exogenous surfactant treatment.
8. Why does the improvement in lung mechanics last after only one or two administrations of exogenous surfactant?
9. How would you assess the effectiveness of exogenous surfactant treatment in a premature newborn with respiratory distress?

Answers to Self-Assessment Questions are found in Appendix A.

CLINICAL SCENARIO

Case courtesy **Robert Harwood, MSA, RRT, Clinical Assistant Professor, Georgia State University.**

A 16-year-old female gave birth to a 25-week, 515-g baby girl by vaginal delivery. The mother had no prenatal care and she had premature rupture of the membranes 12 days before delivery. Immediately at birth the newborn was intubated with a 2.5-mm oral endotracheal tube. Apgar scores after intubation and application of positive-pressure ventilation with a bag and mask were 7 and 9 at 1 and 5 minutes, respectively. After

Continued

transfer to the neonatal intensive care unit (NICU), umbilical venous and arterial catheters (UVC and UAC, respectively) were inserted and the infant was placed on mechanical ventilation with peak inspiratory pressure (PIP), 20 cmH$_2$O; positive end-expiratory pressure (PEEP), 5 cmH$_2$O; respiratory rate (RR), 60 breaths/min; inspiratory time, 0.3 second; and fraction of inspired oxygen (F$_{IO_2}$), 1.0. Physical examination revealed the following: pulse (P), 140 beats/min; blood pressure (BP), 34/22 mmHg; temperature (T), 99.6° F; and oxygen saturation by pulse oximetry (SpO$_2$), 85 to 90%. Laboratory results revealed glucose, 39 mg/dl; white blood cell (WBC) count, 11,900/mm^3; hematocrit, 47%; and platelets, 297,000/mm^3. Chest radiograph showed respiratory distress syndrome, stage II.

Is there an indication for administration of an exogenous surfactant in this case? Support your decision with the available data.

Would this administration of surfactant be a rescue or prophylactic treatment, if given immediately after placement on ventilatory support?

Twelve hours after the dose of surfactant was given, the infant exhibited signs of respiratory distress, with an RR increase from 46 to 78 breaths/min, and a P increase from 140 to 185 beats/min. Periods of desaturation below 90% increased. Exhaled tidal volume decreased to 3 ml/kg body weight, and the F$_{IO_2}$ was increased to 0.80. An arterial blood gas reading was obtained, with the following results: pH, 7.29; arterial carbon dioxide pressure (PaCO$_2$), 58 mmHg; and arterial oxygen pressure (PaO$_2$), 41 mmHg.

What pharmacological treatment is now indicated?

Answers to Clinical Scenario Questions are found in Appendix A.

References

1. Kattwinkel J: Synthetic surfactants: the search goes on, *Pediatrics* 115:1075, 2005.
2. Morton NS: Exogenous surfactant treatment for the adult respiratory distress syndrome? A historical perspective [editorial], *Thorax* 45:825, 1990.
3. Holm BA, Matalon S: Role of pulmonary surfactant in the development and treatment of adult respiratory distress syndrome, *Anesth Analg* 69:805, 1989.
4. Jobe A, Ikegami M: Surfactant for the treatment of respiratory distress syndrome, *Am Rev Respir Dis* 136:1256, 1987.
5. Hamm H, Kroegel C, Hohlfeld J: Surfactant: a review of its functions and relevance in adult respiratory disorders, *Respir Med* 90:251, 1996.
6. Wright JR, Clements JA: Metabolism and turnover of lung surfactant, *Am Rev Respir Dis* 135:427, 1987.
7. Johansson J, Curstedt T, Robertson B: The proteins of the surfactant system, *Eur Respir J* 7:372, 1994.
8. Hawgood S, Poulain FR: Functions of the surfactant proteins: a perspective, *Pediatr Pulmonol* 19:99, 1995.
9. Possmayer F: The role of surfactant-associated proteins [editorial], *Am Rev Respir Dis* 142:749, 1990.
10. Wirtz HR, Dobbs LG: Calcium mobilization and exocytosis after one mechanical stretch of lung epithelial cells, *Science* 250:1266, 1990.
11. Lewis J, Veldhuizen RAW: Surfactant: current and potential therapeutic application in infants and adults, *J Aerosol Med* 9:143, 1996.
12. Wright JR, Wager RE, Hawgood S, Dobbs L, Clements JA: Surfactant apoprotein M$_r$ = 26,000–36,000 enhances uptake of liposomes by type II cells, *J Biol Chem* 262:2888, 1987.
13. Pison U, Max M, Neuendank A, Weissbach S, Pietschmann S: Host defence capacities of pulmonary surfactant: evidence for "non-surfactant" functions of the surfactant system, *Eur J Clin Invest* 24:586, 1994.
14. Fujiwara T, Maeta H, Chida S, Morita T, Watabe Y, Abe T: Artificial surfactant therapy in hyaline membrane disease, *Lancet* 1(8159):55, 1980.
15. Notter RH, Egan EA, Kwong MS, Holm BA, Shapiro DL: Lung surfactant replacement in premature lambs with extracted lipids from bovine lung lavage: effects of dose, dispersion techniques, and gestational age, *Pediatr Res* 19:569, 1985.
16. Gortner L, Bartmann P, Pohlandt F, Bernsau U, Porz F, Hellwege HH, Seitz RC, Hieronimi G, Bremer C, Jorch G, *et al*: Early treatment of respiratory distress syndrome with bovine surfactant in very preterm infants: a multicenter controlled clinical trial, *Pediatr Pulmonol* 14:4, 1992.
17. Moya FR, Gadzinowski J, Bancalari E, Salinas V, Kopelman B, Bancalari A, Kornacka MK, Merritt TA, Segal R, Schaber CJ, Tsai H, Massaro J, d'Agostino R; International Surfaxin Collaborative Study Group: A multicenter, randomized, masked, comparison trial of lucinactant, colfosceril palmitate, and beractant for the prevention of respiratory distress syndrome among very preterm infants, *Pediatrics* 2005 Apr;115(4):1018-29.
18. Sinha SK, Lacaze-Masmonteil T, Valls i Soler A, Wiswell TE, Gadzinowski J, Hajdu J, Bernstein G, Sanchez-Luna M, Segal R, Schaber CJ, Massaro J, d'Agostino R; Surfaxin Therapy Against Respiratory Distress Syndrome Collaborative Group: A multicenter, randomized, controlled trial of lucinactant versus poractant alfa among very premature infants at high risk for respiratory distress syndrome, *Pediatrics* 2005 Apr; 115(4):1030-8.
19. Floros J, Phelps DS, Taeusch HW: Biosynthesis and *in vitro* translation of the major surfactant-associated protein from human lung, *J Biol Chem* 260:495, 1985.
20. Avery ME, Merritt TA: Surfactant-replacement therapy, *N Engl J Med* 324:910, 1991.
21. Rodriguez RJ, Martin RJ: Exogenous surfactant therapy in newborns, *Respir Care Clin N Am* 5:595, 1999.
22. Yamada T, Ikegami M, Tabor BL, Jobe AH: Effects of surfactant protein-A on surfactant function in preterm ventilated rabbits, *Am Rev Respir Dis* 142:754, 1990.

23. Davis JM, Veness-Meehan K, Notter RH, Bhutani VK, Kendig JW, Shapiro DL: Changes in pulmonary mechanics after the administration of surfactant to infants with respiratory distress syndrome, *N Engl J Med* 319:476, 1988.

24. Milner AD: How does exogenous surfactant work? *Arch Dis Childhood* 68:253, 1993.

25. Goldsmith LS, Greenspan JS, Rubenstein SD, Wolfson MR, Shaffer TH: Immediate improvement in lung volume after exogenous surfactant: alveolar recruitment versus increased distention, *J Pediatr* 119:424, 1991.

26. Jobe AH: The role of surfactant therapy in neonatal respiratory distress, *Respir Care* 36:695, 1991.

27. Soll RF, Dargaville P: Surfactant for meconium aspiration syndrome in full term infants, *Cochrane Database Syst Rev* 2:CD002054, 2000.

28. Avery ME: Surfactant deficiency in hyaline membrane disease: the story of discovery, *Am J Respir Crit Care Med* 161:1074, 2000.

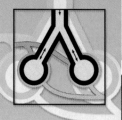

Chapter 11

Corticosteroids in Respiratory Care

DOUGLAS S. GARDENHIRE

CHAPTER OBJECTIVES

After reading this chapter, the reader will be able to:

1. Discuss the indications for inhaled corticosteroid use
2. List all available inhaled corticosteroids used in respiratory therapy
3. Differentiate between specific corticosteroid formulations
4. Describe the route of administration available for corticosteroids
5. Describe the mode of action for corticosteroids
6. Discuss the effect corticosteroids have on the white blood cell count
7. Discuss the effect corticosteroids have on β receptors
8. Differentiate between systemic and local side effects of corticosteroids
9. Discuss the use of corticosteroids in the treatment of asthma and chronic obstructive disease
10. Be able to clinically assess corticosteroid use in patient care

KEY TERMS AND DEFINITIONS

Adrenal cortical hormones — Chemicals secreted by the adrenal cortex, referred to as *steroids*

Endogenous — Refers to *inside*, produced by the body

Exogenous — Refers to *outside*, manufactured to be placed inside the body (e.g., medication)

IgE (immunoglobulin E) — A gamma globulin that is produced by cells in the respiratory tract

Prostaglandin — One of several hormone-type substances circulating throughout the body

Steroids — Also known as *glucocorticoids* or *corticosteroids*, these agents produce an antiinflammatory response in the body

Steroid diabetes — Hyperglycemia (e.g., increased plasma glucose levels) resulting from glucocorticoid therapy; glucocorticoids break down proteins and fats to generate building blocks for gluconeogenesis

---

Chapter 11 presents the use of corticosteroids in respiratory care and provides a brief review of the physiology of endogenous corticosteroid hormones in the body. A summary description of inflammation, and specifically of airway inflammation in asthma, forms the basis for a discussion of the pharmacology of corticosteroids as antiinflammatory drugs. Aerosolized glucocorticoids are presented, along with their uses and side effects.

CLINICAL INDICATIONS FOR USE OF INHALED CORTICOSTEROIDS

Inhaled corticosteroids are available in formulations for oral inhalation (lung delivery) and intranasal delivery. Specific clinical applications are discussed more fully at the end of this chapter. General clinical indications for the use of inhaled corticosteroids are as follows:

- Orally inhaled agents: Maintenance, control therapy of chronic asthma, identified as requiring step 2 care or greater by the National Asthma Education and Prevention Program Expert Panel Report 2 *Guidelines for the Diagnosis and Management of Asthma—Update on Selected Topics*.[1,2]
  - *Step 2 asthma:* Symptoms >2 days/week but <1 time/day and/or >2 nights/month with symptoms, forced expiratory volume in 1 second (FEV_1) or peak expiratory flow (PEF) 80% predicted or greater, but PEF variability at 20 to 30% (see Appendix D).
  - Inhaled agents can be used together with systemic corticosteroids in severe asthma, and may allow systemic dose reduction or elimination for asthma control.
- Inhaled corticosteroids are recommended by the American Thoracic Society (ATS)[3] and the Global Initiative for Chronic Obstructive Lung Disease (GOLD)[4] for chronic obstructive pulmonary disease (COPD).
- Intranasal aerosol agents: Management of seasonal and perennial allergic and nonallergic rhinitis.

IDENTIFICATION OF AEROSOLIZED CORTICOSTEROIDS

Increased numbers of aerosolized corticosteroid preparations are becoming available for both oral inhalation and intranasal delivery. Table 11-1 lists the currently available aerosol formulations of corticosteroids for oral inhalation, and Table 11-2 gives intranasal formulations. Discussion of the rationale for inhaled aerosol agents and a description of the properties of corticosteroids required for success as topical agents are given subsequently, along with additional detail on individual agents.

PHYSIOLOGY OF CORTICOSTEROIDS

> **KEY POINT**
>
> The *physiology* of *endogenous corticosteroids* involves a sequence of stimulation of the adrenal cortex through the *hypothalamic–pituitary–adrenal (HPA)* axis, in which increased blood levels of corticosteroid inhibit the HPA and adrenal cortex from further secretion.

Identification and Source

Corticosteroids are a group of chemicals secreted by the adrenal cortex, and are referred to as **adrenal cortical hormones**. The adrenal or suprarenal gland is composed of two portions (Figure 11-1). The inner zone is the adrenal medulla, and produces epinephrine. The outer zone is the cortex, the source of corticosteroids. Three types of corticosteroid hormone are produced by the adrenal cortex: the glucocorticoids (e.g., cortisol), the mineralocorticoids (e.g., aldosterone), and the sex hormones (e.g., androgens and estrogens). The mineralocorticoid

TABLE 11-1

Corticosteroids Available by Aerosol for Oral Inhalation*

Drug	Brand Name	Formulation and Dosage
Beclomethasone dipropionate HFA	QVAR	MDI: 40 and 80 µg/puff Adults ≥ 12 yr: 40 to 80 µg twice daily,† or 40 to 160 µg twice daily‡ Children ≥5 yr: 40 to 80 µg twice daily
Triamcinolone acetonide	Azmacort	MDI: 100 µg/puff Adults ≥ 12 yr: 2 puffs tid or qid Children ≥ 6 yr: 1 or 2 puffs tid or qid
Flunisolide	AeroBid, AeroBid-M,	MDI: 250 µg/puff Adults and children ≥ 6 yr: 2 puffs bid, adults no more than 4 puffs daily Children ≤ 15 yr: no more than 2 puffs daily
Flunisolide hemihydrate HFA	Aerospan	MDI: 80 µg/puff Adults ≥ 12 yr: 2 puffs bid, adults no more than 4 puffs daily Children 6-11 yr: 1 puff daily, no more than 2 puffs daily
Fluticasone propionate	Flovent HFA	MDI: 44, 110, and 220 µg/puff Adults ≥ 12 yr: 88 µg bid,† 88-220 µg bid,‡ or 880 µg bid¶ Children 4-11 yr: 88 µg bid**
	Flovent Diskus	DPI: 50, 100, and 250 µg Adults: 100 µg bid,† 100-250 µg bid,‡ 1000 µg bid¶ Children 4-11 yr: 50 µg twice daily
Budesonide	Pulmicort Turbuhaler	DPI: 200 µg/actuation Adults: 200-400 µg bid,† 200-400 µg bid,‡ 400-800 µg bid¶ Children ≥ 6 yr: 200 µg bid
	Pulmicort Respules	SVN: 0.25 mg/2 ml, 0.5 mg/2 ml Children 1-8 yr: 0.5-mg total dose given once daily, or twice daily in divided doses†, ‡; 1 mg given as 0.5 mg bid or once daily¶
Mometasone furoate	Asmanex Twisthaler	DPI: 220 µg/actuation Adults and children ≥ 12 yr: 220-440 µg daily,† 220-440 µg daily,‡ 440-880 µg daily¶
Fluticasone propionate/ salmeterol	Advair Diskus	DPI: 100 µg fluticasone/50 µg salmeterol, 250 µg fluticasone/50 µg salmeterol, or 500 µg fluticasone/50 µg salmeterol
	Advair HFA	Adults and children ≥ 12 yr: 100 µg fluticasone/50 µg salmeterol, 1 inhalation twice daily, about 12 hr apart (starting dose if not currently taking inhaled corticosteroids) Maximal recommended dose is 500 µg fluticasone/50 µg salmeterol twice daily Children ≥ 4 yr: 100 µg fluticasone/50 µg salmeterol, 1 inhalation twice daily, about 12 hr apart (for those who are symptomatic while taking an inhaled corticosteroid) MDI: 45 µg fluticasone/21 µg salmeterol, 115 µg fluticasone/21 µg salmeterol, or 230 µg fluticasone/21 µg salmeterol Adults and children ≥ 12 yr: 2 inhalation twice daily, about 12 hr apart
Budesonide/formoterol fumarate HFA	Symbicort	MDI: 80 µg budesonide/4.5 µg formoterol and 160 µg budesonide/4.5 µg formoterol Adults and children ≥ 12 yr: 160 µg budesonide/9 µg formoterol bid, 320 µg budesonide/9 µg formoterol bid; daily maximum: 640 µg budesonide/18 µg formoterol

*Individual agents are discussed in text. Detailed information about each agent should be obtained from the manufacturer's drug insert.
†Recommended starting dose if taking only bronchodilators.
‡Recommended starting dose if previously taking inhaled corticosteroids.
¶Recommended starting dose if previously taking oral corticosteroids.
**This dose should be used regardless of previous therapy.
DPI, Dry powder inhaler; *HFA*, hydrofluoroalkane; *MDI*, metered dose inhaler; *SVN*, small volume nebulizer.

TABLE 11-2

Aerosol Corticosteroid Preparations Available for Intranasal Delivery*

Drug	Brand Name	Formulation and Dosage
Beclomethasone	Beconase AQ	Spray: 42 µg/actuation Adults ≥ 12 yr: 1 or 2 sprays each nostril, twice daily Children 6-11 yr: 1 spray each nostril twice daily, may increase to 2 sprays
Triamcinolone acetonide	Nasacort HFA	MDI: 55 µg/actuation Adults and children ≥ 12 yr: 2 sprays each nostril once daily (starting dose) Children 6-11 yr: 2 sprays each nostril once daily (starting dose)
	Nasacort AQ	Spray: 55 µg/actuation Adults and children ≥ 12 yr: 2 sprays each nostril once daily (starting dose); children 6-11 yr: 1 spray each nostril once daily (starting dose)
Flunisolide	Nasarel Flunisolide	Spray: 29µg/actuation Solution: 25µg/actuation Adults and children ≥ 14 yr: 2 actuations each nostril, bid Children 6–14 yr: 1 actuation each nostril tid or 2 actuations each nostril, bid
Budesonide	Rhinocort Aqua	Spray: 32 µg/actuation Adults and children ≥ 6 yr: 1 sprays each nostril daily (starting dose)
Fluticasone	Flonase	Spray: 50 µg/actuation Adults: 2 sprays each nostril once daily (starting dose) Children ≥ 4 yr: 1 spray each nostril once daily (starting dose)
Mometasone furoate	Nasonex	Spray: 50 µg/actuation Adults and children ≥ 12 yr: 2 sprays each nostril once daily Children 2-11 yr: 1 spray each nostril once daily

*Detailed information about each agent should be obtained from the manufacturer's drug insert.

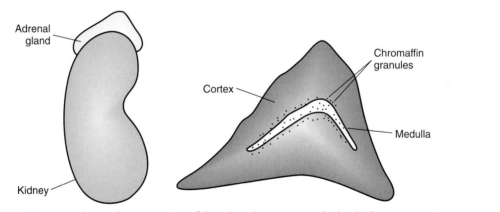

FIGURE 11-1 Location and cross-section of the adrenal, or suprarenal, gland. The outer portion, or cortex, of the adrenal gland is the source of corticosteroid hormones.

aldosterone regulates body water by increasing the amount of sodium reabsorption in the renal tubules. Androgenic corticosteroids, such as testosterone, the male sex hormone, cause secondary sex characteristics to appear and are discussed briefly in the section on androgenic corticosteroids. The corticosteroids used in pulmonary disease are all analogs of cortisol, or *hydrocortisone* as it is also termed. Glucocorticoid agents are referred to as *glucocorticosteroids*, and by the more general term *corticosteroid*, or simply as **steroids**.

KEY POINT

Corticosteroids secreted by the adrenal cortex include the *glucocorticoids* (e.g., cortisol), the *mineralocorticoids* (e.g., aldosterone), and the *androgen/estrogen* hormones.

KEY POINT

Glucocorticoids, often referred to simply as *steroids*, exert an *antiinflammatory effect* in the body.

The Hypothalamic–Pituitary–Adrenal Axis

The side effects of corticosteroids and the rationale for aerosol or alternate-day therapy can be understood if the production and control of **endogenous** (the body's own) corticosteroids are grasped. The pathway for release and control of corticosteroids is the hypothalamic–pituitary–adrenal (HPA) axis (Figure 11-2). Stimulation of the hypothalamus causes impulses to be sent to the area known as the median eminence, where corticotropin-releasing factor (CRF) is released. CRF circulates through the portal vessel to the anterior pituitary gland, which then releases corticotropin, or adrenocorticotropic hormone (ACTH), into the bloodstream. ACTH in turn stimulates the adrenal cortex to secrete glucocorticoids, such as cortisol. Cortisol and glucocorticoids in general regulate the metabolism of carbohydrates, fats, and proteins, generally to increase levels of glucose for body energy. This is the reason cortisol and its analogs are called glucocorticoids. They can also cause lipolysis, redistribution of fat stores, and breakdown of tissue protein stores. These actions are the basis for many of the side effects seen with glucocorticoid drugs. The breakdown of proteins for use of the amino acids (gluconeogenesis) is responsible for muscle wasting, and the effects on glucose metabolism can increase plasma glucose levels. This last is sometimes referred to as **steroid diabetes**.[5]

Hypothalamic–Pituitary–Adrenal Suppression With Steroid Use

> **KEY POINT**
>
> *Exogenous* corticosteroid agents can *suppress the HPA axis* and the adrenal gland.

One of the most significant side effects of treatment with glucocorticoid drugs (**exogenous** corticosteroids) is adrenal suppression or, more generally, HPA suppression. When the body produces endogenous glucocorticoids, there is a normal feedback mechanism within the HPA axis to limit production. As glucocorticoid levels rise, release of CRF and ACTH is inhibited, and further adrenal production of glucocorticoids is stopped. This feedback inhibition of the hypothalamus and the pituitary can be seen in Figure 11-2, and is analogous to the servo mechanism by which a thermostat regulates furnace production of heat by monitoring temperature levels. Unfortunately, the body cannot

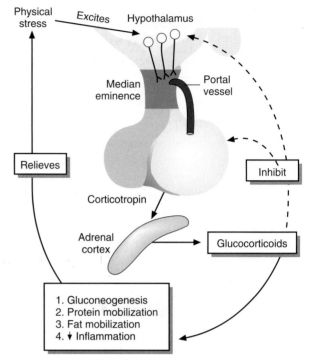

FIGURE 11-2 Hypothalamic–pituitary–adrenal (HPA) axis regulation of corticosteroid secretion (see text for complete description of function).

distinguish between its own endogenous glucocorticoids and exogenous glucocorticoid drugs. Administration of glucocorticoid drugs raises the body's level of these hormones, and this inhibits the hypothalamus and pituitary glands, which in turn decreases adrenal production. This is referred to as *HPA suppression* or, specifically, *adrenal suppression*. It is seen with systemic administration of corticosteroids, begins after a single day, and is significant after a week of oral therapy at usual doses. One of the primary reasons for using aerosolized glucocorticoids is to minimize adrenal, or HPA, suppression by both minimizing the dosage and localizing the site of treatment.

If a patient has received oral corticosteroids and adrenal suppression has occurred, weaning from the exogenous corticosteroids through use of tapered dose therapy allows time for recovery of the body's own adrenal secretion. It should be noted that aerosolized corticosteroids do not deposit sufficient amounts of drug to replace the missing output of a suppressed adrenal gland. Therefore a patient with adrenal suppression cannot be abruptly withdrawn from oral corticosteroids and placed on an aerosol dosage. The aerosol should be started, and the oral agent tapered off slowly at the same time.

The Diurnal Steroid Cycle

KEY POINT

Levels of endogenous corticosteroids follow a daily, or *diurnal*, rhythm.

The production of the body's own glucocorticoids also follows a rhythmic cycle, termed a *diurnal* or *circadian rhythm*. This daily rise and fall of glucocorticoid levels in the body is shown in Figure 11-3. On a daily schedule of daytime work and nighttime sleep, cortisol levels are highest in the morning around 8 A.M. These high plasma levels inhibit further production and release of glucocorticoids and ACTH by the HPA axis because of the feedback mechanism previously presented. During the day, plasma levels of both ACTH (Figure 11-3, *dotted line*) and cortisol (Figure 11-3, *solid line*) gradually fall. As the glucocorticoid level falls, the anterior pituitary is reactivated to begin releasing ACTH, which in turn stimulates production of cortisol by the adrenal cortex. This lag between the increased ACTH and cortisol levels is illustrated in Figure 11-3. One of the reasons for jet lag and the delay in adjusting to night shift from day shift is that this diurnal and regular rhythm of corticosteroid levels becomes out of synchronization with the time zone and the work time. Although the worker needs to sleep at 8 A.M. after working all night, the body is wide awake, with energy stores being released.

Alternate-Day Steroid Therapy

Alternate-day therapy mimics the natural diurnal rhythm by giving a steroid drug early in the morning, when normal tissue levels are high. Thus suppression of the hypothalamic–pituitary system occurs at the same time it normally would with the body's own steroid, and on the alternate day the regular diurnal secretion

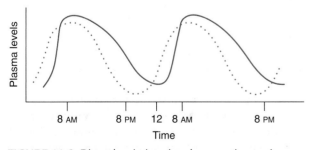

FIGURE 11-3 Diurnal variations in adrenocorticotropic hormone (ACTH; dotted line) and cortisol (solid line) (see text for detailed description).

in the hypothalamic–pituitary–adrenal (HPA) system can resume. Tissue side effects are minimized because the drug is administered at the time when tissues are normally exposed to high corticosteroid levels by the body's rhythm. Use of an intermediate-acting corticosteroid drug, with a duration of 12 to 36 hours, allows drug therapy to be restricted to alternate days.

NATURE OF THE INFLAMMATORY RESPONSE

One of the major therapeutic effects seen with analogs of the natural (endogenous) adrenal cortical hormone hydrocortisone is an antiinflammatory action. Glucocorticoid analogs of natural (endogenous) hydrocortisone are used for this effect in treating asthma, which is an inflammatory process in the lungs. To understand the antiinflammatory activity of the glucocorticoid drugs used in asthma, the nature of inflammation in general, and of airway inflammation in particular, is reviewed briefly.

KEY POINT

Inflammation produces general symptoms of redness, swelling, heat, and pain.

Inflammation

A general definition of inflammation is the response of vascularized tissue to injury. An excellent and still-applicable description of inflammation was given in the first century A.D. by Celsus: *"rubor et tumor cum calore et dolore."* This is translated as "redness and swelling with heat and pain." This is the most general description of an inflammatory reaction to injury, such as a cut, wound infection, splinter, burn, scrape, or bee sting.

An update of Celsus's description occurred in the 1920s with Thomas Lewis's characterization known as the *triple response:*

Redness: The local dilation of blood vessels, occurring in seconds

Flare: A reddish color several centimeters from the site, occurring 15 to 30 seconds after injury

Wheal: Local swelling, occurring in minutes

The process of inflammation producing the visible results described by Celsus, Lewis, and others is caused by the following four major categories of activity:

Increased vascular permeability: An exudate is formed in the surrounding tissues

Leukocytic infiltration: White cells emigrate through capillary walls (diapedesis) in response to attractant chemicals (chemotaxis).

Phagocytosis: White cells and macrophages (in the lungs) ingest and process foreign material such as bacteria.

Mediator cascade: Histamine and chemoattractant factors are released at the site of injury, and various inflammatory mediators such as complement and arachidonic acid products are generated.

Inflammation in the Airway

KEY POINT

In the airway, inflammation is mediated by various cells, such as *eosinophils, basophils, macrophages, mast cells, T lymphocytes,* and *epithelial or endothelial cells* in response to the release of *mediators of inflammation.* This process is complex and involves several mediators, including the *arachidonic acid cascade* (**prostaglandins** and leukotrienes), *histamine,* and a variety of *cytokines,* such as interleukins. These mediators further amplify the inflammatory response by attracting the cells mentioned previously to the airway and inducing the release of *adhesion* factors (e.g., intercellular adhesion molecule [ICAM]) to bind inflammatory cells to the airway surface.

Inflammation can occur in the lungs in response to a variety of causes. These include direct trauma (gunshot wound, stabbing), indirect trauma (blunt chest injury), inhalation of noxious or toxic substances (chlorine gas, smoke), respiratory infections and systemic infections producing septicemia and septic shock with acute respiratory distress syndrome (ARDS), and allergenic or nonallergenic stimulation in asthma. The two most common inflammatory diseases of the airway seen in respiratory care are chronic bronchitis, usually caused by tobacco smoking, and asthma, which can be caused by a range of triggers and involves a complex pathophysiology.

Because glucocorticoids are a mainstay for treating asthma, a brief description of the multiple pathways and mediators for the genesis of airway inflammation seen in asthma is given. Asthma is currently understood as a disease in which there is chronic inflammation of the airway wall, causing airflow limitation and a hyperresponsiveness to a variety of stimuli (Box 11-1).[5,6] The airway inflammation is mediated by inflammatory cells such as the mast cell, eosinophils, T lymphocytes, and macrophages. The mast cell and the eosinophil are considered to be the major effector cells of the inflammatory response, regardless of whether the asthma is

Box 11-1   Operational Definition of Asthma

Asthma is a chronic inflammatory disorder of the airways in which many cells and cellular elements play a role, in particular, mast cells, eosinophils, T lymphocytes, macrophages, neutrophils, and epithelial cells. In susceptible individuals, this inflammation causes recurrent episodes of wheezing, breathlessness, chest tightness, and coughing, particularly at night or in the early morning. These episodes are usually associated with widespread but variable airflow obstruction that is often reversible either spontaneously or with treatment. The inflammation also causes an associated increase in the existing bronchial hyperresponsiveness to a variety of stimuli.

National Asthma Education and Prevention Program, National Heart, Lung, and Blood Institute, National Institutes of Health: Expert Panel Report 2: *Guidelines for the diagnosis and management of asthma,* NIH Publication 97-4051. Bethesda, Md, 1997, National Institutes of Health.

allergic or nonallergic.[6] T lymphocytes may be pivotal in coordinating the inflammatory response by release of numerous proinflammatory cytokines (proteins that regulate immune/inflammatory responses), which in turn act on basophils, epithelial cells, and endothelial cells in the airway to further the inflammatory process. The potent mediators released during an asthmatic reaction cause airway smooth muscle contraction (bronchospasm), increased microvascular leakage and airway wall swelling, mucus secretion, and over the longer term remodeling of the airway wall. In an acute state, asthmatic individuals exhibit wheezing, breathlessness, chest tightness, and cough, especially at night or early morning. The acute symptoms produced by the airway inflammation are at least partly reversible either spontaneously or with pharmacological treatment. Treatment with antiinflammatory agents such as glucocorticoids is important to reduce the basal level of airway inflammation and thereby reduce airway hyperresponsiveness and the predisposition to acute episodes of obstruction.

Asthmatic reactions are biphasic, including an early phase and a late phase. A conceptual representation of the overall process is given in Figure 11-4. After an insult to the asthmatic airway by an allergen, cold air, viral infection, or noxious gas, there is evidence that the early asthmatic response is caused by **immunoglobulin E (IgE)**-dependent activation of airway mast cells, which can release inflammatory mediators such as histamine, prostaglandin D_2 (PGD_2), and leukotriene C_4.[6] The immediate response of the airway to chemicals such

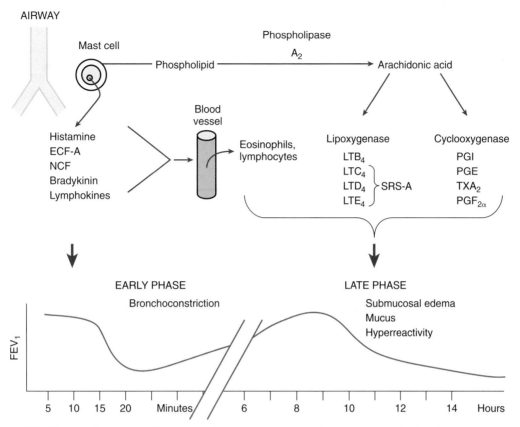

FIGURE 11-4 Conceptual illustration of the inflammatory asthmatic response in the airway, producing a biphasic deterioration in expiratory flow rates described as an early-phase and late-phase response to triggering stimuli. *ECF-A,* Eosinophilic chemotactic factor; *FEV$_1$,* forced expiratory volume in 1 second; *LTB$_4$,* leukotriene B$_4$; *LTC$_4$,* leukotriene C$_4$; *LTD$_4$,* leukotriene D$_4$; *LTE$_4$,* leukotriene E$_4$; *NCF,* neutrophil chemotactic factor; *PGI,* prostaglandin I; *PGE,* prostaglandin E; *PGF$_2$α,* prostaglandin F$_2$α; *SRS-A,* slow-reacting substance of anaphylaxis; *TXA$_2$,* thromboxane A$_2$.

as histamine is bronchospasm. This response peaks at about 15 minutes and then declines over the next hour. This produces the early-phase decrease in expiratory flow rates illustrated in Figure 11-4. Although the early bronchoconstriction of smooth muscle may self-limit or respond to β agonists (described in Chapter 6), the progression of cellular events can continue. Mast cell mediators and the release of cytokines recruit other inflammatory cells (eosinophils, basophils, monocytes/macrophages, and lymphocytes) by activating epithelial cells and endothelial cells to release adhesion molecules (e.g., intercellular adhesion molecule [ICAM]) and other cytokines to cause the late-phase reaction. During the late-phase response, mast cells and recruited eosinophils, lymphocytes, or macrophages that have infiltrated the airway release a range of inflammatory mediators. Neutrophils are not generally associated with asthma and allergic reactions in the absence of infection. The

late asthmatic response occurs 6 to 8 hours after a challenge, and it may last for up to 24 hours. The late-phase reaction is thought to be reflective of the chronic inflammation characterizing asthma between acute episodes.[7]

Phospholipids in the cell membrane of mast cells and other cells are converted by phospholipase A$_2$ to arachidonic acid and then to a variety of bronchoactive and vasoactive substances by the two metabolic paths shown in Figure 11-4: the cyclooxygenase and lipoxygenase pathways. The term *eicosanoid* is used to refer to the products of the two pathways. The migration of eosinophils and lymphocytes and further development of inflammation-producing chemicals such as the arachidonic acid metabolites and cytokines all contribute to build an inflammatory response in the lung.[8] In addition to smooth muscle spasm, mucus secretion occurs, along with mucosal swelling resulting from increased vascular permeability. Shedding of airway cells (desquamation) and goblet cell hyperplasia are seen. The result is mucus plugging of the airway, complicated by the cellular debris in the bronchial lumen. The pathology of bronchial asthma has been described as "chronic desquamating eosinophilic bronchitis."[9] These airway changes lead to further bronchial hyperreactivity seen in asthma. There is evidence of airway remodeling, with increased tenascin (an extracellular matrix protein for cell development), collagens, and fibronectin, all of which can cause thickening of the basement membrane in the airway wall. This deregulates communication between cells, promoting epithelial damage and enhancing the inflammatory response.[10]

AEROSOLIZED CORTICOSTEROIDS

Several corticosteroid preparations are available, such as hydrocortisone, cortisone, prednisone, prednisolone, and methylprednisolone, all of which have antiinflammatory activity. However, they produce undesirable systemic side effects when used to treat asthma, COPD, and inflammation of the lung. As with all inhaled agents, topical application of corticosteroids is intended to provide direct application of the drug to the lung or nasal passages and reduce systemic side effects.

Aerosolized Corticosteroid Agents

Several aerosol steroid agents, all of which are glucocorticoids, are available for inhalational use in the United States at the time of this edition. These are identified in Table 11-1, which summarizes steroids used for oral inhalation, and Table 11-2, which lists agents for intranasal delivery, giving strengths and recommended doses. Originally, in the United States, all of the orally inhaled corticosteroids were available as metered dose inhaler (MDI) formulations. However, three dry powder inhalers (DPIs), the Diskus (fluticasone), the Turbuhaler (budesonide), and the Asmanex Twisthaler (mometasone furoate), have been introduced, along with the only approved small volume nebulizer (SVN) formulation (budesonide [Pulmicort Respules]). At the time of this edition all of the MDI formulations are available with hydrofluoroalkane (HFA) propellant (beclomethasone, flunisolide, fluticasone, and ciclesonide) with the exception of triamcinolone.

These agents possess a high topical-to-systemic potency ratio, which makes them suitable for control of asthma or COPD with minimal systemic side effects. The chemical structures of the aerosol agents available

for oral and nasal inhalation are shown in Figure 11-5. A brief description of each of the aerosol agents is given below.

Beclomethasone dipropionate (QVAR) has been known by several names such as Vanceril and Beclovent; however, with the transition from chlorofluorocarbon (CFC)-propelled MDI formulations, beclomethasone dipropionate has been reformulated with an HFA propellant, in a 40- and 80-µg MDI strength as QVAR (see Table 11-1). Along with the change in propellant, many components of the MDI system were reengineered, significantly increasing the efficiency of this drug delivery system. Lung deposition with QVAR has been measured at 50 to 60% of the emitted dose (see discussion of MDIs in Chapter 3). As seen in Table 11-1, the usual starting dose of QVAR is 40 to 80 µg twice daily.

An aerosol dose of 400 µg is approximately equivalent to 5 to 10 mg of oral prednisone. When inhaled by aerosol, the swallowed drug is slowly absorbed from the gastrointestinal tract, and most of what is absorbed is quickly (half-life in the liver, 10 minutes) broken down in its first passage through the liver, preventing high plasma levels.

Absorption of the drug across the pulmonary epithelium is good, but rapid inactivation prevents systemic accumulation. After inhalation of a 2-mg dose, plasma levels of beclomethasone dipropionate are very low, but the active metabolite, beclomethasone monopropionate (often designated 17-BMP), reaches significant plasma levels of 1.8 to 2.5 ng/ml.[11]

Triamcinolone acetonide (Azmacort) is also topically active and was available as Aristocort and Kenalog before its release as an aerosol. Triamcinolone acetonide is nonpolar and water insoluble, resulting in a lower potential for systemic absorption. This drug is slightly less topically active than beclomethasone dipropionate.[12] High initial doses of 12 to 16 inhalations/day may be needed in severe asthma. This agent is marketed with a built-in spacer device. At the time of this edition Azmacort remains a CFC-driven MDI. Flunisolide (AeroBid, Aerospan) is another topically active aerosol preparation, similar in potency to triamcinolone, and is said to have a longer duration of action. Because of the phase-out of CFC propellant and the increased deposition seen with other HFA MDIs flunisolide, at the time of this edition, is currently available as a CFC MDI (AeroBid) and as an HFA MDI (Aerospan). AeroBid, as the name indicates, is given twice daily at 250 µg/puff. Aerospan is also prescribed twice daily at 80 µg/puff, which is noticeably much less than the AeroBid dosage. This difference between doses is due to the delivery

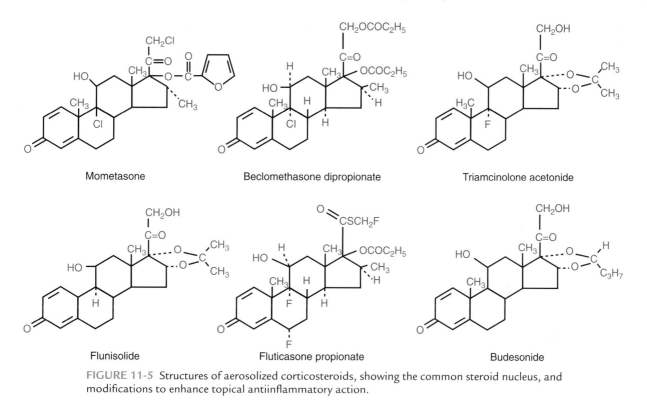

FIGURE 11-5 Structures of aerosolized corticosteroids, showing the common steroid nucleus, and modifications to enhance topical antiinflammatory action.

characteristics of each formulation. Aerospan, like Asmacort, is manufactured with a spacer attached to the actuation device.

Flunisolide shows a peak plasma level after inhalation at between 2 and 60 minutes, indicating good absorption from the lungs, as with beclomethasone. The half-life in plasma with inhalation is approximately 1.8 hours and similar to that with oral or intravenous dosing, indicating a rapid first-pass metabolism.[13]

Fluticasone propionate (Flovent HFA, Flovent Diskus) is a synthetic, trifluorinated glucocorticoid with high topical antiinflammatory potency and is available in MDI and DPI form. The MDI is available in three different strengths: 44, 110, and 220 µg. The DPI form is available in three different strengths as well: 50, 100, and 250 µg. The drug is a further analog of previous agents with high topical potency, synthesized in an attempt to avoid systemic side effects. Fluticasone is derived from the 17β-carbothioate series of androstane analogs, a group that has very weak HPA inhibitory activity but high antiinflammatory effect.[14] Using fluocinolone acetonide as a reference standard, fluticasone propionate was found to have an antiinflammatory potency of 91 in mice, with an HPA-inhibitory activity of only 1, giving a therapeutic index (antiinflammatory potency/HPA potency) of 91. By comparison, beclomethasone dipropionate has an antiinflammatory potency of 21, with an HPA-inhibitory potency of 49 in mice.[15] If given by subcutaneous injection to mice, fluticasone propionate does exhibit HPA inhibition; however, the oral route gives only weak HPA suppression. This is useful with inhaled aerosols, because a portion of the aerosol may be swallowed and contribute to systemic activity of a drug (see Chapter 2, Pharmacokinetics of Inhaled Aerosol Drugs). An explanation for the weak HPA suppression when given orally may be its high first-pass effect, resulting in less than 1% of active drug in the circulation, because fluticasone is rapidly metabolized in the liver to the inactive product, 17β-carboxylic acid.[15]

Budesonide (Pulmicort Respules, Pulmicort Turbuhaler) is available as a DPI (Pulmicort Turbuhaler) or as an inhalation solution (Pulmicort Respules). The Turbuhaler delivers 200 µg/metered dose, whereas Pulmicort Respules is available in doses of 0.25 and 0.5 mg. The benefit of using Respules is that it can be mixed with other agents such as bronchodilators (e.g., albuterol, levalbuterol, and ipratropium). Numerous studies have shown that mixing the agents had no effect on the drugs mixed.[16]

Budesonide is a topically active inhaled corticosteroid with a potency greater than that of beclomethasone dipropionate, triamcinolone, or flunisolide, but less potent than fluticasone, as estimated by skin vaso-constriction assay. With oral administration, only 10% of budesonide enters the systemic circulation because of high (approximately 89%) first-pass metabolism in the liver. After inhalation with a spacer device, peak plasma concentrations occur between 15 and 45 minutes. The plasma half-life is 2 hours. There appears to be minimal metabolism in the lung, with approximately 70% of the inhaled dose reaching the circulation.[17] Budesonide was found to exhibit about half the adrenal suppression of fluticasone, on a microgram equivalent basis in asthmatic patients.[18]

Mometasone furoate (Asmanex Twisthaler) is available as a DPI with 220 µg/actuation dosing. McCormack and Plosker[19] give a review of its use in asthma. Asmanex can be given once or twice daily. The single-day dosing may be a benefit to increase consistency in usage of an inhaled corticosteroid. Karpel and others found that pulmonary function results increased in patients receiving once-daily Asmanex compared with placebo in patients previously using twice-daily doses of inhaled corticosteroids.[20]

Fluticasone propionate/salmeterol (Advair) is a combination product of the corticosteroid fluticasone with the long-acting β_2-agonist bronchodilator salmeterol (see Chapter 6 for a discussion of salmeterol). Advair is available as a DPI and HFA MDI in three different strengths (fluticasone/salmeterol): DPI: 100 µg/50 µg, 250 µg/50 µg, and 500 µg/50 µg, HFA MDI: 45 µg/21 µg, 115 µg/21 µg, and 230 µg/21 µg . The combination of inhaled steroid and long-acting β_2 agonist in a convenient dose package would be useful in patients with asthma requiring step 3 care or higher, needing both types of drug. In a large multicenter clinical study by Shapiro and colleagues,[21] patients with asthma who were taking medium doses of inhaled corticosteroids were treated with 250 µg of fluticasone in combination with 50 µg of salmeterol from the DPI Diskus device for 12 weeks. Patients in the treatment group had significantly better FEV_1 profiles over 12 hours, a significantly greater probability of remaining in the study and not withdrawing because of worsening symptoms, a significantly increased morning peak expiratory flow (PEF), reduced asthma symptom scores, reduced rescue albuterol use, and significantly fewer nights with no awakenings, compared with patients taking salmeterol or fluticasone alone or placebo.

Budesonide/formoterol (Symbicort) is a combination product of the corticosteroid budesonide with the long-acting β_2-agonist bronchodilator formoterol (see Chapter 6 for a discussion of formoterol). Symbicort is available as an MDI in two strengths (budesonide/formoterol: 80 µg/4.5 µg and 160 µg/4.5 µg, respectively). In two large, double-blind, placebo-controlled studies involving more than 100 patients, Symbicort was able to increase lung function as a combination drug better than either drug separately or placebo, plus it was found that the combination therapy was able to increase lung function as quickly as 15 minutes after administration (manufacturer's literature).

Although combination products have the disadvantage of not allowing changes in dose for each drug separately and have been discouraged, there is evidence of a beneficial, complementary interaction between glucocorticoids and β-adrenergic agonists. The addition of long-acting bronchodilators to inhaled corticosteroids has no negative effect and shows improvements in lung function and symptom control, as demonstrated in the clinical trial by Shapiro and associates,[21] Chung for Advair,[22] and Jenkins and colleagues[23] for Symbicort.

The interaction results from the following known or investigational actions of steroids and β agonists:

- Steroids increase β_2-adrenergic receptor transcription (upregulation of β receptors).[22,24]
- Inhaled corticosteroid therapy can provide partial protection against the development of tolerance to β_2-adrenergic agonists.[22]
- Salmeterol has been shown to promote binding of the glucocorticoid receptor to the response element of the cell's nuclear DNA, *without the glucocorticoid present*, in vascular cells, thus initiating the antiinflammatory effect at least partially.[24]

If management of asthma requires both a long-acting β agonist and an inhaled corticosteroid, the combination product of fluticasone propionate/salmeterol or budesonide/formoterol offers the advantage of more convenient, single-formulation dosing.

Intranasal Corticosteroids

All of the steroids available as orally inhaled agents are also available in an intranasal formulation. Exact indications for the intranasal preparations vary by specific agent, but in general, intranasal steroids are used for the treatment of allergic or inflammatory nasal conditions and seasonal or perennial allergic or nonallergic rhinitis and to prevent reoccurrence of nasal polyps. Available preparations are listed in Table 11-2, with strengths and recommended doses. Other agents that are used to treat seasonal allergic rhinitis include H_1-receptor antagonists (e.g., loratadine), cromolyn sodium (see Chapter 12), topical vasoconstrictors (see

Chapter 15) such as oxymetazoline or ephedrine, and anticholinergics such as ipratropium bromide (see Chapter 7).

KEY POINT

Aerosolized glucocorticoids are all topically active drugs and include beclomethasone dipropionate, triamcinolone acetonide, flunisolide, budesonide, fluticasone propionate, and mometasone furoate. Aerosol agents are available for both *oral inhalation* in the control of *asthma and COPD* and *intranasal* administration for *rhinitis*.

PHARMACOLOGY OF CORTICOSTEROIDS

KEY POINT

Glucocorticoids are lipid soluble and act on intracellular receptors to produce their antiinflammatory effects.

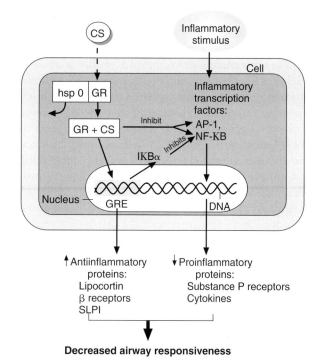

FIGURE 11-6 Proposed mechanism of action by which glucocorticoids exert an antiinflammatory effect. *AP-1*, Activator protein-1; *CS*, corticosteroid; *DNA*, deoxyribonucleic acid; *GR*, glucocorticoid receptor; *GRE*, glucocorticoid response element; *hsp90*, heat shock protein 90; *IκBα*, inhibitor of nuclear factor-κBα; *NF-κB*, nuclear factor-κB; *SLPI*, secretory leukocyte protease inhibitor.

The inflammatory process can be reduced or blocked by the antiinflammatory effects of glucocorticoids. The beneficial effect of glucocorticoids in asthma and other diseases of inflammation is due to their ability to inhibit the activity of inflammatory cells and mediators of inflammation.

Mode of Action

KEY POINT

The *mode of action* of glucocorticoids is through the *upregulation* of antiinflammatory proteins (e.g., β receptors and lipocortin), and the *downregulation* of proinflammatory proteins (e.g., cytokines and substance P).

Glucocorticoids are highly lipophilic and enter airway cells to bind to intracellular receptors.[25] This mechanism of drug signaling action was described briefly in Chapter 2 in the discussion of the pharmacodynamics of lipid-soluble drugs that interact with intracellular receptors. Originally, investigators thought that corticosteroids or, more simply, steroids, exerted antiinflammatory activity by stabilizing lysosomes within neutrophils. This prevented degranulation and an inflammatory response. In the mid-1960s, steroid receptors were discovered, and the realization developed that steroids modify the inflammatory response by inducing

gene expression within the cell. By the 1980s, it was demonstrated that glucocorticoids induce gene expression for the antiinflammatory protein lipocortin, which inhibits the enzyme phospholipase A₂ (PLA₂), preventing the arachidonic acid cascade, which leads to prostaglandin synthesis and lipoxygenase products. However, now it is understood that PLA₂ inhibition is only one of multiple mechanisms by which steroids attenuate the inflammatory response.[7,26-28]

Steroids suppress a local or systemic inflammatory response by at least three general actions. These actions are illustrated in Figure 11-6. In general, steroids diffuse into the cell and bind to a glucocorticoid receptor. Before binding by a steroid, the glucocorticoid receptor is in an inactive state and is bound to a protein complex termed *heat shock protein 90* (hsp90), which prevents the unoccupied receptor from translocating to the nucleus of the cell. When the steroid binds to the receptor, the hsp90 dissociates, and the steroid–receptor complex then translocates to the cell nucleus. One general action (not necessarily the first temporally) of a glucocorticoid is to upregulate the transcription of antiinflammatory genes for substances such as lipocortin, previously described.[26-28] In the nucleus the steroid produces this part of its effect on the cell by binding to portions of the nuclear DNA termed *glucocorticoid response elements*. Binding of the drug–receptor complex to glucocorticoid response elements upregulates, or induces, transcription of antiinflammatory substances such as lipocortin, neutral endopeptidase, secretory leukocyte protease inhibitor (SLPI), or inhibitors of plasminogen activator.[7] These are all antiinflammatory substances. A second general action of glucocorticoids is the suppression of factors such as activator protein-1 (AP-1) and nuclear factor-κB (NF-κB), which cause transcription of genes involved in inflammation. This may be by means of a direct interaction with these transcription factors, by which the transcription factor is inactivated before it induces gene expression in the nucleus.[26] Direct inactivation of AP-1 and NF-κB leads to downregulation of gene expression for proinflammatory mediators such as cytokines. NF-κB regulates genes that have increased expression in asthma, including genes for cytokines such as interleukins (IL-1, IL-3, etc.); chemokines; tumor necrosis factor-α (TNF-α); nitric oxide synthase, which produces nitric oxide in the airway; and adhesion molecules, which promote recruitment and attachment of leukocytes (eosinophils and basophils) from the circulation to the airway endothelium.[15,26,27] A direct inactivation of inflammatory transcription factors such as AP-1 or NF-κB may account for the rapidity with which some cellular effects of steroids are seen and that are not well explained by the time needed for modification of gene expression within a cell. A third action of glucocorticoids is to upregulate the expression of inhibitors of NF-κB, such as the inhibitor protein IκBα. This inhibitor of NF-κB further suppresses gene expression for proinflammatory proteins, such as cytokines.[27-29]

The general result of these actions is to *induce* gene expression for *antiinflammatory* proteins and receptors and to *suppress* gene expression for *proinflammatory* proteins. Overall, glucocorticoids inhibit the cytokine production responsible for recruitment and migration of inflammatory cells such as eosinophils and lymphocytes into the airway. Examples of cytokines that are suppressed through gene suppression activity of steroids are listed in Box 11-2.

Glucocorticoids inhibit many of the cells involved in airway inflammation, including macrophages, T lymphocytes, eosinophils, and mast cells in the

---

Box 11-2 **Cytokines* Involved in Airway Inflammation That Are Suppressed by Glucocorticoids**

Tumor Necrosis Factor-α (TNF-α), Interleukin-1 (IL-1): Released from macrophages, monocytes, and other cells to activate endothelial cells to recruit neutrophils, eosinophils, and basophils from the circulation

Interleukin-4 (IL-4), Interleukin-13 (IL-13): Released from lymphocytes and basophils and associated with allergic diseases; cause the endothelium to bind basophils, eosinophils, monocytes, and lymphocytes

Interleukin-3 (IL-3), Interleukin-5 (IL-5), Granulocyte-Macrophage Colony-stimulating Factor (GM-CSF), Interferon-γ (IFN-): Cause eosinophil priming, resulting in prolonged eosinophil survival and potentiated degranulation to release inflammatory substances

Chemokines: A family of small cytokines (molecules with masses of 8 to 10 kDa) having many chemotactic properties to attract cells to a site. Example: Regulated on activation normal T-cell expressed and secreted (RANTES), one of the most potent chemokines, which induces eosinophil and lymphocyte migration and attraction

---

*Cytokines are proteins secreted by a variety of cells, such as lymphocytes, that regulate local and systemic inflammatory responses.

---

bronchial airway epithelium and submucosa, and reverse the shedding of epithelial cells and goblet cell hyperplasia seen in asthma.[25,30] By decreasing cytokine-mediated survival of eosinophils, apoptosis of eosinophils occurs, reducing the number of eosinophils in the circulation and in the airway of subjects with asthma. Glucocorticoids also reduce the number of mast cells within the airways; mast cells are sources of histamine and other mediators of inflammation, and inhibit plasma exudation as well as mucus secretion in inflamed airways.[25,30]

Effect on White Blood Cell Count

Leukocytes, such as monocytes, macrophages, neutrophils, and basophils, are also essential to the inflammatory response and are attracted to an area of injury by the chemotactic factors identified among the mediators of inflammation. Neutrophils usually adhere ("marginate") to the capillary endothelium of storage sites in the lung. Glucocorticoids cause depletion of these stores and reduce their accumulation at inflammatory sites and in exudates. This is termed *demargination*, and can increase the number of neutrophils in circulation as the cells leave their storage sites. An overall increase in the white cell count can then be seen in patients receiving glucocorticoids. Glucocorticoids affect other leukocytes by inhibiting the number of monocytes, basophils, and eosinophils. This can also be seen in the differential count of these cells. An allergic asthmatic who would otherwise have a higher than normal eosinophil count will show a low count after initiation of drug therapy. Finally, glucocorticoids constrict the microvasculature to reduce leakage of the above-cited cells and fluids into inflammatory sites.

Effect on β Receptors

β-Adrenergic agents are among the most potent inhibitors of mast cell release, yet the asthmatic in an acute episode may be unresponsive to these drugs. A very beneficial effect of glucocorticoids is their ability to restore responsiveness to β-adrenergic stimulation.[24,31] This effect can be seen within 1 to 4 hours after intravenous administration of glucocorticoids and is the rationale for administering a bolus of steroid in status asthmaticus as part of acute treatment. Even though steroid action is slow, the sooner they are given, the sooner the asthmatic will begin to respond to β-adrenergic drugs, and supported ventilation may be avoided. Glucocorticoids enhance β-receptor stimulation by increasing the number and availability of β receptors on the cell surfaces and by increasing affinity of the receptor for β agonists. There is also evidence that glucocorticoids prolong endogenous circulatory catecholamine action by inhibiting the uptake-2 mechanism (extraneuronal uptake), as discussed in Chapter 5. The mechanisms for a positive interaction between β$_2$ agonists and corticosteroids are described in the discussion at the end of the section, Aerosolized Corticosteroid Agents.

HAZARDS AND SIDE EFFECTS OF STEROIDS

Systemic Administration of Steroids

KEY POINT

Hazards to *systemically* administered steroids include HPA suppression, immunosuppression, fluid retention, muscle wasting, and others.

The complicating side effects of systemic steroid treatment are well known and provide the motivation to switch to aerosolized, inhaled steroids when possible. These complications arise from the physiological effects of steroids on the body. These physiological effects are often

---

Box 11-3	**Side Effects Seen With Systemic Administration of Corticosteroids**

- Hypothalamic–pituitary–adrenal suppression
- Immunosuppression
- Psychiatric reactions
- Cataract formation
- Myopathy of skeletal muscle
- Osteoporosis
- Peptic ulcer
- Fluid retention
- Hypertension
- Increased white blood cell count
- Dermatological changes
- Growth restriction
- Increased glucose levels

---

exaggerated with systemic drug therapy, because potency and plasma levels are higher than with the body's own steroids. Complications of systemic therapy are reviewed by Truhan and Ahmed.[32] These complications are summarized in Box 11-3 and are briefly described here.

- Suppression of the HPA axis by exogenous steroids may occur, causing inhibition of ACTH release and cortisol secretion from the adrenal gland. The length of time to recover from this suppression varies with patient, dose, and duration of treatment.
- With sufficient dose and duration, immunosuppression can be caused by systemic use of steroids. This can lead to increased susceptibility to infection by bacterial, viral, or fungal agents.
- Psychiatric reactions can occur, including insomnia, mood changes, and bipolar or schizophrenic psychoses.
- Cataract formation has been noted, and, rarely, intraocular pressure may increase with systemic steroid therapy.
- Myopathy of striated skeletal muscle can occur.
- Steroid-induced osteoporosis is debated, but is thought to be a limitation of extended steroid therapy. Aseptic necrosis of the bone is also caused by steroid therapy.
- Peptic ulcer is thought to be a complication of steroid therapy, but evidence for this is debated. Patients may often be receiving other ulcerogenic medications such as aspirin or nonsteroidal antiinflammatory drugs (NSAIDs).
- Fluid retention can occur as a result of the sodium-sparing effects of glucocorticoids, giving a puffy appearance.
- Hypertension may accompany the fluid retention or be aggravated by it.

- Corticosteroids given systemically can increase the white blood cell count, with an increase in neutrophils and a decrease in lymphocytes and eosinophils.
- Dermatological changes can occur with steroid therapy, including a redistribution of subcutaneous fat causing the cushingoid appearance of central obesity, hump back, and moon face.
- Growth of children can be slowed by prolonged systemic therapy, because corticosteroids retard bone growth and epiphyseal maturation.
- Corticosteroids lead to gluconeogenesis and antagonize glucose uptake, causing hyperglycemia. This can lead to a reversible steroid-induced diabetes.

Systemic Side Effects With Aerosol Administration

KEY POINT

HPA suppression is minimal or absent with inhaled agents, although high doses can cause adrenal suppression in a dose-dependent fashion.

The rationale for the introduction of inhaled aerosol steroids was to eliminate or reduce the side effects seen with systemic therapy. Although the aerosol steroids are administered in low doses because of their high topical activity, local side effects may occur and certain systemic side effects, listed in Box 11-4, are also a concern. Some side effects may occur with transfer from oral therapy to the inhaled route. Three systemic effects of concern with inhaled steroids have been HPA suppression, loss of bone density, and growth restriction in children. A review and brief comment on possible systemic side effects with inhaled steroids is summarized below.

- Adrenal insufficiency may occur after transfer from systemic to inhaled aerosol steroids. Weaning from systemic steroids to allow recovery of adrenal cortex and HPA function and careful monitoring of pulmonary function can help control this problem.
- There may be a recurrence of allergic inflammation in other organs, such as nasal polyps or atopic dermatitis, after cessation of systemic steroids.
- Acute severe episodes of asthma may occur after withdrawal from oral steroids and transfer to inhaled forms. Aerosolized steroids may not be adequate to control asthma, especially during periods of stress, and short courses of oral drug may be necessary ("burst" therapy).
- Suppression of HPA function is nonexistent or low at small doses of inhaled aerosol steroids and increases with higher doses. Clinically significant suppression is rare at inhaled doses below 800 µg/day in adults and

Box 11-4	Potential Hazards and Side Effects With Inhaled Aerosol Corticosteroids
Systemic	**Local (Topical)**
Adrenal insufficiency*	Oropharyngeal fungal infections
Extrapulmonary allergy*	Dysphonia
Acute asthma*	Cough, bronchoconstriction
HPA suppression (minimal, dose dependent)	Incorrect use of MDI (inadequate dose)
Growth restriction (dose dependent)	

*After transfer from systemic corticosteroid therapy.
HPA, Hypothalamic–pituitary–adrenal; MDI, metered dose inhaler.

below 400 µg/day in children.[33] Goldberg and associates[34] investigated MDI beclomethasone administration in children with and without a reservoir. They found that 7 of 15 subjects using the MDI alone (average dose, 474 ± 220 µg/day) showed adrenal suppression as measured by 24-hour urinary free cortisol excretion. Only 2 of 24 subjects using an MDI–reservoir system (average dose, 563 ± 249 µg/day) showed such suppression. Their results indicated that inhalation of low to moderate doses can cause some adrenal suppression and that use of a reservoir can reduce this, probably by reducing the amount of drug swallowed. Although higher inhaled doses of steroid have a greater risk of adrenal suppression, the dose at which the risk for toxicity outweighs the beneficial effect of an inhaled steroid is not known.[33]

- Questions have been raised about the effect of inhaled steroids on growth when used in prepubertal children. A study by Wolthers and Pedersen[35] found a reduction in rate of lower leg growth with inhaled budesonide compared with placebo. Growth restriction was seen in some studies with beclomethasone dipropionate, yet other studies have found no effect on growth with the same drug by inhalation. Results may be confounded by the moderate growth restriction and delay in puberty seen as a result of asthma.[3] The authors cite a meta-analysis that found no association between growth impairment and inhaled beclomethasone dipropionate, even at higher doses.[36] Sharek and Bergman found in a meta-analysis that the use of beclomethasone and fluticasone resulted in a decrease in growth.[37] However, the benefits of inhaled corticosteroids in the treatment of asthma outweigh the possible consequence of growth reduction.

TABLE 11-3

Bioavailability of Oral and Inhaled Corticosteroid Agents

	Oral (%)*	Inhaled (%)†
Beclomethasone dipropionate	<20	≈20
Triamcinolone acetonide	22.5	21.5
Budesonide	1.0	25.0
Fluticasone propionate	<1	20.0

*Figures represent percentages of a 100% oral dose.
†Figures represent the 20% of an inhaled dose that reaches the lungs and indicate complete absorption of that fraction.
Modified from Johnson M: Pharmacodynamics and pharmacokinetics of inhaled glucocorticoids, *J Allergy Clin Immunol* 97(suppl):169, 1996.

- No data have demonstrated clearly the effect of inhaled glucocorticoids on bone density and osteoporosis in asthma. However, Israel and others discovered that the higher the dose of inhaled corticosteroid, the greater the effect on bone density seen in premenopausal, asthmatic women.[38]

In summary, it is logical that the risks of steroid-induced adverse effects are lower with the relatively low doses of inhaled steroids compared with systemic administration. However, the threshold doses by inhalation causing adrenal suppression or other effects are not known. In general, these effects are rare with doses of 800 µg/day or less in adults and 400 µg/day or less in children. Absorption of inhaled steroid leads to systemic bioavailability, from both the swallowed portion and the inhaled portion reaching the lung. Table 11-3 summarizes data on the bioavailability of four agents. When administered orally, bioavailability ranges from less than 1% to more than 20% of the total dose. This is due to the high first-pass metabolism of the swallowed drug. In contrast, all of the inhaled dose reaching the lung is absorbed and enters the systemic circulation, where it is ultimately metabolized in the liver or extrapulmonary tissues.[12] The efficiency of the delivery device in depositing drug in the lungs will therefore determine the amount of drug entering the systemic circulation from the airway. Thorsson and colleagues[39] reported that an MDI of budesonide delivered 18% of the dose to the lungs, whereas a DPI preparation (Turbuhaler) delivered nearly twice as much (32%). Leach and colleagues found that HFA formulations gave more than CFC formulations, with 53% of HFA beclomethasone deposited in the lung.[40]

The higher deposition is related to the particle size distribution of the device. HFA inhalers give a much better particle size distribution than do CFC devices. Unless lower doses are used with HFA devices and DPIs, greater systemic drug levels will result compared with those produced with an equal dose from an MDI. Total bioavailability, and thus the amount of drug that can cause systemic side effects such as HPA suppression, is a function of both the swallowed amount, with its bioavailability, and the inhaled amount, all of which is absorbed into the circulation. You will note that many of the HFA corticosteroid doses are lower than their CFC version. Use of a reservoir device and mouth rinsing can minimize the oropharyngeal loss and amount of swallowed drug contributing to systemic bioavailability and potential side effects. It will be necessary to adjust doses on the basis of the efficiency of the delivery system and the amount reaching the airway.

Topical (Local) Side Effects With Aerosol Administration

KEY POINT

Inhaled agents may cause local *oral candidiasis, hoarseness, cough,* or even bronchoconstriction in some cases.

Two of the most common side effects caused by topical application of inhaled steroids in the respiratory tract are oropharyngeal candidiasis (oral thrush) and dysphonia. Several other complications and precautions with the inhaled route are summarized below.

- Oropharyngeal fungal infections: Infections with *Candida albicans* or *Aspergillus niger* may occur in the mouth, pharynx, or larynx with aerosolized steroid treatment. Some form of this may be seen in up to one-third of patients taking the aerosol formulations, but such an infection responds to topical antifungal agents and seems to diminish with continued aerosol steroid use.[9] Occurrence and severity are dose related and are more likely in patients who are also taking oral steroids. The use of a spacer device and gargling after treatment can reduce oropharyngeal deposition of the steroid and the incidence or severity of such infections.

- Dysphonia: Hoarseness and changes in voice quality also may occur with inhaled steroids in one-third of patients. This can be minimized by use of a spacer and by gargling. The effect is caused primarily by adductor vocal cord paresis, which is thought to be a local steroid-induced myopathy.[41]

• Cough and bronchoconstriction: On occasion, cough or bronchoconstriction may occur after inhalation of an aerosol steroid.[9]
• Incorrect use: Incorrect use of the metered dose inhaler delivery vehicle also represents a possible risk factor, because inadequate amounts of the topical inhaled steroid will be delivered.

With inhaled steroids the following can minimize the risk of adverse effects, both local and systemic:
• Use of minimal doses (400 or 800 μg/day) in children and adults, or the lowest effective dose
• Use of a reservoir device
• Mouth rinsing after treatments

KEY POINT

Side effects with inhaled steroids can be *minimized* by use of a reservoir device, rinsing of the mouth after treatments, and use of minimal doses.

CLINICAL APPLICATION OF AEROSOL STEROIDS

Corticosteroids are used for a wide variety of conditions, with the therapeutic goal of reducing inflammation. These applications include clinical conditions such as contact dermatitis, rheumatoid arthritis, and systemic lupus erythematosus (SLE), as well as asthma and COPD, and include topical cream application and oral, parenteral, and inhaled formulations.

Use in Asthma

KEY POINT

Inhaled steroids are used in asthma as a *first-line therapy* for mild to moderate asthma.

The 2006 Global Initiative for Asthma (GINA),[5] the 1997 National Asthma Education and Prevention Program Expert Panel Report 2 (NAEPP EPR-2): *Guidelines for the Diagnosis and Management of Asthma*,[1] and the 2002 update of the NAEPP guidelines[2] identify corticosteroids as long-term control agents rather than quick-relief agents.

Corticosteroids have traditionally been used in asthma by the oral route for maintenance therapy of severe asthma and by the oral or intravenous route for treatment of status asthmaticus, as well as by inhalation for maintenance of asthma control. However, the increased emphasis on asthma as a disease of inflammation leading to bronchial hyperresponsiveness has shifted the use of inhaled aerosol steroids from second-line or third-line therapy to first-line, primary therapy. Appendix D offers a summary of the pharmacological management of asthma based on the NAEPP EPR-2. The following summarizes the principles of corticosteroid use in asthma, based on those guidelines.
• Bronchial hyperresponsiveness is characteristic of asthma and is related to the degree of airway inflammation.
• The basic pathology of asthma, previously emphasizing bronchospasm, is now understood to be a chronic inflammatory disorder of the airways resulting from a complex interaction among inflammatory cells, mediators, and airway tissue.[1,2] The phrase "chronic desquamating eosinophilic bronchitis" has been used to describe asthma.[9]
• Inhaled corticosteroids are considered to be the most effective long-term therapy for mild, moderate, or severe persistent asthma, and they are well tolerated and safe at recommended dosages.[1,5] Several points are related to the use of inhaled steroids.
  • Barnes suggests starting inhaled steroids at a high enough dose to be effective and then reducing the dose.[42] Alternatively, a short course of systemic corticosteroids can be used to gain control of symptoms followed by a step-down in therapy.[1,2] Loss of patient confidence and compliance with prescribed use of inhaled corticosteroids may be avoided in this way, especially because steroids do not give an immediate effect as a bronchodilator does. Any reduction in pharmacological management should be monitored by symptoms, concomitant need for β₂ agonists, and peak flow rates.
  • An increase in dose of inhaled steroids, such as doubling of the current dose, if peak expiratory flow rates decline 25 to 30%, may avoid the need for oral steroids. However, controlled studies are needed to confirm the effectiveness of such practice.[42]
  • If asthma is not controlled by inhaled steroids and other types of drug therapy, a short burst of oral steroids may be required to regain control of the asthma and to help clear the airways.[1,2,10]

Early Use of Corticosteroids in Asthma

There is evidence that the addition of an inhaled corticosteroid to first-line β-agonist maintenance treatment of asthma reduces morbidity and airway hyperresponsiveness.[1,2,43] Haahtela and associates[44] demonstrated that subjects with mild asthma maintained on inhaled budesonide (1200 μg/day for 2 years, and then

400 μg/day) had decreased bronchial response to histamine challenge compared with subjects taking inhaled terbutaline (375 μg twice daily), over a 2-year period. Perhaps the most significant finding was that the later addition of inhaled budesonide after use of a β_2 agonist was not able to give as high a level of bronchoprotection as achieved by subjects who had started with and continued taking the inhaled steroid. This suggests that irreversible changes had occurred during the 2 years of β_2-agonist therapy and supports earlier use of inhaled steroids. Masoli and colleagues,[45] in a meta-analysis reported that inhaled corticosteroids are best in treating asthma when kept to a therapeutic range of 400 μg/day.

Although inhaled corticosteroids are first-line antiinflammatory agents and acceptable for primary therapy of moderate asthma in children, the antiasthmatic prophylactic agents cromolyn sodium, nedocromil sodium, and leukotriene modifiers may be used as an initial choice for long-term control therapy in mild persistent asthma (step 2 therapy) with children, because these medications have excellent safety profiles.[2]

Inhaled Corticosteroids for Acute Severe Asthma

Inhaled corticosteroids have not been considered useful for treatment of acute, severe asthma episodes, and in fact drug labeling contraindicates this use, because there is no bronchodilator effect. In addition, the dose of inhaled steroids is low compared with oral administration. However, a study by Rodrigo and Rodrigo examined the addition of high, cumulative doses of inhaled flunisolide added to albuterol in emergency room treatment of acute adult asthma.[46] Both drugs were given by MDI with a spacer. Flunisolide was given as 4 puffs (250 μg/actuation) every 10 minutes. Their protocol allowed 3 hours of this treatment, with a cumulative dose of 6 mg of flunisolide each hour, and equally aggressive albuterol dosing. The use of flunisolide resulted in better lung function at 90 minutes and afterward, compared with the use of albuterol alone. Although preliminary, these results suggest that the contraindication to the use of inhaled corticosteroids for treating acute severe asthma may need to be reconsidered.

Clinical Use of Inhaled Corticosteroids

Other considerations in the clinical application of inhaled corticosteroids are as follows:
- High-dose inhaled steroids can be tried in cases of severe, persistent asthma to replace or reduce oral

corticosteroid dependence. High doses of inhaled steroids are two to four times the usual recommended dose. Oral steroid therapy can be reduced slowly while monitoring the patient's pulmonary function.[1,2] (Note that relative inhaled doses considered low, medium, and high are given in the NAEPP guidelines.)
- Although more control may be achieved with high doses of inhaled steroids, side effects, including systemic effects, are also likely to increase with inhaled doses above 1 mg/day. However, if oral steroids can be replaced or even reduced, this can be an overall improvement in the risk-to-benefit ratio.
- MDI-formulated corticosteroids should be administered for oral inhalation using a reservoir device (preferably a holding chamber rather than a spacer) and all formulations should include mouth rinsing, to reduce the risk of oropharyngeal candidiasis or other fungal infections and to reduce systemic absorption from swallowed drug.
- Use of a long-acting β_2 agonist such as salmeterol in subjects with inadequate symptom control, who are already receiving low to moderate doses of inhaled corticosteroids, may prevent the need to increase the inhaled corticosteroid dose.[1,2]
  - The use of long-term agonist with corticosteroid use can improve lung function.[1]
- Compliance with prescribed steroid therapy by inhalation appears to be poor and can be a complicating factor in the management of asthma and COPD. The ability to reduce agents or move to once-a-day dosing may be of benefit.

Use in Chronic Obstructive Pulmonary Disease

KEY POINT

Glucocorticoids may be of use in COPD and are often administered systemically for acute exacerbations. Inhaled glucocorticoids are prescribed for long-term results.

The use of steroids in COPD is recognized as having potential action in relieving symptoms, and exacerbations, but has little to no effect on FEV_1. The use of corticosteroids is described in the 2004 ATS guidelines[3] as well as in the 2005 GOLD guidelines.[4] A review and update on COPD has been provided by Fabbri and colleagues.[47]

COPD is characterized by a different pattern of inflammatory cells than is seen in asthma.[48,49] Whereas eosinophils predominate in asthma, neutrophils are mostly seen in COPD. Oral and inhaled corticosteroids do not influence the inflammatory changes driven by neutrophils.[27,48,49]

Studies that are available demonstrate that corticosteroid use in COPD reduces exacerbations, symptoms, and even mortality,[50] but has little effect on pulmonary function results.[51-54] However, other studies have found that inhaled corticosteroids may slow the decline of FEV_1.[53,55]

In acute exacerbations of COPD, oral or parenteral steroids are often given. Short-term corticosteroid therapy has shown benefit in hospitalized patients.[3,4] Patient with stable COPD should not be given systemic corticosteroids.[3]

RESPIRATORY CARE ASSESSMENT OF INHALED CORTICOSTEROID THERAPY

- Instruct patient in correct use of the aerosol delivery system (MDI, holding chamber, SVN, or DPI), and then verify.
- Assess breathing rate and pattern.
- Assess breath sounds by auscultation, before and after treatment.
- Assess pulse before and after treatment.
- Assess patient's subjective reaction to treatment, for any change in breathing effort or pattern.
- Verify that patient understands that a corticosteroid is a controller agent and is aware of its difference from a rescue bronchodilator (relieving agent); assess patient's understanding of the need for consistent use of an inhaled corticosteroid (compliance with therapy).
- In asthma, instruct patient in use of a peak flow meter, to monitor baseline PEF and changes. Verify that there is a specific action plan, based on symptoms and peak flow results. Subject should be clear on when to contact a physician with deterioration in PEF or exacerbation of symptoms.
- Long term: Assess severity of symptoms (coughing, wheezing, nocturnal awakenings), symptoms during exertion; use of rescue bronchodilator; number of exacerbations, missed work/school days; and pulmonary function. Modify level of therapy with reference to NAEPP and/or GINA guidelines for asthma and ATS and/or GOLD guidelines for COPD.
- Assess for presence of side effects with inhaled steroid therapy (oral thrush, hoarseness or voice changes, cough/wheezing with MDI use); have patient use a reservoir (preferably a holding chamber) with MDI use and verify correct use.

SELF-ASSESSMENT QUESTIONS

1. Identify all corticosteroids approved for clinical use by oral inhalation in the United States, using generic names.
2. What is the major therapeutic effect of corticosteroids?
3. Identify two common respiratory diseases in which inhaled corticosteroids are prescribed.
4. What is the rationale for administering corticosteroids by the inhalation route, rather than by the oral route, in asthma?
5. Contrast the effects of β agonists with those of corticosteroids on the early phase and late phase of asthma.
6. What is the effect of orally administered corticosteroids on growth, bone density, and adrenal function?
7. What is the purpose of alternate-day steroid therapy?
8. Can you transfer an asthmatic patient from oral steroid use to inhaled steroid use? Explain the precautions or reasons, as appropriate.
9. Identify a common side effect with inhaled steroids.
10. Identify two methods of minimizing the side effect identified in question 9.
11. Have inhaled corticosteroids traditionally been used with an asthmatic during an acute episode?

Answers to Self-Assessment Questions are found in Appendix A.

CLINICAL SCENARIO

A 55-year-old white female presents to the emergency department (ED) with a chief complaint of cough, wheezing, shortness of breath, and chest pain. She is well nourished and educated. She is a known asthmatic, with one hospitalization in the previous year for asthma exacerbation. Two days earlier, she reported rhinorrhea, sore throat, sinus congestion, and subsequent increase in dyspnea and wheeze.

Physical examination on admission to the ED exhibited wheezing on auscultation, use of accessory muscles, no cyanosis or diaphoresis, and mild respiratory distress. Vital signs were as follows: temperature (T), 98.4° F; pulse (P), 96 beats/min and regular; respiratory rate (RR), 22 breaths/min; and blood pressure (BP), 92/68 mmHg.

Chest radiograph showed hyperinflation, but no infiltrates or other abnormalities. Electrocardiogram revealed sinus tachycardia. Arterial blood gas determination on room air indicated the following: pH, 7.44; arterial carbon dioxide pressure (Pa_{CO_2}), 38 mmHg; arterial oxygen pressure (Pa_{O_2}), 54 mmHg; base excess (BE), 2.2; bicarbonate (HCO_3^-), 25.9 mEq/L; and arterial oxygen saturation (Sa_{O_2}), 89.4%. Hemoglobin was 13.3 g/dl, and the white blood cell (WBC) count was $8.8 \times 10^3/mm^3$. Administration of metered dose inhaler (MDI) albuterol by reservoir showed little improvement in her peak flow rates.

She was subsequently admitted to the hospital after failing to improve in her flow rates, blood gas values, or symptoms of dyspnea, and albuterol 0.5 cc of a 0.5% solution was administered by small volume nebulizer (SVN), with oxygen at 3 L/min by nasal cannula. She was given theophylline orally, intravenous methylprednisolone 40 mg, and a brand of phenylephrine for nasal decongestion and sinus clearance; ipratropium bromide by MDI was added to her inhaled albuterol. Over a 5-day course in the hospital, her peak flow rates improved to within 80% of her predicted value and her chest sounds were clear to auscultation. A throat culture returned normal flora, and follow-up theophylline levels showed 10 to 12 μg/ml. An arterial sample on day 5 gave the following: pH, 7.45; Pa_{CO_2}, 37 mmHg; Pa_{O_2}, 68 mmHg; HCO_3^-, 26.2 mEq/L; BE, 2.7; and Sa_{O_2}, 94% on room air. Hemoglobin was 12.9 g/dl. In preparation for discharge, respiratory care was consulted for appropriate inhaled medications.

What inhaled aerosol agents would you recommend as appropriate at this time for discharge?

What precautions and recommendations would you make with this subject?

Answers to Clinical Scenario Questions are found in Appendix A.

References

1. National Asthma Education and Prevention Program, National Heart, Lung, and Blood Institute, National Institutes of Health: Expert Panel Report 2: *Guidelines for the diagnosis and management of asthma*, NIH Publication 97–4051. Bethesda, Md, 1997, National Institutes of Health. (Available at http://www.nhlbi.nih.gov/guidelines/asthma/asthgdln.pdf; accessed February 2007.)
2. National Asthma Education and Prevention Program, National Heart, Lung, and Blood Institute, National Institutes of Health: Expert Panel Report: *Guidelines for the diagnosis and management of asthma—update on selected topics 2002*, NIH Publication 02–5074. Bethesda, Md, 2002, National Institutes of Health. (Available at http://www.nhlbi.nih.gov/guidelines/asthma/asthmafullrpt.pdf; accessed March 2007.)
3. Celli BR, MacNee W, ATS/ERS Task Force: Standards for the diagnosis and treatment of patients with COPD: a summary of the ATS/ERS position paper. *Eur Respir J* 23:932, 2004. Available at http://www.thoracic.org/sections/publications/statements/pages/respiratory-disease-adults/copdexecsum.html.accessed March 2007.
4. Global Initiative for Chronic Obstructive Lung Disease: Executive Summary: December 2006, *Global strategy for the diagnosis, management, and prevention of COPD.* National Heart, Lung, and Blood Institute (Bethesda, Md) and World Health Organization (Geneva, Switzerland), 2006. (Available at http://www.goldcopd.org/Guidelineitem.asp?l1=2&12=1&intId=996; accessed March 2007.)
5. Global Initiative for Asthma (GINA), National Heart, Lung, and Blood Institute, National Institutes of Health: *GINA Report, Global Strategy for Asthma Management and Prevention*, November, 2006. Bethesda, MD, 2006, National Institutes of Health (Available at: http://www.ginasthma.com/Guidelineitem.asp??l1=2&l2=1&intId=60, Accessed March 2007.)
6. Holgate ST: The immunopharmacology of mild asthma, *J Allergy Clin Immunol* 98:S7, 1996.
7. Schwiebert LM, Beck LA, Stellato C, Bickel CA, Bochner BS, Schleimer RP: Glucocorticosteroid inhibition of cytokine production: relevance to antiallergic actions, *J Allergy Clin Immunol* 97:143, 1996.
8. Kay AB: Mediators and inflammatory cells in allergic disease, *Ann Allergy* 59:35, 1987.
9. Reed CE: Aerosol glucocorticoid treatment of asthma: adults, *Am Rev Respir Dis* 141(suppl):S82, 1990.
10. Laitinen LA, Laitinen A: Remodeling of asthmatic airways by glucocorticosteroids, *J Allergy Clin Immunol* 97:153, 1996.
11. Johnson M: Pharmacodynamics and pharmacokinetics of inhaled glucocorticoids, *J Allergy Clin Immunol* 97:169, 1996.
12. Check WA, Kaliner MA: Pharmacology and pharmacokinetics of topical corticosteroid derivatives used for asthma therapy, *Am Rev Respir Dis* 141(suppl):S44, 1990.
13. Chaplin MD, Rooks W II, Swenson EW, Cooper WC, Nerenberg C, Chu NI: Flunisolide metabolism and dynamics of a metabolite, *Clin Pharmacol Ther* 27:402, 1980.
14. Holliday SM, Faulds D, Sorkin EM: Inhaled fluticasone propionate: a review of its pharmacodynamic and pharmacokinetic properties, and therapeutic use in asthma, *Drugs* 47:318, 1994.
15. Phillipps GH: Structure–activity relationships of topically active steroids: the selection of fluticasone propionate, *Respir Med* 84(suppl A):19, 1990.
16. McKenzie JE, Cruz-Rivera M: Compatibility of budesonide inhalation suspension with four nebulizing solutions, *Ann Pharmacol* 38:967, 2004.
17. Barnes PJ, Pedersen S: Efficacy and safety of inhaled corticosteroids in asthma: report of a workshop held in Eze, France, October 1992, *Am Rev Respir Dis* 148(suppl):S1, 1993.
18. Clark DJ, Grove A, Cargill RI, Lipworth BJ: Comparative adrenal suppression with inhaled budesonide and

fluticasone propionate in adult asthmatic patients, *Thorax* 51:262, 1996.

19. McCormack PL, Plosker GL: Inhaled mometasone furoate: a review of its use in persistent asthma in adults and adolescents, *Drugs* 66:1151, 2006.

20. Karpel JP, Busse WW, Noonan MJ, Monahan ME, Lutsky B, Staudinger H: Effects of mometasone furoate given once daily in the evening on lung function and symptom control in persistent asthma, *Ann Pharmacother* 39:1977, 2005.

21. Shapiro G, Lumry W, Wolfe J, Given J, White MV, Woodring A, Baitinger L, House K, Prillaman B, Shah T: Combined salmeterol 50 μg and fluticasone propionate 250 μg in the Diskus device for the treatment of asthma, *Am J Respir Crit Care Med* 161:527, 2000.

22. Chung KF: The complementary role of gluco-corticosteroids and long-acting β-adrenergic agonists, *Allergy* 53:7, 1998.

23. Jenkins C, Kolarikova R, Kuna P, Caillaud D, Sanchis J, Popp W, Pettersson E: Efficacy and safety of high-dose budesonide/formoterol (Symbicort®) compared with budesonide administered either concomitantly with formoterol or alone in patients with persistent symptomatic asthma, *Respirology* 11:276, 2006.

24. Anderson GP: Interactions between corticosteroids and β-adrenergic agonists in asthma disease induction, progression, and exacerbation, *Am J Respir Crit Care Med* 161:S188, 2000.

25. Barnes PJ: Inhaled glucocorticoids for asthma, *N Engl J Med* 332:868, 1995.

26. Barnes PJ: Molecular mechanisms of steroid action in asthma, *J Allergy Clin Immunol* 97(suppl):159, 1996.

27. Barnes PJ, Pedersen S, Busse WW: Efficacy and safety of inhaled corticosteroids: new developments, *Am J Respir Crit Care Med* 157:S1, 1998.

28. Barnes NC, Qiu YS, Pavord ID, Parker D, Davis PA, Zhu J, Johnson M, Thomson NC, Jeffery PK: SCO30005 Study Group: Antiinflammatory effects of salmeterol/fluticasone propionate in chronic obstructive lung disease, *Am J Respir Crit Care Med.* 173:736, 2006.

29. Baraniuk JN: Molecular actions of glucocorticoids: an introduction, *J Allergy Clin Immunol* 97:141, 1996.

30. Allen DB, Bielory L, Derendorf H, Dluhy R, Colice GL, Szefler SJ: Inhaled corticosteroids, past lessons and future issues, *J Allergy Clin Immunol* 112(suppl 3):s1, 2003.

31. Svedmyr N: Action of corticosteroids on β-adrenergic receptors, clinical aspects, *Am Rev Respir Dis* 141(suppl):S31, 1990.

32. Truhan AP, Ahmed AR: Corticosteroids: a review with emphasis on complications of prolonged systemic therapy, *Ann Allergy* 62:375, 1989.

33. Kamada AK, Szefler SJ, Martin RJ, Boushey HA, Chinchilli VM, Drazen JM, Fish JE, Israel E, Lazarus SC, Lemanske RF: Issues in the use of inhaled glucocorticoids, *Am J Respir Crit Care Med* 153:1739, 1996.

34. Goldberg S, Algur N, Levi M, Brukheimer E, Hirsch HJ, Branski D, Kerem E: Adrenal suppression among asthmatic children receiving chronic therapy with inhaled corticosteroid with and without spacer device, *Ann Allergy Asthma Immunol* 76:234, 1996.

35. Wolthers OD, Pedersen S: Controlled study of linear growth in asthmatic children during treatment with inhaled glucocorticoids, *Pediatrics* 89:839, 1992.

36. Allen DB, Mullen M, Mullen B: A meta-analysis of the effect of oral and inhaled corticosteroids on growth, *J Allergy Clin Immunol* 93:967, 1994.

37. Sharek PJ, Bergman DA: The effect of inhaled steroids on the linear growth of children with asthma: a meta-analysis, *Pediatrics* 106:e8, 2000.

38. Israel E, Banerjee TR, Fitzmaurice GM, Kotlov TV, LaHive K, LeBoff MS: Effects of inhaled glucocorticoids on bone density in premenopausal women, *N Engl J Med* 345:941, 2001.

39. Thorsson L, Edsbacker S, Conradson T-B: Lung deposition of budesonide from Turbuhaler is twice that from a pressurized metered-dose inhaler P-MDI, *Eur Respir J* 7:1839, 1994.

40. Leach CL, Davidson PJ, Hasselquist BE, Boudreau RJ: Lung deposition of hydrofluoroalkane-134a beclomethasone is greater than that of chlorofluorocarbon fluticasone and chlorofluorocarbon beclomethasone, *Chest* 122:510, 2002.

41. Williams AJ, Baghat MS, Stableforth DE, Cayton RM, Shenoi PM, Skinner C: Dysphonia caused by inhaled steroids: recognition of a characteristic laryngeal abnormality, *Thorax* 38:813, 1983.

42. Barnes PJ: Inhaled glucocorticoids: new developments relevant to updating of the Asthma Management Guidelines, *Respir Med* 90:379, 1996.

43. Kerstjens HA, Brand PL, Hughes MD, Robinson NJ, Postma DS, Sluiter HJ, Bleecker ER, Dekhuijzen PN, de Jong PM, Mengelers HJ, et al.: A comparison of bronchodilator therapy with or without inhaled corticosteroid therapy for obstructive airways disease, *N Engl J Med* 327:1413, 1992.

44. Haahtela T, Jarvinen M, Kava T, Kiviranta K, Koskinen S, Lehtonen K, Nikander K, Persson T, Selroos O, Sovijarvi A, et al.: Effects of reducing or discontinuing inhaled budesonide in patients with mild asthma, *N Engl J Med* 331:700, 1994.

45. Masoli M, Holt S, Weatherall M, Beasley R.: Dose-response relationship of inhaled budesonide in adult asthma: a meta-analysis, *Eur Respir J* 23(4):552–8, 2004.

46. Rodrigo G, Rodrigo C: Inhaled flunisolide for acute severe asthma, *Am J Respir Crit Care Med* 157:698, 1998.

47. Fabbri LM, Luppi F, Beghe B, Rabe KF: Update in chronic obstructive pulmonary disease 2005, *Am J Respir Crit Care Med* 173:1056, 2006.

48. Barnes PJ: Mechanisms in COPD: differences from asthma, *Chest* 117:10S, 2000.

49. Jeffery PK: Remodeling in asthma and chronic obstructive lung disease, *Am J Respir Crit Care Med* 164:s28, 2001.

50. Sin D.D, Man SFP: Inhaled corticosteroids and survival in chronic obstructive pulmonary disease: does the dose matter? *Eur Respir J* 21:260, 2003.

51. Hattotuwa KL, Gizycki MJ, Ansari TW, Jeffery PK, Barnes NC: The effects of inhaled fluticasone on airway inflammation in chronic obstructive pulmonary disease, a double-blind, placebo-controlled biopsy study, *Am J Respir Crit Care Med* 165:1592, 2002.

52. Alsaeedi A, Sin DD, McAlister FA: The effects of inhaled corticosteroids in chronic obstructive pulmonary disease: a systematic review of randomized, placebo-controlled trials, *Am J Med* 113:59, 2002.

53. Highland KB, Strange C, Heffner JE: Long term effects of inhaled corticosteroids on FEV_1 in patients with chronic obstructive disease: a meta-analysis, *Ann Intern Med* 138:969, 2003.

54. Calverley PA: Effect of corticosteroids on exacerbations of asthma and chronic obstructive pulmonary disease, *Am Thorac Soc* 1:161, 2004.

55. Sutherland ER, Allmers H, Ayas NT, Venn AJ, Martin RJ: Inhaled corticosteroids reduce the progression of airflow limitation in chronic obstructive pulmonary disease: a meta-analysis, *Thorax* 58:937, 2003.

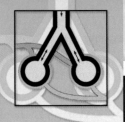

Chapter 12

Nonsteroidal Antiasthma Agents

DOUGLAS S. GARDENHIRE

CHAPTER OUTLINE

CHAPTER OBJECTIVES

After reading this chapter, the reader will be able to:
1. Discuss the indications for nonsteroidal antiasthma agents.
2. List available nonsteroidal antiasthma agents used in respiratory therapy.
3. Differentiate between the specific nonsteroidal antiasthma agents.
4. Describe the routes of administration available for various nonsteroidal antiasthma agents.
5. Describe the mode of action for various nonsteroidal antiasthma agents.
6. Discuss the use of nonsteroidal antiasthma agents in the treatment of asthma.

KEY TERMS AND DEFINITIONS

Antileukotrienes — Agents that block the inflammatory response in asthma
IgE (immunoglobulin E) — A gamma globulin that is produced by cells in the respiratory tract
Leukotrienes — Chemical mediators that cause inflammation

Mast cells — Connective tissue cells that contain heparin and histamine
Mast cell stabilizers — Also known as a *cromolyn-like agents,* these agents are used prophylactically to treat the inflammatory response in asthma

*I*n Chapter 11 the concept of airway inflammation was introduced and some of the numerous cells and chemicals involved in an inflammatory response were described. This was done to present the anti-inflammatory actions of glucocorticoids. Chapter 12 presents drug groups that also have an antiinflammatory effect through mechanisms different from those of the corticosteroids. Three subgroups of agents are included in the nonsteroidal antiasthma group: cromolyn-like drugs **(mast cell stabilizers), antileukotrienes** (anti-LTs), and monoclonal antibodies. A brief summary of the immune mechanisms involved in allergic responses is given as an introduction to the specific mechanisms of action for the drug groups discussed in this chapter.

CLINICAL INDICATION FOR NONSTEROIDAL ANTIASTHMA AGENTS

The general indication for clinical use of nonsteroidal antiasthma agents described in this chapter is *prophylactic* management (control) of mild persistent asthma (asthma requiring step 2 care, according to the classification presented in the 1997 National Asthma Education and Prevention Program [NAEPP] guidelines[1]).

> *Step 2 asthma:* Symptoms more than 2 times/week but less than 1 time/day, nighttime symptoms more than 2 nights/month; forced expiratory volume in 1 second (FEV_1) or peak expiratory flow (PEF) 80% or greater; PEF variability 20 to 30% (see Appendix D).

The following are qualifications to the general indication for use of these agents:

- Cromolyn-like drugs and the antileukotrienes (anti-LTs) are typically recommended as alternatives to low-dose inhaled corticosteroids in asthma requiring step 2 care.[2]
- Cromolyn and nedocromil in particular are often used with infants and young children as alternatives to inhaled corticosteroids in asthma requiring step 2 care because of their safety profiles.[2]
- The anti-LT agents can be useful in combination with inhaled steroids to reduce the dose of steroid.

All of the nonsteroidal antiasthma drugs described in this chapter are controllers, not relievers, and are used in asthma requiring antiinflammatory drug therapy. A summary of agents used in drug therapy for asthma, both relievers and controllers, is presented in Box 12-1 and lists both cromolyn-like agents, antileukotrienes, and monoclonal antibodies as controllers. Use of rescue β_2-agonist agents more than twice a week (i.e., asthma

Box 12-1	Drug Groups Used in the Pharmacological Management of Asthma (Categorized as Controllers or Relievers)

Controllers	Relievers
Inhaled corticosteroids	Short-acting inhaled β_2 agonists
Oral corticosteroids	Systemic corticosteroids (oral burst therapy, intravenous)
Cromolyn sodium and nedocromil	Inhaled anticholinergic bronchodilators
Long-acting inhaled β_2 agonists	
Long-acting oral β_2 agonists	
Leukotriene modifiers	
Sustained-release theophylline	
Monoclonal antibodies (omalizumab)	

requiring step 2 care) is an indicator of the need for initiation of controller drug therapy.

Monoclonal antibodies, specifically omalizumab, are not listed in the NAEPP guidelines[1] because they became available after the guidelines were completed. It is important to understand that the guidelines are just that: a guide. The guidelines do not replace a healthcare provider's responsibility to treat patients and their conditions.[2]

IDENTIFICATION OF NONSTEROIDAL ANTIASTHMA AGENTS

Individual agents in the cromolyn-like group, antileukotriene group, and monoclonal antibody group are identified in Table 12-1, with generic and brand names, formulations and strengths, and usual recommended dosages.

MECHANISMS OF INFLAMMATION IN ASTHMA

KEY POINT

Asthma is an inflammatory disorder of the airways in which *allergic stimuli* often trigger *IgE-mediated mast cell* release of mediators of inflammation. Airway reactivity can be triggered by *nonspecific stimuli* such as cold air or dust as well.

TABLE 12-1

Nonsteroidal Antiasthma Medications: Generic and Brand Names, Formulations, and Usual Recommended Dosages*

Generic Drug	Brand Name	Formulation and Dosage
Cromolyn-like agents (mast cell stabilizers)		
Cromolyn sodium	Intal	MDI: 800 µg/actuation
		Adults and children ≥ 5 yr: 2 inhalations 4 times daily
		SVN: 20 mg/ampoule or 20 mg/2 ml
		Adults and children ≥ 2 yr: 20 mg inhaled 4 times daily
	Nasalcrom	Spray: 40 mg/ml (4%)Adults and children ≥ 2 yr: 1 spray each nostril, 3–6 times daily every 4–6 hr
Nedocromil sodium	Tilade	MDI: 1.75 mg/actuation
		Adults and children ≥ 6 yr: 2 inhalations 4 times daily
Antileukotrienes		
Zafirlukast	Accolate	Tablets: 10 and 20 mg
		Adults and children ≥ 12 yr: 20 mg twice daily, without food
		Children 5–11 yr: 10 mg twice daily
Montelukast	Singulair	Tablets: 10 mg and 4- and 5-mg cherry-flavored chewable; 4-mg packet of granules
		Adults and children ≥ 15 yr: one 10-mg tablet daily
		Children 6–14 yr: one 5-mg chewable tablet daily
		Children 2–5 yr: one 4-mg chewable tablet or one 4-mg packet of granules daily
		6–23 months: one 4-mg packet of granules daily
Zileuton	Zyflo	Tablets: 600 mg
		Adults and children ≥ 12 yr: one 600-mg tablet 4 times per day
Monoclonal Antibody		
Omalizumab	Xolair	Adults and children ≥ 12 yr: Subcutaneous injection every 4 weeks; dose dependent on weight and serum IgE level

*Detailed prescribing information should be obtained from the manufacturer's package insert.

Asthma was previously defined in Chapter 11 as a chronic inflammatory disorder of the airways.[1] Asthma has been distinguished into extrinsic and intrinsic forms on the basis of the triggers for asthma. *Extrinsic* asthma is dependent on allergy, or *atopy,* whereas the *intrinsic* form shows no evidence of sensitization to common inhaled allergens.[3] The allergic, or extrinsic, form of asthma, which is **immunoglobulin E (IgE)** mediated, is associated with younger subjects, and the intrinsic, or nonallergic, form is associated with later onset in adults in whom childhood asthma may not have been present. Holgate[4] describes asthma as an "evolving" disease in early childhood, when viruses are an important trigger, whereas in school and teen years, allergens stimulate an immune response. As asthma progresses, and in adults, the disease becomes intrinsic and may be driven by T cells (lymphocytes) that release various cytokines, as described in Chapter 11. The asthma is chronic and persistent, with continuous inflammation and episodes of acute obstruction. Three components of asthma are described by Drazen and Turino[5] as follows:

1. The acute asthma attack, which resolves spontaneously or with treatment
2. A hyperresponsiveness of the airways to various stimuli
3. Persistent inflammation that becomes worse

In both forms of asthma, intrinsic and extrinsic, mediators and enzymes are released to act on target tissues in the airway, and cells involved in inflammation are recruited and activated in the airway. Airway inflammation is manifested in the responses of bronchoconstriction, airway swelling, mucus secretion and obstruction, and subsequent airway wall remodeling that furthers the responsiveness of the airway.[6]

KEY POINT

The *clinical result* of asthma is chronic persistent airway inflammation and occasional acute episodes of wheezing and airway obstruction caused by *bronchoconstriction, mucosal swelling,* and *mucus secretion.*

The Immunological (Allergic) Response

Most instances of asthma are primarily an allergic response, which involves **mast cells** and immunoglobulin E (IgE).[1] An overview of the immunological response is outlined in Box 12-2. An understanding of the immune response is fundamental to discussing both asthma and the mediator antagonists presented in

Box 12-2   An Overview of the Immune Mechanisms Involved in Allergy and Inflammation

CELL MEDIATED

T lymphocytes (from bone marrow stem cells, processed in the thymus) mediate the immune response by several mechanisms, including cytotoxicity and secretion of cytokines. Members of the family of T lymphocytes, outlined below, are the basis of cellular immunity.

- **Helper/T4 (CD4⁺) cells**, which are subdivided into the following:
  - **Type 1 (Th1) cells:** Regulate classic delayed-type hypersensitivity reactions and other actions related to macrophage activation and T cell–mediated immunity by the production of interferon-γ and interleukin-2 (IL-2).
  - **Type 2 (Th2) cells:** Translate mRNAs for interleukin-4 (IL-4) and interleukin-5 (IL-5) and are involved in atopic allergy. IL-4 is essential for production of IgE by B cells; IL-5 and granulocyte-macrophage colony-stimulating factor (GM-CSF) and interleukin-3 (IL-3) promote eosinophil maturation, activation, and survival.
- **Suppressor/T8 (CD8⁺) cells:** Inhibit the immune response to an antigen after the immune response has begun.

- **Cytotoxic T cells:** Bind to viral antigen on the surface of infected cells, to destroy the cells.
- **Natural killer cells:** Lymphocytes related to cytotoxic T cells; their targets are thought to be tumor cells or cells infected with organisms other than viruses.

ANTIBODY MEDIATED

Antibodies are serum globulins (proteins) modified to specifically combine and react with an antigen (substance capable of provoking antibodies or cellular immunity).

B lymphocytes: Antibody-producing plasma cells; memory cells for later antibody production.

Classes of antibody: The classes of immunoglobulins are as follows:
- Immunoglobulin G (IgG)
- Immunoglobulin A (IgA)
- Immunoglobulin M (IgM)
- Immunoglobulin D (IgD)
- Immunoglobulin E (IgE): Cytophilic antibody (binds to effector cells such as mast cells); termed *reaginic antibody;* involved in allergic responses, atopy

---

this chapter, because allergy is essentially a mistaken immune response. Generation of an immune response, and specifically an allergic asthmatic response, is considered to be *initiated* by the interaction of T lymphocytes with an antigen presented by other cells, such as macrophages or B lymphocytes.[5] Activation of T lymphocytes results in production of IgE by B lymphocytes. Antigen-specific IgE binds to effector cells such as mast cells and is termed a *cytophilic* antibody because of this. When activated by subsequent exposure to an antigen or allergen, mast cells release physiologically active mediators of inflammation such as prostaglandins, **leukotrienes** and proteases, histamine, platelet-activating factor (PAF), and certain cytokines.[5] The cytokines released, which include tumor necrosis factor-α (TNF-α) and interleukin-4 (IL-4), can upregulate endothelial adhesion molecules.[4] This cascade of mediators causes an inflammatory response manifested by vascular leakage, bronchoconstriction, mucus secretion, and mucosal swelling, all of which obstruct airflow in the bronchioles. T lymphocytes also release cytokines (such as interleukins), causing accumulation and activation of eosinophils, which also release chemicals to damage the airway. The process of initiating the inflammatory response and continuing it through amplification, as discussed next, is illustrated in Figure 12-1.

Once initiated by exposure to antigen, the inflammatory response in the airway is *amplified* by chemoattraction

of more lymphocytes, eosinophils, basophils, and neutrophils and by an increase in mast cells. Adhesion molecules increase after stimulation of lymphocytes and mast cells by antigen or allergen. These molecules, found in epithelial cells (intercellular adhesion molecule-1 [ICAM-1]) and vascular endothelial cells (vascular cell adhesion molecule-1 [VCAM-1]) in the airway, are responsible for eosinophil, neutrophil, and lymphocyte recruitment from the microvascular circulation into the airways. The adhesion molecules enable leukocytes to marginate, cross the blood vessel wall, and migrate to the airway mucosa, continuing and further amplifying the inflammation begun.[6] The increase and activation of eosinophils is associated with increased inflammation and severity in asthma.[3]

Nonspecific stimuli such as fog, sulfur dioxide, dust, and cold air can stimulate sensory receptors and cause reflex bronchoconstriction (see Chapter 7).[6] Asthmatic subjects are more sensitive to such stimuli, which reflects either altered neural control or is the result of chronic inflammation sensitizing the airway, or both. Nerve fibers of the noncholinergic nonadrenergic excitatory system, containing potent peptide mediators, contribute to local effects on smooth muscle and mucous glands and reflexly stimulate cholinergic activity. Some of these peptides include substance P (SP), neurokinin A (NKA), and neurokinin B (NKB); they are released from sensory C-fiber nerve endings. These neuropeptides can also contribute to inflammation and the features of asthma previously

than 20 mg/dose. This is typical of the dose ratio of MDIs versus nebulizers, as discussed in Chapter 3.

Nasal Solution (Nasalcrom). Cromolyn is available as a 4% solution for treatment of seasonal and perennial allergic rhinitis. As with the inhaled solution, protection requires prior administration, although the drug does not need to be taken outside of seasonal exposure to allergens. The solution is delivered by means of a metered pump spray device.

Mode of Action

Cromolyn sodium is considered an antiasthmatic, an antiallergic, and a mast cell stabilizer. Pretreatment with inhaled cromolyn sodium results in inhibition of mast cell degranulation, thereby blocking release of the chemical mediators of inflammation (Figure 12-3). By its action, cromolyn is effective in blocking the late-phase reaction in asthma. (The late-phase reaction in asthma is discussed in the review of corticosteroids in Chapter 11.)

Cromolyn prevents the extrusion of granules containing the mediators of inflammation to the cell exterior. For this reason, cromolyn is often classified as a "mast cell stabilizer." The exact mechanism by which this inhibition is accomplished is not completely understood, but the following details of cromolyn activity and mast cell function are known:

- The mode of action of cromolyn sodium is *prophylactic;* pretreatment is necessary for inhibition of mast cell degranulation.
- Cromolyn sodium may inhibit mediator release by preventing calcium influx necessary for microfilament contraction and extrusion of mast cell granules.[9,10]
- Cromolyn sodium does not have an antagonist effect on any of the chemical mediators themselves.
- Cromolyn sodium does not operate through the cyclic adenosine 3′,5′-monophosphate (cAMP) system and does not affect α or β receptors.
- Antibody formation, attachment of antibody (IgE) to the mast cell, and antigen–antibody union are *not* prevented by cromolyn; cromolyn does prevent release of mediators.
- Cromolyn sodium can prevent or attenuate the late-phase response in an asthmatic episode, which can otherwise cause more severe airway obstruction 6 to 8 hours after initial bronchoconstriction.[11,12]

The protective effect of cromolyn in inhibiting mast cell degranulation has been captured by scanning electron microscopy and is shown in the sequence in Figure 12-4. Initial understanding of cromolyn's activity focused on allergy-triggered mast cell release of mediators, and therefore the drug came to be considered useful primarily in allergic asthma. There is evidence that the activity of cromolyn is not limited to preventing allergen-stimulated asthma. Cromolyn inhibits mast cell mediator release caused by nonallergic stimuli and may even reduce reflex-induced asthma. The latter requires about twice the usual dose of cromolyn. Understanding of the broader protection given by cromolyn has supported its successful use in allergic and nonallergic asthma and specifically with exercise-induced asthma. This view of the broader pharmacological activity of cromolyn is discussed by Bernstein.[13,14]

Pharmacokinetics

As with other inhaled aerosols, cromolyn sodium is distributed to the airway and to the stomach via a swallowed portion. Distribution to the stomach (swallowed portion) can be modified by use of reservoir devices with the MDI formulation. The dose reaching the airway is absorbed from the lung and quickly excreted unchanged in the bile and urine. The lung portion does not appear to be metabolized in the airway. The swallowed portion is largely unabsorbed from the gastrointestinal tract (less than 1%) and excreted in the feces.

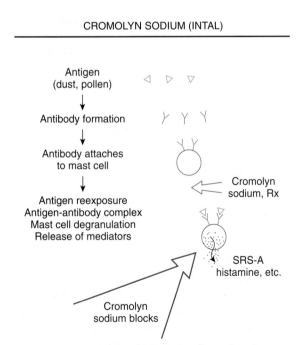

CROMOLYN SODIUM (INTAL)

Antigen (dust, pollen)
↓
Antibody formation
↓
Antibody attaches to mast cell
↓
Antigen reexposure
Antigen-antibody complex
Mast cell degranulation
Release of mediators

Cromolyn sodium, Rx

SRS-A histamine, etc.

Cromolyn sodium blocks

FIGURE 12-3 Mode of action of cromolyn sodium in preventing mast cell degranulation. *SRS-A,* Slow-reacting substance of anaphylaxis, consisting of leukotrienes C_4, D_4, and E_4.

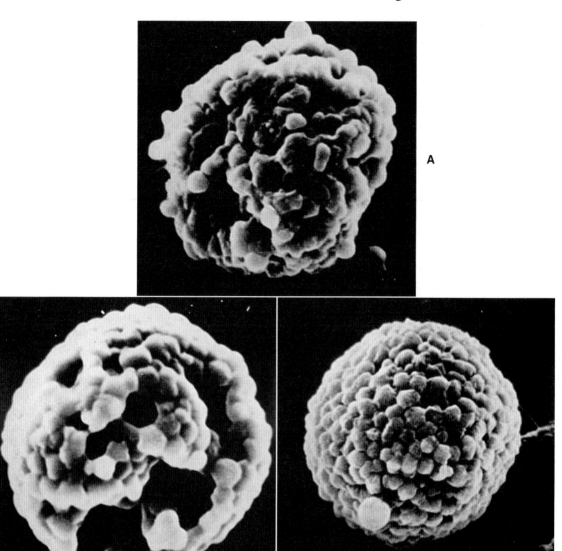

FIGURE 12-4 Degranulation of a mast cell. **A,** Mast cell undergoing gross degranulation shows free granules. **B,** The pores now occupy a large area of the cytoplasm. **C,** A sensitized mast cell fails to degranulate after challenge when pretreated with cromolyn sodium. (Courtesy Rhone-Poulenc Rorer Pharmaceuticals, Inc., Collegeville, PA.)

Side Effects

Cromolyn sodium is a safe drug. It has an effectiveness similar to theophylline in controlling asthma, with a better therapeutic margin than theophylline.[11] In studies comparing the two agents, subjects using theophylline reported more side effects, including nervousness, nausea, school behavioral problems, and more office visits. The overall incidence of adverse effects with cromolyn has been reported at 2%.[15] Nasal congestion may be seen after beginning cromolyn sodium use. Dermatitis, myositis (muscle tissue inflammation), and gastroenteritis occurred in a very few patients.

Use of the *nebulizer solution* has been associated with cough, nasal congestion, wheezing, sneezing, nasal itching, epistaxis, or nose burning. Use of the *nasal solution* has most commonly been associated with sneezing (approximately 10% of patients), as well as nasal stinging or burning (5%), nasal irritation (2.5%), and a bad taste (2%). Side effects with the *oral capsules* for mastocytosis are difficult to differentiate from effects of the disease itself. Adverse events with this use of cromolyn sodium were transient and included headache and diarrhea.

Clinical Efficacy of Cromolyn Sodium

The original trials of cromolyn sodium as a prophylactic agent in asthma were performed with the 20-mg Spinhaler formulation. Studies were conducted in both adult and pediatric subjects and included both intrinsic and extrinsic forms of asthma. The conclusion of these early studies was that inhaled cromolyn sodium is effective as a treatment for approximately 70% of patients.[16] Edwards gives a review of data supporting the use of cromolyn sodium in chronic asthma.[17] In a long-term study by Konig and Shaffer,[18] 175 children were monitored for an average of 8.4 years (2.2 to 16.8 years). Their results showed that pulmonary function improved to normal values in both the group treated with corticosteroids and the group given cromolyn sodium. Cockcroft and Murdock[19] found evidence of protection against antigen challenge, with attenuation of both the early-phase and the late-phase asthmatic response with cromolyn sodium.

MDI Strength. As seen in Table 12-1, the difference between the nebulizer dose (20 mg) and the MDI dose (approximately 1.0 mg/actuation) of cromolyn sodium is 10-fold. If we assume that approximately 10% of an inhaled dose reaches the airway, as seen previously with adrenergic bronchodilators (see Chapter 6), equivalent doses are not available with the usual dose from the nebulizer and the MDI. Although not available in the United States, a 5-mg/actuation MDI strength is used in Great Britain. Holgate[16] cites several studies demonstrating that increased doses using the 5-mg MDI with two actuations give better protection against exercise challenge, with a longer duration of protection in more subjects.

Use in Angiotensin-converting Enzyme Inhibitor Cough. Hargreaves and Benson[20] reported that cromolyn sodium, administered as two actuations, four times daily of the 5-mg MDI formulation, provided protection against the cough often seen as a side effect with use of angiotensin-converting enzyme (ACE) inhibitors.[20] Cromolyn sodium significantly improved cough scores (frequency and severity) in 9 of the 10 patients in the study after 2 weeks. Cough was not completely suppressed in any of the 10 patients.

Anti–sickle Cell Effects. Both the 4% intranasal solution and the 20-mg inhaled powder capsule of cromolyn given as a single dose were observed to cause a striking decrease in sickle cell percentage in nine African children with severe sickle cell disease. Improvement was seen 24 hours after administration of the single dose. The reduction in sickling is hypothesized to be due to the blocking of calcium-activated potassium channels, which play a major part in water loss and erythrocyte dehydration.[21]

Clinical Application of Cromolyn Sodium

Three points should be emphasized concerning the clinical application of cromolyn sodium with asthma and hyperreactive airway states:

1. First, the drug is only prophylactic and should not be used during acute bronchospasm. This is based on its mode of action, because the drug must already be present to prevent mast cell degranulation. *It has no bronchodilating action* and in fact may cause further bronchial irritation as an aerosol.

2. Second, abrupt withdrawal of oral corticosteroids and substitution of cromolyn sodium in asthmatic patients can result in inadequate adrenal function. Cromolyn has no effect on the adrenal system, and tapered withdrawal of corticosteroids is necessary while beginning cromolyn use with patients.

3. Third, it may take from 2 to 4 weeks for improvement in the patient's symptoms, enabling a decrease in concomitant therapy such as bronchodilator or steroid use.

Guidelines for the management of asthma indicate that cromolyn sodium is used in subjects requiring regular use of β agonists for control of symptoms. It is considered an alternative to the use of inhaled corticosteroids, especially in children (see Appendix D).[2]

Dosage Regulation. The protective effect of cromolyn in allergic, nonallergic, or reflex-induced asthma is dose dependent. The usual dosage of 20 mg four times daily (80 mg/day) with the nebulized solution in some cases can be reduced to a maintenance dosage of 40 to 60 mg/day after the patient is stabilized for 1 or 2 months. Likewise, if stimuli for asthma increase in severity (e.g., heavy exercise in cold weather [skiing] as opposed to walking in warm weather), higher dosages or addition of a β agonist may be required. For seasonal allergy, cromolyn should be started at least 1 week before allergen exposure. The drug will protect if given 30 minutes before a specific allergen exposure (e.g., cat fur), and a single dose 15 minutes before exercise on an occasional, rather than a continuous, basis is effective. As stated previously, the degree of exercise and the conditions must be considered in estimating the protection required. Long-term continuous maintenance with cromolyn may be needed for patients with reflex-induced asthma or for those with late-phase reactions or severe bronchial reactivity and lability.[13,14]

Nedocromil Sodium (Tilade)

Nedocromil is marketed as Tilade in an MDI formulation. Nedocromil is considered a second-generation antiasthmatic agent and is a cromolyn-like drug in its action and clinical use. The drug is an inhaled prophylactic antiasthmatic agent and is extensively reviewed by Gonzalez and Brogden.[22] The structure of nedocromil is illustrated in Figure 12-2.

As with cromolyn sodium, nedocromil sodium is indicated as prophylactic therapy in the management of mild persistent asthma.[2] The drug is a controller, not a reliever, has no bronchodilator properties, and is not indicated for use in the reversal of acute bronchospasm. Optimal control of asthma symptoms depends on regular use of the drug, even if symptoms of airway obstruction are not apparent.

Dosage and Administration

Nedocromil is available as an MDI, with 1.75 mg/actuation, with at least 104 metered inhalations per canister. The recommended dosage by MDI for maintenance therapy in asthma is two inhalations four times a day.

Mode of Action

Nedocromil sodium exerts its antiinflammatory and antiasthmatic effect by inhibiting the activation and activity of multiple inflammatory cells, including mast cells, eosinophils, airway epithelial cells, and sensory neurons.[23] Specific activities of nedocromil sodium are listed and illustrated in Figure 12-5.

- Nedocromil sodium inhibits mast cell cytokine release, such as release of histamine, tryptase, and tumor necrosis factor-α (TNF-α).
- Nedocromil sodium modulates the synthesis and release of proinflammatory cytokines such as IL-1β, IL-6, IL-8, granulocyte-macrophage colony-stimulating factor (GM-CSF), TFN-α, and "regulated on activation, normal T cell expressed and secreted" (RANTES, an eosinophil-attracting chemokine), and adhesion molecules from airway epithelial cells.[23]
- Nedocromil sodium can inhibit eosinophil chemotaxis and adhesion in culture media containing the chemoattractive factors released from airway epithelial cells and can block the release of eosinophil cationic protein, which is involved in epithelial cell damage in the airway.[4]
- Nedocromil sodium can prevent neuronally mediated bronchoconstriction by inhibiting afferent sensory

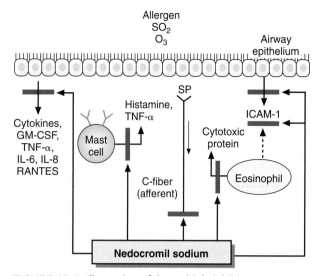

FIGURE 12-5 Illustration of the multiple inhibitory effects by which nedocromil sodium attenuates and prevents inflammation in the airway. *GM-CSF,* Granulocyte-macrophage colony-stimulating factor; *ICAM-1,* intercellular adhesion molecule-1; *IL-6, -8,* interleukin-6, -8; *RANTES,* regulated on activation, normal T cell expressed and secreted; *SP,* substance P; *TNF-α,* tumor necrosis factor-α.

nerve impulses.[4] Nedocromil sodium can also inhibit the cytokines that lead to increased synthesis of neuropeptides, such as substance P, or other tachykinins.

It has been suggested that the activity of nedocromil sodium, as well as cromolyn sodium, in inhibiting activation and activity of inflammatory cells may be through a common pathway of chloride ion transport blockade. An influx of chloride ions is thought to be responsible for some of the high intracellular calcium concentration in mast cells, needed for degranulation. An efflux of chloride mediates in part the regulation of airway *epithelial cell size* and volume decrease with hypotonically induced swelling. Exercise probably leads to the production of hypertonic airway surface fluid. By preventing chloride-regulated cell volume decrease in this instance, nedocromil sodium may alter the availability of afferent sensory nerves in the airways to mechanical or chemical irritants.[24] Finally, chloride efflux from *sensory nerves* produces depolarization and the action potential needed for nerve signal propagation. Evidence suggests that nedocromil sodium inhibits the chloride channels and the transport needed for each of these cell functions. This nonspecific chloride channel–blocking activity may protect the airway from nerve stimulation, which produces bronchospasm and cough, and may inhibit the activity of mast cells and eosinophils in releasing mediators.

In summary, nedocromil sodium can inhibit mast cells, eosinophils, and airway epithelial cells, which taken together can release a wide range of mediators, inflammatory cytokines, and enzymes, all of which would otherwise produce airway inflammation in asthma. Unlike corticosteroids, which downregulate cytokine production to reverse inflammation in the airway, nedocromil sodium blocks further inflammation by blocking the activation of inflammatory cells.[23]

Pharmacokinetics

In asthmatic subjects given nedocromil sodium by inhalation, the peak plasma concentration varied between 5 and 90 minutes, with a terminal half-life of 1.5 hours. It is confined to the extravascular space and does not penetrate the central nervous system well. There is reversible binding to plasma protein (approximately 89% of the drug), and systemic bioavailability is low, although there is good absorption from the airway. Plasma clearance is more rapid than the absorption, at 10 ml/min/kg in humans, with urinary excretion.[25]

Side Effects

Nedocromil is well tolerated in both healthy volunteers and asthmatic subjects. The most commonly reported side effects are as follows[22]:
- Unpleasant taste (13.6%)
- Headache (4.8%)
- Nausea (4.0%)
- Vomiting (1.8%)
- Dizziness (1 to 2%)

Clinical Efficacy

Efficacy in Adults. In adults a dose of 2 MDI actuations two or four times daily has been shown to provide equal or better control of mild to moderate asthma compared with theophylline, based on daytime and nighttime asthma symptoms, need for inhaled bronchodilator, cough, and morning tightness. Nedocromil sodium has also been shown to be of potential use in reducing high-dose inhaled steroid use. Patients taking 2000 μg of inhaled steroid were able to reduce their daily use by 31% after taking 4 mg (approximately two MDI actuations) of nedocromil sodium four times daily. In a large meta-analysis of double-blind, placebo-controlled clinical trials of nedocromil sodium, the drug demonstrated a significant effect compared with placebo on outcome variables of daytime and nighttime asthma symptoms, cough, peak expiratory flow rate, FEV_1, inhaled bronchodilator use, and patient report of control.[26] Doses included both twice-daily and four-times-daily schedules

of two actuations. Clinical improvement was greatest in mild to moderate asthma and with continued bronchodilator treatment.

Efficacy in Children. When nedocromil sodium in a four-times-daily dose was added to current therapy in stable mild asthmatic children in placebo comparisons, there was significant improvement in daily peak expiratory flow and a reduction in daily bronchodilator use.[27] Nedocromil sodium, 4 mg given twice daily, has also been found to be equally effective compared with cromolyn sodium, 5 mg four times daily, in controlling asthma in children, offering a compliance advantage in the reduced dosing frequency. A long-term safety study of 65 chronic asthmatic children receiving nedocromil sodium at 4 mg four times daily for 1 year showed excellent acceptability and only minor expected side effects of headache, cough, or pharyngitis.[28]

ANTILEUKOTRIENE AGENTS

The name leukotriene is based on the fact that these molecules were originally isolated from leukocytes and the carbon backbone has three double bonds in series, termed a *triene*. Chemical structures of the three antileukotriene drugs currently available in the United States are given in Figure 12-6. Two of these agents (zafirlukast and montelukast) attach to and block the receptor for leukotrienes, and a third agent (zileuton) inhibits the synthesis of leukotrienes.

Leukotrienes and Inflammation

The leukotrienes are members of a group of biologically active fatty acids, including prostaglandins, thromboxanes, and lipoxins, that are known as *eicosanoids*. These molecules are lipid mediators of inflammation that are synthesized from the fatty acid precursor arachidonic acid (5,8,11,14-eicosatetraenoic acid). Arachidonic acid is found in cell nuclear membrane phospholipids. The leukotrienes mediate directly or indirectly at least some of the inflammatory process seen in asthma. They are potent bronchoconstrictors and stimulate other cells to cause airway edema, mucus secretion, ciliary beat inhibition, and recruitment of other inflammatory cells into the airway.[29]

Cell Sources of Leukotrienes

The leukotrienes and other lipid mediators are not preformed and stored in cells, but rather are synthesized after a mechanical, chemical, or physical stimulus that activates phospholipase A_2, an enzyme. These stimuli include antigen challenge of sensitized tissues and

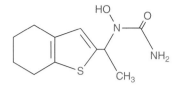

Zileuton

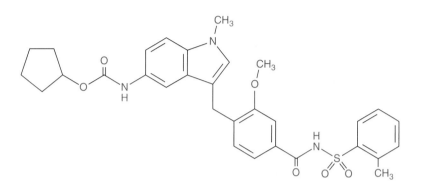

Zafirlukast

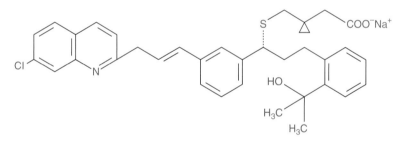

Montelukast

FIGURE 12-6 Chemical structures of the three antileukotriene agents (zileuton, zafirlukast, and montelukast).

exposure to platelet-activating factor (PAF) or other cytokines. Certain cells have the necessary enzymes to synthesize leukotrienes and other mediators. These include eosinophils, mast cells, monocytes, macrophages, basophils, neutrophils, and B lymphocytes.[30] Eosinophils, mast cells, and macrophages are present and recruited to the lung in asthma.[31]

Biochemical Pathways

A simplified diagrammatic view of the arachidonic acid cascade, which results in the various lipid mediators, is given in Figure 12-7. Essentially, free arachidonic acid is converted to various lipid mediators by two routes: the cyclooxygenase and the 5-lipoxygenase pathways. The cyclooxygenase pathway results in the prostaglandins (PGs) and thromboxane, and the 5-lipoxygenase (5-LO) pathway results in the leukotrienes. Aspirin and other nonsteroidal antiinflammatory drugs (NSAIDs; e.g., ibuprofen) inhibit the cyclooxygenase enzyme, blocking prostaglandin and thromboxane production. There are two forms of the cyclooxygenase (COX) enzyme: COX-1 and COX-2. Many NSAIDs are mainly COX-1 selective, such as aspirin, ketoprofen, and indomethacin; some are slightly COX-1 selective, such as ibuprofen and naproxen. Other agents such as celecoxib and rofecoxib, used to treat arthritis, have primarily selective inhibition

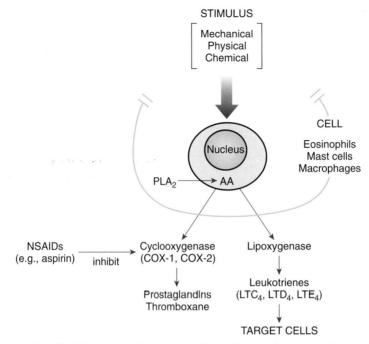

FIGURE 12-7 A simplified diagrammatic overview of stimuli and cell types involved in the arachidonic acid cascade, resulting in cyclooxygenase products such as prostaglandins and lipoxygenase products, the leukotrienes. *AA,* Arachidonic acid; *COX-1, COX-2,* isoenzyme forms of cyclooxygenase; *LTC_4, LTD_4, LTE_4,* leukotrienes C_4, D_4, and E_4; *NSAIDs,* nonsteroidal antiinflammatory drugs; *PLA_2,* phospholipase A_2.

of COX-2. The 5-LO pathway results in the synthesis of leukotrienes; this pathway is the target for drugs in the antileukotriene group.

Leukotriene Production

The lipoxygenase pathway resulting in leukotriene production is illustrated in Figure 12-8. After stimulation of an appropriate cell, the enzyme phospholipase A_2 (PLA$_2$), which is located in the cell cytoplasm, moves to the cell nuclear membrane. In the nuclear membrane, PLA$_2$ hydrolyzes phospholipids to liberate free arachidonic acid. Arachidonic acid (AA) binds to 5-LO–activating protein (FLAP) (AA–FLAP). Another enzyme, 5-LO, moves from both the nucleus and the cell cytoplasm to the nuclear membrane and interacts with the AA–FLAP complex to oxygenate the arachidonic acid. This results in 5-hydroperoxyeicosatetraenoic acid (5-HPETE), which is then converted to the unstable intermediate leukotriene A_4 (LTA$_4$). Leukotriene A_4 is the source of all the other leukotrienes. LTA$_4$ is converted either into leukotriene B_4 (LTB$_4$) or the cysteinyl leukotriene C_4 (LTC$_4$). Both LTB$_4$ and LTC$_4$ are exported from the cell to the extracellular space; LTC$_4$ is converted to leukotrienes D_4 and E_4 (LTD$_4$ and LTE$_4$, respectively).

These three LTs are termed *cysteinyl leukotrienes* because they each have the amino acid cysteine in their chemical structure. This is abbreviated to *CysLTs.* The three CysLTs, LTC$_4$, LTD$_4$, and LTE$_4$, have been identified as the components of the previously termed SRS-A.

CysLT Receptors and Effects of Leukotrienes

Leukotrienes bind to leukotriene receptors to exert their inflammatory effects. There are several different receptor types identified to date. LTB$_4$ binds to a seven transmembrane–spanning receptor, termed the *B leukotriene (BLT) receptor.* The BLT receptor is involved in cellular recruitment (chemotaxis), probably of neutrophils, and may be involved in acute respiratory distress syndrome (ARDS). The cysteinyl LTs (CysLTs) attach to two subtypes of receptors: *CysLT$_1$* and *CysLT$_2$ receptors.* The proasthmatic actions of the cysteinyl LTs are mediated by the CysLT$_1$ receptor, which is located on smooth muscle cells in the airway and other cell types. The human CysLT$_1$ receptor has been cloned and characterized.[32] Stimulation of the CysLT$_1$ receptor causes bronchoconstriction, and the cysteinyl LTs are more potent airway constrictors than histamine.[31] In addition to direct bronchoconstriction,

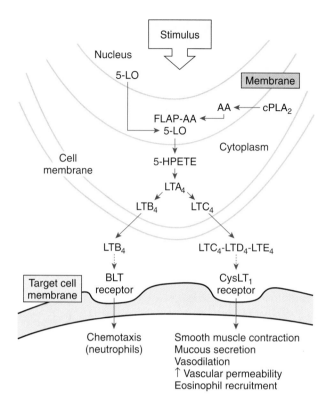

FIGURE 12-8 A detailed model of the synthesis of leukotrienes through the 5-lipoxygenase *(5-LO)* pathway and their effects on target cells. See text for a detailed description. *AA,* Arachidonic acid; *BLT receptor,* B leukotriene (LTB$_4$) receptor; *cPLA$_2$,* cytosolic phospholipase A$_2$; *CysLT$_1$ receptor,* cysteinyl leukotriene receptor subtype 1; *FLAP,* 5-lipoxygenase–activating protein; *5-HPETE,* 5-hydroperoxyeicosatetraenoic acid; *LTA$_4$, LTB$_4$, LTC$_4$, LTD$_4$, LTE$_4$,* leukotrienes A$_4$, B$_4$, C$_4$, D$_4$, and E$_4$.

there is also an increase in bronchial hyperresponsiveness to other irritants such as histamine. Other effects include mucus secretion in the airway, increased vascular permeability causing airway wall edema, and plasma exudation into the airway lumen. The resulting protein and cellular debris in the airway, together with the mucus secretion, increases secretion viscosity and may lead to airway occlusion such as that seen in asthma. The CysLTs may also have an eosinophilic chemoattractant effect. Drugs that block the binding of leukotrienes to CysLT$_1$ receptors are named with the generic suffix *-lukast* (e.g., zafirlukast, montelukast, and pranlukast). The CysLT$_2$ receptor subtype mediates constriction of pulmonary vascular smooth muscle.[33]

The CysLTs are produced largely by eosinophils, mast cells, and macrophages, all of which are cell types seen in the airways of asthmatics. Elevated levels of CysLTs may be markers of asthma. Leukocytes of asthmatics release more CysLTs than do those of nonasthmatics. Plasma levels of LTE$_4$ correlate with asthma severity and are elevated in the urine of patients during an asthma attack, during exercise-induced asthma, and in the presence of nocturnal asthma symptoms.[31] Urinary LTE$_4$ is also elevated after challenge with allergen in atopic asthma or with aspirin in aspirin-sensitive asthmatics.[29]

Zileuton (Zyflo)

Zileuton, also known as Zyflo, is an orally active inhibitor of 5-LO. Its structure is shown in Figure 12-6. This drug is indicated for the prophylaxis and chronic treatment of asthma and is approved for use in adults and children 12 years of age or older. It is considered as a controller agent rather than a reliever and has no indication for use in an acute asthma episode.

Dosage and Administration

Zileuton is available in a single-tablet strength of 600 mg. The recommended dosage for asthma is one 600-mg tablet, four times daily, for a total daily dose of 2400 mg. Zileuton is taken at meals and at bedtime. Hepatic transaminase enzymes should be measured and evaluated before initiation of treatment, once a month for the first 3 months, and every 2 to 3 months thereafter for the first year, with periodic monitoring for longer term therapy. If clinical signs of liver injury (right upper quadrant pain, nausea, fatigue, lethargy, pruritus, jaundice, or flulike symptoms) develop, the drug should be discontinued.

Mode of Action

Taken orally, zileuton inhibits the 5-LO enzyme, which would otherwise catalyze the formation of leukotrienes from arachidonic acid. Specifically, 5-LO in the presence of FLAP catalyzes the conversion of arachidonic acid to the intermediate 5-HPETE, which is converted to LTA$_4$ and ultimately the other leukotrienes. By interrupting the synthesis of these biologically active leukotrienes, their contribution to the inflammatory responses in asthma is effectively blocked. Both the (R)- and the (S)-enantiomers are active as 5-LO inhibitors. The mode of action of zileuton is illustrated along with that of the other antileukotrienes in Figure 12-9.

Pharmacokinetics

Zileuton is rapidly absorbed when taken orally, with an apparent volume of distribution of 1.2 L/kg. The drug is about 93% bound to plasma proteins, including albumin. The drug has a half-life of 2.5 hours, is metabolized

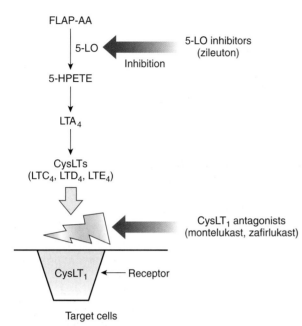

FLAP-AA

5-LO ← 5-LO inhibitors (zileuton)
Inhibition

5-HPETE

LTA$_4$

CysLTs (LTC$_4$, LTD$_4$, LTE$_4$)

CysLT$_1$ antagonists (montelukast, zafirlukast)

CysLT$_1$ ← Receptor

Target cells

FIGURE 12-9 Illustration of the mode and site of action of the antileukotriene agents zileuton, zafirlukast, and montelukast. Zileuton inhibits the 5-lipoxygenase *(5-LO)* enzyme to prevent leukotriene production, and zafirlukast and montelukast antagonize the action of the cysteinyl leukotrienes *(CysLTs)* at the leukotriene receptor, *CysLT$_1$*. *FLAP–AA,* 5-Lipoxygenase–activating protein complexed with arachidonic acid; *5-HPETE,* 5-hydroperoxyeicosatetraenoic acid; *LTA$_4$, LTC$_4$, LTD$_4$, LTE$_4$,* leukotrienes A$_4$, C$_4$, D$_4$, and E$_4$.

to glucuronide conjugates and an N-dehydroxylated metabolite in the liver by cytochrome P450 enzymes, and is eliminated in the urine and feces.

Hazards and Side Effects

Side effects with oral zileuton that are greater than those with placebo include headache, general pain, abdominal pain, loss of strength, and dyspepsia. Elevations of one or more liver function test values have occurred with zileuton, and it is recommended that hepatic transaminases be monitored before and during treatment. Liver enzyme levels may decrease or return to normal either during therapy or after discontinuation. Serum alanine transaminase (ALT, also known as serum glutamate pyruvate transaminase [SGPT]) is a good indicator of liver injury. Zileuton is contraindicated in subjects with acute liver disease or transaminase elevations greater than three times the upper limit of normal.

Zileuton interacts with two important drugs in respiratory care: theophylline and warfarin. Zileuton can increase serum theophylline concentrations and can increase prothrombin time when given concomitantly with warfarin. Dose adjustments of theophylline and oral warfarin may be needed.

Zafirlukast (Accolate)

Zafirlukast, also known as Accolate, is a synthetic asthma prophylactic agent (its structure is illustrated in Figure 12-6). It is indicated for the prophylaxis and chronic treatment of asthma and has been approved for use in those 5 years of age or older. This drug inhibits asthma reactions induced by exercise, cold air, allergen, and aspirin.

Dosage and Administration

Zafirlukast is taken as an oral tablet, 10 mg, twice a day for children 5–11 years of age and 20 mg, twice daily in adults and children 12 years and older. Food reduces the bioavailability of the drug, and it should be taken at least 1 hour before or 2 hours after eating.

Mode of Action

Zafirlukast, and montelukast, are both leukotriene receptor antagonists and thereby block the inflammatory effects of leukotrienes (see Figure 12-9). Specifically, zafirlukast binds to the CysLT$_1$ receptors, with no agonist effect. This causes competitive inhibition of leukotrienes LTC$_4$, LTD$_4$, and LTE$_4$ and subsequent blockade of the inflammatory effects described previously (in the section Leukotrienes and Inflammation).

Pharmacokinetics

Zafirlukast is rapidly absorbed when taken orally. Peak plasma levels are reached 3 hours after dosing, with an elimination half-life of approximately 10 hours. Zafirlukast is metabolized in the liver, with 10% excreted in the urine and the remainder in the feces. Administration of zafirlukast with food reduces mean bioavailability by about 40%.

Hazards and Side Effects

The most common side effects reported in healthy volunteers and patients were headache, infection, nausea, diarrhea, and generalized and abdominal pain. Infections were predominantly respiratory. Because zafirlukast is metabolized by liver enzymes, hepatic impairment (e.g., in cirrhosis) will increase drug plasma levels. Although not noted in 6-month trials of zafirlukast, postmarketing surveillance indicated that doses higher than the 40-mg daily dose can cause elevations in serum aminotransferase concentrations.[33] A case of hepatitis and hyperbilirubinemia with no other attributable cause has been reported in a patient receiving

40 mg a day for 100 days, indicating the possibility of liver enzyme dysfunction with the drug (this case was reported in the manufacturer's drug literature).

Montelukast (Singulair)

Montelukast, also known as Singulair, is an orally active leukotriene receptor antagonist (its structure is illustrated in Figure 12-6). It is indicated for the prophylaxis and chronic treatment of asthma (a controller) and has no bronchodilating effect for use in acute asthma treatment. Montelukast is also approved for allergic rhinitis. Montelukast is the only one of the three currently available antileukotriene agents that is approved for used in children as young as 6 month of age. Montelukast has been shown to have clinical efficacy in treating mild to moderate asthma and exercise-induced bronchoconstriction. Compared with placebo, montelukast significantly improved asthma control in children 12–23 months of age, 2 to 14 years of age, and adults over 15 years of age.[34-38] To date, no safety issues have appeared with pediatric use. The manufacturer states that the drug has not been proven safe and effective in children under 6 months of age. However, Knorr and associates found that the 4-mg dose of granules was just as safe and effective in 3- to 6-month-olds as was found in 6- to 24-month-olds.[39]

Dosage and Administration

Montelukast is available as a 10-mg tablet, as 4- and 5-mg chewable cherry-flavored tablets, and as a 4-mg packet of granules.

Adults and adolescents ≥ 15 years: One 10-mg tablet daily, taken daily

Pediatric patients 6 to 14 years: One 5-mg chewable tablet daily, taken daily

Pediatric patients 2 to 5 years: One 4-mg chewable tablet daily, or one 4-mg packet of oral granules daily

Pediatric patients 12–23 months: One 4-mg packet of oral granules taken every evening

Pediatric patients 6–23 months: One 4-mg packet of oral granules taken daily for *allergic rhinitis*

The drug can be taken with or without meals. Bioavailability when taken orally is not altered by a standard meal.

The oral granules can be directly poured in the mouth of the child or can be mixed with liquid or soft food. Baby formula, breast milk, applesauce, ice cream, and soft foods, such as carrots and rice, were used in studies. The manufacturer suggests only these should be used.

Mode of Action

Like zafirlukast, montelukast is a competitive antagonist for the cysteinyl leukotrienes LTC_4, LTD_4, and LTE_4. It binds with high affinity and selectivity to the $CysLT_1$ receptor subtype (see Figure 12-9). Blockade of the $CysLT_1$ receptor prevents leukotriene stimulation of the receptor on target cells such as airway smooth muscle and secretory glands. Montelukast has been shown to inhibit both early- and late-phase bronchoconstriction caused by antigen challenge.

Pharmacokinetics

Montelukast is rapidly absorbed after oral administration. With a 10-mg dose, peak plasma concentration occurred in 3 to 4 hours, with a mean oral bioavailability of 64%. This bioavailability was not influenced by a standard meal in the morning. Concentration levels were slightly higher with the 5-mg chewable tablet taken while fasting in adults. For the 4-mg chewable tablet, the peak plasma concentration was reached in 2 hours. The drug is metabolized extensively in the liver and excreted via the bile, with little urinary excretion. Mean plasma half-life in adults ranged from 2.7 to 5.5 hours. Mild to moderate hepatic insufficiency will increase plasma levels, but no dosage adjustment is required. Severe hepatic impairment was not evaluated.

Hazards and Side Effects

The safety profile of montelukast was similar to that of placebo in drug testing. Adverse events that occurred in 2% or more of cases included diarrhea, laryngitis, pharyngitis, nausea, otitis, sinusitis, and viral infection. Hypersensitivity reactions were reported. Liver enzymes were not altered compared with placebo. Phenobarbital decreases the plasma level of montelukast, but the manufacturer suggests no dosage adjustment. If potent cytochrome P450 enzyme inducers such as phenobarbital or rifampin are used, appropriate clinical monitoring is suggested.

Role of Antileukotriene Drugs in Asthma Management

Antileukotriene agents are recommended in the NAEPP guidelines for the treatment of mild to moderate asthma.[2] A summary of comparative features for the three currently available antileukotriene agents is given in Table 12-2. An excellent review of asthma management with these agents is given by Drazen and colleagues.[33]

KEY POINT

Drugs that act to *inhibit the mediators* of inflammation include *cromolyn sodium, nedocromil sodium, zafirlukast, montelukast,* and *zileuton*. These agents are *prophylactic* and intended for the management of chronic asthma rather than for relief of acute airway obstruction. They do not provide bronchodilation in an acute asthma episode. *Cromolyn* is available as a dry powder inhaler, a nebulizer solution, and a metered dose inhaler (MDI), and acts as a mast cell stabilizer. *Nedocromil sodium* is available as an MDI, and acts on multiple cell types (mast cells, eosinophils, and airway epithelial cells), sensory neurons, and mediators to inhibit the inflammatory response. These agents are indicated in the management of *mild to moderate asthma,* when more than occasional β-agonist use is needed. *Zafirlukast* and *montelukast* are available as oral agents, and act by competitive antagonism of CysLT$_1$ (cysteinyl leukotriene receptor subtype 1) to prevent bronchoconstriction, vascular permeability, and mucus secretion. *Zileuton* is another oral agent, and acts by inhibiting the 5-lipoxygenase enzyme to prevent generation of leukotrienes.

Protection Against Specific Asthma Triggers

Antileukotrienes are particularly useful in controlling asthma resulting from certain triggers, including exercise-induced asthma, aspirin-induced asthma, and, to a lesser extent, allergen-induced asthma.[33,40]

- *Exercise-induced asthma:* In exercise-induced asthma, cooling and drying of the airway promotes the generation of leukotrienes, resulting in bronchoconstriction. Although protection varies from complete to very little, the antileukotrienes develop no tolerance and may benefit those who want to exercise or whose jobs require exercise under cold, dry conditions, without the use of short-acting rescue β agonists.
- *Aspirin-induced asthma:* In 3 to 8% of asthma cases, aspirin or NSAIDs can cause bronchoconstriction as a result of an increase in leukotriene C$_4$ synthase activity. On the basis of such pathophysiology, which involves leukotriene production, leukotriene modifiers are the treatment of choice of patients with aspirin-induced asthma.
- *Allergen-induced asthma:* Antileukotrienes also block the early asthma response to allergen challenge and attenuate airway obstruction in the late-phase response. They are not completely effective in abolishing the late response that is also due to histamine release.

Chronic Persistent Asthma

The evidence to date supports the use of antileukotriene agents in the management of chronic asthma, including mild, moderate, or severe.[33,41,42] In mild to moderate asthma, antileukotrienes improve lung function, reduce the need for rescue β-agonist use, and decrease asthma symptoms, including nocturnal symptoms. In moderate to severe asthma, the additive effect between antileukotrienes and inhaled corticosteroids is the basis for asthma control with lower steroid doses or without

TABLE 12-2

Summary of Comparative Features of the Three Currently Available Antileukotriene Agents

	Zileuton (Zyflo)	Zafirlukast (Accolate)	Montelukast (Singulair)
Action	5-LO inhibitor	CysLT$_1$ receptor block	CysLT$_1$ receptor block
Age range	≥12 yr	≥6 yr	≥6 mo
Dose	600-mg tablet qid	20-mg tablet bid	Adult: 10-mg tablet q evening Children 6-14 yr: 5-mg tablet q evening Children 2-5 yr: 4-mg tablet q evening
Administration	Can be taken with food	1 hr before or 2 hr after meal	Taken with or without food
Drug interactions	Yes (theophylline, warfarin, propranolol)	Yes (warfarin, theophylline, aspirin)	No
Side effects (common)	Headache, dyspepsia, unspecified pain, liver enzyme elevations	Headache, infection, nausea, possible liver enzyme changes	Headache, influenza, abdominal pain
Contraindications	Active liver disease or elevated liver enzymes; hypersensivity to components	Hypersensivity to components	Hypersensivity to components

CysLT$_1$, Cysteinyl leukotriene receptor subtype 1; *5-LO,* lipoxygenase.

Box 12-3	Advantages and Disadvantages of Antileukotriene Drug Therapy in Managing Asthma

Advantages	Disadvantages
• Oral administration, possible once-daily dosing • Safe, with few side effects to date • Effective in aspirin sensitivity and often in exercise-induced asthma • Systemic distribution reaches entire lung through the circulation • Additive effect with inhaled steroids • May reduce steroid dose, or prevent an increase in steroid dose • A formulation approved for pediatric dosing (montelukast)	• Relatively limited antiinflammatory action limited to one mediator pathway • Unknown long-term toxicity • Variable response—effective in about 50-70% of patients • No predictor of patients who will respond • Systemic drug exposure, not limited to lung • Generally not useful as monotherapy

an increase in steroid dosing (inhaled or oral). There are advantages and disadvantages to antileukotriene drug therapy in asthma, which are summarized in Box 12-3.

Antileukotriene drug therapy is effective in approximately 50% of patients (although this proportion is higher for aspirin-sensitive individuals), but there is no method to predict which patients will be responders.[43,44] Considerable intersubject variability in response has been seen. In a study of exercise challenge, 20 mg of zafirlukast gave complete protection in three subjects, partial protection in four subjects, and no protection in one subject.[45]

Antileukotrienes in Relation to Corticosteroids

Asthma guidelines agree that corticosteroids are the most effective antiinflammatory drugs for use in asthma, and they have broader antiinflammatory activity than the more limited effect of the antileukotrienes. Leukotriene modifiers affect only one biochemical pathway—the lipoxygenase path and resulting leukotriene effects. Two aspects of antileukotriene therapy should be considered in relation to the use of corticosteroids in asthma.

• Choosing between an inhaled steroid and an antileukotriene in mild persistent asthma is based on offsetting advantages: the superior efficacy of inhaled steroids with possibly poor compliance versus the anticipated superior compliance of the orally administered antileukotrienes with their more limited antiinflammatory action.[33]

• There is an additive effect between antileukotriene and inhaled corticosteroid therapy in mild to moderate asthma. A study by Laviolette and colleagues[46] showed a greater response to inhaled beclomethasone alone compared with oral montelukast alone. However, the combination of the two treatments

resulted in the greatest improvement in lung function, as seen in Figure 12-10. In another study, use of montelukast by adult asthmatics taking inhaled steroids chronically resulted in a 47% reduction in steroid dose, compared with a 30% reduction in the placebo group.[47]

Churg-Strauss Syndrome

Churg-Strauss syndrome has been reported in a few patients treated with zafirlukast[48] or montelukast (postmarketing letter).[49] Churg-Strauss syndrome is a vasculitis of unknown etiology, usually occurring in adults between 20 and 40 years of age, marked by peripheral eosinophilia, eosinophilic infiltration of tissues, and necrotizing vasculitis that can result in major organ damage and death if left untreated. The syndrome is rare, with a prevalence of about 1 case per 15,000 to 20,000 patient-years of treatment. Patients to date who developed this syndrome have had difficult-to-control asthma and have been taking oral or high doses of inhaled corticosteroids. It is not completely clear whether this is an effect of antileukotriene treatment or whether the syndrome is unmasked by a reduction in corticosteroid therapy allowed by the antileukotriene therapy.[33] A review by Wechsler and associates[49] of eight patients concluded that the occurrence of Churg-Strauss syndrome in asthmatic patients receiving antileukotriene treatment appeared to be due to unmasking of an underlying vasculitic syndrome diagnosed as moderate to severe asthma and treated with corticosteroids. Nevertheless, experience in humans with antileukotriene drugs, specifically $CysLT_1$ receptor antagonists, is still new, and not all of the processes associated with 5-LO products are completely understood. For example, a type 2 leukotriene receptor ($CysLT_2$), which is *not* blocked by the $CysLT_1$ antagonists such as zafirlukast or

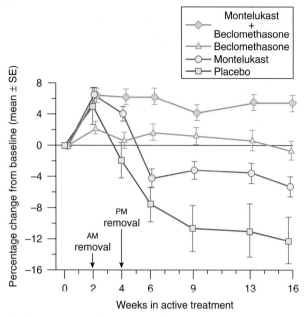

FIGURE 12-10 Mean (±SE) percent change from baseline in four treatment groups receiving combined inhaled beclomethasone and oral montelukast, beclomethasone alone, montelukast alone, or placebo. The A.M. and P.M. beclomethasone inhalers were replaced with placebo in the montelukast and placebo groups during the run-in period. (From Laviolette M and others: Montelukast added to inhaled beclomethasone in treatment of asthma, *Am J Respir Crit Care Med* 160:1862, 1999.)

montelukast, has been identified on human pulmonary vasculature.[31] The effect of introducing a potential imbalance with $CysLT_1$ antileukotriene therapy is not well understood. Although antileukotriene drugs appear safe and effective, additional clinical experience is needed.

Respiratory Syncytial Virus

There appears to be link between respiratory syncytial virus (RSV) and asthma. It is believed that reactive airway disease is a common accompaniment to RSV.[50] One of the thoughts to combat this phenomenon is to use a $CysLT_1$ receptor antagonist, specifically montelukast. In a published report by Bisgaard, it was noted that 22% of patients receiving montelukast had a reduction of symptoms, compared with only 4% receiving placebo.[50] The thought is that the airway's immune response in viral infections is very similar to that after exposure to allergens. CysLTs are inflammatory mediators that are released in both viral and allergic responses. The use of montelukast blocks these mediators in asthma as well as RSV infection.

Summary of Clinical Use of Antileukotriene Therapy

The following points attempt to summarize the current understanding of the role of antileukotriene drug therapy in asthma:

- Antileukotriene agents are prophylactic, controller drugs used in persistent asthma, including mild, moderate, and severe states; they are not indicated for acute relief or rescue therapy.
- Antileukotrienes can be tried as an alternative to inhaled corticosteroids or cromolyn-like agents in mild persistent asthma requiring more than as-needed β_2 agonists.
- Antileukotrienes may not be optimal as monotherapy in persistent asthma.
- Antileukotrienes may allow reduction of high-dose inhaled corticosteroids or prevent an increase in the dose of inhaled corticosteroids, and they reduce or prevent the need for oral corticosteroids.
- Evidence to date shows these agents as safe and often effective choices in managing a wide range of asthma severity.

Monoclonal Antibodies

KEY POINT

Omalizumab (Xolair), a monoclonal antibody, is used to treat moderate to severe asthma.

Omalizumab, also known by the trade name Xolair, is a subcutaneously injected monoclonal antibody. This drug is indicated for the treatment of moderate to severe asthma in adults and adolescents 12 years of age and older who have a positive skin test or *in vitro* reactivity to a perennial aeroallergen. It may be beneficial in treating seasonal allergic rhinitis.[51]

Dosage and Administration

Omalizumab is available as a powder that must be reconstituted; after reconstitution it has a concentration of 150 mg/1.2 ml. Dosing occurs every 2 or 4 weeks and is dependent on the weight and serum IgE level of the patient. Refer to the manufacturer's package insert for specific dosing instructions.

Mode of Action

Omalizumab is a recombinant DNA-derived humanized IgG1(κ) murine monoclonal antibody that selectively binds to human IgE. The drug blocks the binding of IgE to the IgE receptor on the surface of mast cells

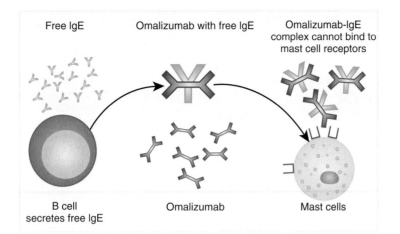

FIGURE 12-11 A model of omalizumab complexing to free IgE to stop attachment to a mast cell, thereby stopping mast cell degranulation. (Modified from Rosenwasser, LJ, Nash, DB: Incorporating omalizumab into asthma treatment guidelines: Consensus Panel recommendations. *Pharmacy & Therapeutics* 28:400-41, 2003.)

and basophils, as noted in Figure 12-11. This allows the reduction of mediators that can be released in an allergic response.

Pharmacokinetics

After parenteral administration, omalizumab is absorbed with an average bioavailability of 62%. Omalizumab is absorbed slowly, reaching peak concentrations after an average of 7–8 days. If doses of greater than 0.5 mg/kg are given a linear correlation exists, meaning the more given the greater the drug availability. Omalizumab is eliminated primarily via the liver. The half-life of the drug averages 26 days and may be weight related: increasing weight increases clearance.[52]

Hazards and Side Effects

The most severe reactions occurring in clinical trials with omalizumab were anaphylaxis and malignancies; however, these were rare. Other, more commonly observed reactions included injection site reactions, viral infection, upper respiratory tract infection, and pharyngitis.

It is important to note that omalizumab is not for acute asthmatic conditions. Patients taking inhaled or systemic corticosteroids and considering omalizumab should note that this drug is not a replacement for regular corticosteroid use.

Role of Omalizumab in Asthma Management

The literature at the time of this edition supports the use of omalizumab in uncontrolled moderate to severe asthma. Busse and colleagues[53] found that omalizumab

reduced asthma exacerbations and decreased corticosteroid and rescue medication use. Soler and colleagues found similar results in that asthma exacerbations per patient were reduced and use of corticosteroids had dropped. Seventy-nine percent of patients taking omalizumab were able to drop their steroid dose by 50% or more, compared with only 55% in the placebo group.[54] In an extension phase of a clinical trial for omalizumab, Buhl and associates found that patients receiving omalizumab had fewer exacerbations and that their corticosteroid use had dropped by approximately 180 µg/day.[55] Lanier and colleagues discovered that patients being treated with omalizumab reduced their corticosteroid use by 108 µg/day compared with those receiving placebo. It was noted that many in the placebo group were given more long-term β agonists and leukotriene inhibitors compared with the omalizumab group.[56]

Summary of Clinical Use of Omalizumab

The following points attempt to summarize the current understanding of the role of omalizumab in asthma:

- Omalizumab is a prophylactic agent used in uncontrolled moderate to severe persistent asthma; it is not indicated for acute relief or rescue therapy.
- Omalizumab is not a replacement for inhaled corticosteroids.
- Omalizumab is not optimal as monotherapy in persistent asthma.
- Omalizumab may allow reduction of high-dose inhaled corticosteroids or prevent an increase in the dose of inhaled corticosteroids.

- Omalizumab may allow reduction of asthmatic rescue agents.

RESPIRATORY CARE ASSESSMENT OF NONSTEROIDAL ANTIASTHMA AGENTS

- Evaluate patient for optimal aerosol delivery formulation for inhaled medications, if more than one delivery system is available (e.g., small volume nebulizer [SVN] or MDI). Note age, ability to understand instructions, and need for reservoir with MDI.
- Initially for aerosol medications: Instruct patient in use of aerosol delivery system selected (MDI, reservoir, SVN) and then verify correct use.
  - Assess breathing rate and pattern.
  - Assess breath sounds by auscultation, before and after treatment.
  - Assess pulse before and after treatment.
  - Assess patient's subjective reaction to treatment, for any change in breathing effort or pattern.
- Verify that patient understands that nonsteroidal antiasthma agents are controller drugs and understands their difference from a rescue bronchodilator (relieving agent); assess patient's understanding of the need for consistent use of these agents (compliance with therapy).
- Instruct patient in use of a peak flow meter, to monitor baseline PEF and changes. Verify that there is a specific action plan based on symptoms and peak flow results. The patient should be clear on when to contact a physician with deterioration in PEF or exacerbation of symptoms.
- Long term: Assess severity of symptoms (coughing, wheezing, nocturnal awakenings, and symptoms during exertion); use of rescue medication; number of exacerbations and missed work/school days; and pulmonary function. Modify level of asthma therapy (up or down, as described in NAEPP Expert Panel Report 2 [EPR-2] guidelines for step therapy).
- Assess for presence of side effects with nonsteroidal antiasthma agents (refer to particular agent and its side effects, as listed previously).

SELF-ASSESSMENT QUESTIONS

1. Identify five nonsteroidal antiasthma drugs used in the management of chronic asthma; give both generic and brand names.
2. Which immunoglobulin is implicated in allergy and is termed *cytophilic*?
3. Which type of asthma involves allergic reaction to an antigenic stimulus?
4. Which type of helper T cell, Th1 or Th2, is involved primarily in the atopic allergic response?
5. A resident wishes to order nebulized cromolyn sodium for a young asthmatic patient in the emergency department who is wheezing and in moderate distress. Would you agree?
6. Which of the following could be recommended as possible choices for the asthmatic patient in question 5: inhaled albuterol, inhaled salmeterol, inhaled ipratropium bromide, theophylline either orally or intravenously?
7. What is the usual dose of nedocromil sodium by inhalation in adults?
8. An asthmatic patient has been taking 40 mg of oral prednisone for 1 week after an acute asthma attack and an emergency department visit. His physician now wants to switch him to inhaled nedocromil and discontinue the oral prednisone. What is the risk in doing this and what would you recommend?
9. Briefly compare and distinguish the mode of action of nedocromil sodium versus cromolyn sodium.
10. How does the mode of action of zafirlukast and montelukast differ from that of zileuton?
11. What is the recommended dose and route of administration for zafirlukast, montelukast, and zileuton?
12. Which of the three antileukotriene agents in question 11 offers the most convenient dosing and the fewest drug interactions?
13. When would you recommend using omalizumab?
14. A 17-year-old asthmatic has been treated for symptoms for the last 12 months. His symptoms have not improved despite the use of the highest inhaled corticosteroid dose and regular use of salmeterol; in addition, trials on montelukast, cromolyn sodium, and oral theophylline have been unsuccessful. What would you recommend for this patient?

Answers to Self-Assessment Questions are found in Appendix A.

CLINICAL SCENARIO

A 45-year-old white female calls her pulmonologist and is seen in the emergency department with a complaint of chest tightness, shortness of breath, and wheezing for the past 1.5 days. She also complains of a cough, with only occasional thin whitish sputum during that period. She denies any fever or chills. She was diagnosed with adult-onset asthma 3 years ago and is aspirin sensitive. She has no history of tobacco use. She had a nasal polypectomy 2 years ago. Since that time she has been maintained on pirbuterol breath-actuated inhaler as needed and since about 4 months ago on oral theophylline 300 mg twice daily. She is alert but mildly anxious.

Her vital signs are as follows: temperature (T), 97° F; pulse (P), 92 beats/min and regular; blood pressure (BP), 90/60 mmHg; and respiratory rate (RR), 22 breaths/min with no laboring. Expiration is slightly prolonged, but there is no use of accessory muscles. No cyanosis is evident. Auscultation reveals diffuse wheezes, greater on expiration than inspiration, and rhonchi bilaterally. Routine blood work later showed the following: hemoglobin, 13.5 g/dl; white blood cell (WBC) count, $6.1 \times 10^3/mm^3$ with 13% eosinophils. Electrolytes were also found to be within normal limits, except for a plasma glucose level of 281 mg/dl. A chest radiograph showed some hyperinflation bilaterally, with no infiltrates, no pneumothorax, and normal heart size. An arterial blood gas measurement on room air revealed the following: pH, 7.38; arterial carbon dioxide pressure (Pa_{CO_2}), 42 mmHg; arterial oxygen pressure (Pa_{O_2}), 72 mmHg; base excess, +0.3 mEq/L; and arterial oxygen saturation (Sa_{O_2}), 96%.

On questioning, she states that she has been using her as-needed pirbuterol, two inhalations, almost every 4 hours over the past 24 hours, with little improvement. She has found it necessary to use her inhaler most days of the week. She also states that she has been experiencing many headaches, upset stomach, some lack of appetite, and insomnia often during the week. It has been 2 to 3 hours since she last used her pirbuterol inhaler.

How would you treat her asthma attack at this point?

What medications would you consider for maintenance of her asthma, given her recent history and prior medications?

Answers to Clinical Scenario Questions are found in Appendix A.

References

1. National Asthma Education and Prevention Program, National Heart, Lung, and Blood Institute, National Institutes of Health: Expert Panel Report 2: *Guidelines for the diagnosis and management of asthma*, NIH Publication 97-4051. Bethesda, Md, 1997, National Institutes of Health. (Available at http://www.nhlbi.nih.gov/guidelines/asthma/asthgdln.pdf; accessed February 2007.)

2. National Asthma Education and Prevention Program, National Heart, Lung, and Blood Institute, National Institutes of Health: Expert Panel Report: *Guidelines for the diagnosis and management of asthma—update on selected topics,* NIH Publication 02-5074. Bethesda, Md, 2003, National Institutes of Health. (Available at http://www.nhlbi.nih.gov/guidelines/asthma/asthmafullrpt.pdf; accessed March 2007.)

3. Platts-Mills TA, Woodfolk JA, Chapman MD, Heymann PW: Changing concepts of allergic disease: the attempt to keep up with real changes in lifestyles, *J Allergy Clin Immunol* 98:S297, 1996.

4. Holgate ST: A rationale for the use of nedocromil sodium in the treatment of asthma, *J Allergy Clin Immunol* 98:S157, 1996.

5. Drazen JM, Turino GM: Progress at the interface of inflammation and asthma: report of an ATS-sponsored workshop November, 1993, *Am J Respir Crit Care Med* 152:386, 1995.

6. Global Initiative for Asthma (GINA), National Heart, Lung, and Blood Institute, National Institutes of Health: NHLBI/WHO Workshop Report: *Global strategy for asthma management and prevention.* NIH Publication 02-3659. Bethesda, Md, 2005, National Institutes of Health. (Available at http://www.ginasthma.com/Guidelineitem.asp?l1=2&l2=1&intId=1169&archived=1; accessed March 2007.)

7. Flak TA, Goldman WE: Autotoxicity of nitric oxide in airway disease, *Am J Respir Crit Care Med* 154:S202, 1996.

8. Liggett SB, Levi R, Metzger H: G-protein coupled receptors, nitric oxide, and the IgE receptor in asthma, *Am J Respir Crit Care Med* 152:394, 1995.

9. Orr TSC: Mast cells and allergic asthma, *Br J Dis Chest* 67:87, 1973.

10. Orr TSC, Hall DE, Allison AC: Role of contractile microfilaments in the release of histamine from mast cells, *Nature* 236:350, 1972.

11. McFadden ER Jr: Cromolyn: first-line therapy for chronic asthma? *J Respir Dis* 8:39, 1987.

12. O'Byrne PM, Dolovich J, Hargeave FE: Late asthmatic responses, *Am Rev Respir Dis* 136:740, 1987.

13. Bernstein IL: Cromolyn sodium, *Chest* 87(suppl):68S, 1985.

14. Bernstein IL: Cromolyn sodium in the treatment of asthma: coming of age in the United States, *J Allergy Clin Immunol* 76:381, 1985.

15. Settipane GA, Klein DE, Boyd GK: Adverse reactions to cromolyn, *JAMA* 241:811, 1979.

16. Holgate ST: Inhaled sodium cromoglycate, *Respir Med* 90:387, 1996.

17. Edwards AM: Sodium cromoglycate (Intal) as an anti-inflammatory agent for the treatment of chronic asthma, *Clin Exp Allergy* 24:612, 1994.

18. Konig P, Shaffer J: Long-term (3–14 years) outcome in children with asthma treated with cromolyn sodium, *Am J Respir Crit Care Med* 149:A210, 1994.

19. Cockcroft DW, Murdock KY: Comparative effects of inhaled salbutamol, sodium cromoglycate, and beclomethasone dipropionate on allergen-induced early asthmatic responses, late asthmatic responses, and increased bronchial responsiveness to histamine, *J Allergy Clin Immunol* 79:734, 1987.

20. Hargreaves MR, Benson MK: Inhaled sodium cromoglycate in angiotensin-converting-enzyme inhibitor cough, *Lancet* 345:13, 1995.

21. Toppet M, Fall AB, Ferster A, Fondu P, Melot C, Vanhaelen-Fastre R, Vanhaelen M: Antisickling activity of sodium cromoglycate in sickle-cell disease [research letter], *Lancet* 356:309, 2000.

22. Gonzalez JP, Brogden RN: Nedocromil sodium: a preliminary review of its pharmacodynamic and pharmacokinetic properties, and therapeutic efficacy in the treatment of reversible obstructive airways disease, *Drugs* 34:560, 1987.

23. Devalia JL, Rusznak C, Abdelaziz MM, Davies RJ: Nedocromil sodium and airway inflammation *in vivo* and *in vitro*, *J Allergy Clin Immunol* 98:S51, 1996.

24. Alton EW, Norris AA: Chloride transport and the actions of nedocromil sodium and cromolyn sodium in asthma, *J Allergy Clin Immunol* 98:S102, 1996.

25. Clark B: General pharmacology, pharmacokinetics, and toxicology of nedocromil sodium, *J Allergy Clin Immunol* 92:200, 1993.

26. Edwards AM, Stevens MT: The clinical efficacy of inhaled nedocromil sodium (Tilade) in the treatment of asthma, *Eur Respir J* 6:35, 1993.

27. Armenio L, Baldini G, Bardare M, Boner A, Burgio R, Cavagni G, La Rosa M, Marcucci F, Miraglia del Giudice M, Pulejo MR, *et al.*: Double blind, placebo controlled study of nedocromil sodium in asthma, *Arch Dis Child* 68:193, 1993.

28. Shields M, McCollum J, Irvine M, Cater J: One year of treatment with flavoured nedocromil sodium in young children, *Eur Respir J* 7(suppl 18):139S, 1994.

29. Busse W: The role and contribution of leukotrienes in asthma, *Ann Allergy Asthma Immunol* 81:17, 1998.

30. Busse W: Leukotrienes and inflammation, *Am J Respir Crit Care Med* 157(suppl):S210, 1998.

31. Bisgaard H: Role of leukotrienes in asthma pathophysiology, *Pediatr Pulmonol* 30:166, 2000.

32. Lynch KR, O'Neill GP, Liu Q, Im DS, Sawyer N, Metters KM, Coulombe N, Abramovitz M, Figueroa DJ, Zeng Z, *et al.*: Characterization of the human cysteinyl leukotriene CysLT$_1$ receptor, *Nature* 399:789, 1999.

33. Drazen JM, Israel E, O'Byrne PM: Treatment of asthma with drugs modifying the leukotriene pathway, *N Engl J Med* 340:197, 1999.

34. Knorr B, Matz J, Bernstein JA, Nguyen H, Seidenberg BC, Reiss TF, Becker A: Montelukast for chronic asthma in 6- to 14-year-old children: a randomized, double-blind trial, *JAMA* 279:1181, 1998.

35. Reiss TF, Chervinsky P, Dockhorn RJ, Shingo S, Seidenberg B, Edwards TB: Montelukast, a once-daily leukotriene receptor antagonist, in the treatment of chronic asthma: a multicenter, randomized, double-blind trial, *Arch Intern Med* 158:1213, 1998.

36. Leff JA, Busse WW, Pearlman D, Bronsky EA, Kemp J, Hendeles L, Dockhorn R, Kundu S, Zhang J, Seidenberg BC, *et al.*: Montelukast, a leukotriene-receptor antagonist, for the treatment of mild asthma and exercise-induced bronchoconstriction, *N Engl J Med* 339:147, 1998.

37. Bisgaard H, Zielen S, Garcia-Garcia ML, Johnston SL, Gilles L, Menten J, Tozzi CA, Polos P: Montelukast reduces asthma exacerbations in 2 to 5 year old children with intermittent asthma, *Am J Respir Crit Care Med* 171:315, 2004.

38. Knorr B, Franchi LM, Bisgaard H, Vermeulen JH, LeSouef P, Santanello N, Michele TM, Reiss TF, Nguyen HH, Bratton DL: Montelukast, a leukotriene receptor antagonist, for the treatment of persistent asthma in children aged 2 to 5 years, *Pediatrics* 108:E48, 2001.

39. Knorr B, Maganti L, Ramakrishnan R, Tozzi CA, Migoya E, Kearns G: Pharmacokinetics and safety of montelukast in children aged 3 to 6 months, *J Clin Pharmacol* 46:620, 2006.

40. Dahlen SE, Malmstrom K, Nizankowska E, Dahlen B, Kuna P, Kowalski M, Lumry WR, Picado C, Stevenson DD, Bousquet J, *et al.*: Improvement of aspirin intolerant asthma by montelukast, a leukotriene antagonist: a randomized, double blind, placebo-controlled trial, *Am J Respir Crit Care Med* 165:9, 2002.

41. Becker A: Leukotriene receptor antagonists: efficacy and safety in children with asthma, *Pediatr Pulmonol* 30:183, 2000.

42. Kemp J: Role of leukotriene receptor antagonists in pediatric asthma, *Pediatr Pulmonol* 30:177, 2000.

43. Ind PW: Anti-leukotriene intervention: is there adequate information for clinical use in asthma? *Respir Med* 90:575, 1996.

44. Smith LJ: Newer asthma therapies, *Ann Intern Med* 130:531, 1999.

45. Finnerty JP, Wood-Baker R, Thomson H, Holgate ST: Role of leukotrienes in exercise-induced asthma, *Am Rev Respir Dis* 145:746, 1992.

46. Laviolette M, Malmstrom K, Lu S, Chervinsky P, Pujet JC, Peszek I, Zhang J, Reiss TF: Montelukast added to inhaled beclomethasone in treatment of asthma, *Am J Respir Crit Care Med* 160:1862, 1999.

47. Lofdahl CG, Reiss TF, Leff JA, Israel E, Noonan MJ, Finn AF, Seidenberg BC, Capizzi T, Kundu S, Godard P: Randomised, placebo controlled trial of effect of a leukotriene receptor antagonist, montelukast, on tapering inhaled corticosteroids in asthmatic patients, *BMJ* 319:87, 1999.

48. Wechsler ME, Garpestad E, Flier SR, Kocher O, Weiland DA, Polito AJ, Klinek MM, Bigby TD, Wong GA, Helmers RA, *et al.*: Pulmonary infiltrates, eosinophilia, and cardiomyopathy following corticosteroid withdrawal in patients with asthma receiving zafirlukast, *JAMA* 279:455, 1998.

49. Wechsler ME, Finn D, Gunawardena D, Westlake R, Barker A, Haranath SP, Pauwels RA, Kips JC, Drazen JM: Churg-Strauss syndrome in patients receiving montelukast as treatment for asthma, *Chest* 117:708, 2000.

50. Bisgaard H; Study Group on Montelukast and Respiratory Syncytial Virus: A randomized trial of montelukast in respiratory syncytial virus postbronchiolitis, *Am J Respir Crit Care Med* 167:379–83, 2003.

51. Kaliner MA: Omalizumab and the treatment of allergic rhinitis [abstract], *Curr Allergy Asthma Rep* 4:237, 2004.

52. Davis LA: Omalizumab: a novel therapy for allergic asthma, *Ann Pharmocother* 38:1236, 2004.

53. Busse W, Corren J, Lanier BQ, McAlary M, Fowler-Taylor A, Cioppa GD, van As A, Gupta N: Omalizumab, anti-IgE recombinant humanized monoclonal antibody, for the treatment of severe allergic asthma, *J Allergy Clin Immunol* 108:184, 2001.

54. Soler M, Matz J, Townley R, Buhl R, O'Brien J, Fox H, Thirlwell J, Gupta N, Della Cioppa G: The anti-IgE antibody omalizumab reduces exacerbations and steroid requirement in allergic asthmatics, *Eur Respir J* 18:254, 2001.

55. Buhl R, Soler M, Matz J, Townley R, O'Brien J, Noga O, Champain K, Fox H, Thirlwell J, Della Cioppa G: Omalizumab provides long-term control in patients with moderate-to-severe allergic asthma, *Eur Respir J* 20:73, 2002.

56. Lanier BQ, Corren J, Lumry W, Liu J, Fowler-Taylor A, Gupta N: Omalizumab is effective in the long-term control of severe allergic asthma, *Ann Allergy Asthma Immunol* 91:154, 2003.

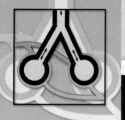

Chapter 13

Aerosolized Antiinfective Agents

DOUGLAS S. GARDENHIRE

CHAPTER OUTLINE

CHAPTER OBJECTIVES

After reading this chapter, the reader will be able to:

1. Discuss the indications for inhaled antiinfective agents.
2. List all available inhaled antiinfective agents used in respiratory therapy.
3. Differentiate between the specific antiinfective agent formulations.
4. Discuss the route of administration available for the various antiinfective agents.
5. Describe the mode of action for the various antiinfective agents.
6. Recognize side effects for the various antiinfective agents.
7. Discuss the use of each antiinfective agent in the treatment of lung disease.

KEY TERMS AND DEFINITIONS

Cystic fibrosis — An inherited disease of the exocrine glands, affecting the pancreas, respiratory system, and apocrine glands. Symptoms usually begin in infancy and are characterized by increased electrolytes in the sweat, chronic respiratory infection, and pancreatic insufficiency

Pneumocystis pneumonia (PCP) — An interstitial plasma cell pneumonia caused by the organism *Pneumocystis carinii (jiroveci)*. This pneumonia is common among patients with lowered immune system response

Respiratory syncytial virus (RSV) — A virus that causes formation of syncytial masses in infected cell structures

Virostatic — Stopping a virus from replicating

Virucidal — Killing a virus

Virus — An obligate intracellular parasite, containing either DNA or RNA, that reproduces by synthesis of subunits within the host cell and causes disease as a consequence of this replication

---

Chapter 13 discusses antiinfective agents currently approved for administration as inhaled aerosols: pentamidine isethionate (NebuPent), ribavirin (Virazole), tobramycin (TOBI), and zanamivir (Relenza). Pentamidine is used to prevent and treat **Pneumocystis pneumonia (PCP)** in patients with acquired immunodeficiency syndrome (AIDS), and ribavirin is used to treat **respiratory syncytial virus (RSV)** infection. A formulation of prepared antibody to RSV, termed *respiratory syncytial virus immune globulin intravenous (RSV-IGIV)*, offers prophylaxis; a monoclonal antibody, palivizumab (Synagis), offers prophylaxis and treatment for RSV infection. Inhaled tobramycin is available for the management of *Pseudomonas aeruginosa* infections in patients with cystic fibrosis. Zanamivir is an inhaled antiviral agent used to treat influenza.

CLINICAL INDICATIONS FOR AEROSOLIZED ANTIINFECTIVE AGENTS

Clinical indications for each of the aerosolized antiinfective agents available at the time of this edition are given. Each agent is discussed separately in detail.

Indication for Aerosolized Pentamidine

Pentamidine by inhalation is indicated for the *prevention* of PCP in high-risk human immunodeficiency virus (HIV)–infected patients who have a history of one or more episodes of PCP or a peripheral CD4+ (T4 helper cell) lymphocyte count of 200/mm^3 or less.

Indication for Aerosolized Ribavirin

Aerosolized ribavirin is indicated for the *treatment* of hospitalized infants with severe lower respiratory tract infection caused by respiratory syncytial virus (RSV).

Indication for Aerosolized Tobramycin

Aerosolized tobramycin is indicated for the *management* (control) of chronic *P. aeruginosa* infection in cystic fibrosis.

Indication for Inhaled Zanamivir

Inhaled zanamivir is indicated for the *treatment* of uncomplicated acute illness caused by influenza virus in adults and children age 7 years or over who have been symptomatic for no more than 2 days.

IDENTIFICATION OF AEROSOLIZED ANTIINFECTIVE AGENTS

Each of the antiinfective agents available for inhalation is listed in Table 13-1, along with details of formulation, usual recommended dosage, and clinical use. These agents are each discussed in more detail.

AEROSOLIZED PENTAMIDINE

Pentamidine isethionate is an antiprotozoal agent that is active against *P. carinii*, the causative organism for PCP. Chemically, it is an aromatic diamidine, whose structure is seen in Figure 13-1. Pentamidine can be given either parenterally or as an inhaled aerosol, but it is not absorbed with oral administration. When given parenterally, either intravenously or intramuscularly, the drug distributes quickly to the major organs (liver, kidneys, lung, and pancreas).

Introduction of Aerosolized Pentamidine (NebuPent)

Both systemic and aerosol administration of pentamidine have been used for the treatment of PCP, which occurs as a common opportunistic respiratory infection

TABLE 13-1

Currently Available Inhaled Antiinfective Agents, Listed by Generic and Brand Name, Along With Formulations, Usual Recommended Dosage, and Clinical Use*

Drug	Brand Name	Formulation and Dosage	Clinical Use
Pentamidine isethionate	NebuPent	300 mg of powder in 6 ml of sterile water; 300 mg once every 4 wk	PCP prophylaxis
Ribavirin	Virazole	6 mg of powder in 300 ml of sterile water (20-mg/ml solution); given 12-18 hr/day for 37 days by SPAG nebulizer	RSV
Tobramycin	TOBI	300 mg/5 ml ampoule Adults and children ≥6 yr: 300 mg bid, 28 days on/28 days off the drug	*Pseudomonas* aeruginosa in CF
Zanamivir	Relenza	DPI: 5 mg/inhalation Adults and children ≥5 yr: 2 inhalations (one 5-mg blister per inhalation) bid <12 hr apart for 5 days	Influenza

*Details on use and administration should be obtained from the manufacturer's drug insert material before use.
CF, Cystic fibrosis; *DPI,* dry powder inhaler; *PCP, Pneumocystis carinii* pneumonia; *RSV,* respiratory syncytial virus; *SPAG,* small particle aerosol generator.

KEY POINT

Aerosolized pentamidine isethionate is approved for use as second-line prophylactic therapy in patients with AIDS to prevent *P. carinii* pneumonia (PCP). Clinical experience with the aerosolized drug has resulted in significant side effects and less efficacy than with the oral agent trimethoprim-sulfamethoxazole (TMP–SMX). TMP–SMX is indicated for prophylaxis of PCP unless side effects are not tolerated, in which case the aerosol drug should be considered.

KEY POINT

The mode of action of pentamidine is not fully understood, but seems to interfere with nuclear metabolism and inhibits DNA, RNA, phospholipids, and protein synthesis.

KEY POINT

Side effects with aerosolized pentamidine include local airway effects such as cough, bronchospasm, dyspnea, and bad taste, as well as systemic effects.

KEY POINT

Aerosolized pentamidine should be administered with a nebulizer capable of producing small particle sizes (mass median aerodynamic diameter [MMAD], 1 to 2 μm),with a scavenging system to protect the environment. Precautions against the spread of tuberculosis (TB) with HIV patients should be taken, such as containment booths or isolation rooms.

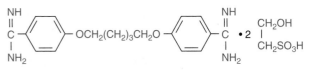

FIGURE 13-1 Chemical structure of pentamidine isethionate (NebuPent).

in individuals with AIDS. In addition to the prophylactic use of aerosolized pentamidine, the aerosol form has also been used for the treatment of acute episodes. The first report by Montgomery and associates was for therapy of acute episodes of PCP.[1]

Rationale for Aerosol Administration

The rationale for aerosol administration of pentamidine to treat or prevent PCP is based on the same rationale for other inhaled aerosol drugs used to treat the pulmonary system: local targeted lung delivery, with fewer or less severe side effects compared with systemic administration. Aerosolized pentamidine produces significantly higher lung concentrations than does intravenous administration.[2] The San Francisco prophylaxis trial showed that 300 mg of aerosolized pentamidine every 4 weeks was effective in preventing PCP in patients with HIV infection.[3] Unfortunately, subsequent clinical experience with aerosolized pentamidine did not show improved clinical efficacy compared with oral drugs such as trimethoprim–sulfamethoxazole (TMP-SMX), brand names Septra and Bactrim, and toxic side effects still occurred.

Description of Pneumocystis carinii Pneumonia

The organism *P. carinii* was first noted in the lungs of guinea pigs by Chagas in 1909 and Carini in 1910. It was named as a new organism by Delanöe and Delanöe in 1912, as *Pneumocystis carinii,* to describe the cystic form in the lungs and its earlier discoverer. Mammals are commonly infected with the organism at an early age, probably through an airborne vector. Disease occurs when there is suppression of the immune system. Before the AIDS pandemic, PCP was reported in malnourished infants in the 1940s and 1950s and in the 1970s in premature infants able to survive.[4] When not contained by a competent immune system, *P. carinii* causes the

pneumonia termed *PCP*. This produces a foamy intraalveolar exudate, which contains cysts of *P. carinii.* The life cycle of *P. carinii* and the resulting pneumonia are illustrated in Figure 13-2. Both pentamidine and TMP-SMX (brand names Septra and Bactrim) are effective against PCP and are usually given parenterally to treat an acute episode.

It should be noted that you may find conflicting names for *Pneumocystis carinii* in your reading. In a paper by Stringer and associates[5] they describe the name change to *Pneumocystis jiroveci* in honor of Otto Jírovec, a Czech parasitologist. However, in a letter to the editor, Hughes[6] pointed out that the name change is not valid or final because it has not been registered in the International Code of Botanical Nomenclature. It is also pointed out that the name change will cause confusion with discussion of *Pneumocystis carinii,* because many still use this terminology. In a letter, Gigliotti[7]

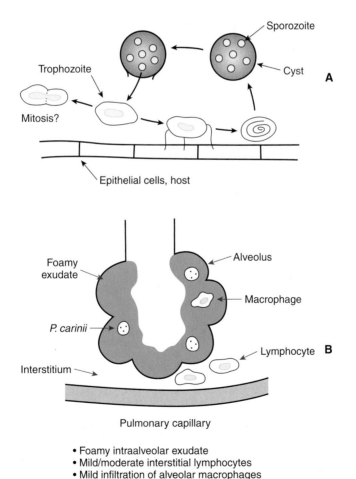

FIGURE 13-2 Pathogenesis of *Pneumocystis carinii,* the organism causing pneumocystis pneumonia (PCP). **A,** Life cycle of *P. carinii.* **B,** Pneumocystis pneumonia pathology.

continues the stance taken by Hughes, that is, that no clear evidence exists that an official name change has occurred.

What is known is that *Pneumocystis carinii* or *Pneumocystis jiroveci* is a fungus. It is also known that the acronym PCP for pneumocystis pneumonia remains the same no matter if you include or exclude "*carinii*."[5]

Dosage and Administration

Details of dose and administration of NebuPent, the aerosolized brand of pentamidine, can be found in the manufacturer's literature. The following summary is not intended to replace the more detailed instructions that accompany the drug.

Dosage

The approved dose of aerosolized pentamidine for prophylaxis of PCP in AIDS subjects is 300 mg, given by inhalation once every 4 weeks. This dose may be altered by physicians in treating individual patients.

NebuPent, the brand of pentamidine approved for inhalation as an aerosol, is supplied as a dry powder, with 300 mg in a single vial. This must be reconstituted with 6 ml of sterile water for injection, USP (not saline, which can cause precipitation), added to the vial. The entire 6 ml of reconstituted solution is placed into a nebulizer.

Administration

Approval of aerosolized pentamidine by the U.S. Food and Drug Administration (FDA) was for administration with the Respirgard II nebulizer. This is a small-volume nebulizer (SVN) system, powered by compressed gas, fitted with a series of one-way valves and an expiratory filter (Figure 13-3). This nebulizer system has been described by Montgomery and associates.[2] The Respirgard II should be powered with a flow rate of 5 to 7 L/min from a 50-psi source or, alternatively, by controlling the flow with a 22- to 25-psi pressure source connected to the small-bore tubing of the nebulizer. Pressures below 20 psi are not sufficient to produce the desired particle size necessary for peripheral delivery of the drug. These requirements with the Respirgard II are found in the manufacturer's literature and further discussed by Corkery and colleagues.[8] It may also be noted that the administration of pentamidine may take place in a room or tent that acts as a "vacuum" to draw any particles that have escaped to a filter. The capturing of these particles will result in less exposure to the respiratory therapist.

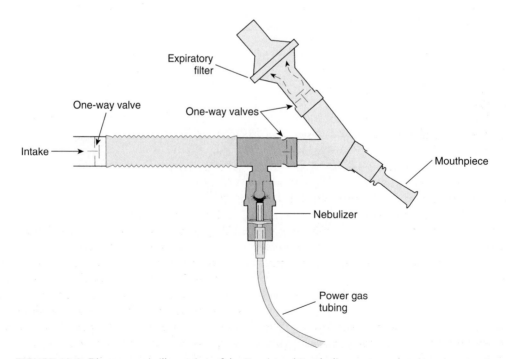

FIGURE 13-3 Diagrammatic illustration of the Respirgard II nebulizer system, showing one-way valves and expiratory filter to scavenge exhaust aerosol.

Nebulizer Performance

Although nebulized pentamidine was approved for general clinical use with the Respirgard II nebulizer system, other nebulizers have been used to administer the drug. At present, the manufacturer recommends use with a Respirgard II nebulizer system.

The general requirement for effective nebulization of pentamidine is a particle size or distribution of sizes with a mass median diameter (MMD) of 1 to 2 microns (μm). This is needed for the following two reasons[5]:

1. To achieve peripheral intraalveolar deposition targeted at the location of the microorganism
2. To reduce or prevent airway irritation seen with larger particle sizes, which will deposit more in larger airways

Studies by Vinciguerra and Smaldone[9] and by Smaldone and associates[10] have examined nebulizer performance and compared treatment time and patient tolerance of aerosolized pentamidine with the Respirgard II versus other nebulizers. Both treatment times and efficiency in drug availability were actually greater with the AeroTech II than the approved Respirgard II.

Mode of Action

The exact mode of action of pentamidine is not known. The drug's toxic effect on *P. carinii* may be due to multiple actions. Pentamidine blocks RNA and DNA synthesis, inhibits oxidative phosphorylation, and interferes with folate transformation.[4,11,12] Resistance to pentamidine by *P. carinii* has not been shown, and this may be due to the multiple effects of the drug on the organism's metabolism.[11]

When given by inhaled aerosol, pentamidine reaches significantly higher concentrations in the lung than when given intravenously.[2] The inhaled drug first binds to lung tissue. Although plasma levels are much less than with parenteral administration, the drug is slowly absorbed into the circulation and distributed to body tissues, as with parenteral administration. As a result, prolonged aerosol administration can result in systemic accumulation. Approximately 75% of the drug is excreted in urine and 25% in feces over the months after administration.

Side Effects

The side effects seen with systemic therapy of PCP using either pentamidine or TMP–SMX provided part of the rationale for aerosol administration of pentamidine. Although both of these drugs are effective in a majority of patients with PCP when given systemically, more than 50% of patients experience adverse side effects.

Side Effects With Parenteral Pentamidine

Side effects with *parenteral* administration of pentamidine have been summarized in several reviews, with numerous references.[8,11] Parenteral use of pentamidine has resulted in the following:

- Pain, swelling, and abscess formation at the site of injection, with intramuscular administration
- Thrombophlebitis and urticarial eruptions, with intravenous administration
- Hypoglycemia (up to 62% of patients), with a cumulative cytotoxic effect on pancreatic beta cells
- Impaired renal function and azotemia
- Hypotension
- Leukopenia
- Hepatic dysfunction

Side Effects With Aerosol Administration

Side effects with aerosol administration can be differentiated into local airway effects and systemic effects. *Local airway effects* with aerosol administration have included the following:

- Cough and bronchial irritation in 36% of patients in one study[3]
- Shortness of breath
- Bad taste (bitter or burning) of the aerosol impacting in the oropharynx
- Bronchospasm and wheezing in 11% of patients[3]
- Spontaneous pneumothoraces[13]

In addition, the following *systemic reactions* have occurred with aerosolized pentamidine:

- Conjunctivitis
- Rash
- Neutropenia
- Pancreatitis[14]
- Renal insufficiency
- Dysglycemia (hypoglycemia and diabetes)
- Digital necrosis in both feet[15]
- Appearance of extrapulmonary *P. carinii* infection

Because of the pharmacokinetics of pentamidine, chronic treatment with the aerosol can lead to tissue accumulation in the body, causing some of the same side effects as with parenteral administration. Suppression of *P. carinii* with local targeting of the lung has resulted in the appearance of infection elsewhere in the body.

Preventing Airway Effects

Use of a β-adrenergic bronchodilator before inhaling aerosolized pentamidine can reduce or prevent local airway reaction, including reduction of coughing or wheezing. Ipratropium has also been shown by Quieffin and colleagues[16] to prevent bronchoconstriction. The airway reaction may be caused by the sulfite moiety in isethionate (see Figure 13-1), which is known to cause airway irritation, or by the drug itself.[17,18] This effect can be reduced by use of a nebulizing system producing very small particle sizes, which will lessen airway deposition and increase alveolar targeting.[8]

Environmental Contamination by Nebulized Pentamidine

The following concerns exist regarding environmental contamination from nebulized pentamidine:

- Exposure to the drug itself from the exhaust aerosol
- Risk of infection with tuberculosis (TB), a disease associated with AIDS, from patients being treated with aerosolized pentamidine

Pentamidine is not known to be teratogenic, based on its use in pregnant women with African sleeping sickness (trypanosomiasis), although detailed clinical data were not kept. The drug is not mutagenic and its carcinogenic potential is considered minimal.[11] Studies have shown that low levels of pentamidine can be detected in health care workers exposed to the drug during treatments.[19,20] The investigators concluded that exposure probably occurred during treatment interruptions, usually caused by coughing episodes. Health care workers have also complained of conjunctivitis and bronchospasm when aerosolizing the drug.[11] On the basis of these reports and the long tissue half-life of pentamidine, contact with the drug should be kept to a minimum or prevented if possible.

The risk of contracting TB when treating AIDS patients with nebulized pentamidine is based on the association of TB and AIDS, the airborne mode of transmission of TB, and the fact that pentamidine aerosol can cause coughing and expulsion of droplet nuclei containing tuberculosis bacilli during aerosol treatments.

Environmental Precautions

The following precautionary measures are suggested when administering the drug, to reduce the risk of both drug exposure and TB infection with aerosolized pentamidine.[21-24]

- Use a nebulizer system with one-way valves and expiratory filter.

- Stop nebulization if the patient takes the mouthpiece out of the mouth (a thumb control on the power gas tubing gives more control).
- Use nebulizers producing an MMD of 1 to 2 μm, to increase alveolar targeting and lessen large airway deposition and cough production.
- Always use a suitable expiratory filter and one-way valves with the nebulizer. Instruct patients to turn off the nebulizer when talking or when taking it out of the mouth.
- Screen patients for cough history and pretreat with a β agonist, with sufficient lead time for effect in reducing the bronchial reactivity.
- Administer aerosol in a negative-pressure room, with six air changes per hour, or consider using an isolation booth/hood assembly with an exhaust fan and air directed through a high-efficiency filter.
- Use barrier protection (gloves, mask, and eyewear) for health care workers.
- Screen patients with HIV infection for TB, and treat where evidence of infection exists.
- Do not allow treatment patients to mix with others until coughing subsides.
- Health care workers should periodically screen themselves for TB.
- Pregnant women and nursing mothers should avoid exposure to the drug, and all practitioners should limit exposure to the extent possible.

Although measures exist to radically limit environmental contamination with aerosolized pentamidine, many of these are expensive, such as negative-pressure rooms and improved ventilation exchange in older buildings. Others are difficult, such as the wearing of effective high-efficiency masks in a busy clinical setting for a prolonged period. The use of room disinfection with ultraviolet light has been reviewed[25] but is debated.[22]

Aerosol Therapy for Prophylaxis of *Pneumocystis carinii* Pneumonia: Clinical Application

Comparisons between the efficacy of aerosolized pentamidine with oral TMP-SMX, together with reports of serious adverse effects with aerosolized pentamidine, caused a reevaluation of aerosol therapy with pentamidine for prophylaxis of PCP. General recommendations for prophylaxis of PCP have been published by the Centers for Disease Control and Prevention (CDC, Atlanta, GA) in *MMWR Recommendations and Reports* for HIV-positive children[26] and for adults.[27] In the 2004 CDC recommendations, oral TMP–SMX was preferred for prophylaxis of PCP, as long as adverse side effects from TMP–SMX were absent or acceptable.[27] Aerosolized pentamidine was not recommended as therapy for prophylaxis of PCP.

RIBAVIRIN

KEY POINT

Ribavirin is an aerosolized antiviral drug used with respiratory syncytial viral (RSV) infections in children and infants at risk for severe or complicated disease.

KEY POINT

Ribavirin acts as a nucleoside analog to terminate viral DNA replication. The aerosol is administered with a small particle aerosol generator (SPAG) unit.

KEY POINT

Side effects with ribavirin include pulmonary deterioration and equipment malfunction (ventilator occlusion and endotracheal tube occlusion). Environmental containment systems are available to protect caregivers.

Ribavirin (Virazole) is classified as an antiviral drug; it is active against RSV, influenza viruses, and herpes simplex virus. Chemically, it is a nucleoside analog and resembles guanosine and inosine.[28] Ribavirin is **virostatic**, not **virucidal**, and inhibits both DNA and RNA (retrovirus) viruses.

Ribavirin has been used throughout the world for a variety of viral infections, including RSV and influenza types A and B. Clinical trials of aerosolized ribavirin for severe RSV infection were conducted by Hall

and associates[29,30] and showed significant improvement with ribavirin treatment compared with placebo.

Clinical Use

Infection with RSV in children results in either bronchiolitis or pneumonia. Guidelines concerning the use of ribavirin were published by the Committee on Infectious Diseases of the American Academy of Pediatrics in 2003. In general, the drug is not recommended for RSV infection.[31] The Agency for Healthcare Research and Quality (AHRQ) has designated the drug as "possibly ineffective."[32]

Ribavirin treatment by aerosol is expensive and risks environmental exposure to the drug by personnel. Studies have given conflicting results on whether the use of ribavirin significantly reduces outcomes such as ventilator days, oxygen needs, intensive care unit days, hospital days, or mortality.[33,34]

Nature of Viral Infection

A short summary of viruses and viral infection is presented to establish key principles and concepts needed for understanding the difficulties in treating viral diseases, as well as the mode of action of ribavirin.

Virus — A virus can be defined as an obligate intracellular parasite, containing either DNA or RNA, that reproduces by synthesis of subunits within the host cell and causes disease as a consequence of this replication.

Figure 13-4 illustrates the simple structure of a virus. These are primitive members of the animal kingdom, submicronic in size, that consist of a strand of DNA or RNA that is surrounded by a protein coat. A virus may or may not be surrounded by an envelope, whose glycoprotein spikes are partially obtained from the host cell.

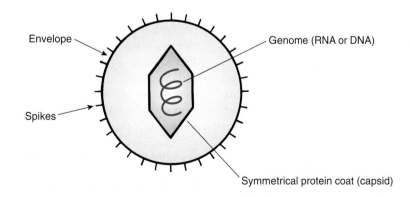

Virion: extracellular virus particle

FIGURE 13-4　Structure of a virus, showing nuclear material (DNA or RNA), protein coat, and an envelope.

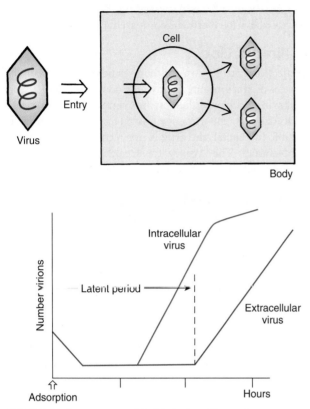

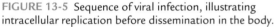

FIGURE 13-5 Sequence of viral infection, illustrating intracellular replication before dissemination in the body.

The concept and sequence of a viral infection are shown in Figure 13-5. A virus enters the body through a variety of routes (oral, inhaled, mucous membranes) and then invades a host cell. This is a multistep process consisting of phases in which the virus adsorbs to the cell, penetrates the cell, uncoats itself, goes through a process of recoding cell DNA (transcription, translation, synthesis), assembles itself, and sheds from the cell. The host cell usually dies in the process. Clinically, signs of a viral infection do not occur until after the initial latent period, when the virus leaves the cell, as illustrated in Figure 13-5. At this point, infection is well established. The diagnosis of viral illness is usually based on clinical signs, including the symptoms, age of the patient, and time of year. Definitive diagnosis requires isolating the virus or demonstrating an antibody titer increase. Diseases produced by viruses include chickenpox, smallpox, fever blisters (herpes simplex virus), genital herpes, poliomyelitis, the common cold, AIDS, influenza, mumps, and measles.

Because of the nature of viral infection, as just outlined, antiviral drug treatment, whether for the common cold or for HIV infection, is difficult. In particular, there are three complications in treating viral disease with drugs, as follows:

1. Attacking the intracellular virus may harm the host cell.
2. Viral replication is maximal before the appearance of symptoms.
3. Viruses have the property of antigenic mutability; that is, they change their appearance to the immune system.

Respiratory Syncytial Virus Infection

Respiratory syncytial virus (RSV) can cause bronchiolitis and pneumonia. Almost all children are exposed to the virus by their second year of life, and in most the infection is mild and self-limiting. Outbreaks of RSV pneumonia are seasonal and peak during winter months (November to March), with some variation according to geographical region.

The name of the virus reflects its effects on cells, which is to cause the formation of large, multinucleated cells, or a *syncytium*. The virus spreads easily by personal contact or hand contamination from surfaces. No effective vaccine exists to prevent RSV respiratory disease. Prepared antibody to RSV is available and is discussed below (RSV immune globulin intravenous).

Dosage and Administration

The following is a descriptive summary of ribavirin dosage and administration. It is not intended to replace detailed instructions contained in the manufacturer's literature, which should be reviewed before administering this drug. This includes the operating manual for the small particle aerosol generator (SPAG) nebulizing system.

Dosage

Ribavirin is given as a 20-mg/ml solution, which is administered by nebulizer (SPAG-2) for 12 to 18 hours per day, for a minimum of 3 days and not more than 7 days. The drug is supplied as 6 g of powder in a 100-ml vial. The powder is reconstituted first in the vial with sterile water for injection/inhalation, transferred to the large-volume (500-ml) reservoir of the nebulizer, and further diluted to a total volume of 300 ml with sterile water. This gives a concentration of 6 g/300 ml, or 20 mg/ml, a 2% strength solution.

Administration

Clinical trials of ribavirin aerosol were carried out with a large volume nebulizing system, known as a small particle aerosol generator (SPAG). The drug was approved

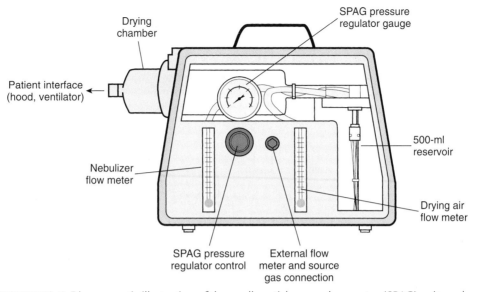

FIGURE 13-6 Diagrammatic illustration of the small particle aerosol generator (SPAG) unit used for nebulizing ribavirin.

for general use with this aerosol generator. A diagram of the SPAG unit is shown in Figure 13-6. It is a large volume, pneumatically powered nebulizer operating on a jet shearing principle, with baffling of aerosol particles and a drying chamber to further reduce particle size to a level of approximately 1.3 μm, MMD. Solutions in the SPAG reservoir should be replaced after 24 hours. Residual solution in the reservoir should be discarded before adding newly reconstituted solution. The drug solution should always be visually inspected for particulate matter or discoloration before use.

The nebulizer is connected to a hood as the patient interface. The manufacturer specifically warns against administration of the drug to infants requiring mechanical ventilation, because of the risk of drug precipitation occluding expiratory valves and sensors or even the endotracheal tube. However, the sickest infants with RSV are likely to need ventilatory support, and there are reports of drug use with mechanical ventilation. Detailed information concerning precautions with ventilator use during administration of the drug have been described by Demers and colleagues.[35] A clinical study of aerosol administration with mechanical ventilation of infants with severe RSV infection was reported by Smith and associates,[33] who showed that treatment reduced duration of ventilation, oxygen support, and hospital stay. Although labor intensive, mechanical ventilatory administration of ribavirin actually simplifies environmental control.

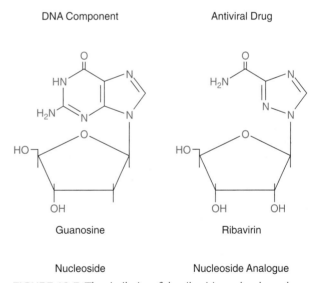

FIGURE 13-7 The similarity of the ribavirin molecule to the DNA precursor component, guanosine, may be the basis for the drug's virostatic effect.

Mode of Action

The mechanism of action by which ribavirin exerts its virostatic effect is not completely understood. Its viral inhibition is probably based on its structural resemblance to the nucleosides used to construct the DNA chain.[28] Figure 13-7 shows the structures of the natural nucleoside guanosine together with that

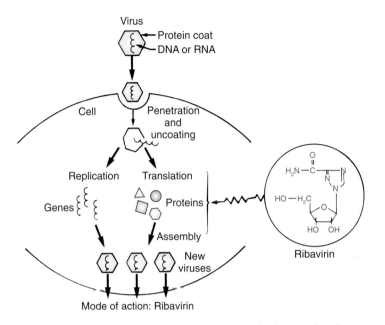

FIGURE 13-8 Illustration of the mode of action of ribavirin in blocking viral replication.

of ribavirin, which is a synthetic nucleoside analog. During the formation and assembly of new viral protein within the cell, ribavirin is most likely taken up instead of the natural nucleoside to form the DNA chain. This prevents construction of viable viral particles and subsequent shedding of virus into the bloodstream. A conceptual illustration of the process is shown in Figure 13-8. Ribavirin does not prevent the attachment or the penetration of respiratory syncytial virus into the cell and does not induce interferon.[28]

When given by inhaled aerosol, ribavirin levels are much greater in respiratory secretions than in the bloodstream. Waskin[11] gives a referenced summary of ribavirin kinetics. With 8 to 20 hours of aerosol treatment, peak plasma levels are 1 to 3 µg/ml, and respiratory secretion levels are greater than 1000 µg/ml. The minimal inhibitory concentration (MIC) for RSV is in the range of 4 to16 µg/ml. The half-life of ribavirin is about 9 hours in plasma and about 1 to 2 hours in respiratory secretions, which is the rationale for the almost continuous administration by aerosol.

Side Effects

Side effects seen with aerosolized ribavirin are listed in the product literature and have been reviewed by Waskin,[11] who gives detailed references. The following list summarizes adverse effects reported, including those seen with adults receiving the drug:

Pulmonary: Deterioration of pulmonary function and worsening of asthma or chronic obstructive disease; pneumothorax, apnea, and bacterial pneumonia have been described.

Cardiovascular: Cardiovascular instability, including hypotension, cardiac arrest, and digitalis toxicity, have been noted.

Hematological: Effects on blood cells have been reported with oral or parenteral administration but not with aerosol use. Reticulocytosis (excess of young erythrocytes in the circulation) has been reported, however, with aerosol use.

Dermatological/topical: Rash, eyelid erythema, and conjunctivitis have also been noted.

Equipment related: Equipment-related adverse effects with ribavirin treatment include occlusion and impairment of expiratory valves and sensors with ventilator use and endotracheal tube blockage from drug precipitate.

Although these effects have been reported, common effects clinically are pulmonary function deterioration, equipment malfunction from drug precipitate, and skin irritation from excess drug precipitation.

Environmental Contamination With Aerosolized Ribavirin

There is concern among health care workers over exposure to ribavirin. The drug has potential for mutagenic and carcinogenic effects, based on in vitro and animal studies.[11] The effect on fertility is uncertain, but the drug has caused testicular lesions in rats. The effect on pregnancy is of particular concern because the drug is teratogenic or embryocidal in animal species. Acute effects from aerosolized ribavirin reported by health care workers have included precipitation on contact lens and conjunctivitis, headache (51%), rhinitis, nausea, rash, dizziness, pharyngitis, and lacrimation (10 to 20%). Several cases of bronchospasm or chest pain have been reported by individuals with reactive airway disease. The symptoms noted have resolved within hours after discontinuing exposure to the drug.[36]

Minimal levels of ribavirin exposure are difficult to specify because of the lack of dose–response data for humans.[37] Corkery and others[38] state that the California Department of Health Services recommended an acceptable occupational airborne concentration for 8 hours of limited exposure to be 1/1000th of the lowest no-observed effect level, which would be 2.5 μg/m³.

Although there are no reports to date of serious effects from drug exposure by aerosol, precautions to limit or avoid exposure to the drug are well indicated, as advocated by Kacmarek.[39] Pregnant females, or those wishing to become pregnant, should avoid exposure to the drug if at all possible. In addition, environmental containment is superior to personnel barrier protection alone. Standard surgical masks do not prevent inhalation of 1- to 2-μm particles. Dermal absorption of ribavirin appears to be negligible.[40] It may be useful to utilize a containment system when the drug is aerosolized to an oxygen hood, several systems have been proposed in the literature.[41–43] All have common features of enclosure around the hood, with vacuum extraction and filtering of gas from the enclosure. Details needed for use can be found in the references given. It is recommended that the drug be administered in well-ventilated areas, that is, six or more air changes per hour.

OTHER AGENTS FOR PREVENTION AND TREATMENT OF RESPIRATORY SYNCYTIAL VIRUS INFECTION

Respiratory Syncytial Virus Immune Globulin Intravenous (Human)—RespiGam

Respiratory syncytial virus immune globulin intravenous (RSV-IGIV) is a sterile liquid formulation of immunoglobulin G (IgG) containing neutralizing antibody to RSV. The immunoglobulin is prepared

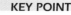

KEY POINT

Respiratory syncytial virus immune globulin intravenous (RSV-IGIV) is available as a monthly infusion of prepared antibody during RSV season, to confer passive immunity protection to children at risk. The humanized monoclonal antibody palivizumab is available for intramuscular injection.

from pooled human plasma containing high titers of neutralizing antibody against RSV. RSV-IGIV is available as RespiGam, and each milliliter contains 50 mg of immunoglobulin, primarily IgG, and trace amounts of IgA and IgM. A vaccine against RSV, which has not been successfully developed yet, would stimulate active immunity against RSV. RSV-IGIV, as prepared antibody against RSV, confers passive immunity. The drug is used on a prophylactic basis against RSV.

Indication for Use

RSV-IGIV is indicated for the prevention of serious lower respiratory tract infection with RSV in children younger than 24 months with bronchopulmonary dysplasia (BPD) or history of premature birth (less than 35 weeks of gestation).

Dosage and Administration

The drug is available in 50-ml vials, containing 2500 mg of RSV immunoglobulin. It is administered as a monthly intravenous infusion of 750 mg/kg. The solution is infused at 1.5 ml/kg/hr for 15 minutes and then increased to 3 ml/kg/hr for 15 minutes if no adverse clinical effects occur. The dose is increased to a maximum rate of 6 ml/kg/hr, which should not be exceeded. Slower infusion rates may be needed in very ill children.

Infusion should begin within 6 hours and be completed by 12 hours after beginning to use the vial. Infuse children at risk (as indicated) each month during RSV season (usually November through April in the northern hemisphere).

Mode of Action

RSV-IGIV is prepared immunoglobulin specific to RSV. As such, it is the antibody to RSV. When given intravenously, the product places antibody to RSV in the bloodstream of the patient, and the patient achieves a level of immunity to RSV. Because the recipient did not develop the antibody in response to RSV infection (which would be active immunity), this is a passive immunity. On exposure to RSV, the subject's immune system is prepared to neutralize the infecting agent.

Adverse Reactions

Side effects with infusion of RSV-IGIV can include fluid volume overload. Fever/pyrexia has also occurred. Immediate allergic, hypersensitivity reactions may occur. Reactions similar to other immunoglobulin infusions may occur, including dizziness, flushing, changes in blood pressure, palpitations, chest tightness, dyspnea, abdominal cramps, pruritus, myalgia, and arthralgia. These may be controlled by the rate of infusion. In general, RSV-IGIV has been well tolerated. RSV-IGIV is treated with a solvent–detergent viral inactivation procedure to guard against possible transmission of blood-borne viruses.

Clinical Efficacy

RSV-IGIV offers a prophylactic alternative to the treatment of acute RSV infection with aerosolized ribavirin. In studies of RSV prophylaxis, monthly RSV-IGIV doses of 750 mg/kg were effective in reducing RSV hospitalization among high-risk children with BPD or prematurity. Groothuis and colleagues noted that RespiGam has proven to be safe and effective, even at the highest dose.[44] In one clinical trial, RSV-IGIV reduced hospitalization resulting from RSV infection by 41% and total days of hospitalization by 53%.[45]

Palivizumab (Synagis)

Palivizumab represents the new drug class of therapeutic monoclonal antibodies.[46] The drug was approved for the prevention and treatment of RSV in premature infants and those with bronchopulmonary dysplasia (BPD).

Indication for Use

Palivizumab is indicated for the prevention of serious lower respiratory tract disease caused by RSV in children and infants at high risk. Safety and efficacy were established for infants with BPD, infants who had been born prematurely (<35 weeks), and children with congenital heart disease (CHD).[47]

Dosage and Administration

The powder for injection is lyophilized and the drug is available at 50 or 100 mg/ml. A premixed injection of 100 mg/ml is also available. The recommended dose is 15 mg/kg, given intramuscularly once a month throughout the RSV season.

Mode of Action

Palivizumab is a humanized monoclonal antibody produced by recombinant DNA techniques, directed against the F protein of the RSV virus. As an antibody against the RSV virus, palivizumab provides neutralizing and fusion-inhibiting activity, preventing viral replication.

Adverse Reactions

The most serious adverse reaction is anaphylaxis; however, this occurs in fewer than 1 per 100,000 cases. Other reactions that occurred in both treatment and placebo groups included fever, upper respiratory infection, otitis media, rhinitis, rash, pain, and hernia, as well as coughing and wheezing.[36]

Clinical Efficacy

In a large multicenter trial of infants at high risk of RSV infection, palivizumab given intravenously at 15 mg/kg reduced the rate of hospitalization resulting from RSV infection to 4.8%, compared with 10.6% in placebo recipients.[48] Adverse events were again similar in placebo and treatment groups.

Feltes and colleagues found that RespiGam is safe and effective for RSV-positive children with congenital heart disease (CHD). In this study 53% of the children experienced reduced hospital stays, and 73% experienced fewer days of supplemental oxygen use.[49]

AEROSOLIZED TOBRAMYCIN

KEY POINT

Nebulized tobramycin is used to manage chronic *Pseudomonas aeruginosa* infection in cystic fibrosis as an alternative to intravenous therapy. The nebulized form is attractive because of poor oral bioavailability for respiratory tract infections.

KEY POINT

Side effects with tobramycin include tinnitus and voice changes. Inhaled tobramycin should be used with caution in the presence of renal impairment, auditory or vestibular problems, or neuromuscular dysfunction.

Clinical Use of Inhaled Tobramycin

One disease state in which aerosolized antibiotics have been used more consistently for pulmonary infections is cystic fibrosis. Patients with **cystic fibrosis** are chronically infected with gram-negative organisms, such as *Pseudomonas aeruginosa,* and the gram-positive bacterium *Staphylococcus aureus,* as well as other microorganisms. In particular, chronic *Pseudomonas* infection leads to recurring acute respiratory infections. With the exception of the quinolone derivatives such as ciprofloxacin, antibiotics that are effective against *Pseudomonas* do not give sufficient lung levels to inhibit bacteria when taken orally. Antibiotics with poor oral bioavailability for lung tissue include the aminoglycosides, penicillin derivatives, and cephalosporins. Consequently, either the intravenous or inhaled aerosol route must be used.

Baran and colleagues administered 40 mg of gentamicin by aerosol to eight children with cystic fibrosis and found high levels of drug (>20 μg/ml) in the bronchial secretions of seven of the children.[50] Blood levels with the inhaled drug were low, supporting the case for minimal systemic toxicity by aerosol. Similar results with nebulized tobramycin (300 mg) were demonstrated by Le Conte and associates.[51] By contrast, intramuscular injection of 1.5 mg/kg gave low levels of less than 2 μg/ml in bronchial secretions and, in some cases, undetectable levels.[50]

Aerosol administration is attractive because of reduced cost potential and ease of use at home compared with intravenous therapy. Furthermore, fluoroquinolones such as ciprofloxacin or norfloxacin, which are active when taken orally, are not as suitable for prolonged maintenance or preventive therapy as the agents given by inhalation, because of the risk of drug-resistant strains of bacteria.[52] A report of the clinical trial establishing the safety and efficacy of inhaled tobramycin (TOBI) in managing *P. aeruginosa* in patients with cystic fibrosis was published by Ramsey and colleagues.[53] The use of TOBI is intended to manage chronic infection with *P. aeruginosa* in cystic fibrosis, as follows:

- Treat or prevent early colonization with *P. aeruginosa*
- Maintain present lung function or reduce the rate of deterioration

Efficacy with *Burkholderia cepacia* has not been demonstrated, using the inhaled route of administration.

Dosage and Administration

TOBI is recommended for those 6 years of age or older. The usual dosage is 300 mg twice daily, approximately 12 hours apart and not less than 6 hours apart, for 28 days consecutively, with the following 28 days off of the drug. This cycle is repeated on a maintenance basis. The drug is formulated as a nebulizer solution with 300 mg in a 5-ml ampoule. In clinical trials it was administered with the PARI LC Plus, with a DeVilbiss Pulmo-Aide compressor. Other nebulizer delivery systems must be tested to ensure adequate drug output and particle size.

Patients should be instructed not to mix dornase alfa or any other drug with tobramycin in the nebulizer. Tobramycin should be inhaled after other therapies

usual in cystic fibrosis, such as chest physiotherapy measures, and other inhaled medications including bronchodilators or dornase alfa.

The drug should be stored at refrigerated temperatures of 2 to 8° C (36 to 46° F). After removal from refrigeration or if refrigeration is not available, the pouches in which the drug is provided can be stored at room temperature less than 25° C for up to 28 days. Drug ampoules should not be exposed to intense light. The solution may darken with aging if not refrigerated, although this does not change the drug activity if the manufacturer's guidelines are followed.

Mode of Action

Tobramycin is a member of the aminoglycoside family of antibiotics, so named because of their structure, which consists of amino sugars with glycosidic linkages. This group of antibiotics is effective in treating gram-negative infections and has a bactericidal effect. Tobramycin binds irreversibly to the 30S subunit of bacterial ribosomes. This binding blocks protein synthesis in the bacteria and causes cellular death. Serum tobramycin levels are approximately 1 μg/ml 1 hour after inhalation in patients with normal renal function.

Side Effects

Side effects for both parenteral and inhaled administration of tobramycin are listed in Box 13-1. The adverse effects with *nebulized* delivery are based on the clinical trial of Ramsey and colleagues,[53] and on 2 years of experience after the approval of inhaled tobramycin.

Parenteral Administration

Adverse effects that can occur with *parenteral* administration of aminoglycosides are reviewed briefly because the presence of impaired renal function or other

---

Box 13-1	Side Effects With Aminoglycosides and Tobramycin

PARENTERAL ADMINISTRATION
- Ototoxicity (auditory and vestibular)
- Nephrotoxicity
- Neuromuscular blockade
- Hypomagnesemia
- Cross-allergenicity
- Fetal harm (deafness)

INHALED NEBULIZED TOBRAMYCIN
- Voice alteration
- Tinnitus
- Nonsignificant increase in bacterial resistance

conditions may increase the risk of these effects with inhaled administration.

Ototoxicity is associated with parenteral use of aminoglycosides. Ototoxicity is manifested as auditory (cochlear) damage with small loss of hearing at the higher frequencies, or vestibular dysfunction with vertigo, nausea, or nystagmus (involuntary movement of eyeball).

Nephrotoxicity is also possible with aminoglycosides, which are excreted as unchanged drug by glomerular filtration. Although toxicity risk increases with dose, it may occur even with conventional doses in prerenal azotemia or impaired renal function. Because excretion is by the renal system, impaired renal function can also increase risk of the other side effects noted.

Neuromuscular blockade is another side effect resulting from the potential curare-like effect of aminoglycosides on the neuromuscular junction. This can aggravate muscle weakness, can cause further worsening of neuromuscular disorders, or prolong and intensify neuromuscular blockade by curare-like paralyzing agents (see Chapter 18). *Hypomagnesemia* can occur in patients who have poor diet or whose diet is restricted.

Cross-allergenicity does exist among the aminoglycosides, and hypersensitivity to one agent in this group constitutes a contraindication to the use of other agents. The side effects cited are more likely with overdosage, poor renal function, and dehydration (resulting from higher renal concentrations with possible nephrotoxicity).

Fetal harm can occur with aminoglycosides, and these drugs can cross the placenta. Irreversible bilateral congenital deafness has been reported in children of mothers who received streptomycin.[36]

Side Effects With Nebulized Tobramycin

The only adverse experiences reported after the 6-month clinical trial of Ramsey and associates[53] were *tinnitus* and *voice alteration*. There was no hearing loss associated with nebulized use of tobramycin, or changes in serum creatinine indicative of renal toxicity. There was a modest decrease in susceptibility of *P. aeruginosa* to tobramycin in the treatment group but not the placebo group, in the study by Ramsey and colleagues. However, this was not associated with a lack of clinical response to inhaled therapy with tobramycin. Use of an alternating schedule of administration may reduce the risk of drug resistance. Ramsey and associates[53,54] noted that their rationale for intermittent administration of tobramycin was the observation

that "drug holidays" allow susceptible pathogens to repopulate the airway in patients with cystic fibrosis. Because tobramycin is delivered by inhalation, the airway concentration can be 100 times as high as systemic levels. Thresholds of pathogen susceptibility with parenteral administration do not apply well to direct inhalation doses.

Precautions in Use of Nebulized Tobramycin

- Inhaled tobramycin should be administered with caution to patients with preexisting renal, auditory, vestibular, or neuromuscular dysfunction.
- Admixture incompatibility exists between β-lactam antibiotics (penicillins and cephalosporins) and aminoglycosides when mixed directly together; tobramycin solution should not be mixed with antibiotics in this group, and in general mixing with other drugs is discouraged.
- Factors that could increase the risk of hearing damage with prolonged tobramycin use are renal impairment, concomitant dosage of parenteral aminoglycosides, dehydration, and concomitant use of ethacrynic acid, furosemide, or other ototoxic drugs.
- Nebulization of antibiotics during hospitalization should be performed under conditions of containment, as previously described for pentamidine and ribavirin, to prevent environmental saturation and development of resistant organisms in the hospital.
- Aminoglycosides can cause fetal harm if administered to pregnant women; exposure to ambient aerosol drug should be avoided by women who are pregnant or trying to become pregnant.
- *Local airway irritation* resulting in cough and bronchospasm with decreased ventilatory flow rates is a possibility with inhaled antibiotics and seems to be related to the osmolality of the solution.[55-58] Peak flow rates and chest auscultation should be used before and after treatments to evaluate airway changes. Pretreatment with a β agonist may be needed.
- *Allergies* in the patient, staff, or family should be considered, if exposure to the aerosolized drug is not controlled. The use of a nebulizing system with scavenging filter, one-way valves, and thumb control could reduce ambient contamination with the drug, as previously described.

Clinical Efficacy

The clinical efficacy of inhaled tobramycin by nebulization was demonstrated in randomized controlled study performed by Ramsey and colleagues.[53] In that study

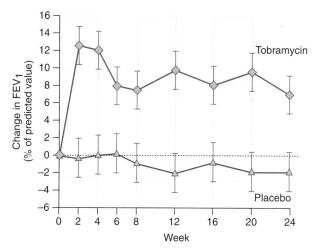

FIGURE 13-9 The mean change in FEV$_1$ from baseline for patients receiving inhaled tobramycin versus placebo. Bars represent 95% confidence intervals. (Modified from Ramsey BW, Pepe MS, Quan JM, Otto KL, Montgomery AB, Williams-Warren J, Vasiljev-KM, Borowitz D, Bowman CM, Marshall BC, Marshall S, Smith AL: Intermittent administration of inhaled tobramycin in patients with cystic fibrosis, *N Engl J Med* 340:23, 1999.)

comparing inhaled tobramycin with placebo in 521 patients with cystic fibrosis, 6 months of alternating inhaled tobramycin together with standard therapy for cystic fibrosis resulted in the following:

- Improved pulmonary function (Figure 13-9)
- Decreased density of *P. aeruginosa* in expectorated sputum
- Reduced need for intravenous antipseudomonal antibiotics and hospitalizations
- No development of significant bacterial resistance

Other studies, such as that by Gibson and colleagues, have produced similar results indicating that inhaled tobramycin is safe and effective in treating *P. aeruginosa* in cystic fibrosis patients.[59]

Because inhaled tobramycin is effective in cystic fibrosis patients, is it effective in other patients with *P. aeruginosa*? LoBue reports that studies to date have been small, or that the drug has not been used long term. Inhaled tobramycin cannot be recommended for treatment other than for cystic fibrosis patients with *P. aeruginosa*.[60]

General Considerations in Aerosolizing Antibiotics

Several points should be noted when nebulizing antibiotic drugs, especially if an injectable formulation is used, although this is *not* recommended for routine clinical use.

- Antibiotic solutions such as gentamicin are more viscous than bronchodilator solutions, and this may affect nebulizer performance. Compressors must be suitably powerful, and high-flow compressors are suggested. Flow rates of 10 to 12 L/min have also been suggested by Newman and associates[61,62] for suitably small particle sizes with antibiotic solutions.
- Environmental contamination in health care agencies and practitioner exposure to aerosolized drug can be reduced by using expiratory filters with one-way valves and a thumb control, as with aerosolized pentamidine.
- Physical incompatibility between some antibiotics has been noted by Hata and Fick.[63] Aminoglycosides such as gentamicin are chemically inactivated by carbenicillin and piperacillin when mixed together. These drugs should be given in separate nebulizer treatments, which has the disadvantage of requiring twice the patient treatment time. Any antibiotic combination, or other drug combinations, should at least be inspected for visible changes such as discoloration or precipitation and not used if this is observed. Ideally, drug mixtures for nebulization should be tested for chemical compatibility in addition to a visual macroinspection.

INHALED ZANAMIVIR

KEY POINT

Zanamivir is available for administration with a dry powder inhaler (DPI) to treat acute symptoms of influenza.

KEY POINT

The mode of action of zanamivir is to inhibit viral neuraminidase, causing viral aggregation to the cell and each other.

KEY POINT

Side effects include possible bronchospasm or lung deterioration, especially in preexisting airways disease and undertreatment or inappropriate treatment of nonviral bacterial respiratory infections.

Clinical Use of Inhaled Zanamivir (Relenza)

Zanamivir (Relenza) is an antiviral agent approved for use in the treatment of uncomplicated influenza illness in adults and children older than 5 years of age,

TABLE 13-2

Comparative Summary of Features for Antiviral Agents Used to Treat or Prevent Influenza

Drug	Brand Name	FDA Approval	Activity	Clinical Use	Route of Administration	Adult Dosage
Amantadine	Symmetrel	1966	Influenza A	Prophylaxis, acute treatment	Oral: tablet, syrup	200 mg/day
Rimantadine	Flumadine	1993	Influenza A	Prophylaxis, acute treatment	Oral: tablet, syrup	100 mg bid
Oseltamivir	Tamiflu	1999	Influenza A and B	Prophylaxis, acute treatment	Oral: capsule, liquid suspension	12 mg,* 75 mg bid, for 5 days
Zanamivir	Relenza	1999	Influenza A and B	Acute treatment	DPI: Diskhaler	10 mg (2 inhalations) bid, for 5 days

*Depends on weight of child; see manufacturer's dosing schedule.
DPI, Dry powder inhaler; *FDA,* U.S. Food and Drug Administration.

during the early onset (within the first 2 days) of infection. An oral antiinfluenza agent, oseltamivir phosphate (Tamiflu) is also available as a 75-mg capsule and oral liquid, 12 mg/ml. In addition, two older drugs, amantadine and rimantadine, have been used both for prophylaxis and treatment of acute symptoms of influenza. Table 13-2 summarizes information about these four agents, only one of which (zanamivir) is available by inhalation. Prophylactic vaccination against influenza, especially in high-risk patients with cardiovascular or respiratory disease, remains the unqualified recommendation, despite the availability of drugs to treat acute infection.

Dosage and Administration

Zanamivir is available in a DPI, the Diskhaler device, for oral inhalation. Each blister contains 5 mg of drug, giving a 5-mg per inhalation dose. There are four blisters in a Rotadisk, and the drug package contains five Rotadisks with one Diskhaler device. The dose for adults and children 5 years of age or older is 2 inhalations (two blisters, for a total of 10 mg) taken twice a day, approximately 12 hours apart, for 5 days. The complete drug package has the equivalent of 5 days of treatment, because each Rotadisk contains 1 day's dosage. Patients should finish the entire 5-day course of drug.

Mode of Action

The general mechanism of viral infection was described previously with ribavirin (see discussion of the nature of viral infection). Zanamivir represents a new class of antiviral agents, termed neuraminidase inhibitors, which act by binding to the viral enzyme neuraminidase and thus blocking the enzyme's action. The influenza virus has an envelope and a protein coat surrounding the viral RNA and targets the respiratory tract. Briefly, as illustrated in Figure 13-10, the virus envelope for both *influenza A* and *B* has two surface glycoproteins, *hemagglutinin (HA)* and *neuraminidase (NA)*. Hemagglutinin binds to a sugary molecule, *sialic acid (SA),* on the surface of a cell to be infected. This binding leads to fusion of virus and cell membranes and allows adsorption and penetration of the virus into the cell. However, when the newly minted viral particles bud from the cell and are ready to be released, the viral envelope acquires sialic acid from the cell, along with its own hemagglutinin and neuraminidase receptors. Without neuraminidase, the viral hemagglutinin would combine with the sialic acid again, "sticking" the viral particles to each other and to the cell surface, preventing further infection. Neuraminidase cleaves part of the sialic acid to prevent HA and SA combination, and prevents viral aggregation (clumping). Neuraminidase is essential for virus release from infected cells, prevents virus aggregation, and may decrease virus inactivation by respiratory mucus. Zanamivir is able to bind to neuraminidase and thereby block the enzyme action. By inhibiting neuraminidase, zanamivir inhibits viral particle separation and cellular release needed for systemic infection to proceed.[64]

Zanamivir is given by inhalation because the drug's binding ability also prevents good absorption when given orally. Inhalation also delivers the drug to the affected organ directly. Approximately 4 to 17% of an inhaled dose is systemically absorbed. Zanamivir has limited plasma protein binding (less than 10%) and is excreted unchanged in the renal system. It is apparently not metabolized to other products *in vivo*. Its serum half-life is 2.5 to 5.1 hours. Any unabsorbed drug is excreted in the feces.

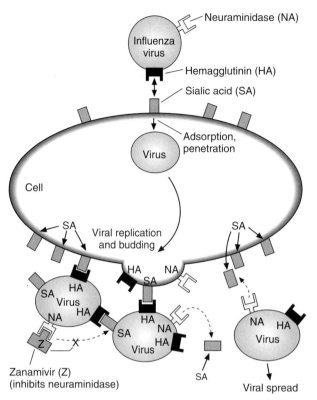

FIGURE 13-10 Simplified illustration of the mode of action by which inhaled zanamivir *(Z)* provides its antiviral effect in influenza viral infection. As a sialic acid *(SA)* analog, zanamivir binds to the enzyme neuraminidase *(NA)* and inhibits its usual inactivation of sialic acid. As a result, the viral hemagglutinin *(HA)* receptor continues to combine with both cell and viral sialic acid, causing viral aggregation and preventing viral release and spread.

Adverse Effects

The side effects discussed in the following sections have been noted during clinical trials and after release of zanamivir.

Bronchospasm and Deterioration of Lung Function

Patients with underlying respiratory disease such as asthma or chronic obstructive lung disease (COPD) may experience bronchospasm after inhaling zanamivir. Respiratory difficulty and wheezing have been reported in a patient with COPD[65] and an asthma patient inhaling zanamivir.[66] Neither patient appeared to have influenza at the time of treatment. A clinical trial of zanamivir by Cass and colleagues[67] in 11 patients with mild to moderate asthma with no influenza showed no symptoms of bronchospasm or airway responsiveness. Such data, however, do not establish the safety of zanamivir in asthmatics with influenza infection, which can cause mucosal damage and airway reactivity from the viral inflammation.[68] In ongoing treatment studies of patients with COPD or asthma who had influenza-like illness, more patients receiving zanamivir, compared with those receiving placebo, had a greater than 20% decline in forced expiratory volume in 1 second (FEV_1) or peak expiratory flow rate.[64] Zanamivir should be discontinued if bronchospasm or a decline in lung function occurs in any patient, and the managing physician should be consulted. The manufacturer recommends that any patient with underlying airway disease not take zanamivir.[36]

Undertreatment of Bacterial Infection

Bacterial respiratory infections can appear with influenza-like symptoms, and viral respiratory infections can progress to serious bacterial secondary infections.[69] Treatment with an antiviral agent such as zanamivir is not effective against bacterial infection and could possibly allow progression of such infection to serious illness such as pneumonia. Two deaths from bacterial infection in subjects taking zanamivir have been reported,[70] although the reasons have not been determined.[69] In a patient with COPD exacerbation who is treated inappropriately, risk of serious complications and the need for hospitalization can result.[69]

Allergic Reactions

As with any drug, patients should be monitored for allergic or allergic-like reactions with zanamivir.

Other Adverse Effects

Adverse reactions occurring in a small percentage of patients included gastrointestinal (diarrhea, nausea, vomiting) and respiratory (bronchitis; cough; sinusitis; ear, nose, and throat infections) effects, as well as dizziness and headaches. These reactions did not differ substantially from those with placebo and may have been caused by the same lactose vehicle used in active drug and the placebo.

Overdosage

There have been no reports of overdosage from use of zanamivir.

Clinical Efficacy and Safety

Clinical efficacy of zanamivir has been established in trials demonstrating that inhaled zanamivir can significantly shorten the duration of influenza symptoms.[68,71,72] With uncomplicated influenza-like illness, treatment with 10 mg of zanamivir twice daily resulted in approximately 1 day of shortening of the median time to improvement in symptoms compared with placebo.[68] The time to improvement in major symptoms was defined as no fever and no or mild headache, myalgia, cough, and sore throat. Among patients who were febrile and began treatment 30 hours or less after onset of symptoms, treatment with zanamivir resulted in a shortening of 3 days in the median time to alleviation of symptoms.[68] There are no data on efficacy when zanamivir is started after more than 2 days of symptoms of influenza.

There was no consistent difference in treatment effect between patients with influenza A versus influenza B. However, the clinical trials of zanamivir enrolled predominantly patients with influenza A (89 to 11% in one clinical trial). Patients with lower temperature and less severe symptoms in general derived less benefit from treatment with zanamivir.

Clinical trials of zanamivir were performed mainly with previously healthy subjects.[68,71,72] The manufacturer's literature states that safety and efficacy of zanamivir for treating influenza have not been demonstrated in patients with chronic pulmonary disease. In fact, zanamivir may carry risk for patients with COPD or asthma, as indicated in the discussion of side effects. Revised labeling for zanamivir adds a warning that zanamivir is *not generally recommended for patients with underlying airways disease* because of the risk of serious adverse effects.[68]

Zanamivir is not approved for prophylaxis to prevent influenza, nor does it reduce the risk of transmission of the virus to others. However, some data suggest a prophylactic benefit with zanamivir in influenza A and B in university and nursing home communities.[73] Results of a controlled study of inhaled zanamivir for both treatment and prevention of influenza in families in which one member developed influenza-like illness showed that zanamivir did reduce the rate of developing influenza in other family members. The proportion of families in which an initially healthy member developed influenza was 4% with zanamivir compared with 19% with placebo.[74] In the trial, treatment of the index cases with zanamivir in families reduced the median duration of symptoms from 7.5 to 5.0 days, a significant reduction. Oseltamivir (Tamiflu) was approved for prevention of influenza A and B in those 1 year of age or older who are in close contact with influenza. Adverse reactions were similar in both groups.[36]

The safety and efficacy of zanamivir have been tested in children. In a study by Hedrick and others, zanamivir was tested on children between 5 and 12 years of age. In the study of 471 children, 224 were given zanamivir, and the remaining children, the control group, were given placebo. Those children taking zanamivir reduced influenza symptoms 1.25 days before those in the placebo group. The zanamivir group returned to normal activities in less time and took less relief medications than placebo.[75]

A final issue with the use of zanamivir or other antiinfluenza agents as acute treatment is the lack of a clinically easy and inexpensive diagnostic tool to confirm the presence of influenza infection. Zanamivir is of no benefit in persons with infections other than influenza. In the clinical trial by Hayden and colleagues, 262 of 417 total patients (63%) with influenza-like illness had confirmed influenza virus infection.[68] As a result, symptoms alone can result in inappropriate use of antiinfluenza drugs, with attendant risks as outlined in the discussion of adverse effects. Inappropriate use contributes to increased cost.

In summary, the cost versus efficacy of zanamivir has been debated. There is modest reduction in symptoms for the cost of the drug; there is no readily available test to confirm the presence of influenza viral infection for use of the drug, resulting in possibly inappropriate use, and the drug carries increased risk for the patients who might benefit most—those with reactive airways disease.

RESPIRATORY CARE ASSESSMENT OF AEROSOLIZED ANTIINFECTIVE AGENTS

The following assessment applies to all of the aerosolized antiinfective agents discussed.

- Assess for the presence of disease indicating appropriate use of the agent:
  - Pentamidine: Risk of PCP
  - Ribavirin: Presence of severe RSV infection in infants or children at risk
  - Tobramycin: Chronic *P. aeruginosa* infection compromising lung function in cystic fibrosis
  - Zanamivir: Symptoms of acute influenza infection within first 2 days of onset
- Assess the correct configuration and function of aerosol equipment for ribavirin; instruct and verify correct use of aerosol delivery device for other agents.

- On initial aerosol treatment, assess respiratory rate and pattern, pulse, and breath sounds; evaluate for the presence of airway irritation resulting in wheezing and bronchospasm.

For pentamidine:

- Monitor for coughing and bronchospasm, and if present provide a short-acting β agonist or an anticholinergic bronchodilator such as ipratropium with inhaled pentamidine.
- Monitor for occurrence rate of PCP, and rate of hospitalizations long term.
- Monitor for presence of side effects (shortness of breath, possible pneumothorax, conjunctivitis, rash, neutropenia, dysglycemia) or appearance of extrapulmonary *P. carinii* infection.

For ribavirin:

- Monitor signs of RSV infection severity for improvement, including vital signs, respiratory pattern and work of breathing (clinically), level of $F_{I_{O_2}}$ (fraction of inspired oxygen) needed, level of ventilatory support, arterial blood gases, body temperature, and other indicators of pulmonary gas exchange.
- Monitor patient for evidence of side effects such as deterioration in lung function, bronchospasm, occlusion of endotracheal tube if present, cardiovascular instability, skin irritation from the aerosol drug, and equipment malfunction caused by drug residue.

For tobramycin:

- Verify that patient understands that nebulized tobramycin should be given after other inhaled medications for cystic fibrosis.
- Check whether patient has renal, auditory, vestibular, or neuromuscular problems or is taking other aminoglycosides or ototoxic drugs. Consider whether tobramycin should be given to the patient, based on severity of preexisting or concomitant risk factors.
- Monitor lung function to note improvement in FEV_1.
- Assess rate of hospitalization before and after institution of inhaled tobramycin.
- Assess need for intravenous antipseudomonal therapy.
- Assess improvement in weight.
- Monitor for occurrence of side effects such as tinnitus or voice alteration; have patient rinse and expectorate after aerosol treatments.
- Evaluate for changes in hearing function or renal function during use of inhaled tobramycin.

For zanamivir:

- Assess improvement in influenza symptoms: fever reduction, less myalgia and headache, reduced coughing and sore throat, and less systemic fatigue.
- Monitor for airway irritation and symptoms of bronchospasm, especially during initial use of the dry powder aerosol. Provide a short-acting β agonist if needed or if patient is at risk for airway reactivity (COPD, asthma).

SELF-ASSESSMENT QUESTIONS

1. Identify the disease states for which each of these drugs is used when inhaled as an aerosol: pentamidine, ribavirin, tobramycin, zanamivir.
2. Briefly, what is the rationale for aerosolizing an antibiotic such as tobramycin in cystic fibrosis?
3. What is the brand name of aerosolized pentamidine?
4. What is the dose and frequency for aerosolized pentamidine?
5. What device is approved for aerosolization of pentamidine?
6. Identify the common airway effects with aerosolized pentamidine, and suggest a method for preventing or lessening these effects.
7. What is a major risk to the caregiver when aerosolizing pentamidine to a patient with AIDS?
8. What is the current Centers for Disease Control and Prevention (CDC) recommended prophylactic treatment for PCP in AIDS patients?
9. What is the brand name and dose for aerosol ribavirin?
10. What is the mode of action of ribavirin?
11. Identify two serious hazards when ribavirin is given to a patient undergoing mechanical ventilation.
12. How, in general, can you prevent environmental contamination when delivering ribavirin to an oxygen hood?
13. What is the recommended dosage for inhaled tobramycin?
14. What common side effects have been observed with aerosolized tobramycin?
15. Identify two potential hazards to family members with aerosolized tobramycin at home.
16. Give the brand name and dosage for zanamivir.
17. In one sentence, describe the mode of action of zanamivir.
18. What are common hazards in the use of inhaled zanamivir?
19. What factors cause debate over the use of zanamivir in treating influenza?

Answers to Self-Assessment Questions are found in Appendix A.

CLINICAL SCENARIO

Mr. P. is a 29-year-old adult male with cystic fibrosis. The history of his disease and its previous treatment are well known to his pulmonary physician. He has been admitted to the hospital with complaints of increasing cough, shortness of breath, and sputum production. He reports that his sputum is greenish. His recent history reveals that his last admission for exacerbation of cystic fibrosis was approximately 6 months ago. He has used albuterol by metered dose inhaler (MDI), with 2 puffs qid, and recently began to use salmeterol, 2 puffs bid. He maintains himself on a regular regimen of cystic fibrosis medications, including iron and vitamin supplements and pancrelipase (Pancrease). Approximately 3 weeks ago, he complained of increasing pulmonary secretions and noted a mild elevation of his temperature (99.1° F). At that time, his physician prescribed ciprofloxacin, 500 mg orally bid, and he completed a course of 14 days, ending 5 days ago.

He is alert, oriented, and in no acute distress at this time. His skin is warm and dry. His vital signs are as follows: blood pressure (BP), 106/66 mmHg; pulse (P), 88 beats/min and regular; respiratory rate (RR), 20 breaths/min; and temperature (T), 98.9° F. His respiratory pattern is normal, and there is no use of accessory muscles. Auscultation reveals scattered rales and wheezes bilaterally, both anteriorly and posteriorly. His cough is nonproductive during the examination.

Chest radiograph shows hyperexpanded lung fields, with linear fibrotic changes bilaterally over the lung fields. Cardiac silhouette shows mild right atrial hypertrophy. No consolidation or pleural effusion is seen. Complete blood count (CBC) results are as follows: hemoglobin, 13.2 g/dl; hematocrit, 38.6%; and white blood cell (WBC) count, $13.5 \times 10^3/mm^3$. Remaining blood values are within normal limits. Pulse oximetry measures 89% saturation on room air. His pulmonary function, measured approximately 2 months ago and available in his chart, shows the following:

	Observed	Predicted	Percent Predicted
Total lung capacity (TLC), L	7.66	6.67	115
Forced vital capacity (FVC), L	3.52	5.23	67
Forced expiratory volume in 1 s (FEV$_1$), L	1.41	3.51	40
Mean forced expiratory flow during middle half of FVC (FEF$_{25-75}$), L/s	0.49	2.93	17
Expiratory reserve volume (ERV), L	0.94	1.69	56
Residual volume (RV), L	4.0	1.54	260

A sputum culture is taken and sent to the laboratory. Mr. P. is admitted for acute exacerbation of his pulmonary symptoms.

What would you suggest as key elements of his respiratory care plan?

What is the risk of using ciprofloxacin as an antibiotic to treat his symptoms of infection?

His physician decides to institute a course of tobramycin rather than repeating the ciprofloxacin. Can this antibiotic be given orally as an effective antibacterial agent for Mr. P.'s respiratory infection?

Identify two alternative routes of administration for tobramycin, in this case.

Mr. P.'s physician orders intravenous tobramycin as well as by aerosol, 300 mg bid, and he asks you to make a detailed suggestion on administration by nebulizer. What would you suggest?

How would you evaluate (1) the aerosolized antibiotic therapy, and (2) the treatment plan for Mr. P.?

Answers to Clinical Scenario Questions are found in Appendix A.

References

1. Montgomery AB, Debs RJ, Luce JM, Corkery KJ, Turner J, Brunette EN, Lin ET, Hopewell PC: Aerosolized pentamidine as sole therapy for *Pneumocystis carinii* pneumonia in patients with acquired immunodeficiency syndrome, *Lancet* 2:480, 1987.
2. Montgomery AB, Debs RJ, Luce JM, Corkery KJ, Turner J, Brunette EN, Lin ET, Hopewell PC: Selective delivery of pentamidine to the lung by aerosol, *Am Rev Respir Dis* 137:477, 1988.
3. Leoung GS, Feigal DW Jr, Montgomery AB, Corkery K, Wardlaw L, Adams M, Busch D, Gordon S, Jacobson MA, Volberding PA, et al.: Aerosolized pentamidine for prophylaxis against *Pneumocystis carinii* pneumonia, *N Engl J Med* 323:769, 1990.
4. Levine SJ, White DA: *Pneumocystis carinii*, *Clin Chest Med* 9:395, 1988.
5. Stringer JR, Beard CB, Miller RF, Wakefield AE: A new name *(Pneumocystis jiroveci)* for pneumocystis from humans, *Emerg Infect Dis* 8:891, 2002.
6. Hughes WT: *Pneumocystis carinii* vs. *Pneumocystis jiroveci*: another misnomer [response to Stringer et al.], *Emerg Infect Dis* 9:276, 2003.
7. Gigliotti F: *Pneumocystis carinii*: has the name really changed? *Clin Infect Dis* 41:1752, 2005.
8. Corkery KJ, Luce JM, Montgomery AB: Aerosolized pentamidine for treatment and prophylaxis of

Pneumocystis carinii pneumonia: an update, *Respir Care* 33:676, 1988.

9. Vinciguerra C, Smaldone G: Treatment time and patient tolerance for pentamidine delivery by Respirgard II and AeroTech II, *Respir Care* 35:1037, 1990.

10. Smaldone GC, Perry RJ, Deutsch DG: Characteristics of nebulizers used in the treatment of AIDS-related *Pneumocystis carinii* pneumonia, *J Aerosol Med* 1:113, 1988.

11. Waskin H: Toxicology of antimicrobial aerosols: a review of aerosolized ribavirin and pentamidine, *Respir Care* 36:1026, 1991.

12. Mathewson HS: *Pneumocystis carinii* pneumonia: chemotherapy and prophylaxis, *Respir Care* 34:360, 1989.

13. Martinez CM, Romanelli A, Mullen MP, et al.: Spontaneous pneumothoraces in AIDS patients receiving aerosolized pentamidine [letter]. *Chest* 94:1317–18, 1988.

14. Hart CC: Aerosolized pentamidine and pancreatitis [letter], *Ann Intern Med* 111:691, 1989.

15. Davey RT Jr, Margolis D, Kleiner D, Deyton L, Travis W: Digital necrosis and disseminated *Pneumocystis carinii* infection after aerosolized pentamidine prophylaxis, *Ann Intern Med* 111:681, 1989.

16. Quieffin J, Hunter J, Schechter MT, Lawson L, Ruedy J, Pare P, Montaner JS: Aerosol pentamidine–induced bronchoconstriction: predictive factors and preventive therapy, *Chest* 100:624, 1991.

17. Fine JM, Gordon T, Sheppard D: The roles of pH and ionic species in sulfur dioxide and sulfite-induced bronchoconstriction, *Am Rev Respir Dis* 136:1122, 1987.

18. Corkery KJ, Montgomery AB, Montanti R, Fine JM: Airway effects of aerosolized pentamidine isethionate [abstract], *Am Rev Respir Dis* 141:A152, 1990.

19. Smaldone GC, Vinciguerra C, Marchese J: Detection of inhaled pentamidine in health care workers, *N Engl J Med* 325:891, 1991.

20. O'Riordan TG, Smaldone GC: Exposure of health care workers to aerosolized pentamidine, *Chest* 101:494, 1992.

21. Fallat RJ, Kandal K: Aerosol exhaust: escape of aerosolized medication into the patient and caregiver's environment, *Respir Care* 36:1008, 1991.

22. Chaisson RE, McAvinue S: Control of tuberculosis during aerosol therapy administration, *Respir Care* 36:1017, 1991.

23. Centers for Disease Control: Guidelines for preventing the transmission of tuberculosis in health-care settings, with special focus on HIV-related issues, *MMWR Recomm Rep* 39(RR-17):1, 1990.

24. American Respiratory Care Foundation: *Pentamidine aerosols and care giver safety*, Dallas, Tx, 1992, American Association for Respiratory Care.

25. Riley RL, Nardell EA: Clearing the air: the theory and application of ultraviolet air disinfection, *Am Rev Respir Dis* 139:1286, 1989.

26. Mofenson LM, Oleske J, Serchuck L, Van Dyke R, Wilfert C; CDC; National Institutes of Health: Infectious Diseases Society of America: Treating opportunistic infections among HIV-exposed and infected children: recommendations from CDC, the National Institutes of Health, and the Infectious Diseases Society of America, *MMWR Recomm Rep* 53(RR-14):1, 2004.

27. Benson CA, Kaplan JE, Masur H, Pau A, Holmes KK; CDC; National Institutes of Health, Infectious Diseases Society of America: Treating opportunistic infections among HIV-infected adults and adolescents, *MMWR Recomm Rep* 53(RR-15):1, 2004.

28. Reines ED, Gross PA: Antiviral agents, *Med Clin North Am* 72:691, 1988.

29. Hall CB, McBride JT, Walsh EE, Bell DM, Gala CL, Hildreth S, Ten Eyck LG, Hall WJ: Aerosolized ribavirin treatment of infants with respiratory syncytial viral infection: a randomized double-blind study, *N Engl J Med* 308:1443, 1983.

30. Hall CB, McBride JT, Gala CL, Hildreth SW, Schnabel KC: Ribavirin treatment of respiratory syncytial viral infection in infants with underlying cardiopulmonary disease, *JAMA* 254:3047, 1985.

31. American Academy of Pediatrics Committee on Infectious Diseases: Respiratory syncytial virus, In Pickering LK, editor: *Red book: 2003 report of the Committee on Infectious Diseases.* ed 26, Elk Grove Village, Ill, 2003, American Academy of Pediatrics.

32. Agency for Healthcare Research and Quality: Management of bronchiolitis in infants and children. Evidence report/technology assessment: number 69. AHRQ publication no. 03-E014. Rockville, Md, 2003, Agency for Healthcare Research and Quality. (Available at http://www.ahrq.gov/clinic/epcsums/broncsum. htm; accessed March 2007.)

33. Smith DW, Frankel LR, Mathers LH, Tang AT, Ariagno RL, Prober CG: A controlled trial of aerosolized ribavirin in infants receiving mechanical ventilation for severe respiratory syncytial virus infection, *N Engl J Med* 325:24, 1991.

34. Meert KL, Sarnaik AP, Gelmini MJ, Lieh-Lai MW: Aerosolized ribavirin in mechanically ventilated children with respiratory syncytial virus lower respiratory tract disease: a prospective, double-blind, randomized trial, *Crit Care Med* 22:566, 1994.

35. Demers RR, Parker J, Frankel LR, Smith DW: Administration of ribavirin to neonatal and pediatric patients during mechanical ventilation, *Respir Care* 31:1188, 1986.

36. *Drug Facts and Comparisons*, St. Louis, Mo, 2006, Facts and Comparisons, Wolters Kluwer Health.

37. Centers for Disease Control: Assessing exposures of health-care personnel to aerosols of ribavirin: California, *MMWR Morb Mortal Wkly Rep* 37:560, 1988.

38. Corkery K, Eckman D, Charney W: Environmental exposure of aerosolized ribavirin [abstract], *Respir Care* 34:1027, 1989.

39. Kacmarek RM: Ribavirin and pentamidine aerosols: caregiver beware! [editorial], *Respir Care* 35:1034, 1990.

40. American Academy of Pediatrics Committee on Infectious Diseases: Use of ribavirin in the treatment of respiratory syncytial virus infection, *Pediatrics* 92:501, 1993.

41. Cefaratt JL, Steinberg EA: An alternative method for delivery of ribavirin to nonventilated pediatric patients, *Respir Care* 37:877, 1992.

42. Kacmarek RM, Kratohvil J: Evaluation of a double-enclosure double-vacuum unit scavenging system for ribavirin administration, *Respir Care* 37:37, 1992.

43. Charney W, Corkery KJ, Kraemer R, Wugofski L: Engineering and administrative controls to contain aerosolized ribavirin: results of simulation and application to one patient, *Respir Care* 35:1042, 1990.

44. Groothuis JR, Simoes EA, Levin MJ, Hall CB, Long CE, Rodriguez WJ, Arrobio J, Meissner HC, Fulton DR, Welliver RC, *et al.* Respiratory Syncytial Virus Immune Globulin Study Group: Prophylactic administration of respiratory syncytial virus immune globulin to high-risk infants and young children, *N Engl J Med* 329:1524, 1993.

45. PREVENT Study Group: Reduction of respiratory syncytial virus hospitalization among premature infants with bronchopulmonary dysplasia using respiratory syncytial virus immune globulin prophylaxis, *Pediatrics* 99:93, 1997.

46. Breedveld FC: Therapeutic monoclonal antibodies, *Lancet* 355:735, 2000.

47. American Academy of Pediatrics Committee on Infectious Diseases and Committee on Fetus and Newborn: Revised indications for the use of palivizumab and respiratory syncytial virus immune globulin intravenous for the prevention of respiratory syncytial virus infections, *Pediatrics* 112:1442, 2003.

48. Impact-RSV Study Group: Palivizumab, a humanized respiratory syncytial virus monoclonal antibody, reduces hospitalization from respiratory syncytial virus infection in high-risk infants, *Pediatrics* 102:531, 1998.

49. Feltes TF, Cabalka AK, Meissner HC, Piazza FM, Carlin DA, Top FH Jr, Connor EM, Sondheimer HM, Cardiac Synagis Study Group: Palivizumab prophylaxis reduces hospitalizations due to respiratory syncytial virus in young children with hemodynamically significant congenital heart disease, *J Pediatr* 143:532, 2003.

50. Baran D, Dachy A, Klastersky J: Concentration of gentamicin in bronchial secretions of children with cystic fibrosis or tracheostomy, *Int J Clin Pharmacol Biopharm* 12:336, 1975.

51. Le Conte P, Potel G, Peltier P, Horeau D, Caillon J, Juvin ME, Kergueris MF, Bugnon D, Baron D: Lung distribution and pharmacokinetics of aerosolized tobramycin, *Am Rev Respir Dis* 147:1279, 1993.

52. Neu HC: Quinolones: a new class of antimicrobial agents with wide potential uses, *Med Clin North Am* 72:623, 1988.

53. Ramsey BW, Pepe MS, Quan JM, Otto KL, Montgomery AB, Williams-Warren J, Vasiljev KM, Borowitz D, Bowman CM, Marshall BC: *et al.*: Intermittent administration of inhaled tobramycin in patients with cystic fibrosis, *N Engl J Med* 340:23, 1999.

54. Smith AL, Ramsey B: Aerosol administration of antibiotics, *Respiration* 62(suppl 1):19, 1995.

55. Littlewood JM, Smye SW, Cunliffe H: Aerosol antibiotic treatment in cystic fibrosis, *Arch Dis Child* 68:788, 1993.

56. Dickie KJ, de Groot WJ: Ventilatory effects of aerosolized kanamycin and polymyxin, *Chest* 63:694, 1973.

57. Dally MB, Kurrle S, Breslin ABX: Ventilatory effects of aerosol gentamicin, *Thorax* 33:54, 1978.

58. Wilson FE: Acute respiratory failure secondary to polymyxin-B inhalation, *Chest* 79:237, 1981.

59. Gibson RL, Emerson J, McNamara S, Burns JL, Rosenfeld M, Yunker A, Hamblett N, Accurso F, Dovey M, Hiatt P, *et al.* Significant microbiological effect of inhaled tobramycin in young children with cystic fibrosis, *Am J Respir Crit Care Med* 167:841–849, 2003.

60. LoBue PA: Inhaled tobramycin not just for cystic fibrosis anymore?, *Chest* 127:1098, 2005.

61. Newman SP, Pellow PG, Clay MM, Clarke SW: Evaluation of jet nebulisers for use with gentamicin solution, *Thorax* 40:671, 1985.

62. Newman SP, Pellow PGD, Clarke SW: Choice of nebulisers and compressors for delivery of carbenicillin aerosol, *Eur J Respir Dis* 69:160, 1986.

63. Hata JS, Fick RB Jr: *Pseudomonas aeruginosa* and the airways disease of cystic fibrosis, *Clin Chest Med* 9:679, 1988.

64. Gubareva LV, Kaiser L, Hayden FG: Influenza virus neuraminidase inhibitors, *Lancet* 355:827, 2000.

65. Williamson JC, Pegram PS: Respiratory distress associated with zanamivir, *N Engl J Med* 342:661, 2000.

66. Winquist AG, Fukuda K, Bridges CB, Cox NJ, Centers for Disease Control and Prevention: Neuraminidase inhibitors for treatment of influenza A and B infections, *MMWR Recomm Rep* 1999 48(RR-14):1. Available at http://www.cdc.gov/mmwr/preview/mmwrhtml/rr4814a1.htm. (Accessed March 2007).

67. Cass LM, Gunawardena KA, Macmahon MM, Bye A: Pulmonary function and airway responsiveness in mild to moderate asthmatics given repeated inhaled doses of zanamivir, *Respir Med* 94:166, 2000.

68. Hayden FG, Osterhaus AD, Treanor JJ, Fleming DM, Aoki FY, Nicholson KG, Bohnen AM, Hirst HM, Keene O, Wightman K: Efficacy and safety of the neuraminidase inhibitor zanamivir in the treatment of influenza-virus infections, *N Engl J Med* 337:874, 1997.

69. U.S. Food and Drug Administration: Revised labeling for zanamivir, *JAMA* 284:1234, 2000.

70. Yamey G: Drug company issues warning about flu drug, *Brit Med J* 320:334, 2000.

71. O'Riordan TG: Inhaled antimicrobial therapy: from cystic fibrosis to the flu, *Respir Care* 45:836, 2000.

72. MIST (Management of Influenza in the Southern Hemisphere Trialists) Study Group: Randomised trial of efficacy and safety of inhaled zanamivir in treatment of influenza A and B virus infections, *Lancet* 352:1877, 1998.

73. Dunn CJ, Goa KL: Zanamivir: a review of its use in influenza, *Drugs* 58:761, 1999.

74. Hayden FG, Gubareva LV, Monto AS, Klein TC, Elliot MJ, Hammond JM, Sharp SJ, Ossi MJ; Zanamivir Family Study Group: Inhaled zanamivir for the prevention of influenza in families, *N Engl J Med* 343:1282, 2000.

75. Hedrick JA, Barzilai A, Behre U, Henderson FW, Hammond J, Reilly L, Keene O: Zanamivir for treatment of symptomatic influenza A and B infection in children five to twelve years of age: a randomized controlled trial, *Pediatr Infect Dis J* 19:410, 2000.

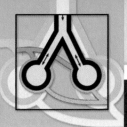

Chapter 14

Antimicrobial Agents

CHRISTOPHER A. SCHRIEVER, MANJUNATH P. PAI, SUSAN L. PENDLAND

CHAPTER OUTLINE

CHAPTER OBJECTIVES

After reading this chapter, the reader will be able to:

1. Define antibiotic
2. Describe the process involved in bacterial suscepti- bility testing
3. Discuss possible outcomes of antimicrobial combi- nations
4. List the various classes of the penicillins
5. List the various classes of the cephalosporins
6. Recognize similarities between members of the macrolides
7. Recognize similarities between members of the quinolones
8. List four mechanisms of action of antibacterials
9. List five commonly used antimycobacterials
10. Describe the commonly used azole antifungals and how they differ in spectrum of activity
11. Discuss similarities between members of the echi- nocandins
12. Describe the mechanism of action of the antiretro- virals

KEY TERMS AND DEFINITIONS

Antagonism — When the effect of the combination is lower than the effect expected from either agent alone (i.e., $1 + 1 < 1$)

Antibiotics — Natural compounds produced by microor- ganisms that either inhibit or kill other microorganisms

Antimicrobials — Include both natural and synthetic compounds that either inhibit or kill microorganisms

Synergy — When the combined effect of two antimicrobi- als is greater than their added effect (i.e., $1 + 1 > 2$)

The antimicrobial properties of fermented bev- erages, moldy soybean curd, and spices were first described by the Chinese more than 2500 years ago.[1] However, dissemination and acceptance of such knowledge did not take root until the early 1900s. The discovery of microscopic "little animals" by Anton van Leeuwenhoek paved the way for Robert Koch to validate that these "little animals," or germs, caused disease. Before Koch's work, almost no one believed that germs caused human disease. Despite the discovery of this important relationship, it would take numerous paradigm shifts and incredible luck before the discovery and usage of antimicrobials transpired.[2]

The sulfanilamides, azo compounds used in the German dye industry, were the first class of agents seren- dipitously discovered to have antibacterial activity. These compounds were initially unsuccessful and required mul- tiple modifications to reduce their unpleasant side effects. In 1928, Alexander Fleming discovered the first antibiotic, which he named *penicillin*. However, Fleming, like other sci- entists of the time, did not realize the utility of penicillin for systemic infections. It took a historic 1940 publication entitled "Penicillin as a Chemotherapeutic Agent," by Chain and colleagues,[3] to set into motion what we now refer to as the "golden age" of antimicrobial chemotherapy.

The realization that living organisms may pro- duce compounds that kill microbes is a relatively new concept. Since this realization, more than 30 classes of

compounds have been identified from natural sources or created synthetically to treat infections resulting from bacteria, fungi, protozoa, and viruses. Techniques to identify organisms and to determine their suscepti- bility have also evolved over the years and are vital to the choice of the proper antimicrobial agent. In addition, other factors such as the host, antimicrobial pharmaco- dynamics, antimicrobial combinations, and methods of monitoring therapy are important parameters that need consideration before selecting an antimicrobial agent. This chapter focuses on these basic principles of antimi- crobial therapy, provides a synopsis of the mechanism of action and adverse effects, and emphasizes the clini- cal use of the various antimicrobial classes for the treat- ment of respiratory illnesses.[1]

PRINCIPLES OF ANTIMICROBIAL THERAPY

Several factors require careful consideration before choosing a particular antimicrobial agent. Identification of the organism or organisms responsible for the infec- tion is the first step toward treatment. Once the organ- ism is isolated, antimicrobial susceptibility is determined according to standardized methods that can be repli- cated between laboratories. The susceptibility pattern of the organism narrows the choice of potential agents. Consideration must then be given to host factors such as age, pregnancy, organ function, and site of infection. In addition, drug factors such as available dosage forms, ease of administration, pharmacokinetics, potential adverse events, and economic considerations influence the choice of a specific agent.[4]

Identification of the Pathogen

The first step to identification of the organism is the collection of potentially infected material for culture. Specimens commonly collected for culture include blood, urine, sputum, cerebrospinal fluid, pleural fluid, synovial fluid, and peritoneal fluid. Several methods are then employed to rapidly identify the pathogens, using various chemical stains, immunological assays,

and microscopic examination. The simplest and most common preparation is the Gram stain. This stain designates bacteria into two major classes: gram positive (stain purple) or gram negative (stain pink). Bacteria stain differently depending on the structural components of their cell wall. These structural components also affect their susceptibility to antimicrobials. Other bacteria such as *Mycobacterium tuberculosis* require the use of an acid-fast stain to penetrate their waxlike cell walls. Mycobacteria require up to 6 weeks for growth on cultures, which makes the acid-fast stain vital for the rapid diagnosis of tuberculosis. Immunological methods such as the enzyme-linked immunosorbent assay (ELISA) and latex agglutination have also been developed to identify

TABLE 14-1

Common Pathogens and Treatment of Respiratory Infections in Adults*

Respiratory Infection	Common Pathogens	Potential Antibiotic Regimens
Sinusitis		
Acute (community acquired)	*Streptococcus pneumoniae, Haemophilus influenzae, Moraxella catarrhalis*	Amoxicillin–clavulanate or cefuroxime axetil or trimethoprim–sulfamethoxazole (TMP-SMX)
Acute (hospital acquired)	*Pseudomonas aeruginosa, Acinetobacter* spp., *Staphylococcus aureus*	Ceftazidime or a carbapenem and vancomycin
Chronic	*Bacteroides* spp., *Peptostreptococcus* spp., *Fusobacterium* spp.	Antibiotics are usually unsuccessful; sinus drainage may be required
Bronchitis		
Acute	*Mycoplasma pneumoniae, Chlamydia pneumoniae, Bordetella pertussis*	Antibiotics are usually not indicated
Exacerbation of chronic bronchitis	*S. pneumoniae, H. influenzae, M. catarrhalis*	Value of antibiotics is controversial; doxycycline may be considered
Pneumonia		
Community acquired	*S. pneumoniae, H. influenzae, M. catarrhalis, M. pneumoniae, C. pneumoniae, Legionella pneumophila*	Azithromycin or clarithromycin or levofloxacin or telithromycin or moxifloxacin or (cefuroxime and erythromycin) or gemifloxacin
Hospital acquired (nonneutropenic patient)	*S. pneumoniae, P. aeruginosa*	(Cefepime or a carbapenem or ceftazidime or piperacillin) + an aminoglycoside or ciprofloxacin
Hospital acquired (neutropenic patient)	As listed for nonneutropenic patients and fungi such as *Aspergillus* spp., *Pneumocystis carinii* (especially if HIV positive)	[(Cefepime or a carbapenem or ceftazidime or piperacillin) + an aminoglycoside or ciprofloxacin] ± vancomycin ± amphotericin B ± TMP-SMX
Aspiration suspected	*S. pneumoniae, Bacteroides fragilis, Peptostreptococcus* spp., *Fusobacterium* spp.	Clindamycin
Patient with cystic fibrosis	*S. aureus, P. aeruginosa, Burkholderia cepacia*	Aminoglycoside + piperacillin or ceftazidime, ciprofloxacin, TMP-SMX (*B. cepacia*)
Empyema	*Streptococcus milleri, B. fragilis,* Enterobacteriaceae, *Mycobacterium tuberculosis*	Third-generation cephalosporin + clindamycin[†]

*The potential treatments listed here are not listed in order of superiority. The choice of antimicrobials depends on the individual susceptibility pattern of the suspected organisms within the specific institution.
†See Table 14-7 for antimycobacterial regimens.
HIV, Human immunodeficiency virus.

pathogens such as viruses, molds, certain bacteria, and protozoa. In many clinical cases the exact identity of the infecting organism is not known. As a result, patients are empirically treated with an antimicrobial agent active against the organism or organisms that are most likely causing the infection. For example, 30 to 40% of patients with community-acquired pneumonia fail to expectorate sputum, which prevents identification of a specific pathogen. However, research has shown that the most common pathogens responsible for community-acquired pneumonia include *Streptococcus pneumoniae,* *Haemophilus influenzae,* and atypical (intracellular) organisms such as *Mycoplasma pneumoniae, Chlamydia pneumoniae,* and *Legionella pneumophila.* As a result, empiric therapy for community-acquired pneumonia involves antimicrobials active against this spectrum of organisms. Conversely, identification of an organism from culture material does not necessarily indicate an infection. For example, hospitalized patients often have growth of gram-negative bacilli (rods) in sputum samples. However, these organisms may only represent colonization and not hospital-acquired *(nosocomial)* pneumonia. Common pathogens and treatment of specific respiratory infections are listed in Table 14-1.[5]

Susceptibility Testing and Resistance

KEY POINT

The susceptibility of an organism to an antimicrobial is quantified as the *minimal inhibitory concentration (MIC)* and the *minimal bactericidal concentration (MBC).* The science of understanding the optimal effect of an antimicrobial as a function of its concentration to the MIC against the microorganism is known as *pharmacodynamics.*

Once an organism is isolated, susceptibility test results can usually be obtained within 24 hours. Several methods are commonly used to determine the susceptibility of isolated pathogens. The Kirby-Bauer disk diffusion test involves the use of antibiotic-impregnated disks that are placed on an agar plate heavily inoculated (10^5 colony-forming units [cfu]/ml) with the isolated bacteria. If the organism is susceptible to the antibiotic, then a clear zone of inhibition (no growth of the organism) develops around the disk. The degree of susceptibility or resistance of the organism depends on the diameter of this circular zone of inhibition; that is, a larger diameter indicates greater sensitivity. Another disk diffusion test is the E-test, or elliptical test. The E-test strip is placed on an agar plate heavily inoculated with the isolated organism. The

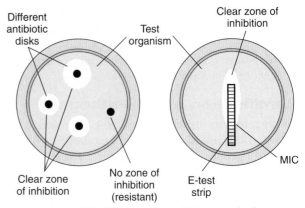

FIGURE 14-1 Disk diffusion test and E-test methods.

strip creates an antimicrobial gradient, which results in a clear elliptical zone of inhibition. This method allows the determination of the *minimal inhibitory concentration* (MIC). The MIC is defined as the least concentration of antimicrobial that prevents visible growth. The Kirby-Bauer and E-test methods are illustrated in Figure 14-1.

Other methods include inoculation of the organism into serial dilutions of an antimicrobial in agar or, more commonly, in broth culture media (Figure 14-2). Automated systems such as Vitek and MicroScan take advantage of broth microdilution methods to provide efficient and rapid susceptibility results. When susceptibility testing is performed in broth media, a small sample can be removed from the test tubes or microwells with no growth and used to inoculate agar plates. The lowest concentration of antimicrobial agent that prevents growth of the organism on the agar plate after a 24-hour incubation is termed the *minimal bactericidal concentration* (MBC). Drugs that inhibit the growth of bacteria but do not kill them are termed *bacteriostatic.* A *bactericidal* drug is one that kills the bacteria. Examples of bacteriostatic and bactericidal drugs are listed in Box 14-1.

Susceptibility testing is a critical part of antimicrobial therapy because the empiric regimen may fail when used to treat infections with resistant organisms. Microorganisms, like all living things, have genetic variability that affects their susceptibility to antimicrobials. Selective pressure from extensive clinical and agricultural use of antibiotics is thought to play a primary role in the emergence of resistant bacteria. Mechanisms of bacterial resistance include the production of enzymes that degrade or modify antibiotics, alteration of bacterial cell walls or membranes, up-regulation of antimicrobial efflux pumps, and alteration of the site of antimicrobial action. Examples of important emerging resistant bacteria are listed in Table 14-2.[4]

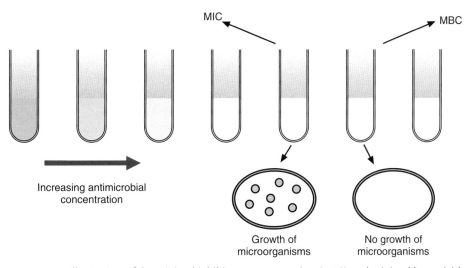

FIGURE 14-2 Illustration of the minimal inhibitory concentration (MIC) and minimal bactericidal concentration (MBC) by broth macrodilution.

Host Factors

KEY POINT

The outcome of antimicrobial therapy is dependent on *host factors, susceptibility/resistance* to the antimicrobial, and *pharmacodynamics.*

The safety and efficacy of an antimicrobial agent vary, based on the population of patients being treated.[5] For example, bone marrow transplant recipients with an active infection may not improve despite use of the ideal antimicrobial agent because of their impaired immune function. Similarly, other immunocompromised hosts such as patients with acquired immunodeficiency syndrome (AIDS), recipients of cancer chemotherapy or steroids, and solid organ transplant recipients are also at risk of failing to improve on antimicrobial therapy. Other factors such as the altered pharmacokinetics of an antimicrobial can affect response to therapy. For example, the absorption of certain antimicrobials such as itraconazole (an antifungal agent) is increased in the presence of gastric acid, others, such as penicillin G, are degraded in the presence of acid. The pH of the stomach varies with age; older patients tend to have achlorhydria and young children tend to have a higher gastric pH. As a result, these two populations may have enhanced absorption of penicillin and decreased absorption of itraconazole relative to the rest of the population.

The function of the liver and the kidney also changes with age. These two organs play a major role in the metabolism and elimination of drugs from the body.

Premature and newborn children have diminished renal function at birth. Drugs such as the β-lactams and aminoglycosides that are eliminated unchanged in the urine require less frequent dosing because of their reduced clearance. Similarly, renal function declines with age, necessitating dosage reductions in the elderly to prevent potential toxicities from antimicrobial accumulation.

Prevention of toxicity to the fetus or infant while treating a pregnant or nursing mother is also a crucial consideration. In general, most β-lactams and macrolides appear to be safe in pregnancy. The teratogenic potential of most other antimicrobials is simply unknown. However, the tetracyclines have been shown to affect fetal dentition and to adversely affect pregnant women. Antimicrobials are often eliminated in breast milk and so have the potential to adversely affect nursing infants. For example, premature babies are often jaundiced at birth because they are unable to efficiently conjugate and eliminate bilirubin. Even a small dose of sulfonamides ingested through breast milk from a treated mother can displace the albumin-bound bilirubin and predispose the child to kernicterus. Kernicterus is marked by a pattern of cerebral palsy with uncoordinated movements, deafness, disturbed vision, and speech difficulties resulting from deposition of bilirubin in the developing brain.

Antimicrobials concentrate in varying degrees within organ systems and can influence the outcome of therapy. Clindamycin achieves excellent bone concentrations and is very useful for treatment of osteomyelitis resulting from susceptible organisms. Similarly, drugs such as the aminoglycosides, most fluoroquinolones, and penicillins achieve very high concentrations in the

Box 14-1 — Examples of Bacteriostatic/Fungistatic and Bactericidal/Fungicidal Antimicrobials

CIDAL

- Aminoglycosides
- Carbapenems
- Cephalosporins
- Colistin
- Daptomycin
- Isoniazid
- Metronidazole
- Penicillins
- Polyenes
- Quinolones
- Rifampin, rifabutin
- Vancomycin*

Static

- Azoles
- Chloramphenicol
- Clindamycin
- Ketolides (telithromycin)
- Linezolid*
- Macrolides
- Nitrofurantoin
- Quinupristin/dalfopristin*
- Tetracyclines
- Tigecycline
- Trimethoprim–sulfamethoxazole

*Agents that are bactericidal against *Staphylococcus aureus* but bacteriostatic against *Enterococcus* species.

TABLE 14-2

Emerging Resistant Bacterial Pathogens

Class of Bacteria	Name
Gram positive	Methicillin-resistant *Staphylococcus aureus* (MRSA)
	Vancomycin–intermediate susceptible *Staphylococcus aureus* (VISA)
	Vancomycin-resistant *Staphylococcus aureus* (VRSA)
	Penicillin-resistant *Streptococcus pneumoniae*
	Vancomycin-resistant *Enterococcus* (VRE)
Gram negative	Multidrug-resistant (MDR) nonenteric bacilli (*Pseudomonas aeruginosa, Stenotrophomonas maltophilia, Acinetobacter* spp.)
	Third-generation cephalosporin-resistant *Enterobacter* and *Citrobacter* spp.
	Extended-spectrum β-lactamase (ESBL)-producing *Escherichia coli* and *Klebsiella* spp.
	Ampicillin-resistant *Haemophilus* spp.

urine and are useful for the treatment of urinary tract infections. Conversely, certain drugs, although active against the organism *in vitro,* cannot achieve adequate concentrations at the site of infection. For example, aminoglycosides cannot penetrate the blood–brain barrier to adequately treat meningitis in adults. The blood–brain barrier is the result of tight junctions between the epithelial cells of the capillary wall that prevent drugs from entering the central nervous system.[4]

Pharmacodynamics

Pharmacodynamics refers to the science of understanding the optimal effect of a drug as a function of its concentration and the *in vitro* activity (MIC) against an organism. The pharmacodynamic properties of an antimicrobial are measured *in vitro* by using time–kill studies. These studies measure the rate and extent of microorganism killing when exposed to varying concentrations of antimicrobials. If the microbial kill rate increases proportionally with drug concentration, the antimicrobial is said to have a *concentration-dependent* effect. If the microbial kill rate is influenced by the time of drug concentration above the MIC, the antimicrobial is defined as *time dependent* (or *concentration independent*). Another pharmacodynamic phenomenon exhibited by antimicrobials is known as the *postantibiotic effect* (PAE). The PAE refers to the sustained suppression of bacterial growth even after the concentration of the antibiotic drops below detectable levels. The length of the PAE varies by the type of organism and the drug. In general, time-dependent drugs, such as the β-lactams, have short PAEs; whereas concentration-dependent drugs, such as the aminoglycosides, metronidazole, and the quinolones, have longer PAEs. Agents with a short PAE should be dosed frequently, and longer dosing intervals should be used for antimicrobials having a long PAE. These pharmacodynamic properties have been demonstrated both *in vitro* and in numerous animal studies. Clinical trials validating these principles and practical guidelines to incorporate pharmacodynamics in clinical practice are still under study.[4]

Antimicrobial Combinations

Empiric regimens must often cover a broad spectrum of organisms, which occasionally requires the use of two or more classes of antimicrobials. Ideally, the regimen should be narrowed once the specific organism has been isolated and susceptibilities are determined. Certain infections are polymicrobial, and in certain settings the use of antimicrobial combinations is justified. When antimicrobials are used in combination, it is important to know whether these agents act synergistically or are antagonistic. **Synergy** is demonstrated *in vitro* when the combined effect of two antimicrobials is greater then their added effect (i.e., $1 + 1 > 2$). **Antagonism** occurs when the effect of the combined drug is lower than the effect expected from either agent alone (i.e., $1 + 1 < 1$). Clearly, antagonism may result in an unfavorable response and such drug combinations should be avoided. A classic example of antagonism was the use of tetracycline and penicillin in children with pneumococcal meningitis. The mortality associated with the use of combination therapy was three times higher than for patients treated with penicillin alone. Conversely, synergistic combinations have played a vital role in the treatment of resistant *Pseudomonas* infections in patients with cystic fibrosis. These patients have recurrent bouts of pseudomonal pneumonia and are often colonized with resistant species. Certain synergistic combinations of β-lactams and aminoglycosides have been shown to curb the development of resistance and to improve outcomes.[4]

Monitoring Response to Therapy

KEY POINT

Treatment failure may manifest as continued fever spikes, elevated white blood cell (WBC) count, repeated positive cultures, and nonresolution of symptoms.

Certain laboratory parameters can be monitored to assess the efficacy of an antimicrobial regimen, but ultimately the clinical assessment of the patient is the best measure of response to therapy. Treatment failure may manifest as continued fever spikes, elevated white blood cell (WBC) count, repeated positive cultures, nonresolution of symptoms, and so on. The reasons for failure can be multifactorial and require consideration of all the aforementioned factors. In addition, noncompliance with the treatment regimen can also play a significant role in treatment failure.

The use of antimicrobials can be associated with significant toxicities. The agent amphotericin B, which is used to treat fungal infections such as pulmonary aspergillosis, can cause significant renal dysfunction. Similarly, other agents can have adverse effects on the liver, gastrointestinal tract, neuromuscular system, hematological system, heart, and lungs. The incidence of these adverse events varies between agents and is often reversible. Careful monitoring of patients receiving antimicrobials can prevent serious and potentially life-threatening adverse events.[4]

ANTIBIOTICS

Numerous antibiotics have been discovered and developed over the last 50 years. A synopsis of the mechanism of action, clinical uses, and adverse reactions of each class is described in the following sections.

Penicillins

KEY POINT

The β-*lactams* are a large class of antibiotics that includes the *penicillins, cephalosporins, carbapenems,* and the *monobactams (aztreonam).*

The discovery of penicillin in 1928 by Alexander Fleming ultimately led to the creation of a broad class of antibiotics commonly referred to as the β-*lactams.* The β-lactam antibiotics include the penicillins, cephalosporins, monobactams, and carbapenems.[6] The main constituent of these antibiotics is the β-lactam ring structure. Chemical manipulation of β-lactam side chains led to the development of new agents with enhanced spectrums of antimicrobial activity compared with penicillin. Specific side-chain modifications of penicillin have resulted in a broad class that includes the natural penicillins, aminopenicillins, penicillinase-resistant penicillins, carboxypenicillins, and ureidopenicillins (Table 14-3). Penicillins have also been combined with β-lactamase inhibitors to overcome a common mechanism of bacterial resistance. In general, the penicillins are widely distributed throughout the body and are associated with relatively low levels of toxicity. Most penicillins are acid labile (destroyed in the stomach) and therefore are not readily absorbed orally. The majority of agents in this class are not metabolized, but are excreted unchanged in the urine. Therefore most penicillins require reductions in dosage for patients with renal dysfunction.[7]

Mechanism of Action

The penicillins exert their pharmacological activity by inhibiting cell wall synthesis. Penicillins bind to enzymes (penicillin-binding proteins) located within the cell wall, and prevent cross-linking of the peptidoglycan structure necessary for cell wall development. In addition, penicillins activate an endogenous autolytic system within bacteria, which subsequently leads to cell lysis and death. Penicillins are bactericidal, demonstrate time-dependent killing, and can act synergistically with aminoglycosides against some bacteria (i.e., *Pseudomonas aeruginosa* and enterococci).[8]

TABLE 14-3

Classification and Clinical Uses of Penicillins

β-Lactam Class (Generic Name)	Brand Name	Route	Common Uses (Microorganism)
Natural Penicillins			
Penicillin G (benzylpenicillin)	Pfizerpen	IM, IV	*Streptococcus pyogenes, Neisseria meningitidis,*
Penicillin G (procaine)	Wycillin	IM	*Bacillus anthracis* (anthrax), *Clostridium*
Penicillin G (benzathine)	Bicillin L-A	IM	*perfringens* (gangrene), *Pasteurella multocida,*
Penicillin V	Pen Vee K	PO	*Treponema pallidum* (syphilis)
Penicillinase-Resistant Penicillins			
Oxacillin	Prostaphlin	PO, IM, IV	Methicillin-sensitive *Staphylococcus aureus*
Nafcillin	Unipen	PO	(MSSA), methicillin-sensitive *Staphylococcus*
Dicloxacillin	Dynapen	PO	*epidermidis* (MSSE)
Aminopenicillins			
Ampicillin	Omnipen	PO, IM, IV	*Listeria monocytogenes, Proteus mirabilis, Eikenella*
Amoxicillin	Amoxil, Wymox	PO	*corrodens, Borrelia burgdorferi*
Carboxypenicillins			
Carbenicillin	Geopen	PO, IM, IV	*Pseudomonas aeruginosa,* Enterobacteriaceae
Ticarcillin	Ticar	IV, IM	
Ureidopenicillins			
Mezlocillin	Mezlin	IM, IV	*P. aeruginosa,* Enterobacteriaceae
Piperacillin	Pipracil	IM, IV	
Penicillin Plus β-Lactamase Inhibitors			
Amoxicillin–clavulanic acid	Augmentin	PO	Increased activity against β-lactamase-
Ampicillin–sulbactam	Unasyn	IM, IV	producing strains *S. aureus, Haemophilus influenzae, Moraxella catarrhalis, Proteus* spp., *Bacteroides* spp.
Ticarcillin–clavulanic acid	Timentin	IV	*P. aeruginosa,* Enterobacteriaceae
Piperacillin–tazobactam	Zosyn	IV	

IM, Intramuscular; *IV,* intravenous; *PO,* oral.

Clinical Uses

Natural Penicillins. Benzylpenicillin (penicillin G) is the parent compound of this class. This agent may be administered by the parenteral (IV) or intramuscular (IM) route. Penicillin G procaine is used for intramuscular dosing only and provides a less painful alternative when sustained serum concentrations are required. Phenoxymethyl penicillin (penicillin V) resists degradation by gastric acid and can be administered orally (PO). The natural penicillins are effective primarily against gram-positive bacteria and anaerobes. Penicillin G is the drug of choice for the treatment of primary and secondary syphilis *(Treponema pallidum),* along with pharyngitis caused by group A streptococci *(Streptococcus pyogenes).* Because of the increasing frequency of resistance in *Staphylococcus aureus, S. pneumoniae,* and *Neisseria gonorrhoeae,* penicillin G should no longer be considered the agent of choice for infections caused by these organisms.[7]

Penicillinase-resistant Penicillins. In an attempt to overcome the emergence of penicillinase (β-lactamase)–producing staphylococci, semisynthetic penicillinase-resistant antibiotics were developed. These agents are commonly referred to as *antistaphylococcal* agents because of their excellent activity against *S. aureus.* Methicillin was the first agent in this class of antibiotics, followed by oxacillin, nafcillin, cloxacillin, and dicloxacillin. Chemical modification of penicillin by the addition of an acyl side chain prevents hydrolysis of the agents in the presence of penicillinase. This class has activity against gram-positive cocci (staphylococci and streptococci) and is routinely used in skin and soft tissue infections. They are not effective in the treatment of infections caused by gram-negative organisms or anaerobes. Until the 1980s, these antibiotics were the mainstay of treatment against staphylococci. However, the emergence of methicillin-resistant staphylococci has greatly reduced the clinical effectiveness of these agents.[7]

Aminopenicillins. Ampicillin and amoxicillin are the primary antibiotics in this class. The aminopenicillins were the first penicillin class developed that were considered clinically active against some gram-negative bacteria *(Escherichia coli, H. influenzae).* Unlike penicillin, ampicillin and amoxicillin are both stable in gastric acid and therefore are suitable for oral administration. Both ampicillin and amoxicillin are frequently used in infections with susceptible organisms of the respiratory *(S. pneumoniae, H. influenzae)* and urinary tracts *(E. coli).*[7]

Carboxypenicillins. With the emergence of more resistant gram-negative bacilli, penicillins with increased gram-negative activity were needed. Carbenicillin was the first penicillin to have activity against *Pseudomonas aeruginosa.* It was also active against most members of the family Enterobacteriaceae, including *E. coli, Enterobacter, Proteus, Morganella,* and *Serratia.* Subsequent modification of carbenicillin resulted in ticarcillin, which has even greater *in vitro* activity against *P. aeruginosa* and members of the Enterobacteriaceae (including *Klebsiella).* Neither of these agents is considered to have appreciable activity against gram-positive organisms (staphylococci or streptococci). These agents are administered primarily in the intravenous form, because high serum concentrations cannot be achieved with the oral formulations.[7]

Ureidopenicillins. Even though carbenicillin and ticarcillin provided increased gram-negative coverage, antimicrobial agents with enhanced antipseudomonal activity were still needed. The ureidopenicillins were developed to fill this need. Piperacillin is a penicillin antibiotic with enhanced gram-negative activity (especially against *P. aeruginosa*) and with fewer adverse reactions than the carboxypenicillins. In addition, the ureidopenicillins also exhibit activity against streptococci and enterococci, as well as activity against many anaerobes. Piperacillin is the primary agent of this class and has been efficacious in the treatment of pneumonia, bacteremia, infections of the urinary tract, osteomyelitis, and soft tissue infections.[7]

β-Lactam and β-Lactamase Inhibitor Combinations. Certain bacteria have the ability to produce enzymes (β-lactamases) that destroy the activity of penicillins by disrupting the β-lactam structure. β-Lactamase inhibitors were developed to overcome this form of resistance. Consequently, combination β-lactam and β-lactamase inhibitors have a large spectrum of activity, making them particularly useful in polymicrobial infections. At present there are three β-lactamase inhibitors approved for combination with penicillins: clavulanic acid, sulbactam, and tazobactam. The β-lactamase inhibitors enhance the activity of β-lactams against β-lactamase–producing strains of *S. aureus, Moraxella catarrhalis, E. coli, H. influenzae, Klebsiella* species, and *Bacteroides* species.[7]

Adverse Reactions and Precautions for the Penicillins

The most common adverse reaction to penicillins is hypersensitivity. Approximately 3 to 10% of the population are allergic to penicillin. Reactions may vary in severity from a mild rash to life-threatening anaphylaxis. Patients allergic to a penicillin could be potentially allergic to all classes of β-lactams (cephalosporins, carbapenems). In addition to allergic reactions, hematological reactions such as thrombocytopenia and increased bleeding times have been reported. Hematological disturbances are thought to be higher with carboxypenicillins than with ureidopenicillins. Gastrointestinal disturbances (nausea, vomiting, and diarrhea) are more common with oral dosage forms of the penicillins, especially ampicillin. Interstitial nephritis occurred most commonly with methicillin (not commercially available) but may occur with other penicillins as well. Central nervous system toxicities (i.e., seizures) have been reported with the penicillins. Patients with an underlying seizure disorder and those with renal insufficiency are at greatest risk for developing this complication.[7]

Cephalosporins

KEY POINT

Cephalosporins have been loosely grouped into *"generations"* based on their spectrum of activities. At present there are four generations (classes) of cephalosporins.

The cephalosporins include a large group of antimicrobials that are structurally related to the penicillins. This class, discovered in the 1940s as a microbial by-product of the fungus *Cephalosporium acremonium,* is now widely used in clinical practice. Like the penicillins, this class exhibits bactericidal activity, is distributed throughout the body, and produces relatively few adverse effects. Cephalosporins are used for a variety of clinical indications and are available in both oral and intravenous formulations (Table 14-4). Agents from this class have been loosely grouped into "generations" based on their spectrum of activities. At present there are four generations (classes) of cephalosporins.

Mechanism of Action

Cephalosporins inhibit bacterial cell wall synthesis in a manner similar to the penicillins. The cephalosporins bind to the penicillin-binding proteins within the cell

TABLE 14-4

Classification and Clinical Uses of Cephalosporins

Cephalosporin (Generic Name)	Brand Name	Route	Common Uses (Microorganism)
First Generation			
Cefadroxil	Duricef	PO	MSSA, streptococci
Cephalexin	Keflex, Biocef	PO	
Cephradine	Velosef	IM, IV	
Cefazolin	Ancef, Kefzol	IM, IV	
Second Generation			
Cefaclor	Ceclor	PO	MSSA, MSSE, *Streptococcus*
Cefprozil	Cefzil	PO	*pneumoniae, Klebsiella* spp.,
Cefuroxime axetil	Ceftin	PO	*Escherichia coli, Proteus* spp.,
Cefuroxime	Zinacef, Kefurox	IM, IV	*Haemophilus influenzae*
Cefotetan	Cefotan	IM, IV	As above and *Bacteroides fragilis*
Cefoxitin	Mefoxin	IM, IV	
Third Generation			
Cefixime	Suprax	PO	Better activity than second-
Cefpodoxime proxetil	Vantin	PO	generation cephalosporins
Ceftibuten	Cedax	PO	against *Klebsiella, E. coli,*
Cefdinir	Omnicef	PO	*Proteus* spp., *H. influenzae,*
Cefotaxime	Claforan	IM, IV	*Enterobacter* spp.
Ceftriaxone	Rocephin	IM, IV	
Ceftizoxime	Cefizox	IM, IV	
Ceftazidime	Fortaz, Tazidime	IM, IV	As above and *P. aeruginosa*
Cefoperazone	Cefobid	IM, IV	
Fourth Generation			
Cefepime	Maxipime	IM, IV	MSSA, *S. pneumoniae, Klebsiella, E. coli, Proteus* spp., *H. influenzae, P. aeruginosa, Enterobacter* spp.

IM, Intramuscular; *IV,* intravenous; *MSSA,* methicillin-sensistive *Staphylococcus aureus; MSSE,* methicillin-sensitive *Staphylococcus epidermidis; PO,* oral.

wall and inhibit the cross-linking of peptidoglycan. This compromises the structural integrity of the bacterial cell wall, resulting in cell lysis (bactericidal).

Clinical Uses

As a class the cephalosporins are active against a wide variety of organisms. Because of their broad spectrum of activity and low level of toxicity, these agents are commonly used for a wide variety of infections. The spectrum of activity differs for each cephalosporin generation. Notably, all cephalosporins are ineffective against enterococci.[9]

First-generation Cephalosporins. The first-generation cephalosporin agents are very active against a wide variety of gram-positive organisms, including methicillin-sensitive *S. aureus* (MSSA) and streptococci. They have moderate activity against community-acquired gram-negative organisms such as *E. coli, Klebsiella pneumoniae, H. influenzae, M. catarrhalis,* and some *Proteus*

species. They are also considered effective against many oral anaerobes (such as *Peptostreptococcus*). Commonly used agents within this class are cephalexin, cefazolin, and cefadroxil. These agents are not active against *Bacteroides fragilis, P. aeruginosa,* and most members of the family Enterobacteriaceae. In general, first-generation cephalosporins are appropriate for treatment of infections of skin and soft tissue, uncomplicated community-acquired urinary tract infections, streptococcal pharyngitis, and surgical prophylaxis.

Second-generation Cephalosporins. Second-generation cephalosporins comprise two groups: the true cephalosporins and the synthetic cephamycins. Cefuroxime and cefaclor, are some of the more widely used true cephalosporins. In contrast to the first-generation cephalosporins, these agents display enhanced gram-negative activity while maintaining comparable gram-positive activity. This group provides improved activity against *H. influenzae, M. catarrhalis, Neisseria* *meningitidis, N. gonorrhoeae,* and some members of the Enterobacteriaceae. These agents are considered effective in treating the following: community-acquired pneumonia, otitis media, pharyngitis, skin and soft tissue infections, and uncomplicated urinary tract infections. The cephamycins, consisting of cefotetan and cefoxitin, have enhanced activity against gram-negative members of the Enterobacteriaceae, along with anaerobic activity against many *Bacteroides* species. They are not considered effective against gram-positive organisms such as staphylococci and streptococci. The cephamycins are also useful in the treatment of the following infections: intraabdominal, pelvic, and gynecological infections; decubitus ulcers; diabetic foot; and mixed aerobic–anaerobic soft tissue infections.

Third-generation Cephalosporins. Commonly used agents within the class of third-generation cephalosporins are cefixime, cefpodoxime, ceftibuten, cefoperazone, cefotaxime, ceftazidime, ceftriaxone, and ceftizoxime. These agents are active against most gram-negative organisms. However, only ceftazidime, and to a lesser extent cefoperazone, have activity against *P. aeruginosa.* The third-generation cephalosporins display excellent activity against *S. pneumoniae, S. pyogenes, H. influenzae, N. meningitidis, N. gonorrhoeae,* and *M. catarrhalis.* Although activity varies with individual agents, this group is not considered to have significant activity against anaerobes. Ceftriaxone, cefotaxime, and, to a lesser extent, ceftizoxime achieve clinically significant concentrations within the meninges, making them ideal agents for the treatment of meningitis. In addition, ceftriaxone has replaced penicillin as the agent of choice in treating all forms of gonococcal *(N. gonorrhoeae)* infection because of the increased prevalence of penicillinase (a β-lactamase)–producing strains. Third-generation cephalosporins are commonly used to treat nosocomial pneumonia, bacteremia, urinary tract infections, osteomyelitis, and soft tissue infections.

Fourth-generation Cephalosporins. The latest group, the fourth-generation cephalosporins, has extended gram-positive and gram-negative coverage. Cefepime is presently the only agent available in the United States. It is parentally administered and active against most gram-negative aerobic organisms, including *P. aeruginosa.* In addition, it has excellent activity against methicillin-sensitive *S. aureus* (MSSA), *Neisseria* species, *H. influenzae, S. pneumoniae,* and *S. pyogenes.* Cefepime has been used primarily for the treatment of patients with uncomplicated and complicated urinary tract infections and those with skin and soft tissue infections, and for the empiric treatment of patients with neutropenic fever, nosocomial pneumonia, and other serious bacterial infections.

Adverse Reactions and Precautions for the Cephalosporins

Similar to the penicillins, the cephalosporins as a group are well tolerated. Hypersensitivity reactions occur in 1 to 3% of patients, with cross-reactivity of cephalosporins in patients with penicillin allergy ranging between 5 and 15%. In general, patients with a penicillin allergy (limited to a rash) may be challenged with a cephalosporin. However, cephalosporin use is contraindicated in patients with a history of anaphylaxis to β-lactams.[10] The process of desensitization should be performed if no therapeutic alternative exists for the use of a cephalosporin. Oral cephalosporins have been associated with minor gastrointestinal complaints such as nausea, vomiting, and diarrhea. Hypoprothrombinemia has been reported, especially with those agents (cefotetan and cefoperazone) with a methylthiotetrazole (MTT) side chain. The MTT side chain may also induce a disulfiram-like reaction in patients who concurrently ingest alcohol (disulfiram inhibits the metabolism of alcohol). The symptoms of this uncomfortable reaction include flushing, nausea, thirst, palpitations, chest pain, vertigo, and in some cases even death. Most cephalosporins are eliminated through the kidneys and require dosage adjustment in the presence of renal insufficiency.[11]

Carbapenems

The carbapenems are the newest class of β-lactam antibiotics. At present, three carbapenems, imipenem–cilastatin, meropenem, and ertapenem, are available for use in the United States. Cilastatin is used to inhibit the metabolism of imipenem within the kidney to prolong the half-life of this agent. Carbapenems are broad-spectrum antibiotics, displaying activity against a wide variety of gram-positive, gram-negative, and anaerobic bacteria.[12]

Mechanism of Action

The mechanism of action of the carbapenems is similar to that of other β-lactam antibiotics. These agents demonstrate bactericidal activity.

Clinical Uses

Imipenem and meropenem are both active against *P. aeruginosa,* multidrug-resistant gram-negative bacilli, and most anaerobes. Ertapenem differs from the other carbapenems in that it possesses no activity against *P. aeruginosa.*[13] All three carbapenems have activity against gram-positive organisms such as MSSA and *Streptococcus* species, including pneumococci *(S. pneumoniae).* Imipenem and meropenem have been used clinically for empiric treatment of bacteremia and sepsis, community-acquired and nosocomial pneumonia, skin and skin structure infections, complicated urinary tract infections, intraabdominal infections, obstetrical and gynecological infections, osteomyelitis, and infections in patients with cancer and neutropenia. Because ertapenem is not effective against *P. aeruginosa,* it should not be used in the treatment of nosocomial pneumonia, neutropenic fever, or any other infection in which *P. aeruginosa* is a likely pathogen.[13] Because of their excellent *in vitro* activity and broad spectrum of coverage, these agents are often reserved to treat infections that are caused by bacteria resistant to most other agents.

Adverse Reactions and Precautions

Carbapenems are generally well tolerated, with a low incidence of adverse reactions. Because the carbapenems are structurally related to other β-lactam antibiotics, cross-reactivity may occur when used in patients with allergies to β-lactams. The occurrence of seizures has been reported with the carbapenems, more frequently with imipenem than with meropenem or ertapenem. They are most commonly seen in patients with decreased renal function and those with an underlying seizure disorder. Dosage adjustment is necessary in the presence of renal insufficiency to prevent accumulation of the drug and to reduce the potential for seizures.

Monobactams (Aztreonam)

Aztreonam is a synthetic monocyclic β-lactam antibiotic. This is the only commercially available agent belonging to the class of antibiotics known as the *monobactams.*[14]

Mechanism of Action

Aztreonam has a mechanism of action similar to that of other β-lactam antibiotics and demonstrates bactericidal activity.

Clinical Uses

Aztreonam is active only against gram-negative aerobic bacilli (most Enterobacteriaceae and *P. aeruginosa*). It is not effective against gram-positive and anaerobic bacteria. The strict gram-negative spectrum of aztreonam limits its use as a single agent. It has been used for the treatment of serious urinary tract infections and bacteremia. Aztreonam has more extensive use in combination therapy for treatment of intraabdominal infections, spontaneous bacterial peritonitis, gram-negative osteomyelitis, and hospital-acquired pneumonia and in patients with neutropenic fever.

TABLE 14-5

Clinical Uses of Aminoglycosides

Aminoglycoside Generic Name (Trade Name)	Most Common Clinical Uses
Streptomycin	Brucellosis, tuberculosis, endocarditis caused by gentamicin-resistant enterococci
Gentamicin (Garamycin) Tobramycin (Nebcin)	Nosocomial Enterobacteriaceae and *Pseudomonas aeruginosa* infections, tularemia, brucellosis; endocarditis caused by susceptibleenterococci or viridans streptococci, *Staphylococcus aureus*, *Corynebacterium* spp., penicillin-susceptible *Streptococcus*
Amikacin (Amikin)	Similar to gentamicin and tobramycin but useful against *Acinetobacter* spp., *Nocardia* spp., *Mycobacterium avium-intracellulare, M. chelonae, M. fortium*
Neomycin (Neosporin)	Prevention of wound infections, preoperative gastrointestinal sterilization
Netilmicin (Netromycin)	Similar to gentamicin and tobramycin
Paromomycin (Humatin)	Intestinal amebiasis, tapeworm infestation, *Cryptosporidium* diarrhea

Adverse Reactions and Precautions

Aztreonam is well tolerated and is thought to have little to no cross-reactivity to β-lactams. However, rare cases of rashes and even anaphylactic reactions have been reported when aztreonam was used in patients with a β-lactam allergy.

Aminoglycosides

Streptomycin was discovered in 1943 and was the first chemotherapeutic agent available to treat tuberculosis. Numerous other aminoglycosides have been developed since and include gentamicin, tobramycin, netilmicin, and amikacin. These agents are used for gram-negative infections, including those caused by *P. aeru2giosa.* These antimicrobials have poor gastrointestinal absorption and so require parenteral administration.[15] Table 14-5 lists aminoglycosides and their clinical uses.

Mechanism of Action

Aminoglycosides bind irreversibly to the 30S bacterial ribosome and inhibit the translation of ribonucleic acid (RNA) into proteins. Aminoglycosides also competitively displace cations that link lipopolysaccharides in the outer cell wall of gram-negative bacteria. This destabilization of the cell wall results in increased cell permeability and lysis. Aminoglycosides are bactericidal agents and demonstrate concentration-dependent killing. They are often synergistic when used in combination with β-lactam antibiotics.[16]

Clinical Uses

Gentamicin and tobramycin have been used for nosocomial gram-negative infections such as ventilator-associated pneumonias. However, aminoglycosides do not achieve high concentrations in bronchial secretions when administered systemically. This is thought to be particularly problematic for patients infected with resistant gram-negative organisms. As a result, aminoglycosides (particularly tobramycin) have been administered by inhalation to control *P. aeruginosa* infections in patients with cystic fibrosis (see Chapter 13, Aerosolized Antiinfective Agents). Amikacin is currently more expensive and is generally reserved for organisms resistant to the other aminoglycosides. Aminoglycosides are used synergistically with β-lactams when treating endocarditis caused by *Streptococcus* species and *Enterococcus* species. Aminoglycosides are also used extensively to treat intraabdominal infections. Streptomycin is used in combination with other antitubercular antimicrobials, especially for multidrug-resistant (MDR) tuberculosis.

Adverse Reactions and Precautions

KEY POINT

Primary toxicities associated with the use of aminoglycosides are nephrotoxicity and ototoxicity.

The primary toxicities associated with the use of aminoglycosides are nephrotoxicity and ototoxicity. Nephrotoxicity usually develops after at least 5 to 7 days of therapy and occurs more commonly in patients with hypotension, liver disease, advanced age, and coadministration of other nephrotoxic agents. Ototoxicity (both cochleotoxicity and vestibular toxicity) may be irreversible because significant damage must occur before it can be detected. The most common symptoms associated with the development of cochleotoxicity include tinnitus (ringing in the ears); vestibular toxicity manifests as dizziness and nausea. Another serious but rare toxicity is neuromuscular blockade associated with peritoneal irrigation and rapid high-dose aminoglycoside use. Underlying conditions such as myasthenia gravis or concomitant use of neuromuscular blockers may potentiate this side effect, requiring supportive measures such as intubation and possible ventilation support.[17]

Tetracyclines

KEY POINT

Tetracyclines are broad-spectrum antibiotics with activity against gram-positive and gram-negative microorganisms, as well as many rickettsiae, chlamydiae, mycoplasmas, spirochetes, protozoa, and mycobacteria.

The tetracyclines are broad-spectrum antibiotics with activity against gram-positive and gram-negative microorganisms, as well as many rickettsiae, chlamydiae, mycoplasmas, spirochetes, protozoa, and mycobacteria. The most commonly used agent in this class is doxycycline because it can be administered twice daily and is relatively inexpensive. Other available tetracyclines include demeclocycline, minocycline, oxytetracycline, and tetracycline. The agents are available in oral and parenteral formulations.[18]

Mechanism of Action

Tetracyclines bind reversibly on the 30S ribosome and inhibit the attachment of transfer RNA to an acceptor site on the messenger RNA–ribosome complex. This inhibition blocks protein synthesis and results in a bacteriostatic effect.

Clinical Uses

Clinical conditions in which tetracyclines are used include respiratory tract infections and other systemic infections. Acute exacerbation of chronic bronchitis and community-acquired pneumonia caused by typical (*S. pneumoniae, H. influenzae*) and atypical (*C. pneumoniae, M. pneumoniae, L. pneumophila*) bacteria can be treated with a tetracycline. Tetracyclines are also useful for the treatment of *Chlamydia trachomatis* (sexually transmitted disease), Rocky Mountain spotted fever, Q fever, typhus, brucellosis, Lyme disease, ehrlichiosis, relapsing fever, and cholera. Tetracyclines tend to concentrate in the skin and are useful for the treatment of acne. In addition, tetracyclines have also been used as sclerosing agents for the treatment of malignant and refractory pleural effusions.

Adverse Reactions and Precautions

Gastrointestinal symptoms such as nausea, vomiting, and diarrhea are the most common side effects associated with the tetracyclines. Tetracyclines bind to growing bone and can temporarily inhibit their growth. The latter side effect makes its use a contraindication during pregnancy, when breast-feeding, and in children less than 8 years of age. Tetracyclines bind to divalent and trivalent cations (calcium, magnesium, aluminum, and iron), which decrease their gastrointestinal absorption when given with antacids, iron supplements, and dairy products. Avoiding the coadministration of tetracyclines with these agents by 1 to 2 hours can prevent this interaction. The prolonged use of minocycline has been associated with vestibular side effects, a blue-black oral pigmentation, and lupus-like symptoms.

Tigecycline

Tigecycline, a member of the glycylcycline antibiotics, is similar in structure to the tetracycline antibiotics. Because of substitution of a central four-ring carbocyclic nucleus, tigecycline has a greater spectrum of activity than tetracyclines. Tigecycline is active against most gram-positive bacteria including *S. pneumoniae*, vancomycin-susceptible and -resistant enterococci, coagulase-negative staphylococci, and methicillin-susceptible and -resistant *S. aureus*. Tigecycline also has activity against most gram-negative bacteria including *H. influenzae, M. catarrhalis*, most members of the Enterobacteriaceae family (including extended-spectrum β-lactamase [ESBL]-producing organisms) and *Acinetobacter* species. It is also active against many anaerobic bacteria. However, tigecycline is not active against *P. aeruginosa* and *Proteus* species.[19]

Mechanism of Action

Tigecycline displays a similar mechanism to tetracycline antibiotics by inhibiting bacterial protein synthesis at the 30S ribosome. Because of the large, bulky constituent at ring position 9, tigecycline maintains antimicrobial activity against organisms that carry resistance to tetracycline antibiotics. Tigecycline is generally considered to be bacteriostatic against most organisms, except *S. pneumoniae*, to which it is bactericidal.

Clinical Uses

Tigecycline is currently approved for the treatment of complicated skin and skin structure infections, and complicated intraabdominal infections. Tigecycline is available only as an intravenous formulation and is typically dosed at 100 mg initially, followed by 50 mg every 12 hours thereafter.

Adverse Reactions and Precautions

During clinical trials the most common side effects observed with the use of tigecycline were gastrointestinal and included nausea, vomiting, diarrhea, and abdominal pain. Other frequently reported adverse effects were headache, thrombocytopenia, and elevations of liver enzymes. Because tigecycline is a structural derivative of minocycline, it is appropriate to monitor for side effects associated with other tetracycline antibiotics such as phototoxicity and dental disorders.[20]. Tigecycline should not be used in individuals with hypersensitivity reactions to tetracycline antibiotics.

Macrolides

> **KEY POINT**
>
> *Macrolides* exhibit activity against gram-positive bacteria (streptococci, methicillin-sensitive *Staphylococcus aureus* [MSSA]), gram-negative bacteria *(Haemophilus influenzae and Moraxella catarrhalis),* and atypical bacteria (mycoplasmas, rickettsiae, *Legionella, and Chlamydia).*

Erythromycin was introduced in 1952 and was the first agent of this class to be used for infections with atypical organisms and for infections in patients intolerant to penicillin G. Early work with erythromycin involved production of various salt derivatives to improve its gastrointestinal tolerability and absorption. In the last decade, clarithromycin and azithromycin (an azalide) have been introduced. Macrolides exhibit activity against gram-positive bacteria (streptococci, MSSA), gram-negative bacteria *(H. influenzae, M. catarrhalis),* and atypical bacteria (mycoplasmas, rickettsiae, *Legionella,* and *Chlamydia).* In addition, clarithromycin and azithromycin are active against *Mycobacterium avium.*[21]

Mechanism of Action

Macrolides inhibit protein synthesis by reversibly binding to the 50S ribosomal subunit and induce the dissociation of transfer RNA from the ribosome during the elongation phase. As a result, bacterial growth is inhibited (bacteriostatic).

Clinical Uses

Erythromycin is considered the drug of choice for the treatment of pneumonia caused by the atypical pathogens *C. pneumoniae, M. pneumoniae,* and *L. pneumophila.*

TABLE 14-6

Classification and Clinical Uses of Quinolones

Quinolones (Generic Name)	Brand Name	Route	Common Uses (Microorganism)
Ciprofloxacin	Cipro	IV, PO	*Pseudomonas aeruginosa*, Enterobacteriaceae, *Neisseria gonorrhoeae, Mycoplasma pneumoniae, Legionella pneumophila*
Ofloxacin	Oflox	IV, PO	*P. aeruginosa*, Enterobacteriaceae, *N. gonorrhoeae, M. pneumoniae, Chlamydia pneumoniae, L. pneumophila*
Lomefloxacin	Maxaquin	PO	Enterobacteriaceae, *N. gonorrhoeae, C. pneumoniae*
Levofloxacin	Levaquin	IV, PO	*P. aeruginosa*, Enterobacteriaceae, *S. pyogenes*, methicillin-susceptible *S. aureus* (MSSA), *Haemophilus influenzae, Moraxella catarrhalis*, penicillin-resistant *Streptococcus pneumoniae, M. pneumoniae, C. pneumoniae, L. pneumophila*
Moxifloxacin	Avelox	PO	Enterobacteriaceae, *S. pyogenes*, MSSA, *H. influenzae, M. catarrhalis*, penicillin-resistant *S. pneumoniae, M. pneumoniae, C. pneumoniae, L. pneumophila*
Gemifloxacin	Factive	PO	*H. influenzae, C. pneumoniae, Klebsiella pneumoniae, S. pneumoniae, M. catarrhalis, M. pneumoniae, L. pneumophila, S. pyogenes, S. aureus, Klebsiella oxytoca*
Trovafloxacin	Trovan	IV, PO	Enterobacteriaceae, *S. pyogenes*, MSSA, *H. influenzae, M. catarrhalis*, penicillin-resistant *S. pneumoniae, M. pneumoniae, C. pneumoniae, L. pneumophila, Bacteroides fragilis*
Norfloxacin	Noroxin	PO	Enterobacteriaceae (only used in treatment of urinary tract infections)
Enoxacin	Penetrex	PO	Enterobacteriaceae, *N. gonorrhoeae* (used only in treatment of urinary tract infections, including uncomplicated urethral or cervical gonorrhea)
Cinoxacin	Cinobac	PO	Enterobacteriaceae (only used in treatment of urinary tract infections)

IV, Intravenous; *PO*, oral.

Erythromycin is considered a safer alternative to the tetracyclines for the treatment of chlamydial *(C. trachomatis)* pelvic infections in pregnant women. Clarithromycin is the preferred agent in combination with ethambutol or rifabutin for the treatment of *M. avium* complex (MAC) in patients with human immunodeficiency virus (HIV) infection. Azithromycin has a superior pharmacokinetic profile compared with the latter agents by maintaining prolonged intracellular concentrations (long half-life). As a result, azithromycin can be administered once weekly for the prophylaxis of MAC in patients with HIV, compared with clarithromycin, which must be administered twice daily. Similarly, a 5-day regimen of azithromycin has been found to be as effective as a 10-day regimen of erythromycin for the treatment of community-acquired pneumonia.

Adverse Reactions and Precautions

Clarithromycin and azithromycin are generally better tolerated than erythromycin. The most common adverse reactions of macrolides include gastrointestinal complaints such as nausea, vomiting, abdominal cramps, and diarrhea (up to 30% of patients taking erythromycin). The use of intravenous erythromycin is associated with thrombophlebitis. Ventricular tachycardia and Q–T prolongation have been reported with the use of the macrolides. Erythromycin and clarithromycin are potent inhibitors of the hepatic drug metabolism system known as the *cytochrome P450 system (CYP)*. As a result, erythromycin and clarithromycin can increase the systemic concentrations of drugs metabolized through CYP. For drugs with narrow therapeutic indices such as theophylline, warfarin, and triazolam, this interaction can lead to potential life-threatening complications. Abnormalities in liver function, tinnitus, dizziness, and reversible hearing loss have also been associated with the use of macrolides.[22]

Telithromycin

Telithromycin is the first member of the ketolide group of antimicrobials, which are structurally related to the macrolide antibiotics. It has good antimicrobial activity against respiratory pathogens typically responsible for community-acquired pneumonia such as *S. pneumoniae, H. influenzae, M. pneumoniae, C. pneumoniae,*

L. pneumophila, and *M. catarrhalis*. Telithromycin has improved acid stability compared with erythromycin and therefore has good oral absorption.[23]

Mechanism of Action

Similar to the macrolides, telithromycin also inhibits bacterial protein synthesis by interacting with the peptidyltransferase site of the 50S ribosome. In addition, it has also been shown to inhibit the formation of both the 50S subunit, and at higher concentrations the 30S unit, of ribosomes.

Clinical Uses

At present, telithromycin is indicated for the treatment of acute exacerbation of chronic bronchitis (AECB), acute bacterial sinusitis, and community-acquired pneumonia (CAP). For AECB and acute bacterial sinusitis, a 5-day course of telithromycin was shown to have comparable efficacy to comparator agents (amoxicillin–clavulanate, cefuroxime, or clarithromycin). Longer courses of telithromycin, 7-10 days, are required for treatment of CAP. It is not currently approved for the treatment of streptococcal pharyngitis; however, it has been shown to be equally as effective as clarithromycin or penicillin V. It appears that telithromycin may serve as an alternative agent for patients at risk of infection with penicillin-resistant or macrolide-resistant *S. pneumoniae*.[23] It is also an alternative treatment in patients with penicillin allergies. Telithromycin is available only in oral formulation and is typically dosed as 800 mg daily.

Adverse Reactions and Precautions

Telithromycin is generally well tolerated, with most side effects being mild to moderate. The most commonly occurring adverse effects were gastrointestinal, with nausea and diarrhea occurring in 7% to 13% of patients. Visual disturbances (blurred vision, difficulty focusing, and diplopia) were reported in slightly higher than 1% of patients. These effects often occurred after the first or second dose and resolved on discontinuation of the medication. Telithromycin has the potential to prolong the Q–T interval; however, clinical trials to date have not reported a significant incidence. Of note, telithromycin is a competitive inhibitor of certain cytochrome P450 enzymes including 3A4 and 2D6. Therefore, care should be used when administering other medications metabolized through these pathways.

Quinolones (Fluoroquinolones)

The fluoroquinolones (Table 14-6) are a semisynthetic group of antimicrobials structurally related to nalidixic acid (quinolone), one of the by-products of chloroquine synthesis. They are widely distributed into most body fluids and tissues (achieving high respiratory tract concentrations). The quinolones are eliminated primarily through the kidneys and achieve high concentrations in the urine. Agents from this class have variable activity against gram-negative gram-positive bacteria, anaerobes, atypical bacteria, and mycobacteria.[24] Ciprofloxacin, levofloxacin, gatifloxacin, and moxifloxacin are the fluoroquinolones most commonly used in the United States. However, gatifloxacin has recently been removed from the market because of the high incidence of diabetes and other blood sugar irregularities.

Mechanism of Action

> **KEY POINT**
>
> Quinolones exert their antibacterial effect through inhibition of DNA synthesis and are considered bactericidal agents, demonstrating concentration-dependent killing.

The quinolones exert their antibacterial effect through inhibition of DNA synthesis. They act to inhibit topoisomerase II (DNA gyrase) and topoisomerase IV, which are necessary for bacterial replication. Quinolones are considered bactericidal agents and demonstrate concentration-dependent killing.

Clinical Uses

Most of the quinolones (excluding norfloxacin, cinoxacin, enoxacin, and lomefloxacin) have activity against the common respiratory pathogens, including *S. pneumoniae, H. influenzae, M. catarrhalis, C. pneumoniae, M. pneumoniae,* and *L. pneumophila*. The quinolones have been shown to be effective in the treatment of upper and lower respiratory tract infections, genitourinary tract infections, and skin and skin structure infections, with results comparable to those found with other antiinfective agents such as cephalosporins, macrolides, and trimethoprim-sulfamethoxazole. The currently available quinolones (except trovafloxacin) do not penetrate the cerebrospinal fluid to any significant extent. Ciprofloxacin has been shown to have the best *in vitro* activity of the quinolones against *P. aeruginosa* and other gram-negative aerobes. Ciprofloxacin, levofloxacin, and gatifloxacin have been used for the treatment of nosocomial pneumonia.

Adverse Reactions and Precautions

The quinolones are well tolerated and are considered one of the safest antimicrobial classes. Gastrointestinal side effects such as nausea, vomiting, and diarrhea occur in less than 5% of patients treated with quinolones. Prolongation of the Q–T interval (especially in female patients) has been reported with the use of quinolones. Seizures have been reported with ciprofloxacin in elderly patients and those with diminished renal function. Trovafloxacin use has been associated with fatal cases of liver toxicity. At present, trovafloxacin use outside the hospital setting for greater than 14 days is not recommended. Studies in immature laboratory animals have demonstrated changes in weight-bearing joints subsequent to quinolone exposure. Although quinolone-induced arthropathy has not been documented in humans, use of quinolones in children (≤18 years of age) should be reserved for cases in which the benefits outweigh the risks. Dosage adjustment of the quinolones (except trovafloxacin) is necessary in the presence of renal insufficiency. Concomitant use of antacids and iron supplements reduces the absorption of quinolones (as with the tetracyclines).

Other Antibiotics

The following agents belong to various classes of antimicrobials with different mechanisms of action and spectrums of activity. The individual agents are discussed as they represent the clinically used agents of their antimicrobial class.

Chloramphenicol

Chloramphenicol has been available for use in the United States since 1949. This agent has a broad spectrum of activity against gram-positive, gram-negative, and anaerobic bacteria. Chloramphenicol distributes well into various tissues including the brain. Use of this antibiotic has declined with the availability of less toxic agents.[25]

Mechanism of Action. Chloramphenicol inhibits protein synthesis by reversibly binding to the 50S ribosome subunit and essentially has a bacteriostatic effect. With prolonged exposure, chloramphenicol demonstrates bactericidal activity against some organisms by inducing bacterial cell lysis.

Clinical Uses. Chloramphenicol is highly active against *Salmonella* and has been used for the treatment of gastroenteritis with sepsis, as well as *Salmonella* meningitis. Chloramphenicol has excellent activity against rickettsial diseases such as scrub typhus, murine typhus, and Rocky Mountain spotted fever. However, these diseases are usually treated with tetracyclines, with chloramphenicol reserved for pregnant patients. Anaerobic infections and mixed anaerobic–aerobic infections such as peritonitis and aspiration pneumonia can be treated with chloramphenicol. In addition, chloramphenicol can be used to treat bacteremias caused by *Enterococcus* species, including some isolates that are resistant to vancomycin.

Adverse Reactions and Precautions. Because of the possibility of irreversible bone marrow suppression that may lead to serious and fatal blood dyscrasias (aplastic anemia), this agent should not be used when other effective agents are available. Aplastic anemia is a life-threatening complication reported in 1 of every 20,000 patients treated with chloramphenicol. This agent should not be used in premature and newborn infants, who cannot adequately metabolize this drug. The decreased metabolism of chloramphenicol results in high serum concentrations that can lead to gray baby syndrome (vomiting, pallor, cyanosis, circulatory collapse), which has an attributable mortality of 60%. The prolonged use of chloramphenicol in children with cystic fibrosis has been associated with optic neuritis leading to blindness.

Colistin (colistimethate)

Colistin, a member of the polymyxin family, was used in the early 1960s for serious gram-negative infections, including those caused by *P. aeruginosa*. It was approved in 1968 by the U.S. Food and Drug Administration (FDA), but was later abandoned for drugs with similar gram-negative efficacy and more favorable side-effect profiles.[26] However, there has been a resurgence in the use of colistin because of the emergence of multidrug-resistant gram-negative bacteria including *P. aeruginosa* and *Acinetobacter* species.

Mechanism of Action. Colistin is a surface-active, antipathic agent with a mechanism of action similar to that of a detergent. Because colistin has both hydrophilic and hydrophobic portions, it is relatively easy for the molecule to incorporate into bacterial cell membranes, causing disruption. Colistin exhibits bactericidal activity against most gram-negative bacteria.

Clinical Uses. Colistin has a broad range of activity against most gram-negative bacteria including multidrug-resistant *P. aeruginosa* and *Acinetobacter* species. Its use is often reserved for severe systemic infections, including ventilator-associated pneumonias. *Proteus* and *Neisseria* species are generally resistant to colistin, along with most anaerobes and gram-positive bacteria. Colistin is administered in an inactive form (colistimethate) either intravenously, intramuscularly, or by nebulization. Once administered, inactive colistimethate is converted *in vivo* to the active form colistin.[26] Nebulized colistin is used often in patients with cystic fibrosis who harbor MDR *P. aeruginosa*.

Adverse Reactions and Precautions. The most serious side effect associated with intravenously administered colistin is nephrotoxicity, which appears to be dose related and reversible. Nephrotoxicity has been reported to occur in up to 20% of patients given colistin. Neuromuscular blockage, seizures, and respiratory paralysis have also been reported and appear to be a dose-dependent phenomenon as well. Caution should be used when coadministering colistin with other agents capable of causing nephrotoxicity, neuromuscular blockage, or respiratory failure, such as the aminoglycosides.

Daptomycin

> **KEY POINT**
>
> *Daptomycin* is a novel cyclic lipopeptide that has activity against a wide range of gram-positive bacteria, including multidrug-resistant staphylococci and enterococci.

Daptomycin is a novel cyclic lipopeptide that has activity against a wide range of gram-positive bacteria, including multidrug-resistant staphylococci and enterococci.

However, daptomycin is inactive against gram-negative bacteria.

Mechanism of Action. The exact mechanism of daptomycin has not been completely elucidated; however, it is believed to occur by irreversible binding to the cytoplasmic membrane of bacterial cells and subsequent disruption of the membrane potential. This disruption appears to cause leakage of intracellular ions, leading to rapid cell death.[27]

Clinical Uses. Daptomycin is currently approved for use in complicated skin and skin structure infections caused by susceptible gram-positive bacteria and *S. aureus* bacteremia. It has excellent activity against resistant staphylococci and enterococci, including vancomycin-resistant strains, although not approved for this use. Of note, in a phase 3 trial involving daptomycin for the treatment of community-acquired pneumonia, daptomycin was inferior to the comparator agent (ceftriaxone), especially in patients with more serious infections. This poor response in pulmonary infections has been attributed to inactivation of daptomycin by pulmonary surfactants.[27] Consequently, daptomycin in not indicated for use in the treatment of pneumonia. Daptomycin is typically dosed at 4 to 6 mg/kg every 24 hours. It is available only as an intravenous infusion.

Adverse Reactions and Precautions. In earlier clinical studies involving daptomycin dosed every 8-12 hours, creatine phosphokinase (CPK) elevations and myalgias were noted that resulted in temporary suspension of drug development of this agent in the early 1990s. Once-daily administration of daptomycin has minimized these abnormalities noted in earlier studies. Clinical data have reported CPK elevations as a rare occurrence; however, the manufacturer recommends stopping hydroxymethylglutaryl-coenzyme A (HMG-CoA) reductase inhibitors and other drugs associated with rhabdomyolysis during daptomycin therapy. In addition, daptomycin should be discontinued in patients with myalgias associated with CPK elevations or in asymptomatic patients with CPK elevations greater that 10 times the upper limit of normal.

Trimethoprim–Sulfamethoxazole

Sulfamethoxazole belongs to the class of antibiotics known as the sulfonamides. Trimethoprim is a pyrimidine found to potentiate the activity of sulfamethoxazole. The combination of trimethoprim and sulfamethoxazole (TMP–SMX, or Bactrim) was introduced in 1968 and has since gained a place in the treatment of numerous infections. This combination is active against gram-positive (streptococci, MSSA) and gram-negative *(H. influenzae, Burkholderia cepacia, Stenotrophomonas maltophilia)* bacteria. In addition, it is active against *Pneumocystis jiroveci* (formerly known as *Pneumocystis carinii*).[28]

Mechanism of Action. TMP–SMX exerts antibacterial effects by sequentially blocking bacterial dihydropteroate synthetase and dihydrofolate reductase. These enzymes are responsible for the production of folic acid. Without folic acid, bacteria are unable to synthesize nucleic acid and proteins necessary for growth. TMP–SMX acts synergistically and is considered bacteriostatic.

Clinical Uses. TMP–SMX is used for the treatment and prophylaxis of *Pneumocystis* pneumonia (PCP) in patients infected with HIV. TMP–SMX is widely distributed in the body, achieving detectable levels in most tissues. High concentrations are achieved in the urine, making it an ideal agent for the treatment of urinary tract infections (UTIs). In addition, it has been used for treatment of acute exacerbations of bronchitis, traveler's diarrhea caused by enterotoxigenic *E. coli,* otitis media, and shigellosis. In recent years, bacterial resistance to TMP–SMX has increased, creating controversy over the continued use of this combination as a first-line agent for UTIs.

Adverse Reactions and Precautions. TMP–SMX is relatively well tolerated, with nausea, vomiting, diarrhea, and hypersensitivity being the most common adverse effects. In addition, sulfamethoxazole has side effects that are common to all sulfonamides such as neutropenia, thrombocytopenia, hemolytic anemia, jaundice, hepatic necrosis, and drug-induced lupus. TMP–SMX should be avoided in all patients with "sulfa" allergies or hypersensitivities. Patients who are deficient in the enzyme glucose-6-phosphate dehydrogenase (G6PD) should not receive TMP–SMX, because this combination can increase the risk of hemolytic anemia. The daily dosage of TMP–SMX should be reduced in the presence of renal insufficiency because both agents are eliminated through the kidneys.

Clindamycin

Clindamycin, a member of the lincosamide class of antibiotics, has activity against gram-positive and anaerobic bacteria. In addition, this agent is active against *Toxoplasma gondii* and *P. carinii.*[25,29]

Mechanism of Action. Like chloramphenicol, clindamycin binds to the bacterial 50S ribosomal subunit to inhibit protein synthesis, resulting in a bacteriostatic effect. This suppression of protein synthesis has been shown to reduce toxin production in certain strains of *S. aureus* (toxic shock syndrome) and *S. pyogenes* (necrotizing fasciitis).

Clinical Uses. Clindamycin distributes well in body tissues, but has minimal penetration into cerebrospinal fluid even in the presence of meningitis. Clindamycin is used as an adjunct to agents with gram-negative activity for intraabdominal, pelvic, and diabetic foot infections, all of which tend to be polymicrobial. Anaerobic infections of the respiratory tract such as necrotizing pneumonia, lung abscess, empyema, and aspiration pneumonia are often treated with clindamycin. AIDS-related illnesses such as *Toxoplasma* encephalitis and PCP can also be treated with clindamycin.

Adverse Reactions and Precautions. Nausea, vomiting, and diarrhea are the most common side effects associated with clindamycin. This diarrhea may be a consequence of *Clostridium difficile.* Discontinuing the offending antibiotic and initiating oral vancomycin or metronidazole therapy treats this mild to life-threatening diarrhea. Prolongation of the neuromuscular blocking effects of pancuronium with the concomitant use of clindamycin has also been reported.

Metronidazole

Metronidazole is a nitroimidazole that was used initially for its antiprotozoal effects against pathogens such as *Trichomonas vaginalis, Giardia lamblia,* and *Entamoeba histolytica.* Its anaerobic properties were discovered after an observation that acute ulcerative gingivitis improved in patients being treated for trichomonal vaginitis.[25]

Mechanism of Action. The exact mechanism of action of metronidazole is unknown, although it is thought to have different effects in protozoa versus anaerobic bacteria. It is postulated that the microorganisms convert metronidazole into its reduced form. This reduced form causes a loss of the helical structure of DNA and results in DNA strand breaks. Metronidazole is bactericidal against anaerobic pathogens such as *B. fragilis.*

Clinical Uses. Anaerobic infections have been implicated in abscesses within the brain, lung, and intraabdominal cavity. Metronidazole is often added as an adjunct, especially when surgical drainage of the abscess is not possible. Unlike clindamycin, metronidazole penetrates well into the central nervous system and therefore is useful for the treatment of brain abscesses. A key anaerobic pathogen, *B. fragilis* is part of the normal enteric flora and can contribute to sepsis in the event of gastrointestinal disease, surgery, or penetrating trauma. Metronidazole is often added to treat polymicrobial infections, especially where *B. fragilis* is suspected. Bacterial vaginosis caused by *Gardnerella, Trichomonas,* and *Bacteroides* species is also treated with metronidazole. In addition, diarrhea caused by *C. difficile* can be treated with metronidazole.

Adverse Reactions and Precautions. An unpleasant metallic taste, nausea, and vomiting are common complaints associated with the use of metronidazole. The prolonged use of this agent, especially with high doses, can lead to peripheral neuropathy. In some rare situations, seizures, encephalopathy, and cerebellar dysfunction have also been noted. Metronidazole can interact with warfarin to potentiate its hypoprothrombinemic effect and lead to significant bleeding. In addition, patients should avoid the use of alcohol while taking metronidazole (inhibits alcohol dehydrogenase) because the concomitant use can result in a disulfiram-like reaction.

Nitrofurantoin

Multiple nitrofuran compounds have been synthesized since their discovery in the early 1940s. The most widely used agent of this class has been nitrofurantoin. This antibacterial does not achieve therapeutic concentrations in body tissues other than the kidney. As a result, it is used only for UTIs.[30]

Mechanism of Action. Mechanisms such as inhibition of bacterial enzymes, protein synthesis, and damage to bacterial DNA have been implicated. The presence of these multiple inhibitory mechanisms may explain the infrequency of resistance. Nitrofurantoin is bactericidal at the high concentrations achieved in the urine.

Clinical Uses. Nitrofurantoin is effective for UTIs such as urethritis (urethral infection), cystitis (bladder infection), and pyelonephritis (kidney infection). The most common pathogen associated with these infections is the gram-negative bacterium *E. coli*.

Adverse Reactions and Precautions. Nausea and vomiting are common side effects that can require cessation of therapy. Hypersensitivity syndromes such as skin rashes, drug fever, and even asthma have been observed. Nitrofurantoin can accumulate in patients with renal dysfunction and result in serious complications such as peripheral neuritis. In addition, pneumonitis mimicking acute respiratory infection has been reported, but is rapidly reversible with discontinuation of this drug. Chronic pulmonary disease marked by interstitial fibrosis has been reported. This reversible condition may occur in patients who receive nitrofurantoin for longer than 6 months. Hemolytic anemia in patients with glucose-6-phosphate dehydrogenase (G6PD) deficiency can be precipitated with this agent. A disulfiram-like reaction can also occur in patients who consume alcohol while being treated with nitrofurantoin.

Vancomycin

Vancomycin is a glycopeptide antibiotic with activity against gram-positive bacteria. It is not active against gram-negative bacteria. Its use in recent years has escalated as a result of the emergence of methicillin-resistant *S. aureus* (MRSA).[31]

KEY POINT

Vancomycin is a glycopeptide antibiotic with activity against gram-positive bacteria. It is not active against gram-negative bacteria.

Mechanism of Action. Vancomycin inhibits transglycosylation of peptidoglycan by binding to the precursor D-alanine–D-alanine portion. This process prevents the formation of a rigid cell wall structure and results in bacterial cell lysis. Vancomycin is considered bactericidal against gram-positive organisms with the exception of enterococci (bacteriostatic).

Clinical Uses. Vancomycin is used for infections caused by MRSA, such as bacteremias, endocarditis, pneumonia, peritonitis, and skin and soft tissue infections. Vancomycin also serves as the alternative agent to penicillin for the treatment of viridans streptococcal endocarditis. Vancomycin does not cross the blood–brain barrier efficiently, even in the presence of acute meningeal inflammation. However, pneumococcal meningitis resistant to penicillin can still be treated by these low concentrations of vancomycin. An oral formulation of vancomycin can be used to treat *C. difficile* diarrhea that is refractory to metronidazole.

Adverse Reactions and Precautions. A common reaction known as red man or red neck syndrome has been associated with the rapid infusion of vancomycin (related to histamine release). Increasing the time of infusion can prevent this syndrome of skin itch, flushing, angioedema, and hypotension. Ototoxicity and nephrotoxicity have been noted to occur more frequently in patients who receive vancomycin concomitantly with aminoglycosides. Vancomycin is renally excreted and therefore requires dosage adjustment in patients with renal impairment.

Quinupristin and Dalfopristin

Quinupristin and dalfopristin are streptogramins that act synergistically when used together (as in the product Synercid). These agents are active against gram-positive bacteria and are used primarily to treat infections caused by vancomycin-resistant *Enterococcus faecium* (VREF).[31]

Mechanism of Action. Dalfopristin blocks peptide bond formation and distorts the ribosome to enhance the binding of quinupristin. The ribosome-bound quinupristin inhibits the binding of aminoacyl-transfer RNA to inhibit protein synthesis. The combination is bactericidal against MRSA, but is bacteriostatic against VREF.

Clinical Uses. Quinupristin–dalfopristin is used primarily for life-threatening VREF infections, but is also indicated for skin and soft tissue infections and pneumonias caused by susceptible gram-positive pathogens. Quinupristin–dalfopristin is not active against most gram-negative bacteria and anaerobes. However, quinupristin–dalfopristin has good *in vitro* activity against *M. pneumoniae* and *L. pneumophila*.

Adverse Reactions and Precautions. Quinupristin–dalfopristin is available only as a parenteral formulation and must be administered through a central line (catheter inserted and threaded to the superior or inferior vena cava) because peripheral administration is associated with a high incidence of thrombophlebitis. Arthralgias and myalgias of varying severity have also been reported with the use of these agents in up to 40% of patients. Like erythromycin, quinupristin–dalfopristin is an inhibitor of the CYP system. Therefore drugs (metabolized through the CYP system) with a narrow therapeutic index should be used cautiously in patients receiving quinupristin–dalfopristin.

Linezolid

The antibiotic linezolid belongs to a novel class of antibiotics known as the oxazolidinones. Linezolid, like quinupristin–dalfopristin, is active against gram-positive bacteria and is approved for the treatment of severe life-threatening VREF infections. Unlike vancomycin and quinupristin–dalfopristin, linezolid is available as an oral formulation that is completely absorbed from the gastrointestinal tract.[32]

Mechanism of Action. Linezolid prevents RNA translation by binding to the 23S ribosomal RNA of the 50S subunit to prevent the formation of a functional 70S initiation complex. Use of this novel antimicrobial target for the inhibition of protein synthesis has not been previously exploited.

Clinical Uses. Linezolid is indicated for the treatment of VREF infections, including cases with concurrent bacteremia. Nosocomial pneumonias and complicated skin and skin structure infections caused by *S. aureus*, including MRSA, may be treated with linezolid. Linezolid lacks significant activity against gram-negative bacteria.

Adverse Reactions and Precautions. The most common adverse events reported with linezolid include diarrhea, nausea, and headaches. Thrombocytopenia has been reported with the use of linezolid but is associated with prolonged use of the antibiotic (≥ 2 weeks). Linezolid is a reversible, nonselective inhibitor of monamine oxidase and has the potential to interact with adrenergic (e.g., dopamine, norepinephrine) and serotonergic (e.g., selective serotonin reuptake inhibitors) agents.

ANTIMYCOBACTERIALS

Tuberculosis has received heightened attention largely because of the increase in cases attributed to the HIV epidemic. Each year millions of individuals are exposed to tuberculosis, many through casual contact. More than 3 million new cases of tuberculosis were reported in the United States for 1996. The Centers for Disease Control and Prevention (CDC, Atlanta, GA) makes annual recommendations for the prevention and treatment of tuberculosis infection. Nosocomial transmission can be prevented by placing patients with suspected or confirmed tuberculosis in respiratory isolation (negative-pressure room) until they are (1) determined to not have tuberculosis, (2) discharged from the hospital, or (3) confirmed to be noninfectious. Other measures such as use of fitted respiratory masks (by health care personnel) can prevent transmission of *Mycobacterium tuberculosis* by aerosolization to caregivers. Treatment consists of multiple antibiotic regimens for 6 to 12 months in duration. Single-agent regimens should never be used for treatment because the likelihood of developing resistance is high. Treatment failures often result from poor patient compliance, as well as from resistance to antibiotics. Drugs used in the treatment of tuberculosis can be categorized as either first-line or second-line agents depending on their efficacy and side-effect profiles. Initial therapy generally involves a combination of isoniazid, pyrazinamide, rifampin, and ethambutol. A summary of the clinically used antimycobacterial agents, doses, routes of administration, and side effects is given in Table 14-7. Addition or subtraction of agents from this regimen is usually based on culture and sensitivity data, along with patient response to treatment. Guidelines for the treatment of active pulmonary tuberculosis are provided in Table 14-8.[33,34] or may be viewed directly at: http://www.cdc.gov/mmwr/preview/mmwrhtml/rr5211a1.htm (accessed April 2007).

KEY POINT

The most commonly used *antimycobacterials* in the treatment of tuberculosis include *isoniazid, rifampin, rifabutin, pyrazinamide, ethambutol,* and *streptomycin.*

TABLE 14-7

Commonly Used Antimycobacterials Including Dose, Route, and Side-Effect Profile

Antimycobacterial	Adult Dose	Route	Side Effects
Isoniazid	5 mg/kg/day; maximum of 300 mg/day	PO, IM	Hepatotoxicity (symptoms include nausea, loss of appetite, abdominal pain), peripheral neuritis, rash, fever, anemia
Rifampin	10 mg/kg/day; maximum of 600 mg/day	PO, IV	Hepatotoxicity, flulike symptoms, discolorations of body secretions to an orange color
Rifabutin	300 mg/day	PO	Hepatotoxicity, flulike symptoms, discolorations of body secretions to an orange color
Pyrazinamide	15-30 mg/kg/day; maximum of 2000 mg/day	PO	Hepatotoxicity, arthralgia, hyperuricemia
Ethambutol	15-25 mg/kg/day; maximum of 2500 mg/day	PO	Optic neuritis (higher in patients receiving >15 mg/kg/day)
Streptomycin	15 mg/kg/day; maximum of 1000 mg/day	IM	Ototoxicity (high-frequency hearing loss, vertigo), nephrotoxicity

IM, Intramuscular; *IV,* intravenous; *PO,* oral.

TABLE 14-8	

Guidelines for the Treatment of Active Pulmonary Tuberculosis

Clinical Scenario	Treatment Regimen
1. INH resistance rate < 4%	INH + RIF (or RFB) + PZA + B$_6$ daily for 2 mo, then INH + RIF (or RFB) + B$_6$ daily for an additional 4 mo
2. INH resistance rate > 4%	INH + RIF (or RFB) + PZA + ETB or SM + B$_6$ daily for 2 mo, then INH + RIF or unknown (or RFB) + B$_6$ daily for an additional 4 mo
3. Noncompliant or unreliable patient	Requires directly observed therapy (DOT) INH + RIF (or RFB) + PZA + ETB + B$_6$ or SM daily for 2 wk, then 2-3 times/wk for 6 wk, then INH + RIF (or RFB) + B$_6$ 2-3 times/wk for 6 mo
4. Patient known to be INH resistant or unable to tolerate INH	DOT for RIF (or RFB) + PZA + ETB daily for 6 mo
5. Patient known to be RIF resistant or unable to tolerate RIF	INH + FQN + ETB + B$_6$ daily for 12-18 mo; supplement with PZA the first 2 mo
6. Pregnancy	INH + RIF + ETB daily for 9 mo
7. HIV infection or AIDS	Treatment as in clinical scenarios 1 and 2 for the first 2 mo, then extend the INH + RIF (or RFB) + B$_6$ daily for an additional 7 mo

Data from American Thoracic Society, CDC, Infectious Diseases Society of America: Treatment of tuberculosis, *MMWR Recomm Rep* 52(RR-11):1, 2003.

AIDS, acquired immunodeficiency syndrome; *B$_6$,* Pyridoxine; *DOT,* directly observed therapy; *ETB,* ethambutol; *FQN,* fluoroquinolone; *HIV,* human immunodeficiency virus; *INH,* isoniazid; *PZA,* pyrazinamide; *RIF,* rifampin; *RFB,* rifabutin; *SM,* streptomycin.

Isoniazid

Isoniazid (INH) is well absorbed orally and is distributed throughout the body, especially in the cerebrospinal fluid. Isoniazid is metabolized by the liver, and its metabolite is eliminated by the kidneys.

Mechanism of Action

Isoniazid inhibits cell wall synthesis by inhibiting synthesis of mycolic acid, a primary component of the mycobacterial cell wall. This agent is bactericidal against replicating tuberculosis bacilli and bacteriostatic against nonreplicating organisms.

Adverse Reactions and Precautions

An elevation in liver enzymes has been reported in patients receiving isoniazid and is reversible with discontinuation of the drug. Rare cases of serious hepatitis and death also have been reported. Hepatotoxicity usually occurs between the fourth and eighth weeks of treatment but may occur at any time. Tests used to measure hepatocellular injury should be performed and include monitoring liver transaminases such as alanine aminotransferase (ALT) and aspartate aminotransferase (AST). In addition, patients should be monitored for the development of symptoms of hepatitis such as nausea, loss of appetite, and abdominal pain. Neurotoxicity has also been reported and occurs more frequently in patients receiving higher dose therapy. Supplementation with pyridoxine (vitamin B$_6$) has been shown to reduce the frequency of this adverse reaction. Rare miscellaneous reactions such as rash, anemia, and fever also have been reported.

Rifampin and Rifabutin

Rifampin and rifabutin are semisynthetic antibiotics referred to as *rifamycins*. Rifampin and rifabutin have similar structures, as well as spectrums of activity. They are well absorbed orally, with good penetration into most tissues. They do not penetrate the central nervous system well in the absence of inflammation. Rifampin is extensively metabolized through the liver and is an inducer of the CYP system. Rifabutin is also metabolized hepatically; however, it is a weaker enzyme inducer than rifampin. CYP induction is known to decrease plasma concentrations of drugs hepatically metabolized; therefore dosage adjustments of agents metabolized by this system are necessary.

Mechanism of Action

The rifamycins inhibit bacterial DNA–dependent RNA polymerase. They are bactericidal against actively dividing bacteria.

Adverse Reactions and Precautions

Hepatotoxicity is the major adverse reaction associated with the rifamycins. Elevations of liver transaminases are commonly reported and are usually reversible on discontinuation of the drug. Patients with preexisting liver damage are more prone to rifamycin-induced hepatotoxicity. Rifamycins are known to change the color of body fluids to a deep orange hue. Patients should be warned that urine, feces, tears, saliva, sputum, and semen might turn an orange color. Uveitis (inflammation of the iris), which manifests as blurry vision, has also been reported. Rare reports of flulike symptoms such as fever, chills, nausea, and vomiting have been reported during rifamycin therapy.

Pyrazinamide

Pyrazinamide is a nicotinic acid derivative that is well distributed into most tissues, including the cerebrospinal fluid. Pyrazinamide is hepatically metabolized and excreted by the kidneys.

Mechanism of Action

The precise mechanism of action is not known. Mycobacteria convert pyrazinamide to pyrazinoic acid. It is speculated that pyrazinoic acid accumulates in macrophages to lower the intracellular pH and increase the antimycobacterial activity of macrophages in combination with pyrazinamide. Pyrazinamide is bactericidal against mycobacteria when tested in an acidic environment.

Adverse Reactions and Precautions

Nausea and vomiting are the most common side effect with pyrazinamide treatment. Hepatotoxicity has also been reported in patients receiving pyrazinamide; therefore liver transaminases should be frequently monitored. Patients with preexisting liver abnormalities should be monitored closely. It is not known to induce or inhibit the CYP system to any significant extent.

Ethambutol

Ethambutol is a synthetic, orally administered agent that distributes extensively throughout the body, including the cerebrospinal fluid. Most of it is eliminated unchanged in the urine.

Mechanism of Action

Ethambutol decreases the synthesis of cell wall polysaccharides such as arabinogalactan to inhibit mycobacterial cell growth. It is a bacteriostatic agent.

Adverse Reactions and Precautions

Optic neuropathy is the major toxicity associated with the use of ethambutol. Patients usually complain of blurred vision in conjunction with altered color (red–green) perception. Optic neuritis is usually seen with the use of high doses of ethambutol and is slowly reversible on discontinuation of the drug. Baseline optometric evaluation, followed by periodic examinations, is advisable to help monitor for visual changes during treatment. The dose of ethambutol should be adjusted in patients with renal insufficiency.

Streptomycin

Streptomycin is an aminoglycoside antibiotic that has been in use since the 1940s for the treatment of tuberculosis. It is available for use intravenously and intramuscularly and indicated as an add-on agent in patients with documented or suspected drug-resistant tuberculosis.

Mechanism of Action

Streptomycin has a mechanism of action similar to that of other aminoglycosides.

Adverse Reactions and Precautions

Streptomycin, like other aminoglycosides, is associated with nephrotoxicity and ototoxicity. It is eliminated unchanged in the urine and requires dosage adjustment in patients with renal insufficiency.

ANTIFUNGALS

> **KEY POINT**
>
> The use of *antifungals*, such as the *polyenes*, *azoles*, and *echinocandins*, is increasing with the number of immunocompromised patients.

The incidence of fungal infections has increased dramatically. *Candida* species are now the fourth most commonly isolated bloodstream pathogens. Candidemia has an attributable mortality of up to 40%. The number of patients immunocompromised as a result of AIDS, cancer chemotherapy, and organ transplantation has been increasing. These patient populations have diminished cell-mediated immunity and are predisposed to numerous fungal pathogens that vary in incidence geographically. The treatment of choice for most of these infections has been the polyene amphotericin B. The high incidence of nephrotoxicity associated with this agent served as the impetus for the development of the azoles. Ketoconazole was the first agent of this class, but it has largely been replaced by the triazoles fluconazole and itraconazole. Newer triazoles with improved activity against molds are being developed. In addition, a new class of antifungals known as the *echinocandins* is now available. A summary of systemically used antifungals,

TABLE 14-9

Classification of the Systemically Used Antifungals

Antifungal Class (Generic Name)	Brand Name	Route	Common Uses (Microorganism)
Polyenes			
Amphotericin B	Fungizone	IV, PO*	*Candida* spp., *Aspergillus* spp., *Cryptococcus neoformans*, *Histoplasma capsulatum*, *Blastomyces dermatitidis*, *Coccidioides immitis*
Amphotericin B colloidal dispersion	Amphotec	IV	*Candida* spp., *Aspergillus* spp., mucormycosis, *C. neoformans*
Amphotericin B lipid complex	Abelcet	IV	*Candida* spp., *Aspergillus* spp., mucormycosis, *C. neoformans*
Liposomal amphotericin B	AmBisome	IV	*Candida* spp., *Aspergillus* spp., mucormycosis, *C. neoforms*, leishmaniasis
Azoles			
Ketoconazole	Nizoral	PO	*Candida* spp.,† *C. neoformans*, *H. capsulatum*, *B. dermatitidis*
Fluconazole	Diflucan	IV, PO	*Candida* spp.,† *C. neoformans*
Itraconazole	Sporanox	IV, PO	*Candida* spp.,† *Aspergillus* spp., *C. neoformans*, *H. capsulatum*, *B. dermatitidis*, *C. immitis*, *Sporothrix schenckii*
Voriconazole	Vfend	IV, PO	*Candida* spp.,† *Aspergillus* spp., *C. neoformans*, *C. immitis*, *H. capsulatum*, *B. dermatitidis*, *Fusarium* spp., *Scedosporium* spp.
Posaconazole	Noxafil	IV, PO	*Candida* spp.,† *Aspergillus* spp., *C. neoformans*, *C. immitis*, *H. capsulatum*, *B. dermatitidis*, *Fusarium* spp., *Scedosporium* spp.
Echinocandins			
Caspofungin	Cancidas	IV	*Aspergillus* spp., *Candida* spp.
Micafungin	Mycamine	IV	*Aspergillus* spp., *Candida* spp.
Anidulafungin	ERAXIS	IV	*Aspergillus* spp., *Candida* spp.
Other Antifungals			
Flucytosine	Ancobon	PO	*Aspergillus* spp., *Candida* spp., *C. neoformans*
Griseofulvin	Fulvicin	PO	Tinea corporis, tinea cruris, tinea barbae, tinea capitis, and tinea unguium
Terbinafine	Lamisil	PO	Tinea corporis, tinea pedis, tinea manuum, tinea cruris, tinea imbricata, tinea capitis, and tinea unguium

*The oral form of amphotericin B is not absorbed through the gastrointestinal tract.
†*Candida krusei* is intrinsically resistant to all azoles.
IV, Intravenous; *PO*, oral.

including route and clinical uses, is provided in Table 14-9.[35-37]

Polyenes

The polyenes include amphotericin B and nystatin. Amphotericin B has been available for more than 50 years and remains the drug of choice for most systemic fungal infections. In more recent years, amphotericin B has been formulated into lipid-based products. These lipid-based products alter the distribution of amphotericin B, resulting in a higher uptake of the agent into the reticuloendothelial system (liver, spleen, lymphatics) relative to the kidneys.[38] The net effect of this shift in distribution has been shown to reduce the incidence of nephrotoxicity. Nystatin is only used topically for oral and intertriginous (between skin surfaces) candidiasis. However, a lipid-based formulation of nystatin is currently under investigation.

Mechanism of Action

The polyenes bind to ergosterol (a type of cholesterol) in the fungal cell membrane, creating pores that increase cell membrane permeability. Intracellular potassium and other components escape through the pores, resulting in cell death (fungicidal).

Clinical Uses

The fungicidal activity of amphotericin B has made it the first-line agent for several pathogens causing pulmonary infections, including aspergillosis, blastomycosis, coccidioidomycosis, histoplasmosis, and cryptococcosis. These infections are associated with a high mortality, especially in patients who are neutropenic. Consequently, preventive measures such as amphotericin B prophylaxis and high-dose treatment (through the use of lipid-based formulations) have been sought. However, the optimal dose and treatment duration have been difficult to define because the successful outcome of a systemic fungal infection is largely dependent on recovery of the host immune system.

Adverse Reactions and Precautions

The parenteral administration of amphotericin B is associated with two major types of toxicity. The first is infusion-related and includes flushing, fever, and chills. Pretreating patients (who manifested these symptoms) with antipyretics and antihistamines may minimize these effects. The second major toxicity is renal impairment thought to be a result of diminished renal perfusion. Hydrating the patient with normal saline boluses before and after amphotericin B infusion has been attempted to prevent this toxicity. The liposomal products, such as amphotericin B lipid complex and liposomal amphotericin B, have been shown to be less nephrotoxic than the traditional product and allow the administration of higher doses of amphotericin B.

Azoles

The systemically used azoles include ketoconazole, fluconazole, itraconazole, voriconazole and posaconazole. Ketoconazole was the first oral agent available to treat systemic fungal infections. This agent is poorly absorbed from the gastrointestinal tract (when an acidic environment is not present) and has potential for substantial toxicity. As a result, ketoconazole has largely been replaced by the newer triazoles fluconazole, itraconazole, and voriconazole. Fluconazole, for example, is available in oral and intravenous formulations, is widely distributed into the tissues, and is relatively nontoxic. But compared with ketoconazole, it has a narrow spectrum of activity. Itraconazole has an enhanced spectrum of activity compared with fluconazole, but slightly less than that of voriconazole. Itraconazole and voriconazole are also available in oral and intravenous formulations. Posaconazole, available only for compassionate use, is intended for patients failing or refractory to other therapies and has been documented to be active against zygomycetes.[37]

Mechanism of Action

Fungal cell growth is impaired because of the reduced production of ergosterol. Azoles prevent the conversion of lanosterol to ergosterol by inhibiting the fungal CYP system and, therefore, producing their fungistatic effect.

Clinical Uses

Ketoconazole has largely been replaced by the more potent and better tolerated triazoles. The primary indication for fluconazole is for candidiasis (nonneutropenic patients) and as suppressive therapy for patients with cryptococcal meningitis, but it may also be used to treat coccidioidomycosis. Itraconazole is considered the drug of choice for the treatment of cutaneous and lymphangitic sporotrichosis. Itraconazole is also used as prophylaxis and suppressive therapy for pulmonary aspergillosis, histoplasmosis, blastomycosis, cryptococcosis, coccidioidomycosis, paracoccidioidomycosis, and candidiasis. Voriconazole is considered the drug of choice as primary therapy for invasive aspergillosis and has been approved for the management of candidemia and infections cause by rare pathogens such as *Fusarium* and *Scedosporium apiospermum*. Of note, candidiasis caused by *Candida krusei* (lacks the CYP system) may be intrinsically resistant to this class of agents although *in vitro* activity has been documented with voriconazole and posaconazole.

Adverse Reactions and Precautions

Fluconazole is well tolerated and has minimal side effects. Common adverse effects with ketoconazole, itraconazole, and voriconazole are anorexia, nausea, and vomiting. In addition, transaminase and bilirubin elevations have been reported. Impotence, decreased libido, and gynecomastia are also known to occur with ketoconazole and are attributed to its inhibition of sex steroid synthesis, and consequently it is used clinically for certain endocrine disorders. Voriconazole can cause visual disturbances such as photopsia and chromatopsia, which occur in up to 30% of all patients.[36,39] Ketoconazole, itraconazole, and voriconazole are metabolized in the liver and are potent inhibitors of the CYP3A4 system, so each has a significant potential for drug interactions. Conversely, fluconazole does not undergo significant hepatic metabolism and has the lowest drug interaction potential of the triazoles. Fluconazole is, however, eliminated unchanged in the urine and so requires dosage adjustment in patients with impaired renal function. Renal function is also important when administering the intravenous formulations of itraconazole and voriconazole. These drugs should be avoided in patients with creatinine clearances less than 30 ml/min to prevent the accumulation of cyclodextrin, an intravenous solubilizing agent. Cyclodextrin is also used to formulate oral itraconazole solution and has been cited as the cause of the high incidence of adverse gastrointestinal intolerance relative to itraconazole capsules, which do not contain this agent.

Echinocandins

Caspofungin was the first echinocandin to receive FDA approval in early 2001. Both micafungin and anidulafungin received FDA approval in 2004 and 2006, respectively. These agents have similar pharmacokinetic and pharmacodynamic properties. They have poor gastrointestinal absorption and all require parenteral administration.[40]

Mechanism of Action

These agents inhibit fungal cell wall synthesis by inhibiting (1,3)-β-D-glucan synthase.[37] Echinocandins may be either fungicidal or fungistatic against fungi depending on the isolate.

Clinical Uses

All echinocandins have demonstrated *in vitro* and *in vivo* (animal studies) activity against *Candida* and *Aspergillus* species. Caspofungin is currently indicated for the treatment of febrile neutropenia, candidemia, esophageal candidiasis, and aspergillosis in patients refractory or intolerant to amphotericin B, lipid-based amphotericin B, and itraconazole. Micafungin is indicated only for esophageal candidiasis treatment and prophylaxis after hematopoietic stem cell transplants. Anidulafungin, the most recently approved agent, is indicated for the treatment of candidemia, nonneutropenic candidiasis, and esophageal candidiasis. All echinocandins are considered ineffective against *Cryptococcus* species, as these organisms lack (1,3)-β-D-glucan in their cell wall.

Adverse Reactions and Precautions

The echinocandins appear to be well tolerated, although most of the safety data are for caspofungin and micafungin. In most studies, common adverse reactions were infusion related and included fever, rash, flushing, and thrombophlebitis. Infusion-related reactions reached approximately 10% for caspofungin and slightly less for micafungin. Anidulafungin has produced infusion-related reactions in up to 15% of patients. Nausea and vomiting were also frequently reported for all three agents. Elevations in liver transaminase (AST and ALT) levels and hyperbilirubinemia were noted with the echinocandins, but these were mild and reversible on drug discontinuation. The echinocandins are not metabolized through the CYP450 system, thus reducing the potential for drug interactions.[41] All echinocandins can increase the area under the curve (AUC) of cyclosporine when coadministered, with caspofungin creating the most significant changes in AUC. The mechanism of this interaction is unknown. Concurrent use of cyclosporine and the echinocandins may warrant careful monitoring.

Flucytosine

Flucytosine acts as an antimetabolite and is used primarily as adjunctive therapy for susceptible fungal pathogens. It is active against *Candida, Cryptococcus,* and *Aspergillus.*[35]

Mechanism of Action

Flucytosine is converted to fluorouracil and competes with uracil during the formation of fungal RNA. Inhibition of RNA formation decreases protein synthesis and prevents cell growth (fungistatic).

Clinical Use

Resistance to flucytosine develops rapidly when it is used as a single agent for systemic fungal infections. As a result, flucytosine has been used in combination with amphotericin B for the treatment of cryptococcal meningitis and aspergillosis.

Adverse Reactions and Precautions

The most common adverse event associated with this agent is bone marrow suppression leading to anemia, leukopenia, and thrombocytopenia. This toxicity usually results when serum concentrations of this agent exceed 100 μg/ml. Dosage reduction in patients with renal impairment is imperative to prevent this serious complication.

Griseofulvin and Terbinafine

Griseofulvin was one of the first antifungals discovered; however, only dermatophytes (skin fungi) are susceptible to this agent. The absorption of this agent is greatly increased when taken with a high-fat meal. Terbinafine, which was developed more recently, has demonstrated more potent activity against dermatophytes. Terbinafine is a highly lipophilic allylamine that concentrates in the stratum corneum, sebum, and hair follicles. This property makes it an excellent agent for cutaneous dermatophytosis ("ring-worm" infection, athlete's foot, etc.) and onychomycosis (fungal infection in nails).[35]

Mechanism of Action

Griseofulvin is active only against growing dermatophytes. It interferes with microtubule formation of the mitotic spindle, preventing the growth of hyphae. Terbinafine inhibits squalene epoxidase, which reduces ergosterol production and inhibits fungal cell growth.

Clinical Uses

Griseofulvin and terbinafine are used for fungal infections (tinea) of the skin, hair, and nails. However, the recurrence rates of these infections tend to be higher with griseofulvin relative to terbinafine. Treatment for 12 to 16 weeks with terbinafine has been demonstrated to be superior to griseofulvin for the eradication of fingernail and toenail fungus.

Adverse Reactions and Precautions

Heartburn, flatulence, angular stomatitis, glossodynia, and a black-furred tongue are common gastrointestinal side effects of griseofulvin. Headache, also a common side effect of griseofulvin, subsides during the course of therapy. Terbinafine is well tolerated, with the most common side effects reported to be nausea, vomiting, and abdominal cramps. Terbinafine has been associated with transient increases in hepatic transaminases, which revert to normal on discontinuation of the agent. Rash and hypersensitivity reactions have been reported with both of these agents.

ANTIVIRAL AGENTS

KEY POINT

Antivirals (excluding antiretrovirals) mimic nucleosides and inhibit DNA synthesis.

Several agents are available for treating viral infections (Table 14-10). All of these agents act by inhibiting steps involved in viral replication, with none inhibiting non-replicating viruses. *Antivirals* (excluding antiretrovirals) mimic nucleosides and inhibit DNA synthesis. Agents used to treat HIV are not discussed.[42]

Acyclovir and Valacyclovir

Acyclovir is available in intravenous, oral, and topical formulations. Oral acyclovir is not readily absorbed and so requires frequent daily dosing. Valacyclovir, a prodrug of acyclovir, was developed to improve gastrointestinal absorption of acyclovir. Valacyclovir is available only in oral formulation.[42]

Mechanism of Action

Acyclovir is a nucleoside analog, which is phosphorylated and inserted into the replicating viral DNA. Once inserted in the growing chain, viral replication is terminated. Valacyclovir is converted to the active drug acyclovir by enzymatic hydrolysis in the liver and intestine.

Clinical Uses

Acyclovir and valacyclovir are effective against members of the herpesvirus family. They are most effective against herpes simplex virus (HSV)-1 and HSV-2. In addition, they also have activity against Epstein-Barr virus (EBV), cytomegalovirus (CMV), and varicella-zoster virus (VZV). Acyclovir and valacyclovir are clinically used for the treatment of genital infections caused by HSV and VZV.

Adverse Reactions and Precautions

Acyclovir is eliminated unchanged in the urine; therefore dosage adjustment is required for acyclovir and valacyclovir in individuals with renal impairment. Cases of nephropathy secondary to acyclovir have been reported in individuals with renal impairment. This adverse event occurs primarily in patients taking high doses of acyclovir. Keeping patients well hydrated can prevent nephropathy. The oral formulations are generally well tolerated. The topical formulation of acyclovir may cause transient burning and irritation at the site of application.

Penciclovir and Famciclovir

Penciclovir and famciclovir are similar in structure and activity to acyclovir. Famciclovir, the prodrug of penciclovir, is converted to its active form (penciclovir) in the gastrointestinal tract. Famciclovir is available in oral formulation, and penciclovir is available only in a 1% topical cream. Penciclovir and famciclovir appear to have greater *in vitro* activity against HSV and VZV than does acyclovir.[42]

Mechanism of Action

Penciclovir and the prodrug famciclovir are guanine nucleoside analogs, which exert their antiviral effects by incorporating into growing DNA chains, subsequently interfering with viral DNA synthesis and replication.

Clinical Uses

Penciclovir has activity against viruses from the herpes family. It is effective against HSV-1, HSV-2, and VZV. Like acyclovir, it is less effective against EBV and CMV. *In vitro* studies have demonstrated some activity against hepatitis B virus (HBV). Penciclovir and famciclovir are clinically used for the treatment of genital infections caused by HSV and VZV.

Adverse Reactions and Precautions

Both penciclovir and famciclovir are considerably well tolerated. Use of famciclovir has been associated with nausea, vomiting, diarrhea, and headaches. Rare cases

TABLE 14-10			
Classification of Antivirals			
Antiviral (Generic Name)	Brand Name	Route	Common Uses (Microorganism)
Acyclovir	Zovirax	IV, PO, TOP	Herpes simplex (HSV-1 and HSV-2), herpes zoster (HZV), varicella-zoster (VZV)
Valacyclovir	Valtrex	PO	HSV-1 and HSV-2, HZV, VZV
Penciclovir	Denavir	TOP	HSV-1, HSV-2, HZV, VZV
Famciclovir	Famvir	PO	HSV-1, HSV-2, HZV, VZV
Ganciclovir	Cytovene	IV, PO, IO	Cytomegalovirus (CMV)
Valganciclovir	Valcyte	PO	CMV
Cidofovir	Vistide	IV	CMV
Foscarnet	Foscavir	IV	HSV-1, HSV-2, VZV, and CMV that are suspected to be resistant to acyclovir and ganciclovir
Fomivirsen	Vitravene	IVit	CMV
Amantadine	Symadine	PO	Influenza A
Rimantadine	Flumadine	PO	Influenza A
Oseltamivir	Tamiflu	PO	Influenza A and B

IO, Intraocular; *IV*, Intravenous; *IVit*, intravitreal injection; *PO*, oral; *TOP*, topical.

of neutropenia have been reported. Penciclovir is eliminated through the kidneys; therefore dosage adjustment of famciclovir is required in patients with moderate to severe renal insufficiency.

Ganciclovir and Valganciclovir

Ganciclovir is a guanine nucleoside analog with a mechanism of action similar to that of acyclovir. Valganciclovir is a newly approved prodrug of ganciclovir that improves ganciclovir absorption. Ganciclovir has a higher affinity for DNA transferase than does acyclovir, which increases the intracellular half-life of the drug and allows less frequent dosing. Valganciclovir is available only in oral formulation; ganciclovir is available in oral, intravenous, and intraocular (eye implant) formulations.[42]

Mechanism of Action

Ganciclovir and the prodrug valganciclovir are both guanine nucleoside analogs. They have a similar mechanism of action as acyclovir. Both agents will incorporate into growing DNA chains, consequently terminating viral DNA synthesis and replication.[43]

Clinical Uses

Ganciclovir resembles acyclovir in its activity against members of the herpesvirus family and VZV. However, ganciclovir has much higher activity against CMV *in vitro* and *in vivo*. Ganciclovir is indicated for the treatment and chronic suppression of CMV retinitis and prevention of CMV disease in AIDS and posttransplantation patients.

Adverse Reactions and Precautions

The most common adverse reaction associated with the use of ganciclovir is bone marrow suppression. In patients with AIDS the incidence of thrombocytopenia and neutropenia may be as high as 20 and 40%, respectively. Dosages should be reduced in the presence of renal insufficiency. In addition to the side effects of myelosuppression, headache, nausea, rash, fever, and liver transaminase elevations have also been reported.

Cidofovir

Cidofovir is an acyclic phosphonate nucleoside analog that has potent antiviral activity against a wide variety of viruses. Unlike the guanine nucleoside analogs, cidofovir has enhanced activity against HSV, EBV, VZV, and CMV. Cidofovir is available only in intravenous formulation.[42]

Mechanism of Action

Cidofovir exerts its mechanism of action by inhibition of viral replication. Cidofovir is phosphorylated and inserted into the growing DNA chain. Once inserted, viral replication is terminated by inhibition of viral polymerases.

Clinical Uses

Cidofovir has potent activity against members of the herpesvirus family, EBV, and CMV. It is indicated for use in patients with CMV who failed previous treatments of ganciclovir or foscarnet. It has been used extensively in the treatment of CMV retinitis in patients with AIDS.[44]

Adverse Reactions and Precautions

Severe dose-dependent nephrotoxicity has been associated with the use of cidofovir. It is contraindicated for use in individuals with renal insufficiency. Saline infusions before and concomitant probenecid administration during cidofovir treatment have been used to help reduce nephrotoxicity. In addition to nephrotoxicity, neutropenia, fever, headache, emesis, rash, and diarrhea have also been reported with cidofovir use.

Foscarnet

Foscarnet is a pyrophosphonate nucleoside analog that has potent antiviral activity against HSV, EBV, VZV, and CMV. In addition, foscarnet has demonstrated activity against the hepatitis B and influenza viruses. It is poorly absorbed; therefore it is available only in intravenous formulation.[42]

Mechanism of Action

Because foscarnet is a pyrophosphate analog, it does not require phosphorylation to become active. Foscarnet works by reversibly blocking viral polymerase phosphorylation, which inhibits viral replication.

Clinical Uses

Foscarnet has activity against herpesvirus family, along with VZV, EBV, and influenza A and B. Foscarnet is used mainly for the treatment of CMV retinitis in patients with AIDS who are unable to tolerate ganciclovir therapy. However, it is also used for treatment of CMV infections in other immunosuppressed individuals (organ transplantation). In addition, foscarnet has been used to treat HSV and VZV infections that are resistant to acyclovir and ganciclovir. Ganciclovir or acyclovir may act synergistically with foscarnet against some strains of CMV.

Adverse Reactions and Precautions

Nephrotoxicity is a relatively common side effect occurring in approximately 25% of patients treated. Adequate hydration during foscarnet infusion may reduce the incidence of nephrotoxicity. Dosage reduction is required in those individuals with renal insufficiency. Other adverse reactions include fever, nausea, electrolyte imbalances, vomiting, diarrhea, and headache.

Fomivirsen

Fomivirsen is the first member of a new class of antiretrovirals termed *antisense oligonucleotides*. It is available only as an intravitreal preparation.[45]

Mechanism of Action

Antisense oligonucleotides are short stretches of DNA or RNA that bind to complementary sequences within the viral nucleic acid. Once bound, viral transcription is terminated. Fomivirsen acts by specifically binding to complementary regions of CMV RNA.

Clinical Uses

Fomivirsen is indicated only for the treatment of CMV retinitis in patients with AIDS. Fomivirsen has been shown to significantly delay the progression of CMV retinitis in AIDS patients. Fomivirsen is administered by intravitreal (into the vitreous humor) injection every week for 3 weeks, and then every other week thereafter.

Adverse Reactions and Precautions

Transient increases in intraocular pressure have been reported along with intraocular inflammation of the anterior and posterior chambers. Topical steroids (eye drops) may be used to alleviate this adverse reaction.

Amantadine and Rimantadine

Amantadine and rimantadine are closely related antivirals with activity only against influenza A. In addition, amantadine has also been used in the treatment of Parkinson's disease. Both agents are well absorbed from the gastrointestinal tract and suitable for oral administration.[42]

Mechanism of Action

Amantadine and rimantadine act by inhibiting viral replication and viral assembly. It is also thought that these agents inhibit the influenza virus from uncoating and entering the mucosal cells of the respiratory tract.

Clinical Uses

Amantadine and rimantadine have a narrow spectrum of activity because they are active only against influenza A virus. Both agents may be used prophylactically in high-risk (i.e., immunocompromised) patients who are unable to tolerate or benefit from influenza vaccination. In addition, they may also be used in conjunction with vaccination in the same high-risk patient populations. These agents should be initiated within the first 48 hours of onset of symptoms to be effective.

Adverse Reactions

Amantadine and rimantadine are well tolerated. Central nervous system side effects such as tremor, insomnia, lightheadedness, seizure, cardiac arrhythmias, and agitation have been reported with both drugs (more often with amantadine) and appear to be related to higher serum concentrations of these agents. A dosage adjustment of amantadine, but not rimantadine, is required in the presence of renal insufficiency.

Oseltamivir

Oseltamivir belongs to a new class of antivirals known as the *neuraminidase inhibitors*. Oseltamivir is a prodrug, which is converted to its active form (oseltamivir carboxylate) once it is absorbed. It is available only as an oral formulation.[42]

Mechanism of Action

Oseltamivir specifically inhibits influenza A and B neuraminidase, which prevents influenza viruses from leaving the host cell to infect other cells.

Clinical Uses

Oseltamivir is effective only for the treatment of influenza A and B infection. It has been shown to clinically reduce the duration of influenza infection. However, therapy must be initiated within 40 hours of the initiation of symptoms to be effective.

Adverse Reactions and Precautions

Oseltamivir is well tolerated, with nausea and vomiting reported as the most frequent adverse reaction. These symptoms usually occur on the first 2 days of therapy. Dosage adjustment is required in patients with renal insufficiency.

SELF-ASSESSMENT QUESTIONS

1. What is the difference between bacteriostatic and bactericidal antimicrobial agents?
2. Describe the difference between antimicrobial agents that act in a concentration-dependent manner and agents that act in a time-dependent manner.
3. Describe at least three parameters that may indicate antibiotic failure in a patient.
4. Why is it useful to use combination antibiotic therapy? (Be specific.)
5. Describe the mechanism of action of penicillin antibiotics. Name at least two additional antibiotic classes with similar mechanisms of action.
6. Which β-lactam antibiotic is least likely to cause an allergic reaction in a patient with a penicillin allergy?
7. Name three antimicrobial agents that would be useful in the treatment of community-acquired pneumonia.

SELF-ASSESSMENT QUESTIONS —cont'd

8. What is the antimicrobial agent of choice for the treatment of *Pneumocystis carinii* pneumonia (PCP)?
9. What agents are considered first-line therapy for the treatment of pulmonary tuberculosis?
10. Which antimicrobial agents are useful for the treatment of nosocomial pneumonia caused by *Pseudomonas aeruginosa*?

Answers to Self-Assessment Questions are found in Appendix A.

CLINICAL SCENARIO

C.S. is a 61-year-old white male with a history of chronic obstructive pulmonary disease (COPD) and recurrent pneumonia admitted to University Hospital from the community, with complaints of cough with productive yellow-green sputum, fever, chills, and worsening shortness of breath (SOB). The patient states that he has felt relatively well the past 3 to 4 weeks, except for occasional night sweats.

COPD was diagnosed in 1995. He also has hypertension (HTN), mild benign prostatic hypertrophy (BPH), and a left below-the-knee amputation (BKA). C.S. is also allergic to penicillin (anaphylactic reaction).

C.S.'s medications (before admission) are as follows:

Ipratropium 2 puffs q6h (COPD)

Albuterol 2 puffs q4-6h (COPD)

Lisinopril 10 mg qd (HTN)

Terazosin 2 mg hs (BPH)

His vital signs are as follows: temperature (T), 101.2° F; blood pressure (BP), 158/92 mmHg; heart rate (HR), 104 beats/min; respiratory rate (RR), 28 breaths/min; weight, 130 lb; height, 65 in; oxygen saturation by pulse oximetry (Spo_2, 92% on 4 L O_2, 68% on room air).

C.S.'s physical examination revealed the following (remarkable findings): elderly cachectic male in acute distress; tachycardic, with a regular rhythm; bilateral respiratory crackles; and clubbing and cyanotic nailbeds.

His white blood cell (WBC) count is 15.6×10^3 cells/mm^3. Sputum demonstrated many WBCs, few epithelial cells, many gram-positive cocci in chains/pairs; a culture is pending. His chest X-ray film revealed left lower lobe (LLL) infiltrate.

What signs and symptoms of infection in this patient are consistent with the diagnosis of community-acquired pneumonia (CAP)?

What is the most likely pathogen responsible for CAP in this patient?

Name two antibiotics that can be used to treat this patient's CAP.

If the sputum stains are acid-fast positive, what precautions should be taken and what drug therapy should be initiated?

Answers to Clinical Scenario Questions are found in Appendix A.

References

1. Chambers HF, Sande MA: General considerations. In Goodman LS, Gilman A, editors: *The pharmacologic basis of therapeutics*, ed 9, New York, 1995, McGraw-Hill.
2. Meyer F, Friendland GW: *Medicine's 10 greatest discoveries*, New Haven, 1998, Yale University Press.
3. Chain E, Florey HW, Gardner AD, Heatley NG, Jennings MA, Orr-Ewing J, Sanders AG: Penicillin as a chemotherapeutic agent, *Lancet* 2:226, 1940.
4. Thompson RL, Wright AJ: General principles of antimicrobial therapy, *Mayo Clin Proc* 73:995, 1998.
5. Mandell LA, Campbell GD: Nosocomial pneumonia guidelines: an international perspective, *Chest* 113(suppl 3):188S, 1998.
6. Tomasz A: From penicillin-binding proteins to the lysis and death of bacteria: a 1979 view, *Rev Infect Dis* 1:434, 1979.
7. Wright AJ: The penicillins, *Mayo Clin Proc* 74:290, 1999.
8. Selwyn S: The evolution of the broad-spectrum penicillins, *J Antimicrobial Chemother* 9(suppl B):1, 1982.
9. Sanders CC: Cefepime: the next generation? *Clin Infect Dis* 17:369, 1993.
10. Anne S, Relsman RE: Risk of administering cephalosporin antibiotics to patients with histories of penicillin allergy, *Ann Allergy Asthma Immunol* 74:167, 1995.
11. Norrby SR: Side effects of cephalosporins, *Drugs* 34(suppl 2):105, 1987.
12. Hellinger WC, Brewer NS: Carbapenems and monobactams: imipenem, meropenem, and aztreonam, *Mayo Clin Proc* 74:420, 1999.
13. Keating GM, Perry CM: Ertapenem: a review of its use in the treatment of bacterial infections, *Drugs* 65:2151, 2005.
14. Asbel LE, Levison ME: Cephalosporins, carbapenems, and monobactams, *Infect Dis Clin North Am* 14:435, 2000.
15. Gilbert DN: Aminoglycosides. In Mandell GL, Bennet JE, Dolin R, editors: *Mandell, Douglas and Bennett's principles and practices of infectious disease*, vol 1, ed 6, vol. 1 New York, 2005, Elsevier, Churchill Livingstone.
16. Davis BD: Mechanism of bactericidal action of aminoglycosides, *Microbiol Rev* 51:341, 1987.
17. Kahlmeter G, Dahlager JL: Aminoglycoside toxicity: a review of clinical studies published between 1975 and 1982, *J Antimicrob Chemother* 13(suppl A):9, 1984.
18. Smilack JD: The tetracyclines, *Mayo Clin Proc* 74:727, 1999.
19. Pankey GA: Tigecycline, *J Antimicrobial Chemother* 56:470, 2005.
20. Guay DR: Tigecycline, In Yu VL, Edwards G, McKinnon PS, Peloquin C, Morse GD, editors: *Antimicrobial therapy and vaccines, vol 2: Antimicrobial agents*, ed 2, Pittsburg, Pa, 2005, ESun Technologies.
21. Piscitelli SC, Danziger LH, Rodvold KA: Clarithromycin and azithromycin: new macrolide antibiotics, *Clin Pharm* 11:137, 1992.
22. Pai MP, Graci DM, Amsden GW: Macrolide drug interaction: an update, *Ann Pharmacother* 34:495, 2000.
23. Willington K, Noble S: Telithromycin, *Drugs* 64:1683, 2004.
24. O'Donnell JA, Gelone SP: Fluoroquinolones, *Infect Dis Clin North Am* 14:498, 2000.
25. Kasten MJ: Clindamycin, metronidazole, and chloramphenicol, *Mayo Clin Proc* 74:825, 1999.
26. Kaye KS, Kaye D: Polymyxins (polymyxin B and colistin). In Mandell GL, Bennet JE, Dolin R, editors: *Mandell, Douglas and Bennett's principles and practices of infectious disease*, vol 1 ed 6, New York, 2005, Elsevier, Churchill Livingstone.
27. Schriever CA, Fernandez C, Rodvold KA, Danziger LH: Daptomycin, *Am J Health Syst Pharm* 62:1145, 2005.
28. Smilack JD: Trimethoprim–sulfamethoxazole, *Mayo Clin Proc* 74:730, 1999.
29. Akins RL, Coyle EA, Levison ME, Verhoef J: Clindamycin. In Yu VL, Edwards G, McKinnon PS, Peloquin C, Morse GD, editors: *Antimicrobial therapy and vaccines, vol 2: ed 2, Antimicrobial agents*, Pittsburg, Pa, 2005, ESun Technologies.
30. Cunha BA: Nitrofurantoin: an update, *Obstet Gynecol Surv* 44:399, 1989.
31. Murray BE, Nannini EC: Glycopeptides (vancomycin and teichoplanin), streptogramins (quinupristin-dalfopristin), and lipopeptides (daptomycin). In Mandell GL, Bennet JE, Dolin R, editors: *Mandell, Douglas and Bennett's principles and practices of infectious disease*, vol 1 ed 6, New York, 2005, Elsevier, Churchill Livingstone.
32. Clemett D, Markham A: Linezolid, *Drugs* 59:815, 2000.
33. American Thoracic Society: Targeted tuberculin testing and treatment of latent tuberculosis infection, *MMWR Recomm Rep* 49(RR-6):1, 2000.
34. Van Scoy RE, Wilkowske CJ: Antimycobacterial therapy, *Mayo Clin Proc* 74:1038, 1999.
35. Kauffman CA, Carver PL: Antifungal agents in the 1990s: current status and future developments, *Drugs* 53:539, 1997.
36. Groll AH, Kolve H: Antifungal agents: *in vitro* susceptibility testing, pharmacodynamics, and prospects for combination therapy. In Yu VL, Edwards G, McKinnon PS, Peloquin C, Morse GD, editors: *Antimicrobial therapy and vaccines, vol 2: Antimicrobial agents*, ed 2, Pittsburg, Pa, 2005, ESun Technologies.
37. Herbrecht R, Nivoix Y, Fohrer C, Nataarajan-Ame S, Letscher-Bru V: Management of systemic fungal infections: alternatives to itraconazole, *J Antimicrobial Chemother* 56:39, 2005.

38. Dupont B: Overview of the lipid formulations of amphotericin B, *J Antimicrobial Chemother* 49(suppl 1):31, 2002.

39. Courtney R, Radwanski E, Lim J, Laughlin M: Pharmacokinetics of posaconazole coadministered with antacid in fasting and nonfasting healthy men, *Antimicrob Agents Chemother* 48:799, 2004.

40. Walsh TJ, Viviani MA, Arathoon E, Chiou C, Ghannoum M, Groll AH, Odds FC: New targets and delivery systems for antifungal therapy, *Med Mycol* 38(suppl 1):335, 2000.

41. Krause DS, Reinhardt J, Vazquez JA, Reboli A, Goldstein BP, Wible M, Hinkel T: Phase 2, randomized, dose-ranging study evaluating the safety and efficacy of anidulafungin in invasive candidiasis and candidemia, *Antimicrob Agents Chemother,* 48:2021, 2004.

42. Keating MR: Antiviral agents for non-human immunodeficiency virus infections, *Mayo Clin Proc* 74:1266, 1999.

43. Freeman RB: Valganciclovir: oral prevention and treatment of cytomegalovirus in the immuno-compromised host, *Expert Opin Pharmacother* 5:2007, 2004.

44. Plosker GL, Noble S: Cidofovir: a review of its use in cytomegalovirus retinitis in patients with AIDS, *Drugs* 58:325, 1999.

45. Perry CM, Barman-Balfour JA: Fomivirsen, *Drugs* 57:375, 1999.

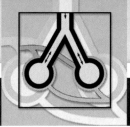

Chapter 15

Cold and Cough Agents

DOUGLAS S. GARDENHIRE

CHAPTER OUTLINE

CHAPTER OBJECTIVES

After reading this chapter, the reader will be able to:
1. Differentiate between the common cold and the flu
2. Differentiate between the specific types of cold and cough agents
3. Discuss the mode of action for each specific cold and cough agent

KEY TERMS AND DEFINITIONS

Antihistamines — Drugs that reduce the effects mediated by histamine, a chemical released by the body during allergic reactions. It is often administered to reduce secretions (e.g., runny nose and sneezing), but can cause drowsiness and impaired responses. *Note:* Drying of secretion, whether caused by antimuscarinic or antihistamine action, may suppress a needed defense reaction of the airways. Nocturnal use is more indicated than around-the-clock use

Antitussives — Drugs that suppress the cough reflex. *Note:* Productive coughs should not be suppressed, and the logic therefore of an expectorant-antitussive combination is questionable

Common cold — A nonbacterial respiratory tract infection, characterized by malaise and a runny nose

Expectorants — Drugs that increase the stimulation of mucus. Many have questionable efficacy in a cold. The best expectorant, especially with colds, is plain water and juices, avoiding caffeinated beverages such as tea or colas and beer or other alcoholic mixtures

Flu — A nonbacterial infection with rapid onset of symptoms, including fever, headache, and fatigue

Mucolytic expectorants — Agents that facilitate removal of mucus by a lysing, or *mucolytic,* action. *Example:* dornase alfa

Stimulant expectorants — Agents that increase the production and therefore presumably the clearance of mucus secretions in the respiratory tract. *Example:* guaifenesin

Sympathomimetics — Drugs that partially or completely mimic the effects of the sympathetic nervous system. *Note:* Tremor, tachycardia, and increased blood pressure can occur with their use, especially when taken orally. Rebound congestion can occur if used for longer than a day

---

Bewildering and in some cases irrational numbers of compounds, both prescription and over-the-counter (OTC), are available for treating symptoms of the common cold.

Common cold: The term "common cold" is used to describe nonbacterial upper respiratory tract infections (URIs), usually characterized by a mild general malaise, and a runny, stuffy nose.

Other symptoms include sneezing, possible sore throat, cough, and possibly some chest discomfort. Allergic rhinitis is *not* included in this discussion, nor are serious illnesses such as influenza, acute bronchitis, or infections of the lower respiratory tract. Influenza, or the **"flu,"** caused by the influenza virus is associated with symptoms of fever, headache, general muscle ache, and extreme fatigue or weakness. Onset of symptoms is usually rapid. The fever and systemic symptoms with influenza are contrasted with symptoms of the common cold in Table 15-1.

Four classes of agents can be distinguished in cold remedies, used individually or in combination, as follows:

Sympathomimetics: For decongestion
Antihistamines: To reduce (dry) secretions
Expectorants: To increase mucus clearance
Antitussives: To suppress the cough reflex

These four classes of cold medications target the primary symptoms caused by the cold virus in the respiratory tract. This is illustrated conceptually in Figure 15-1. Each class is discussed briefly, with representative agents listed. In addition to these four types of ingredients, an analgesic such as acetaminophen may be included, as in Sinutab, which consists of 30 mg of pseudoephedrine (decongestant) and 325 mg of acetaminophen (analgesic).

SYMPATHOMIMETIC (ADRENERGIC) DECONGESTANTS

KEY POINT

Adrenergic agents act to vasoconstrict and relieve *nasal congestion.*

Sympathomimetic (adrenergic) agents are discussed in their use as bronchodilators in Chapter 6, and the general effects of sympathetic stimulation are outlined in Chapter 5. In cold remedies, sympathomimetics are intended for a *decongestant* effect, which is based on their α-stimulating property and resulting vasoconstriction.

TABLE 15-1		
Differences in Symptoms Between the Common Cold and Influenza		
Signs and Symptoms	Cold	Influenza
Fever	Rare	Typical, high
Chills	None	Typical
Cough	Present, hacking	Nonproductive, may be severe
Headache	Rare	Prominent
Fatigue	Mild	Early and severe
Myalgia	None or slight	Usual, may be severe
Nasal congestion	Common	Occasional
Sneezing	Common	Occasional
Sore throat	Common	Occasional

TABLE 15-2	
Examples of Adrenergic Agents Used as Nasal Decongestants	
Drug	Route
Phenylephrine (Neo-Synephrine)	Topical, oral
Pseudoephedrine HCl (Sudafed, various)	Oral
Pseudoephedrine sulfate (Drixoral)	Oral
Xylometazoline (Otrivin)	Topical
Naphazoline (Privine)	Topical
Tetrahydrozoline (Tyzine)	Topical
Oxymetazoline (Afrin)	Topical

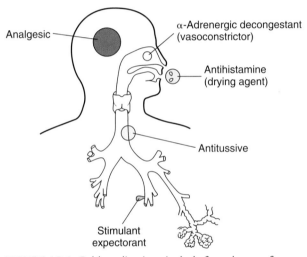

FIGURE 15-1 Cold medications include four classes of drugs, targeted at the symptoms produced by this upper respiratory viral infection, along with analgesics.

Sympathomimetics such as pseudoephedrine are found under brand names such as Sudafed and Dimetap and can be taken orally. Because of changes in the U.S. Patriot Act single agents or combination drugs using pseudoephedrine will be placed behind the counter and regulated sales will be documented, because the drug was being overpurchased for use in methamphetamines. Manufacturers have turned to phenylephrine as a substitute; however, the U.S. Food and Drug Administration (FDA)-approved dose of 10 mg has little effect on nasal decongestion when used orally because of the drug's high first-pass effect. In a study by McLaurin and associates[1] it was found that 10 mg of phenylephrine was no more effective than placebo. Oxymethazoline, a sympathomimetic with brand names such as Afrin and Vicks Sinex,

can be used topically for the nasal mucosa. In general, topical applications require lower dosages than oral use. Problems can occur with either route of administration. Table 15-2 lists sympathomimetic agents used as nasal decongestants in cold remedies.

Topical Application

Topical sympathomimetic decongestant sprays or drops produce results faster than oral applications. However, repeated use can cause the mucosa to swell, which is known as *rebound congestion*. Rebound nasal congestion occurs with overuse of these agents, the result of which is that the vasoconstriction does not occur.

Systemic Application

Systemic, compared with topical, application has the advantage of giving more extensive decongestant effects involving deeper blood vessels. However, producing nasal vasoconstriction through systemic routes will often lead to other systemic effects of sympathomimetics, such as a rise in blood pressure and increased heart rate.

ANTIHISTAMINE AGENTS

Histamine occurs naturally in the body, and is contained in tissue mast cells and blood basophils. The role of the mast cell in releasing histamine with allergic asthma is discussed in Chapters 11 and 12.

Effect of Histamine

Histamine is an important mediator of local inflammatory responses. Histamine can cause smooth muscle contraction, increased capillary permeability and dilation, itching, and pain. Scraping a tongue depressor or blunt pencil across the sensitive skin of the inner arm can illustrate a local inflammatory reaction at least partly mediated by histamine. The result is a *wheal and flare* reaction, also called a *triple response* (local redness, welt formation, and a reddish-white border). The redness and wheal (welt) are caused by dilation and leakage of plasma proteins from skin capillaries. The exudation of plasma causes the swelling. The flare, or reddish-white area surrounding the wheal, is probably due to local axon reflexes from sensory fibers causing dilation of neighboring arterioles.

Histamine Receptors

Histamine (H) produces its inflammatory effects by stimulating specific cell surface receptors. Three types of histamine receptors have been discovered. Two of the receptors are distinguished in mediating local inflammatory responses.

H_1 **receptors:** Located on nerve endings and smooth muscle and glandular cells. These receptors are involved in inflammation and allergic reactions, producing wheal and flare reactions in the skin, bronchoconstriction and mucus secretion, nasal congestion and irritation, and hypotension in anaphylaxis.

H_2 **receptors:** Located in the gastric region. These receptors regulate gastric acid secretion, as well as feedback control of histamine release.[2]

H_3 **receptors:** Located primarily in the central nervous system. These receptors may be autoreceptors for cholinergic neurotransmission in the airway at the autonomic ganglia, involved in central nervous system functioning and feedback control of histamine synthesis and release.[2,3]

The typical antihistamine found in cold medications is an H_1-receptor antagonist. Examples of these are pyrilamine and chlorpheniramine. H_1-receptor antagonists block the bronchopulmonary and vascular actions of histamine, to prevent rhinitis and urticaria. H_2-receptor antagonists are exemplified by cimetidine (Tagamet) or ranitidine (Zantac), which are used to block gastric acid secretion when treating ulcers.

Antihistamine Agents

KEY POINT

Antihistamines *dry secretions* through an anticholinergic effect, as well as by blockade of H_1 receptors.

All of the antihistamines considered in this chapter are H_1-receptor antagonists. These antihistamine agents are further classified into the major groups given in Table 15-3. The first five groups of antihistamines listed in Table 15-3 are all first-generation agents and can be found in cold preparations. Some of the brand

TABLE 15-3

Major Groups of Antihistamines With Representative Agents by Nonproprietary and Brand Names

Group	Drug
First Generation (Nonselective)	
Ethanolamine derivatives	Diphenhydramine HCl (Benadryl)
	Clemastine (Tavist)
	Carbinoxamine (Histex, Palgic)
Piperazine	Hydroxyzine (Vistaril)
Piperidine derivatives	Cyproheptadine
	Phenindamine (Nolahist)
Phenothiazine derivatives	Promethazine HCl (Phenergan)
Alkylamine derivatives	Chlorpheniramine (Chlor-Trimeton)
	Brompheniramine (LoHist, Bidhist)
	Dexchlorpheniramine maleate (various)
	Triprolidine (Zymine)
Second Generation (Peripherally Selective)	
Nonsedating, Long Acting	
Phthalazinone	Azelastine (Astelin)
Piperidines	Loratadine (Claritin)
	Fexofenadine (Allegra)
	Desloratadine (Clarinex)
Piperazine	Cetirizine (Zyrtec)

names given may be familiar from OTC preparations readily available in drugstores. Others are found in combination products; these are discussed and listed subsequently. Second-generation antihistamines, which are longer acting and nonsedating, are also listed in Table 15-3.

Effects of Antihistamines

Antihistamines have three major classes of effects: antihistaminic, sedative, and anticholinergic activity. Second-generation agents are selective for H_1 receptors and are less sedating than first-generation agents. Antihistaminic activity blocks the increased vascular permeability, pruritus, and bronchial smooth muscle constriction caused by histamine. These actions are the reason antihistamines are used to treat allergic disorders such as rhinoconjunctivitis, allergic rhinitis, and urticaria.

The sedative effect of antihistamines is thought to be caused by penetration of the agents into the brain, where inhibition of histamine *N*-methyltransferase and blockage of central histaminergic receptors occurs. There is also antagonism of other central nervous system receptors, such as serotonin and acetylcholine.[2] The effect of drowsiness with the classic (older) antihistamines can be a major hazard if alertness is required, such as in operating heavy machinery (e.g., a car) or monitoring a patient. This effect can be so pronounced that diphenhydramine HCl is added to acetaminophen in Tylenol PM, and the compound is described as a non-prescription sleep aid.

Finally, the anticholinergic effect produces considerable upper airway drying, just as would occur with an antimuscarinic agent such as atropine sulfate. In addition, effects seen with cholinergic blockade may occur, including central nervous system effects of stimulation, anxiety, and nervousness, as well as peripheral effects of dilated pupils, blurred vision, urinary retention, and constipation.[3] These effects are less likely in occasional use with a cold, but they may be significant with greater use (and dose) for allergic rhinitis or other conditions (e.g., urticaria).

KEY POINT

Antihistamines dry secretions, but can cause *impaction of secretions* and possible sinus blockage, and should be used sparingly. Use during work should be avoided because of the side effect of *drowsiness*.

The duration of action of the older antihistamines is generally 4 to 6 hours. However, newer, second-generation agents, often termed "nonsedating," are effective for up to 12 hours or more, depending on dose, and lack the sedating and anticholinergic effects. These newer agents are exemplified by fexofenadine (Allegra) and cetirizine (Zyrtec). These agents are also listed in Table 15-3. The second-generation agents have little affinity for muscarinic cholinergic receptors and therefore do not cause dry mouth or gastrointestinal side effects. They also lack antiserotonin activity and do not cause appetite stimulation and weight gain, although astemizole and ketotifen may differ in this.[3] These newer drugs may inhibit mediator release from allergic inflammatory cells, in addition to blocking the histamine receptor. Allergic symptoms of sneezing and rhinorrhea are equally well controlled with first-generation and second-generation H_1 antagonists.[3]

Structure–Activity Relations

H_1-receptor antagonists were first discovered in 1937.[4] The chemical structure of histamine, the general structure of the H_1-receptor antagonists, and two examples of H_1-receptor antagonists are given in Figure 15-2. Chlorpheniramine is an antihistamine found in many cold remedies; it represents one of the older, classic H_1-receptor antagonists. Fexofenadine is a newer, nonsedating H_1-receptor antagonist.

The resemblance between histamine and the general formula for the H_1-blocking agents can be seen in the structures shown. In the older agents, exemplified by chlorpheniramine, the R_1 and R_2 attachments are usually a ring structure connected to an ethylamine (C–C–N) group. The presence of the ring structures and other substitutions on the structure makes the older antihistamines lipophilic. As a result, the classic first-generation antihistamines readily penetrate into the central nervous system and produce the effect of sedation and drowsiness previously discussed. The newer, nonsedating agents, such as terfenadine, do not readily cross the blood–brain barrier and therefore do not block central H_1 receptors.[4]

Use With Colds

One of the beneficial effects of antihistamine use with a cold is the drying of upper airway secretions, which lessens the rhinitis and accompanying sneezing. There is some question whether the drying of secretions is due to histamine antagonism or to the anticholinergic effect of these agents. How much histamine release occurs with colds is debated. In allergic rhinitis, there is no question that histamine causes much of the inflammatory response, and in fact the newer long-acting agents are particularly helpful with this condition. Blockade of H_1 receptors prevents the histamine contribution to the symptoms of nasal itching, congestion, sneezing, rhinorrhea, and ocular irritation.

KEY POINT

Adrenergic decongestants are useful for nasal clearing, but *rebound congestion* can occur.

Regardless of the exact effect, the drying of runny nasal secretions is welcomed by cold sufferers, and this coupled with drowsiness can be useful to produce needed rest and sleep at night. Secretions, however, are a defense mechanism with an upper airway viral infection. Antihistamines may cause harm as a result of suppressed secretion clearance and impacted secretions with sinus blockage. Adequate hydration with a cold is always helpful, with or without use of antihistamines.

An alternative to antihistamines for rhinorrhea in a cold is the anticholinergic nasal spray *ipratropium*

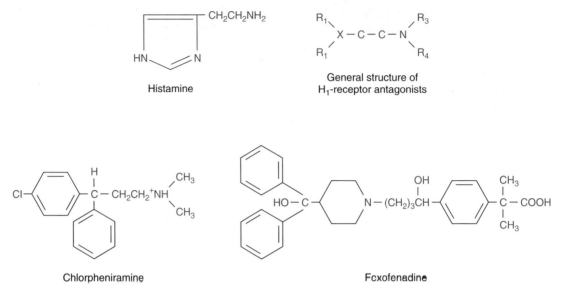

FIGURE 15-2 The structure of histamine, an inflammatory mediator; the general structure of H_1-receptor antagonists; and the structure of two antihistamines, chlorpheniramine and fexofenadine, are shown. R_1 to R_4 indicate the sites of attachments, with R_1 and R_2 being ring structures in most H_1 antagonists.

bromide (Atrovent), which is discussed in Chapter 7. Ipratropium has been shown to be effective in reducing nasal discharge in viral infectious rhinitis (colds), as well as allergic and nonallergic rhinitis.[5] There is no evidence of rebound congestion, mucosal irritation, or significant systemic effects. It can be effective for 4 to 8 hours. An anticholinergic agent applied topically offers an attractive alternative to both vasoconstricting decongestants and antihistamine H_1 antagonists.

Treatment of Seasonal Allergic Rhinitis

The second-generation H_1-receptor antagonists are more useful in the treatment of seasonal allergic rhinitis, as well as other disorders requiring antihistamine treatment, than in the treatment of colds. They are also better tolerated in treating allergic rhinitis than the first-generation agents, because side effects of drowsiness are minimal and duration of action is longer. Agents such as astemizole, loratadine, fexofenadine, and cetirizine are indicated for use in seasonal allergic rhinitis and chronic urticaria. They are intended to relieve symptoms of sneezing; rhinorrhea; itchy nose, palate, and throat; itchy, watery eyes; and pruritus. Categories and examples of agents used in the treatment of seasonal allergic rhinitis are summarized in Table 15-4.[6] Other uses of antihistamines include the treatment of symptoms seen with motion sickness and control of nausea.

TABLE 15-4

Categories of Agents Used in Treating Seasonal Allergic Rhinitis

Category	Example
H_1-Receptor antagonists	Cetirizine
Corticosteroids	Budesonide, ciclesonide
Mediator antagonist	Cromolyn sodium
Anticholinergics	Ipratropium bromide
Vasoconstrictors	Pseudoephedrine
Specific immunotherapy	Standardized extracts

EXPECTORANTS

Expectorants are defined as agents that facilitate removal of mucus from the lower respiratory tract. A distinction is made in Chapter 9 (Mucus-controlling Drug Therapy) between the following types of expectorants:

Mucolytic expectorants: Agents that facilitate removal of mucus by a lysing, or mucolytic, action. *Example:* dornase alfa

Stimulant expectorants: Agents that increase the production and therefore presumably the clearance of mucus secretions in the respiratory tract. *Example:* guaifenesin

In general, the expectorants considered here are stimulants, although the action does not always allow clear distinction. An example is guaifenesin, which is thought to reduce the adhesiveness and surface tension of mucus, and thus increase *mucokinesis*, that is, movement and clearance of the secretion. Another term used with these agents is *mucoevacuant*.

Efficacy and Use

There is controversy over the effectiveness and use of expectorants. The issue is clouded by the following:

- Difficulty in assessing the effectiveness of expectorants and, in particular, lack of objective criteria to demonstrate effectiveness
- In conjunction with the first point, who would benefit from the use of expectorants? In particular, should expectorants be included in the treatment of cold symptoms, if a cold involves the upper respiratory tract?

KEY POINT

Expectorants *stimulate mucus* production, and cough suppressants *depress the cough* reflex. The use of expectorants is questionable in the uncomplicated cold, because the lower respiratory tract is not involved.

Use in Chronic Bronchitis

Petty reported the results of a national study evaluating use of the expectorant iodinated glycerol (Organidin).[7] Patients had chronic bronchitis, which is quite different from a common cold. The study concluded that in chronic obstructive bronchitis, iodinated glycerol was safe and effective. Its use improved cough symptoms, chest discomfort, ease in bringing up sputum, and sense of well-being. The duration of acute exacerbations of chronic bronchitis was decreased. It is reasonable that in bronchitis, symptoms and airflow will improve and further infection will be reduced if mucus clearance can be improved. However, in a study by Rubin and associates they found no change in lung function or sputum in patients with chronic bronchitis.[8]

Irwin and associates have released evidence-based guidelines in the diagnosis and management of cough.[9] The guidelines cover acute and chronic cough as well as specific diseases such as chronic bronchitis and cystic fibrosis. For specific guidelines access the above citation (available at http://www.chestjournal.org/cgi/content/full/129/1_suppl/1S; accessed April 2007).

Mode of Action

Stimulant expectorants are thought to work by a variety of means, depending on the agent. These mechanisms include the following:

- Vagal gastric reflex stimulation
- Absorption into respiratory glands to directly increase mucus production
- Topical stimulation with inhaled volatile agents

Guaifenesin, also known as glycerol guaiacolate, is classified as a category I agent, which is safe and effective.[10] Ziment[11] has reviewed the mechanisms of action with iodides, such as iodinated glycerol. Other agents, such as terpin hydrate, sodium citrate, ammonium chloride, and menthols, have no demonstrated efficacy.[10]

Because mucus incorporates water as it is produced, an adequate intake of plain water or other nondiuresing liquids (milk, fruit juices) can help preserve mucus viscosity and clearance, especially with a simple cold.

Expectorant Agents

Table 15-5 lists available expectorant agents. Major agents or groups of agents are briefly characterized.

Iodine Products

Potassium iodide is a very old agent that has been used as an expectorant in asthma and chronic bronchitis.[12] It has a direct mucolytic effect in sufficient concentrations. It also has an indirect effect on mucus viscosity by stimulating submucosal glands to produce new, lower viscosity secretions.

The exact mechanism of action with iodine products is unclear. Iodide appears to distribute to mucous glands, where it is secreted along with increased mucus. Iodide also stimulates the gastropulmonary reflex, has a mucolytic effect, and can stimulate ciliary activity.[11] Iodides are associated with hypersensitivity reactions in some individuals, and a case of pulmonary edema has been reported with its use.[13]

Guaifenesin (Glycerol Guaiacolate)

Guaifenesin by inhalation is also considered to be an emollient. In experimental animals, doses larger than those used in humans caused an increase in bronchial secretions. Guaifenesin taken orally is thought to reduce the adhesiveness and surface tension of mucus secretions, thereby enhancing mucus clearance. It is considered safe and effective by the FDA.

Topical Agents

Topical agents usually evoke memories of the heated humidifier (vaporizer) with clouds of steam scented with camphor, menthol, or (in the past) chloroform. These agents may still be found in use, but efficacy as an expectorant has not been shown. The burn risk of a hot vaporizer should preclude its use with the young or the old and debilitated.

Some research has shown that so-called bland aerosols of saline do increase sputum volume, possibly

TABLE 15-5	
A Partial List of Expectorants With Representative Brand Names	
Drug	**Representative Brand**
Guaifenesin (glycerol guaiacolate)	Robitussin, Mucinex
Iodinated glycerol	Iophen
Potassium iodide	SSKI, various

through reflex irritation of the bronchi and with increased secretion clearance as a result of coughing.[14] Certainly a particulate suspension may have the potential to function as an irritant to the upper airways.

Parasympathomimetics (Cholinergic Agents)

Using parasympathomimetic agents will stimulate mucous gland secretion, but the effect on other muscarinic receptors is too diffuse for practical use as an expectorant. For this reason, a drug such as pilocarpine is not used as an expectorant. Likewise, stimulation of the medulla can increase respiratory tract secretions, but stimulation of the central nervous system is hazardous (see discussion of central nervous system stimulants in Chapter 22).

COUGH SUPPRESSANTS (ANTITUSSIVES)

KEY POINT

Cough suppressants are useful for the treatment of a nonproductive, irritating, *dry, hacking cough.*

A fourth category of drugs used with colds and cold symptoms is the cough suppressant. Coughing is a defense mechanism to protect the upper airway from irritants such as dust particles or aerosols, liquids, and other foreign objects. This mechanism is a reflex, coordinated by a postulated cough center in the medulla. For detailed cough management guidelines refer to Irwin and associates.[9]

Agents and Mode of Action

Cough suppressants act by depressing the cough center in the medulla. Narcotics (see Chapter 22) exert powerful depressant effects on the medullary centers, including the CO_2 chemoreceptors, and are often used for this purpose. Common agents are codeine or hydrocodone. A commonly used nonnarcotic is dextromethorphan.

Box 15-1	Cough Suppressant Drugs

- Codeine sulfate (various brand names)
- Hydrocodone (Hycodan Syrup)
- Dextromethorphan (Hold DM, Trocal, Robitussin Cough Calmers, Benylin DM)
- Diphenhydramine (Bydramine, Tusstat)
- Benzonatate (Tessalon Perles)

Benzonatate (Tessalon), a nonnarcotic, is chemically related to the local anesthetic tetracaine and anesthetizes stretch receptors in the lungs and pleura. This inhibits the cough reflex at its source. There is no inhibitory effect on the central nervous system. The effect begins in 15 to 20 minutes and lasts between 3 and 8 hours.[15] The antihistamine *diphenhydramine* (Benadryl), available as a syrup, in liquid form, and in combination with other products, may be an effective cough suppressant. Diphenhydramine is becoming more common in the market because of increased abuse of dextromethorphan. It should be noted that persons taking any agent with diphenhydramine should be warned of the effect of drowsiness.

Some cough suppressants, or antitussives, contain *codeine*. In a dose below 15 mg, codeine does not produce analgesia in the adult. In the 10- to 20-mg range, there is an antitussive action. Above 30 mg, codeine produces analgesia. *Hydrocodone* produces an antitussive effect with a dose of approximately 5 mg. Box 15-1 lists common antitussive agents, many of which are used in cold compounds. Both dextromethorphan and codeine are available in OTC preparations. These two agents are considered to be preferred cough suppressants, based on both safety and efficacy. The need for a prescription antitussive is unusual, especially in a cold, with the availability of OTC preparations.

Use of Cough Suppressants

Several principles apply to the use of antitussives:
- They are helpful and indicated to suppress dry, hacking, nonproductive irritating coughs, especially if the coughing causes sleep loss. Furthermore, a constant nonproductive cough can cause irritation of the trachea, leading to more coughing.
- Do not suppress the cough reflex in the presence of copious bronchial secretions that need to be cleared. This includes situations of cystic fibrosis and other chronic obstructive lung diseases such as bronchitis. Excess mucus secretions from the lower respiratory tract are not present in an uncomplicated cold (see the definition of a *common cold* at the beginning of the

chapter) and indicate the need for further evaluation and possible treatment with an antibiotic.

- The combination of an expectorant and an antitussive in a cold medication is questionable. This amounts to suppressing the clearance mechanism while stimulating secretions to be cleared. Use of a single-entity cough preparation, such as Benylin DM (10 mg dextromethorphan per 5 ml) or Robitussin Pediatric (7.5 mg of dextromethorphan per 5 ml), to treat a dry, irritating cough is recommended.

The combination of expectorant and antitussive is based on the rationale that a dry, hacking, frequent cough can be better replaced by a less frequent but productive cough. It can be questioned whether this is needed in an uncomplicated cold. Also, many cold compounds combine an antihistamine to dry secretions with the expectorant that is to stimulate mucus production. The rationale for this is open to question.

COLD COMPOUNDS

A list of selected cold remedies, with the classes of agents included in the compounds, is given in Table 15-6. Table 15-6 includes single-ingredient products, such

as Neo-Synephrine, as well as examples of compounds with multiple drug classes, such as Pediacof Syrup. Some of the preparations in elixir form use significant amounts of alcohol as a solvent. For example, Nyquil Nighttime Cold/Flu liquid contains 25% alcohol, and Contac Severe Cold & Flu Nighttime Liquid has 18.5% alcohol. Another aspect of cold remedies that adds to their confusion is the variation in ingredients, all under the same basic brand name with suffixed initials to indicate substituted or deleted ingredients. For example, Robitussin Cold and Cough, Robitussin A-C Syrup, and Robitussin DAC all vary in ingredients, as seen in Table 15-6. Because these compounds change fairly rapidly, no list remains current in terms of what is on the market. However, the basic principle of the typical four classes of ingredients remains, and new compounds can be evaluated for particular uses by considering the effects of these four classes of agents.

Many of these compounds are available as OTC preparations, thus requiring no prescription. The possibility of overdosing and abuse by combining prescribed compounds and OTC compounds is very real. Often OTC preparations have the same classes of ingredients but in lower concentrations.

TABLE 15-6

Categories of Ingredients Found in Selected Cold Multicompound Medications

Trade Name	Adrenergic	Antihistamine	Expectorant	Antitussive
Sudafed (tablets)	Pseudoephedrine, 30 and 60 mg			
Neo-Synephrine	Phenylephrine, 1%			
Chlor-Trimeton Allergy (4-hr tablets)		Chlorpheniramine, 4 mg		
Robitussin			Guaifenesin, 100 mg/5 ml	
Benylin Adult				Dextromethorphan, 15 mg/5 ml
Dimetane (decongestant, caplets)	Phenylephrine, 10 mg	Brompheniramine, 4 mg		
Mytussin DM (liquid)			Guaifenesin, 100 mg	Dextromethorphan, 10 mg
Polaramine (expectorant, liquid)	Pseudoephedrine, 20 mg	Dexchlorpheniramine, 2 mg	Guaifenesin, 100 mg	
Hycomine (compound, tablets)	Phenylephrine, 10 mg	Chlorpheniramine, 2 mg		Hydrocodone bitartrate, 5 mg
Novahistine DMX	Pseudoephedrine, 30 mg		Guaifenesin, 100 mg	
Pediacof (syrup)	Phenylephrine, 2.5 mg	Chlorpheniramine, 0.75 mg	Potassium iodide, 75 mg	Codeine, 5 mg
Robitussin Cold and Cough	Pseudoephedrine, 30 mg		Guaifenesin, 200 mg	Dextromethorphan, 10 mg
Robitussin-DAC	Pseudoephedrine, 30 mg		Guaifenesin, 100 mg	Codeine, 10 mg
Robitussin A-C Syrup			Guaifenesin, 100 mg	Codeine, 10 mg

Treating a Cold

There is no cure for the common cold, and the four classes of drugs used in cold remedies treat only symptoms. Furthermore, their potentially undesirable effects should be considered:

Sympathomimetics: Tremor, tachycardia, and increased blood pressure can be seen, especially when used orally. Rebound congestion can occur if used for longer than a day.

Antihistamines: Can cause drowsiness and impaired responses. Drying of secretions, whether caused by antimuscarinic or antihistamine action, may suppress a needed defense reaction of the airways. Nocturnal use is more indicated than around-the-clock use.

Expectorants: Many have questionable efficacy in a cold. The best expectorant, especially with colds, is plain water and juices, avoiding caffeinated beverages such as tea or colas and beer or other alcoholic mixtures.

Antitussives: Useful in the presence of an irritating, persistent, nonproductive cough. However, productive coughs should not be suppressed, and the logic therefore of an expectorant–antitussive combination is questionable.

A combination of all four classes of drugs in one compound does not allow acute or occasional use of the sympathomimetic for decongestion, nocturnal use of antihistamines, and separate use of an expectorant or antitussive, as indicated by symptoms. Single-entity cold medications, such as Sudafed for decongestion or Benylin Adult for cough suppression, are available to treat specific symptoms based on the principles outlined. Fluids and rest remain a basic and rational approach to surviving colds and preventing spread of the rhinovirus, but is probably the least feasible for current lifestyles.

SELF-ASSESSMENT QUESTIONS

1. Identify the four classes of ingredients found in cold medications.
2. For each of the following agents, identify the category (e.g., adrenergic, antitussive, etc.): codeine, chlorpheniramine, phenylephrine, dextromethorphan, pseudoephedrine.
3. What is the intended purpose of α-adrenergic agents in cold medications?
4. What is the intended effect of antihistamines (H_1 blockers) in cold medications?
5. Are antihistamines in cold remedies H_1 or H_2 blockers?

SELF-ASSESSMENT QUESTIONS —cont'd

6. You drink several beers at a friend's house after taking a dose of Chlor-Trimeton. Should you drive home, and why or why not?
7. Identify the most common expectorant in over-the-counter (OTC) cold remedies.
8. Briefly explain how guaifenesin stimulates mucus production.
9. List some specific fluids you would recommend to someone with a cold.
10. Differentiate a "cold" from the "flu."

Answers to Self-Assessment Questions are found in Appendix A.

CLINICAL SCENARIO

A 24-year-old respiratory therapy student approaches you after class. He is a previously healthy male, within normal weight limits, and with mild but irregular physical activity. He complains of mild malaise, a runny stuffy nose, sneezing, and a slight sore throat.

What other symptoms would you ask about to differentiate his complaint as a cold versus the flu?

What is your conclusion, at this point?

Based on your information, what would you suggest to him for self-treatment?

Two days later, he complains of a productive cough with yellowish sputum, and his temperature is 99° F. He has chest ache on a deep breath and is feeling very tired. He reports that he had stayed up late the last two nights studying for a pharmacology examination.

What is your assessment now?

Answers to Clinical Scenario Questions are found in Appendix A.

References

1. McLaurin JW, Shipman WF, Rosedale R Jr: Oral decongestants: a double blind comparison study of the effectiveness of four sympathomimetic drugs: objective and subjective, *Laryngoscope* 71:54–67, 1961.
2. Simons FER, Simons KJ: Second-generation H_1-receptor antagonists, *Ann Allergy* 66:5, 1991.
3. Du Buske LM: Clinical comparison of histamine H_1-receptor antagonist drugs, *J Allergy Clin Immunol* 98:S307, 1996.
4. Woodward JK: Pharmacology of antihistamines, *J Allergy Clin Immunol* 86:606, 1990.

5. Meltzer EO: Intranasal anticholinergic therapy of rhinorrhea, *J Allergy Clin Immunol* 90:1055, 1992.

6. Bousquet J, Chanez P, Michel FB: Pathophysiology and treatment of seasonal allergic rhinitis, *Respir Med* 84(suppl A):11, 1990.

7. Petty TL: The National Mucolytic Study: results of a randomized, double-blind, placebo-controlled study of iodinated glycerol in chronic obstructive bronchitis, *Chest* 97:75, 1990.

8. Rubin BK, Ramirez O, Ohar JA: Iodinated glycerol has no effect on pulmonary function, symptom score, or sputum properties in patients with stable chronic bronchitis, *Chest* 109:348, 1996.

9. Irwin RS, Baumann MH, Bolser DC, Boulet LP, Braman SS, Brightling CE, Brown KK, Canning BJ, Chang AB, Dicpinigaitis PV, et al.; American College of Chest Physicians (ACCP): Diagnosis and management of cough executive summary: ACCP evidence-based clinical practice guidelines, *Chest* 129:1S, 2006.

10. Covington TR: OTC cough suppressants/expectorants, *Facts and Comparisons Drug Newsletter* 10:4, 1991.

11. Ziment I: Inorganic and organic iodides, In Braga PC, Allegra L, editors: *Drugs in bronchial mucology*, New York, 1989, Raven Press.

12. Alstead S: Potassium iodide and ipecacuanha as expectorants, *Lancet* 2:932, 1939.

13. Huang T, Peterson GH: Pulmonary edema and iododerma induced by potassium iodide in the treatment of asthma, *Ann Allergy* 46:264, 1981.

14. Pavia D, Thomason ML, Clarke SW: Enhanced clearance of secretions from the human lung after the administration of hypertonic saline aerosol, *Am Rev Respir Dis* 117:199, 1978.

15. *Drug Facts and Comparisons*, St. Louis, Mo, 2006, Facts and Comparisons, Wolters Kluwer Health.

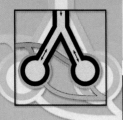

Chapter 16

Selected Agents of Pulmonary Value

DOUGLAS S. GARDENHIRE

CHAPTER OBJECTIVES

After reading this chapter, the reader will be able to:

1. Discuss the indication for α₁-proteinase inhibitor
2. Recognize α₁-proteinase inhibitor deficiency in a patient
3. List the α₁-proteinase inhibitors that are available
4. List three types of formulations for nicotine replacement
5. Recognize the advantages and disadvantages of nicotine replacement
6. Discuss the indication for nitric oxide
7. Describe the effect of inhaled nitric oxide on a patient
8. List the two toxic products of nitric oxide
9. List the only inhaled antidiabetic agent available in the United States

KEY TERMS AND DEFINITIONS

α_1-**Antitrypsin** — Also known as α_1-*proteinase inhibitor (API)*. An inhibitor of trypsin that may be deficient in patients with emphysema

API deficient — Individual has low serum levels of API possessing altered electrophoretic properties

API dysfunctional — Individual has normal serum levels of API that does not function normally

API normal — Individual has normal serum levels of API that functions normally

API null — Individual has undetectable serum levels of API

Chapter 16 presents three groups of drugs that are used for the direct treatment or prevention of respiratory disease. These include α_1-proteinase inhibitors, used in the treatment of congenital α_1-antitrypsin deficiency; nicotine replacement and other agents used in smoking cessation; and pulmonary vasiodilators, used for pulmonary hypertension states in newborns and in acute respiratory distress syndrome (ARDS) in adults. An orally inhaled insulin for the treatment of diabetes is described as well.

α_1-PROTEINASE INHIBITOR (HUMAN)

KEY POINT

α_1-Proteinase inhibitor is given intravenously to individuals with *congenital* α_1-*antitrypsin deficiency* and who exhibit panacinar emphysema at a prematurely early age.

α_1-Proteinase inhibitor (abbreviated as α_1-PI or simply API) is also known as **α_1-antitrypsin (α_1-AT)** and is intended for therapy of congenital α_1-antitrypsin deficiency, which leads to emphysema. The product is prepared from pooled human plasma from normal donors, with purification and treatment to remove potentially infectious agents. The disease state is usually termed *α_1-antitrypsin deficiency,* and the deficient protein is termed *α_1-proteinase inhibitor.* However, the terms *α_1-antitrypsin* and *α_1-proteinase inhibitor* are used interchangeably and refer to the same protein.

α_1-Antitrypsin Deficiency

α_1-Antitrypsin deficiency is a genetic defect that can lead to the development of severe panacinar emphysema. This autosomal recessive disorder is characterized by serum API levels below 35% of normal and presents as panacinar emphysema at age 30 to 50 years. It is estimated that API deficiency accounts for approximately 2% of all emphysema in the United States. It is estimated that there are 60,000 to 100,000 Americans with severe α_1-AT deficiency.[1,2]

Studies done in the United States vary in their estimates of the prevalence among newborns of α_1-AT deficiency, ranging from 1 in 2857 to 1 in 5097.[3] Among white individuals, α_1-AT deficiency is as common a genetic disorder as cystic fibrosis.[4] In about 50% of emphysema that results from API deficiency, there is accompanying chronic bronchitis with mucus hypersecretion, perhaps as a result of secretory cell metaplasia caused by unchecked proteases in the epithelial lining fluid.[5] Emphysema caused by API deficiency is worse in the lower lung zones and can be markedly accelerated by cigarette smoking.[1]

The basic pathology of emphysema resulting from API deficiency is an imbalance between proteases, especially neutrophil elastase (NE) and antiproteases, especially α_1-proteinase inhibitor. The main substrate for API is neutrophil elastase. The pathogenesis of emphysema is described as a process of alveolar wall destruction caused by insufficient protection from the protease neutrophil elastase, an enzyme that can cleave all forms of connective tissue and degrade elastic fiber in the lungs by solubilizing elastin. With inadequate API levels in the lung to balance the protease activity, emphysema results at a significantly earlier age than is normally seen. A presentation of severe emphysema at an unexpectedly young age, such as the third or fourth decade, leads to a high suspicion of a genetic defect causing inadequate API levels in the blood and subsequently in the lungs. The main role of another protease inhibitor, secretory leukocyte protease inhibitor (SLPI), which is secreted by bronchial glands and goblet cells, is to protect the airway epithelium against proteolytic injury. However, Wewers and associates[6] have provided evidence that α_1-proteinase inhibitor (α_1-antitrypsin) is the predominant antiprotease protecting against neutrophil elastase.

KEY POINT

Individuals who are homozygous (have both recessive alleles) for the defective gene that expresses *α_1-proteinase inhibitor (API)* lack this enzyme to balance the action of *neutrophil elastase (NE),* another enzyme in the lung that solubilizes connective tissue, causing alveolar wall destruction.

Genetics

α_1-Proteinase inhibitor is a 54-kDa glycoprotein, encoded by a single gene on chromosome 14. The alleles of the API gene can be categorized as follows[5]:

API normal: Normal serum levels of normal-functioning API
API deficient: Lower than normal serum concentrations of API with altered electrophoretic properties
API null: Undetectable API levels in the serum
API dysfunctional: Normal amounts of abnormally functioning API

Persons with normal alleles for API (designated by the letter *M* for the alleles) are termed *PI*MM,* for protease inhibitor with a pair of the normal alleles. They are homozygous for the normal allele. Normal values for serum API are 150 to 350 mg/dl, based on comparison with a commercial standard preparation, and 20 to 48 μM (micromolar) based on comparison with a purified laboratory standard. The commercially available preparations are about 40% higher in comparison with the purified laboratory standards. Results referenced to the commercial standard are expressed as milligrams per deciliter, whereas comparisons with the highly purified (true) standard are given in micromolar units. Commercial standard values can be converted to true standard values by multiplying the commercial value by 0.71.[5,6]

About 95% of persons in the severely deficient category are homozygous for the Z allele, and are designated as PI*ZZ. Serum levels of API in these individuals range from 2.5 to 7 μM, or a mean of about 16% of normal.[5] The Z allele is rare in Asians and African Americans. Alleles that do not express API at all are quite rare and such individuals are designated as PI type null-null. PI type null-null individuals have an absence of measurable API in the serum. Wewers and colleagues[6] describe the treatment of a patient with the null-null phenotype and no measurable API serum levels. They were able to show that intravenously administered augmentation therapy with α_1-AT (API) led to normal API levels in the blood, as well as in the lung epithelial lining fluid.

The major risk factor for developing emphysema among PI*ZZ subjects appears to be cigarette smoking, in which emphysema appears much earlier than in non-susceptible individuals, as previously noted. Other features seen with airflow obstruction in PI*ZZ individuals include a history of pneumonia, episodes of increased cough and sputum production, and a parental history of emphysema.[2]

Indication for Drug Therapy

α_1-Proteinase inhibitor therapy is indicated for chronic replacement therapy in individuals with congenital deficiency of API, with clinically demonstrable panacinar emphysema. At present there are three agents available: Aralast, Prolastin, and Zemaira. Aralast and Zemaira are indicated only for patients who have established α_1-proteinase deficiency. Prolastin is not indicated for use in patients other than those with the PI*ZZ, PI*Z-null, or PI*null-null phenotype. Subjects with the PI*MZ or PI*MS phenotype appear to be at low risk for panacinar emphysema.[7] Results from controlled, long-term trials are not available to show that chronic therapy halts the progression of emphysema because of inherent difficulties in such trials, including the need for large numbers of patients.[1] α_1-Proteinase inhibitor therapy has been provided only to adult subjects. Given the nature of the disease and the action of the drugs, the drugs cannot reverse damage or improve lung function. The drugs are extremely expensive, costing in the range of $25,000 to $40,000 per year for therapy. A cost-effectiveness analysis of Prolastin concluded that α_1-AT replacement therapy is cost effective in individuals who have severe α_1-AT deficiency and severe chronic obstructive pulmonary disease (COPD).[8]

The American Thoracic Society (ATS) states that API augmentation therapy should be used for patients with a serum concentration of API less than 11 μM, or 80 mg/dl.[2,9] It is not indicated for patients with cigarette smoking–related emphysema who have normal or heterozygous phenotypes.[5] It is not indicated for individuals with liver disease associated with API deficiency, unless they also have lung disease. The ATS guidelines suggest using augmentation therapy if lung function studies become abnormal and if serial studies show deterioration.

Dosage and Administration

The recommended dosage of API is 60 mg/kg of body weight, given once weekly. The dose is given intravenously at a rate of 0.08 ml/kg/min or greater, depending on patient comfort, and usually takes about 15-30 minutes for total infusion. A summary of Aralast, Prolastin, and Zemaira is given in Table 16-1.

Warnings and Adverse Reactions

Because API agents are derived from human plasma there is a risk of disease transmission. Although there was some variation in reactions to each API agent, fever, exacerbation, and flulike symptoms were most common.

TABLE 16-1

α₁-Proteinase Inhibitors Currently Available*

Brand Name	Strength
Aralast	400 and 800 mg
Prolastin	500 and 1000 mg
Zemaira	1000 mg†

*All agents are in powder form; reconstitution must take place before administration.
†Must be administered through a filter.

Respiratory Care Assessment of Therapy

Respiratory care assessment of α_1-AT replacement therapy is directed primarily at lung function and the rate of change of airflow obstruction in patients.

- Pulmonary function testing of flow rates is used to monitor the degree of airflow obstruction over long-term use of the drug.
- Smoking status should be monitored, and α_1-AT–deficient individuals who smoke should receive both education on the effect of smoking with this disease and direction to resources to aid in smoking cessation (drug therapy and behavior modification assistance).
- Overall pulmonary health should be assessed, based on frequency and severity of respiratory infections, cough, sputum production if present, and hospitalization rate.

SMOKING CESSATION DRUG THERAPY

> ### KEY POINT
>
> Smoking cessation agents include nicotine as a transdermal patch, chewing gum, nasal spray, or inhaler as substitute therapy for *smoking cessation* in those with a strong physical addiction and withdrawal symptoms from nicotine absorbed during smoking. A tapered dose regimen allows withdrawal with minimal symptoms and assists in reducing the craving for cigarettes. *Bupropion,* an antidepressant, and *varenicline* have been found to be helpful in smoking cessation.

Nicotine, along with lobeline, are naturally occurring alkaloids that are capable of stimulating acetylcholine receptors at the autonomic ganglia of both the sympathetic and parasympathetic systems, as well as cholinergic nicotinic receptors at skeletal muscle sites (see Chapter 5) and in the brain. The structures of these two agents are shown in Figure 16-1. It is the affinity

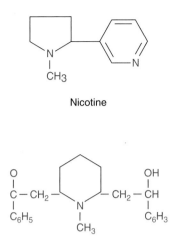

FIGURE 16-1 The chemical structures of nicotine and lobeline, both of which are nicotinic agonists.

of nicotine for ganglionic and neuromuscular receptor sites that led to the use of the term *nicotinic* to distinguish them from *muscarinic* receptors, because all of these receptors utilize acetylcholine as a neurotransmitter.

Lobeline is a plant derivative that has less potency than nicotine but a similar spectrum of action. Nicotine itself has greater affinity for ganglionic receptors than for skeletal muscle nicotinic receptors. The response to nicotine stimulation involves simultaneous discharge of both sympathetic and parasympathetic systems. The sympathetic effect predominates in the cardiovascular system, with hypertension, tachycardia, and peripheral vasoconstriction. Part of the sympathomimetic effect is mediated by nicotinic stimulation of receptors on the adrenal medulla, leading to release of epinephrine and norepinephrine. Nicotine produces a parasympathetic effect in the gastrointestinal and urinary tracts, with nausea, vomiting, diarrhea, and urination. Response to nicotine is dose dependent, and increasing or toxic doses can produce a depolarizing blockade of receptors. Stimulation of neuromuscular receptors causes tremor and loss of hand steadiness.

In addition to stimulating nicotinic receptors at the autonomic ganglia, neuromuscular junctions, and the adrenal medulla, nicotine binds to receptors in the central nervous system. This causes respiratory stimulation, tremors, convulsions, nausea, and emesis. The last two effects are often seen when nicotine is first inhaled as tobacco smoke, although tolerance rapidly occurs. Nicotine is the chief alkaloid in tobacco products, and addiction to nicotine is the basis for tobacco dependence. In the seasoned smoker, within seconds of inhaling from a cigarette, the internal carotid arteries carry a large bolus of nicotine to the brain, where it binds to nicotine receptors.[10] This binding causes secretion of dopamine, which causes a feeling of pleasure and cognitive arousal. Nicotine also increases levels of norepinephrine, β-endorphin, acetylcholine, serotonin, and other substances in the central nervous system, all of which increase the sensation of euphoria and well-being; enhance concentration, alertness, and memory; and decrease tension and anxiety. Sensitivity and responsiveness to nicotine in the central nervous system are genetically determined and constitute the basis for forming the physiological addiction to nicotine. Without the proper genetic substrate, a smoker cannot become nicotine dependent. About 10% of smokers lack this substrate and are not physiologically dependent; whereas 90% have the substrate and are nicotine addicted to various degrees.[10]

Cigarette smoking is a preventable cause of cardiovascular and lung disease and accelerates the rate of decline of lung function that occurs with aging, as shown in the Lung Health Study.[11] The Lung Health Study concluded that aggressive smoking intervention and cessation reduce the age-related decline in forced expiratory volume in 1 second (FEV_1) among middle-age smokers. Withdrawal from the nicotine in tobacco products is difficult because the stimulatory and reward effects are lost and physical symptoms occur. The latter include craving for nicotine, nervousness, irritability, anxiety, drowsiness, sleep disturbance, impaired concentration, and increased appetite with attendant weight gain. Nicotine replacement therapy, in various dosing formulations, is intended to aid with smoking cessation by allowing initial replacement and then gradual withdrawal of the nicotine found in tobacco. Because nicotine is well absorbed from the skin and mucosa, a transdermal patch, a chewable gum formulation, a nasal spray, and an inhaler have been developed.

Indication for Use

Nicotine replacement agents are indicated as an aid to smoking cessation to relieve nicotine withdrawal symptoms. Replacement therapy should be used as part of a comprehensive smoking cessation program to increase compliance and reduce relapse. Smokers with signs of a high physical dependence on nicotine may benefit the most from nicotine replacement therapy. Signs of strong physical dependence are listed in Box 16-1.[10]

| Box 16-1 | Signs of High Physical Addiction/Dependence on Nicotine |

- Smokes more than 15 cigarettes per day
- Prefers brands with nicotine levels above 0.9 mg
- Has habit of inhaling smoke frequently and deeply
- Smokes within 30 minutes of rising
- Finds it difficult to give up the first morning cigarette and smokes more frequently in the morning
- Smokes most frequently in the morning
- Finds it difficult to refrain from smoking in smoke-free environments
- Smokes even when ill enough to be bed-ridden

Drug Formulations

Smoking cessation drug therapy includes various formulations of nicotine and bupropion, an antidepressant found to be useful as an aid to smoking cessation. Table 16-2 lists pharmaceutical details on the various agents in use at the time of this edition. Ferrill[12] offers a survey and review of smoking cessation agents. Details on the nicotine substitute agents can be found in manufacturers' literature.[13]

Nicotine Polacrilex (Nicotine Resin Complex)

Nicotine polacrilex, a resin complex, is available as a chewing gum, as a lozenge, as a nasal spray, and as an inhaler.

Nicotine polacrilex gum contains nicotine bound to an ion-exchange resin in a chewing gum base. The gum can be difficult to chew, causing jaw ache, and has a bad taste. Absorption of the active nicotine can be inconsistent although it is faster than with the transdermal patch. The absorption of nicotine is reduced if acidic beverages such as coffee, soda, or orange juice are taken simultaneously. Users are instructed to chew the gum until malleable, then "park" it between the cheek and gum, repeating this every few minutes each time the taste is gone. Chewing slowly titrates the dose of nicotine received. Intermittent rather than continuous chewing slows the buccal absorption of the nicotine released. This will also slow the amount of nicotine swallowed, which is not well absorbed from the stomach and can cause gastrointestinal irritation. Each piece of gum (2 mg, 4 mg) delivers about 50% of its nicotine.

The *nicotine lozenge* is a hard resin complex that is bound with nicotine. The lozenge is to be placed in the user's mouth to slowly dissolve, with occasional transfer from side to side until dissolved. Users should refrain

TABLE 16-2

Smoking Cessation Drug Formulations

Category	Brand Name	Dosage
Nicotine transdermal system	NicoDermCQ	21 mg/day for first 6 wk, 14 mg/day for next 2 wk, 7 mg/day for last 2 wk
	Nicotrol	15 mg/day for first 12 wk, 10 mg/day for next 2 wk, 5 mg/day for last 2 wk
Nicotine polacrilex	Nicorette (gum)	2 mg if fewer than 25 cigarettes/day: 9 pieces/day; maximum 24 pieces/day; 4 mg if 25 or more cigarettes/day: 9 pieces/day; maximum of 24 pieces/day
	Commit (lozenge)	2 and 4 mg, no more than 5 lozenges in 6 hr, maximum 20 lozenges/day
	Nicotrol NS	0.5 mg/spray, one each nostril (1.0 mg); 1 or 2 doses/hr (2 sprays with nasal spray, 1 each nostril, is 1 dose), up to 5 doses/hr, or 40 doses/day
	Nicotrol Inhaler	4 mg/use; recommended dosage is 24 to 64 mg (6 to 16 cartridges) per day, up to 12 wk, with gradual reduction over a period up to 12 wk
Bupropion	Zyban	150-mg sustained-release tablets; begin at 150 mg/day for 3 days; increase to 150 mg/day bid, with maximum of 300 mg/day, interval of 8 hr between doses; continue treatment for 7-12 wk
Varenicline	CHANTIX	1 week titration of 0.5 mg once daily for first 3 days, twice daily for remainder of week. Begin 1 mg twice daily for 11 weeks

from drinking liquids 15 minutes before or during use, and should not chew or swallow the lozenge.

The *nicotine nasal spray* offers the advantage of producing rapid peak plasma levels of nicotine, by delivering the spray directly to the nasal membranes. This may help to reduce or control cravings to smoke. Irritant effects with the nasal spray may include runny nose and nasal irritation, sneezing, cough, and watery eyes. Although rapid relief may be obtained, administration is more obtrusive than with the patch or the gum formulations.

The *nicotine inhaler* offers smokers a "simulated cigarette"; the kit contains a 10-mg/cartridge unit dose, which delivers 4 mg/use, a mouthpiece, blister trays of nicotine cartridges, and a plastic case. The use of a mouthpiece resembling a cigarette holder allows delivery of the nicotine in a manner similar to smoking a cigarette, with oral gratification. This system delivers less nicotine than the other systems. All of the nicotine is absorbed across the oropharyngeal membranes.[10] The inhaler may be most useful in the low-dependency smoker, as an adjunct to the patch to treat sudden cravings, or in combination with bupropion.

Nicotine Transdermal System

The nicotine transdermal system is a multilayered unit that delivers nicotine for 24 hours after application to the skin. Approximately 68% of the nicotine released from the system enters the circulation. Products may differ in their kinetics. The transdermal product provides a more consistent level of nicotine than does the gum or lozenge. This is an easy, convenient, and

inconspicuous method of nicotine replacement delivery. A common side effect is skin irritation at the site, but this is minimized by alternating sites. Any skin site that is clean, dry, and hairless can be used. The largest patch (21 mg) is equal to approximately half a pack of cigarettes per day.

Bupropion (Zyban)

Bupropion is an antidepressant found in Wellbutrin; it is also a nonnicotine aid to smoking cessation. The drug is a relatively weak inhibitor of neuronal uptake of norepinephrine, serotonin, and dopamine, which is the basis for its antidepressant effect. The exact mechanism by which bupropion aids in smoking cessation is not known. Bupropion may relieve nicotine withdrawal by slowing the normal reuptake of dopamine or preventing its breakdown in the central nervous system. It has been shown that mood and emotional state are related to the need for smoking and nicotine, although bupropion is effective in smoking cessation even if the smoker is not depressed.[10] Symptoms of nicotine dependence among smokers are correlated with the magnitude of symptoms of depression. Subjects who are negative or depressed are less likely to be able to quit smoking. This would indicate that the antidepressant effect of bupropion assists in smoking cessation. Jorenby and associates[14] found little difference between a placebo group and a nicotine patch group in smoking cessation at 12 months (15.6 vs. 16.4%). However, a group receiving bupropion alone achieved a 30.3% cessation rate, and the combination of bupropion and nicotine patch gave the highest cessation rate of 35.5%.

This suggests that bupropion added to nicotine substitutes in a program of smoking cessation is helpful. Only about 6% of smokers succeed in quitting with no replacement therapy.[14]

If a patient has not made significant progress toward abstinence from smoking by week 7, it is unlikely that the effort will be successful and bupropion should be discontinued for that attempt. Dose tapering for discontinuation is not required.

Use of bupropion is associated with a dose-dependent risk of seizure. Doses below 300 mg/day are generally safer and have a risk of about 0.1% for seizure.

Coadministration of bupropion with a monoamine oxidase inhibitor (MAOI) or other medications containing bupropion is contraindicated. The drug should not be used by individuals with seizure disorders or with bulimia or anorexia nervosa, which have a higher incidence of seizures.

Varenicline (CHANTIX)

Varenicline is a selective $\alpha_4\beta_2$ nicotinic acetylcholine receptor partial agonist developed for explicit use in smoking cessation. Varenicline works by attaching to $\alpha_4\beta_2$ receptors, inhibiting the activation of this receptor by nicotine. This blocks the sensation produced by smoking, thereby breaking the cycle of nicotine addition.

In clinical trials, varenicline produced a 39% quit rate compared with bupropion (20%) and 11% for placebo after 12 weeks.[15] In another study, varenicline produced quit rates of 44 and 49%, respectively, at lower and higher doses of the drug compared with placebo at 12%.[16]

Varenicline is administered in a 12-week-long treatment process that begins with a 1-week titration process. The most common adverse reactions found with varenicline were nausea, insomnia, constipation, and vomiting.

Precautions

Individuals undergoing nicotine replacement therapy should be informed that the replacement formulations do contain active nicotine. If taken while still using tobacco products, potentially toxic concentrations of nicotine can occur in the blood. Individuals should stop smoking when initiating therapy. Transference of nicotine dependency from the tobacco product to the replacement product can occur. Use within a program of smoking cessation is encouraged to achieve complete withdrawal. Replacement formulations should be gradually withdrawn and stopped by 3 months. Use of nicotine replacement therapy should be carefully weighed in patients with cardiovascular disease, including coronary artery disease, cardiac arrhythmias, or vasospastic disease, and in patients with hypertension.

Health care workers should avoid handling active nicotine products, such as patches, because nicotine is easily absorbed through the skin. Washing with soap will increase absorption; so only water should be used. Used products must be disposed of properly, so that children or pets are not exposed.

Respiratory Care Assessment of Therapy

The primary outcome of interest with smoking cessation drug therapy is success in quitting over the long term.

- Monitor abstinence rates at intervals such as 3, 6, or 12 months.
- Monitor for symptoms of nicotine overdosage (possible if subjects continue smoking while using nicotine substitutes), such as nausea, salivation, abdominal pain, vomiting, diarrhea, cold sweat, headache, dizziness, disturbed vision and hearing, mental confusion, or marked weakness.
- Assess bupropion use for improvement in emotional attitude, including reduction in irritability, anxiety, difficulty in concentrating, or depression.
- Assess varenicline use for improvement in nicotine withdrawal symptoms.
- Assess patients for weight gain, and encourage a program of exercise to prevent relapse caused by desire for appetite control.
- Continue to provide counseling and support throughout treatment for smoking cessation.

NITRIC OXIDE

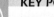

KEY POINT

Nitric oxide is approved for *pulmonary vascular relaxation* and is used in the treatment of *persistent pulmonary hypertension of the newborn* and investigationally in *acute respiratory distress syndrome (ARDS)* of the adult.

Nitric oxide (NO) is a product of endothelial cells that acts as a nitrovasodilator. It was investigated for its ability to lower pulmonary vascular resistance in various disease states, such as persistent pulmonary hypertension of the newborn (PPHN) and ARDS. Furchgott and Zawadzki have shown that endothelial cells in blood vessels elaborate a short-lived vasodilator, which was termed endothelium-derived relaxing factor (EDRF).[17] The neurotransmitter acetylcholine, which can normally dilate blood vessels, has no effect or even vasoconstricts if applied to blood vessels without endothelium. Subsequently, the substance EDRF was identified by Palmer and colleagues[18] and Ignarro and colleagues[19] as nitric oxide. This endogenously produced vasodilator can be inhaled as a gas to cause pulmonary vasodilation.

Indication for Use

Nitric oxide is approved for use in neonates with hypoxic respiratory failure, to reduce pulmonary artery pressure and to increase oxygenation in newborns with pulmonary hypertension and hypoxia. Off-label use for nitric oxide have been made to adults; however, data on its effectiveness are conflicting.[13]

- *Nitric oxide (INOmax)* is used in conjunction with ventilatory support and other critical care in the treatment of term and near-term (>34 weeks) neonates with hypoxic respiratory failure associated with clinical or echocardiographic evidence of pulmonary hypertension.

Off-label uses of nitric oxide include reduction of pulmonary vascular resistance and pulmonary artery pressure during neonatal cardiac surgery, treatment of hypoxemia or pulmonary hypertension after lung transplantation, and treatment of ARDS. Nitric oxide has been approved with an orphan drug designation.

Dosage and Administration

Nitric oxide, supplied in two sizes of gas cylinder, is available at 100 and 800 ppm. The recommended dose is 20 ppm. The treatment should be maintained up to 14 days or until the underlying oxygenation problem has resolved and the neonate can be successfully weaned from nitric oxide. In the Neonatal Inhaled Nitric Oxide Study (NINOS) trial, the majority of patients who failed to improve on 20 ppm, and whose dose was increased to 80 ppm, had no response at the higher concentration.[20] The risk of methemoglobinemia and elevated nitrogen dioxide (NO_2) levels increases significantly above 20 ppm, as discussed below.

The safety and effectiveness of nitric oxide were established in patients receiving other critical care support for hypoxic respiratory failure, including vasodilators, intravenous fluids, bicarbonate therapy, and mechanical ventilation. Additional therapies might be needed to maximize oxygen delivery, such as surfactant administration and high-frequency oscillatory ventilation. Information about the effectiveness of nitric oxide therapy in infants older than 14 days or adults is not available.

In the clinical trials of nitric oxide, the delivery system used was the INOvent system, which gives a constant concentration of nitric oxide during the respiratory cycle, with minimal nitrogen dioxide generation.

The following summarizes guidelines for the safe administration of nitric oxide, based on several sources listed in the references, including a statement by the American Academy of Pediatrics.[3,21,22]

- Blending and delivery systems should be designed and tested for accurate nitric oxide delivery, minimum nitrogen dioxide production, and capability of administering nitric oxide in constant concentration ranges in parts per million or less throughout the respiratory cycle.
- The delivery system should be calibrated using a precisely defined mixture of nitric oxide and nitrogen dioxide.
- Sample gas for analysis should be drawn before the Y-piece, proximal to the patient.
- Inhaled nitric oxide and nitrogen dioxide should be monitored continuously, using chemiluminescence or electrochemical analyzers.
- Oxygen levels in the inspired gas should be measured.
- Blood methemoglobin levels should be measured frequently.
- The minimal effective concentration of nitric oxide should be used.
- Weaning from nitric oxide should be gradual to prevent arterial desaturation and pulmonary hypertension.
- Because inhaled nitric oxide is used in respiratory failure, institutions that offer nitric oxide therapy generally should have extracorporeal membrane oxygenation (ECMO) capability in the event nitric oxide therapy fails. Alternatively, a plan for timely transfer of infants to a collaborating ECMO center should be established prospectively, and transfer should be accomplished without interruption of nitric oxide therapy.

The second-to-last point is particularly significant in the clinical use of nitric oxide to manage pulmonary hypertension. When withdrawing nitric oxide, rebound hypertension occurs; this can be severe and cause oxygen desaturation. This may be due to a downregulating effect on endogenous nitric oxide production in the pulmonary endothelium. The vasodilating effect of inhaled nitric oxide ends with the removal of the gas because of its short half-life (as subsequently described), a result of its binding to hemoglobin. An increase in the fractional concentration of oxygen in inspired gas (FIO_2) up to 1.0

may be needed as the inhaled nitric oxide is terminated. The FiO_2 can then be reduced over the next few hours as pulmonary hemodynamics restabilize. Close monitoring of arterial oxygenation is critical when weaning from nitric oxide.

KEY POINT

Nitric oxide is administered as an inhaled gas; it readily diffuses into the vascular endothelium, where it *stimulates guanylyl cyclase* in the cell, *increases cGMP*, and produces *smooth muscle relaxation*. Nitric oxide also quickly diffuses into the bloodstream, where it is *inactivated by binding to hemoglobin*, producing methemoglobin. Nitric oxide has a *short half-life* of less than 5 seconds because it is quickly bound by hemoglobin. In the presence of oxygen, nitric oxide is converted to *nitrogen dioxide*, a nitrite toxic to the lung.

Pharmacology of Nitric Oxide

The formation, mode of action, and fate of endogenous nitric oxide are diagrammed in Figure 16-2. Nitric oxide is formed endogenously in vascular endothelial cells of the respiratory tract from the precursor amino acid L-arginine by several isoforms of the enzyme nitric oxide synthase (NOS). Nitric oxide synthase requires the cosubstrates nicotinamide adenine dinucleotide phosphate (NADPH) and oxygen (O_2). In the reaction, nitrogen is contributed by the arginine, oxygen by the oxygen molecule, and a free electron by NADPH. Nitric oxide synthase is categorized as constitutive NOS (cNOS),

including that found in endothelial cells (ecNOS) and in neurons (nNOS), and as inducible NOS (iNOS).[21] The vascular relaxation caused by acetylcholine is due to stimulation of cNOS, which results in an increase in nitric oxide. Histamine, leukotrienes, and bradykinin are other mediators that increase cNOS-mediated nitric oxide and promote vasodilation and lowering of blood pressure. Proinflammatory cytokines, such as interferon-γ (IFN-γ), tumor necrosis factor-α (TNF-α), and interleukin-1 (IL-1), can all induce iNOS to increase endogenous levels of nitric oxide. Glucocorticoids block the induction of iNOS and inhibit the formation of NO.[22] Nitric oxide is the active form of nitrovasodilators such as nitroglycerin and sodium nitroprusside.[17] Nitric oxide has also been identified as at least one of the neurotransmitters in the nonadrenergic, noncholinergic (NANC) inhibitory nervous system (see Chapter 5).[23] The endogenous production of nitric oxide can be inhibited by L arginine analogs, which inhibit NOS, for example, N-nitro-L-arginine. The nitric oxide molecule is small and lipophilic, and it has a very short duration of action of 0.1 to 5 seconds in physiological systems.[19,23]

Nitric oxide is generated in vascular endothelial cells and diffuses rapidly into myocytes in the endothelium, binding to guanylyl cyclase. Guanylyl cyclase (also termed guanylate cyclase) stimulates the production of cyclic guanosine-3′,5′-monophosphate (cGMP), which causes a decrease in intracellular calcium, and consequent vascular or nonvascular smooth muscle relaxation. The nitric oxide–induced increase in cGMP within the cells also inhibits platelet adherence and aggregation, as well as polymorphonuclear leukocyte chemotaxis.[24] Nitric oxide readily diffuses into the blood vessel itself, as well as into endothelial cells, and enters the red blood cells to bind rapidly with hemoglobin, forming methemoglobin and becoming inactivated in the process. Nitric oxide is also converted in the red blood cells to nitrate, and some endogenous nitric oxide is exhaled from the lung.[24] Because nitric oxide diffuses so readily into the bloodstream and is inactivated by being bound to hemoglobin, its action is limited to the pulmonary vascular endothelium, whether generated endogenously within the lung or inhaled as an exogenous gas. It is thus a selective pulmonary vasodilator. The end products of nitric oxide that enter the systemic circulation are predominantly methemoglobin and nitrate. Nitrite is the predominant nitric oxide metabolite excreted in the urine, accounting for more than 70% of the inhaled dose. A more detailed review of the biology of nitric oxide is given by Aranda and Pearl.[25]

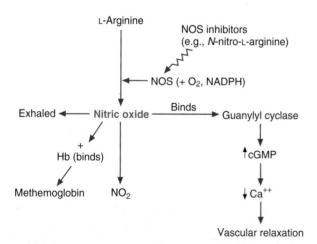

FIGURE 16-2 Production, physiological effect, and metabolism of endogenous nitric oxide. *cGMP*, cyclic guanosine 3′,5′-monophosphate; *Hb*, hemoglobin; *NADPH*, nicotinamide adenine dinucleotide phosphate; *NO₂*, nitrogen dioxide; *NOS*, nitric oxide synthase.

Effect on Pulmonary Circulation

With normal pulmonary hemodynamics (normal vascular resistance), inhalation of NO produces no effect on pulmonary artery pressure or gas exchange.[17] However, Frostell and associates[26] reported that hypoxic pulmonary vasoconstriction caused by breathing 12% oxygen in healthy adults increased mean pulmonary artery pressure from 14.7 ± 0.8 to 19.8 ± 0.9 mmHg.[24] This was reversed by adding 40 ppm of nitric oxide to the gas mixture. No change occurred in systemic vascular resistance because nitric oxide was inactivated locally by hemoglobin. Taylor and associates found that 5 ppm of NO was successful in improving oxygenation in the short term for patients with acute lung injury.[27]

In persistent pulmonary hypertension of the newborn (PPHN), pulmonary vascular resistance is high, which causes right-to-left shunting through the patent ductus arteriosus and foramen ovale. Inhaled nitric oxide dilates pulmonary blood vessels in regions of the lung where ventilation is delivered. This redistributes pulmonary blood flow from areas of low ventilation to those with better ventilation. The improved ventilation-perfusion matching leads to an improved partial pressure of oxygen in arterial blood (Pa_{O_2}). Because nitric oxide is rapidly and locally inactivated by hemoglobin, no systemic vasodilation or hypotension occurs.[28]

Toxicity

Toxicity with exposure to nitric oxide can be caused by the nitric oxide itself, by the formation of the nitrite, nitrogen dioxide, and the formation of methemoglobin. Nitric oxide can be a mediator of lung injury, for example, with paraquat poisoning, in which inhibition of nitric oxide synthetase actually reduces the amount of lung injury.[29] Nitrogen dioxide is a strong oxidizer that causes lipid peroxidation in cells. The amount of nitrogen dioxide produced depends on the amount of nitric oxide and the amount of surrounding oxygen. The higher the Fi_{O_2}, the greater the amount of oxidation of nitric oxide to nitrogen dioxide. Similarly, the higher the concentration of nitric oxide, the shorter the time to achieve oxidation to nitrogen dioxide. The lethal effect of nitrogen dioxide is due to pulmonary edema, and short-term exposure to more than 150 ppm of nitrogen dioxide is usually fatal.[24] In the usual doses of nitric oxide, such as 0.5% to 4%, methemoglobinemia is not usually a problem, although this should be monitored.

It is not known whether nitric oxide can cause fetal harm when given to pregnant women, and the manufacturer notes that it is not intended for adults. It is not known whether nitric oxide is excreted in human milk. Occupational exposure to nitric oxide is set by the Occupational Safety and Health Administration (OSHA) at 25 ppm and for nitrogen dioxide at 5 ppm (manufacturer's literature).

Contraindications

Nitric oxide should not be used in neonates who are known to be dependent on right-to-left shunt.

Respiratory Care Assessment of Therapy

- Because nitric oxide is administered in conjunction with ventilatory support, the usual measures of critical care assessment and in particular ventilator monitoring should be followed.
- Evaluate therapy for a reduction in the oxygenation index (OI = mean airway pressure in $cmH_2O \times Fi_{O_2}$/Pa_{O_2}).
- Evaluate the effect of nitric oxide and monitor the Pa_{O_2} and the overall level of ventilatory support (Fi_{O_2}, inspiratory pressure and time, end-expiratory pressure, rate).
- Monitor preductal and postductal pulse oximetry (Sp_{O_2}) to evaluate shunting.
- If available, review the echocardiogram to evaluate right-to-left shunting.
- Monitor inspired nitric oxide and nitrogen dioxide, along with methemoglobin.
- Monitor cardiovascular status and stability, including the level of intravenous fluids and vasoactive medications needed.

INSULIN HUMAN (rDNA ORIGIN)

KEY POINT

Exubera is an inhaled form of insulin and is not recommend for use in patients with lung disease.

Individuals diagnosed with diabetes had two common formulations to regulate insulin production and control sugar: oral medications or injectable insulin. However, with the release of Exubera, an orally inhaled insulin is available. Although this is not a respiratory medication, side effects such as bronchospasm and reduction in lung function are possible. The respiratory therapist should be aware of its use and inhaled formulation.

Indication for Use

Exubera is indicated for type 1 and 2 diabetes mellitus in adult patients needing to control hyperglycemia. Exubera is not intended for pediatric use; it is intended for adults 18 years of age and older.

Dosage and Administration

Exubera is available in 1- and 3-mg blisters of powdered insulin for inhalation. The blisters should be used only with the Exubera inhaler. Exubera should be taken immediately before meals. The dose required will need to be calculated. This is done by weight or using equivalent dosing from subcutaneous injections. However, titration may be necessary because of glucose concentrations, meal size, and exercise.

Patients with type 1 diabetes should use a long-acting insulin with Exubera. Exubera is not intended as monotherapy in this type of diabetes. However, Exubera may be used as monotherapy in type 2 diabetes or in combination with other agents. Rosenstock and colleagues studied more than 300 subjects and found that Exubera improved and controlled blood sugar when substituted for orally therapy.[30]

Precautions

Exubera is not recommended for patients with underlying lung disease (e.g., asthma, COPD) and is contraindicated in uncontrolled lung disease. Patients that elect to start Exubera should be comprehensively tested for pulmonary function before therapy begins. In studies, Exubera has been shown to decrease lung function, especially FEV_1 and diffusing capacity of the lung for carbon monoxide (DL_{CO}).

Although bronchospasm was rarely reported in studies it is important to recognize that the adverse event is possible. Patients prescribed bronchodilators should take a prescribed dose 30 minutes before use of Exubera. Patients experiencing a respiratory illness (e.g., bronchitis, rhinitis) can continue to take Exubera.

Exubera is contraindicated in smokers or patients who have quit smoking less than 6 months before starting therapy. In studies, smokers experienced a much higher level of insulin, increasing the lowering effect of the agent.

Respiratory Care Assessment of Therapy

Respiratory care assessment of inhaled insulin therapy is directed primarily at lung function and the rate of change of airflow obstruction in patients.

- Pulmonary function testing of flow rates is used to monitor the degree of airflow obstruction over longterm use of the drug.
- Smoking status should be monitored, and Exubera patients who smoke or have not quit within 6 months of therapy should not take the medication.
- Overall pulmonary health should be assessed on the basis of frequency and severity of respiratory infections, cough, and bronchospasm.

SELF-ASSESSMENT QUESTIONS

1. What is the disease state in which an α_1-proteinase inhibitor (API) is indicated?
2. What is the route of administration for α_1-proteinase inhibitor?
3. What is the mode of action of α_1-proteinase inhibitor in treating emphysema associated with inadequate API levels?
4. Is treatment with API indicated for age-related emphysema or in general for those who smoke and have emphysema later in life?
5. Identify three pharmaceutical formulations of nicotine that are used as smoking cessation aids.
6. What is the usual effect of nicotine, whether in a smoking cessation aid or in cigarettes, on blood pressure?
7. Name two nonnicotine agents used in the treatment of smoking cessation.
8. What is the effect of inhaled nitric oxide?
9. Identify two potentially toxic by-products of inhaled nitric oxide.
10. What is the usual dose of inhaled nitric oxide?
11. Identify two disease states in which nitric oxide has been used to reverse pulmonary hypertension.
12. Can insulin be inhaled? Explain.

Answers to Self-Assessment Questions are found in Appendix A.

CLINICAL SCENARIO

A 42-year-old white female was referred by her family physician to Dr. G., a pulmonologist, with complaints of shortness of breath on exertion and increasing fatigue during her usual activities. On questioning, she reported that she had an uncle who had died "many years previously" in middle age with lung disease, but he had also smoked cigarettes. She admitted that she had been a heavy smoker (around a pack per day) for 5 or 6 years but had quit more than 8 years ago. She denied any use of alcohol. She described having several attacks of "bronchitis" in the past year, for which her family physician had prescribed antibiotics, with subsequent resolution each time. She also described a small, but increasing, production of sputum during the past year, usually clear unless she had an episode of bronchitis. She currently has a cough, with production of a slight amount of greenish sputum on occasion. Her medications include albuterol by metered dose inhaler (MDI), prescribed by her family physician last year.

On physical examination, she is a well-developed, well-nourished appearing individual who exhibits mild respiratory distress. Auscultation of her chest reveals expiratory wheezing, diminished breath sounds bilaterally, and a somewhat prolonged expiratory phase. There is no digital clubbing, cyanosis, pedal edema, or jugular distention. Her vital signs are as follows: temperature (T), 37.1° C; blood pressure (BP), 110/76 mmHg; pulse (P), 76 beats/min; and respiratory rate (RR), 24 breaths/min and regular. On room air, her reading on pulse oximetry is 91%.

Given this presenting scenario, what laboratory tests would you recommend Dr. G. obtain to further evaluate her respiratory status?

Based on her clinical picture and the laboratory results, what further test would Dr. G. want now?

With these results, would the use of α_1-proteinase inhibitor therapy be indicated?

Answers to Clinical Scenario Questions are found in Appendix A.

References

1. Wewers MD, Casolaro MA, Sellers SE, Swayze SC, McPhaul KM, Wittes JT, Crystal RG: Replacement therapy for α_1-antitrypsin deficiency associated with emphysema, *N Engl J Med* 316:1055, 1987.
2. Stoller JK: Clinical features and natural history of severe α_1-antitrypsin deficiency, *Chest* 111:123S, 1997.
3. American Thoracic Society, European Respiratory Society: Standards for the diagnosis and management of individuals with alpha-1 antitrypsin deficiency, *Am J Respir Crit Care Med* 168:818, 2003. (Available at www.alphaone.org/healthcare/?c=03-ATSERS-Standards-PDFs; accessed April 2007.)
4. Memorandum: α_1-Antitrypsin deficiency: memorandum from a WHO meeting, *Bull WHO* 75:397, 1997.
5. Snider GL: α1-Protease inhibitor deficiency and the preventive therapy of emphysema, In Leff AR, editor: *Pulmonary and critical care pharmacology and therapeutics*, New York, 2000, McGraw-Hill.
6. Wewers MD, Casolaro MA, Crystal RG: Comparison of alpha-1-antitrypsin levels and antineutrophil elastase capacity of blood and lung in a patient with the alpha-1-antitrypsin phenotype null-null before and during alpha-1-antitrypsin augmentation therapy, *Am Rev Respir Dis* 135:539, 1987.
7. Cohen AB: Unraveling the mysteries of α_1-antitrypsin deficiency, *N Engl J Med* 314:778, 1986.
8. Alkins SA, O'Malley P: Should health-care systems pay for replacement therapy in patients with α_1-antitrypsin deficiency? *Chest* 117:875, 2000.
9. American Thoracic Society: Guidelines for the approach to the patient with severe hereditary alpha-1-antitrypsin deficiency, *Am Rev Respir Dis* 140:1494, 1989.
10. Lillington GA, Leonard CT, Sachs DPL: Smoking cessation: techniques and benefits, *Clin Chest Med* 21:199, 2000.
11. Anthonisen NR, Connett JE, Kiley JP, Altose MD, Bailey WC, Buist AS, Conway WA Jr, Enright PL, Kanner RE, O'Hara P, et al.: Effects of smoking intervention and the use of an inhaled anticholinergic bronchodilator on the rate of decline of FEV$_1$: the Lung Health Study, *JAMA* 272:1497, 1994.
12. Ferrill MJ: Snuffed out: smoking deterrents, *Drug Newsletter* 15:83, 1996.
13. *Drug Facts and Comparisons*, St. Louis, Mo, 2006, Facts and Comparisons, Wolters Kluwer Health.
14. Jorenby DE, Leischow SJ, Nides MA, Rennard SI, Johnston JA, Hughes AR, Smith SS, Muramoto ML, Daughton DM, Doan K, et al.: A controlled trial of sustained-release bupropion, a nicotine patch, or both for smoking cessation, *N Engl J Med* 340:685, 1999.
15. Nides M, Oncken C, Gonzales D, Rennard S, Watsky EJ, Anziano R, Reeves KR: Smoking cessation with varenicline, a selective $\alpha_4\beta_2$ nicotinic receptor partial agonist, *Arch Intern Med* 166:1561, 2006.
16. Oncken C, Gonzales D, Nides M, Rennard S, Watsky E, Billing CB, Anziano R, Reeves K: Efficacy and safety of the novel selective nicotinic acetylcholine receptor partial agonist, varenicline, for smoking cessation, *Arch Intern Med* 166:1571, 2006.
17. Furchgott RF, Zawadzki JV: The obligatory role of endothelial cells in the relaxation of arterial smooth muscle by acetylcholine, *Nature* 288:373, 1980.
18. Palmer RMJ, Ferrige AG, Moncada S: Nitric oxide release accounts for the biological activity of endothelium-derived relaxing factor, *Nature* 327:524, 1987.
19. Ignarro LJ, Buga GM, Wood KS, Byrns RE, Chaudhuri G: Endothelium derived relaxing factor produced and released from artery and vein is nitric oxide, *Proc Natl Acad Sci USA* 84:9265, 1987.
20. Neonatal Inhaled Nitric Oxide Study Group: Inhaled nitric oxide in full-term and nearly full-term infants with hypoxic respiratory failure, *N Engl J Med* 336:597, 1997.
21. Zapol WM, Rimar S, Gillis N, Marletta M, Bosken CH: Nitric oxide and the lung, *Am J Respir Crit Care Med* 149:1375, 1994.
22. American Academy of Pediatrics Committee on Fetus and Newborn: Use of inhaled nitric oxide, *Pediatrics* 106:344, 2000.
23. Barnes PJ, Kharitonov SA: Exhaled nitric oxide: a new lung function test, *Thorax* 51:233, 1996.
24. Mizutani T, Layon AJ: Clinical applications of nitric oxide, *Chest* 110:506, 1996.

25. Aranda M, Pearl RG: The biology of nitric oxide, *Respir Care* 44:156, 1999.

26. Frostell CG, Blomqvist H, Hedenstierna G, Lundberg J, Zapol WM: Inhaled nitric oxide selectively reverses human hypoxic pulmonary vasoconstriction without causing systemic vasodilation, *Anesthesiology* 78:427, 1993.

27. Taylor RW, Zimmerman JL, Dellinger RP, Straube RC, Criner GJ, Davis K Jr, Kelly KM, Smith TC, Small RJ; Inhaled Nitric Oxide in ARDS Study Group: Low dose inhaled nitric oxide in patients with acute lung injury, *JAMA* 291:1603, 2004.

28. Palevsky HI: Treatment of pulmonary hypertension, In Leff AR, editor: *Pulmonary and critical care pharmacology and therapeutics*, New York, 2000, McGraw-Hill.

29. Martin WJ, Rehm S: Toxic injury of the lung parenchyma, In Leff AR, editor: *Pulmonary and critical care pharmacology and therapeutics*, New York, 2000, McGraw-Hill.

30. Rosenstock J, Zinman B, Murphy LJ, Clement SC, Moore P, Bowering CK, Hendler R, Lan SP, Cefalu WT: Inhaled insulin improves glycemic control when substituted for or added to oral combination therapy in type 2 diabetes, *Ann Intern Med* 143:549, 2005.

Chapter 17

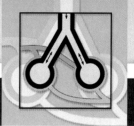

Neonatal and Pediatric Aerosolized Drug Therapy

RUBEN D. RESTREPO

CHAPTER OUTLINE

CHAPTER OBJECTIVES

After reading this chapter, the reader will be able to:

1. Explain off-label use of aerosolized medications
2. Describe the advantages and disadvantages of aerosol delivery
3. List and describe the most important factors affecting neonatal and pediatric aerosol drug delivery
4. Describe the clinical response of neonatal and pediatric patients to aerosolized drugs
5. Describe special situations related to selection of delivery devices for neonatal and pediatric patients
6. Explain lung deposition of inhaled drugs in pediatric and neonatal intubated patients

KEY TERMS AND DEFINITIONS

Emitted dose — Dose released by an aerosol device

Infant — A child between the ages of 1 month and 1 year

Inhaled or delivered dose — Dose reaching the patient's mouth or artificial airway

Lung dose — Dose actually reaching the trachea and beyond

Neonatal — Refers to the period of time between birth and the first month of life

Nominal dose — Dose in the delivery device

Off-label — Use of drugs with no U.S. Food and Drug Administration–approved labeling

Pediatric — Refers to the period of time between 1 month and 18 years of age

Target concentration — Administering a drug until a certain blood level is reached; therapeutic effects and side effects are therefore related to the drug concentration in the blood

Target effect — Administering a drug until the desired effect is achieved or unacceptable side effects or toxicity occur

---

Substantial differences exist between the adult and **neonatal/pediatric** airway environment that affect aerosolized drug therapy. The lack of neonatal and pediatric dose labeling for many drugs given by inhaled aerosol complicates aerosol drug dosing for clinicians and can lead to varied dosing among centers. The differences between aerosol drug delivery as a form of topical administration and systemic administration of drugs is not clearly appreciated in many instances, causing aerosol doses to be modified in neonates and children as if they were given systemically. Data on lung deposition and clinical response, especially to bronchodilators, in this population support the use of aerosol drug therapy in young subjects. Differences among aerosol delivery devices should be considered in relation to the age of the subject. All of the considerations in this chapter relate to use of inhaled aerosols for therapeutic use in the lung and not for systemic treatment. The data cited also are based largely on traditional aerosol delivery devices. New and highly efficient delivery systems may lead to different results in the future. Terms used for different age ranges are given in Box 17-1.

OFF-LABEL USE OF DRUGS IN NEONATAL AND PEDIATRIC PATIENTS

KEY POINT

Pediatric patients are the most common group for which off-label use medications are prescribed.

The term **off-label** is used to refer to drugs lacking U.S. Food and Drug Administration (FDA)-approved dosing information for a specific age group or condition.[1]

Off-label prescribing is a commonly used and accepted medical practice. Although these drugs do have FDA approval, it is for a different use. While aspirin has been a common pain reliever for more than 100 years, in 1988 doctors began prescribing its use in preventing heart attacks. Its use for the prophylaxis of heart attack is considered an off-label use. It has been estimated that nearly half of all prescriptions today are written for off-label uses. Infants, children, and pregnant women are the most common groups in which off-label use medications are prescribed. More than 70% of the entire *Physicians' Desk Reference (PDR)* entries have either no existing dosing information for pediatric patients or specific statements that the safety and efficacy in children have not been determined. It has been reported that when a "suitable alternative" does not exist, doctors prescribe unlicensed or "off-label" medicine for 90% of babies in neonatal intensive care units, 70% of children in pediatric intensive care units, and two-thirds of children in general medical and surgical pediatric wards in the United Kingdom.

Even though the drug labeling often states that safety and efficacy in children have not been determined, many of the inhaled aerosol drugs reviewed in this chapter have clinical indications and uses in the neonatal and pediatric population. Virtually all

Box 17-1	Terms and Age Ranges Defining Periods From Birth to Adult

- Premature neonate: <37 weeks of gestational age
- Neonate: First month of postnatal life
- Infant: 1 to 12 months
- Child: 1 to 12 years
- Adolescent: 12 to 18 years
- Adult: >18 years

TABLE 17-1

Pediatric Drug Labeling for Inhaled Aerosols and Leukotriene Modifiers*

Drug Name	Formulation	Age Labeling (FDA Approved)
β-Adrenergic Agents		
Albuterol	MDI	≥4 yr: 2 inhalations q4-6h
	SVN[†]	2-12 yr: 0.63 mg or 1.25-mg unit dose tid-qid[††]
Epinephrine	SVN	≥4 yr: 0.5 ml of 2.25% solution in 3.0 ml diluent; q3-4h
Metaproterenol	SVN	≥6 yr: 0.1 to 0.2 ml of 5% solution tid-qid
Salmeterol	DPI	≥4 yr: 1 inhalation (50 µg) bid
Formoterol	DPI	≥5 yr: 1 inhalation (12 µg) bid
Levalbuterol	MDI	≥4 yr: 2 inhalations (90 µg) q4-6h
	SVN	6-11 yr: 0.31 mg tid; maximum 0.63 mg tid
Corticosteroids		
Beclomethasone	MDI	6-12 yr: 1 or 2 inhalations qid
Budesonide	DPI	≥6 yr: 200 µg (1 inhalation) bid; maximum 400 µg bid
	SVN	12 mo-8 yr: 0.5-mg total daily dose given once, or twice daily, in divided doses; maximum 1-mg total daily dose given once or 0.5 mg twice daily
Flunisolide	MDI	6-15 yr: 2 inhalations twice daily
Fluticasone	DPI	≥4 yr: 50 µg twice daily up to 100 µg twice daily
Triamcinolone	MDI	6-12 yr: 1 or 2 inhalations tid-qid or 2-4 inhalations bid
Mucolytic agent		
Dornase alfa	SVN	Safety and efficacy in children <5 yr have not been studied; usual dose: one 2.5-mg dose daily
Nonsteroidal Antiasthma Agents		
Cromolyn sodium	MDI	≥5 yr: 1 or 2 puffs tid-qid
	SVN	≥2 yr: 20 mg tid-qid
Nedocromil	MDI	6-11 yr: 1 or 2 puffs bid-qid
Inhaled Antiinfectives		
Ribavirin	SPAG	Infants and young children: a 20-mg/ml solution nebulized for 12-18 hr/day for 3-7 days
Tobramycin	SVN	≥6 yr: 300 mg bid, alternate 28 days on, 28 days off
Leukotriene Modifiers		
Montelukast	PO	12-23 mo: one packet of 4-mg oral granules daily in the evening
		2-5 yr: one 4-mg chewable tablet daily in evening or one packet of 4-mg oral granules daily in the evening
		6-14 yr: one 5-mg chewable tablet daily in evening
Zafirlukast	PO	5-11 yr: one 10-mg tablet bid

DPI, Dry powder inhaler; *MDI*, metered dose inhaler; *SPAG*, small particle aerosol generator; *SVN*, small volume nebulizer; *PO*, by mouth.

*Additional detail on dosing for adults can be found in previous chapters. Manufacturers' information and other sources on drug administration and dosing should be consulted before use. Drug labeling is current at the time of this edition.

[†]The NAEPP guideline[15] still suggests dosification of albuterol via SVN on the basis of weight (0.05 mg/kg q4-6h).

[††]Most frequent administration is not recommended. Patients 6 to 12 years of age with more severe asthma (baseline FEV_1 less than 60% predicted), weight >40 kg, or patients 11 to 12 years of age may achieve a better initial response with the 1.25-mg dose.

inhaled β agonists and corticosteroid formulations have been approved by the FDA for patients over 12 years of age.

Table 17-1 lists inhaled aerosol drugs and leukotriene modifiers that currently have approved age labeling for pediatric use at the time of this edition. Drugs that are not listed in Table 17-1 do not yet have labeling for pediatric use. The process can take time; for example,

only in March 2004 did the U.S. Patent and Trademark Office issue a patent covering AccuNeb, the only FDA-approved (in 2001) lower concentration, unit-dose albuterol sulfate for the treatment of asthma in children aged 2 to 12 years.

In 1994, the FDA's Center for Drug Evaluation and Research issued guidelines encouraging pediatric testing of drugs.[2] A subsequent FDA ruling mandated that drugs submitted for FDA approval after December 2000 be evaluated in children. Waivers can be given if the drug has no meaningful application in children or is likely to be unsafe or ineffective in pediatric patients.[3] There is a substantial cost associated with additional studies to document safety and efficacy in pediatric patients. Therefore, the creation of the "pediatric rule" has provided the pharmaceutical companies that carry out studies with pediatric patients an economic incentive by allowing extended time for marketing before generic formulations of the product are marketed.[4] The FDA cannot, by law, regulate how a drug is used medically or "interfere with the practice of medicine."[1] When a drug is prescribed by a duly licensed physician for any indication deemed appropriate, the following points generally apply[1]:

• The drug is prescribed in a manner that conforms to the community's standard of care.
• The therapy is considered reasonable (i.e., the drug use is based on sound physiological principles and pathological need).
• The therapy is safe—the clinician is aware of known side effects, there are means for assessing toxicity, and generally any risk is acceptable and appropriate given the patient situation.
• Parameters to be used in monitoring for side effects and safety, as well as frequency of monitoring, must be decided before drug dosing begins.

Although it is legal for physicians to prescribe off-label use of drugs, drug dosing becomes much more problematic when standardized dose guidelines have not been previously developed during drug clinical trials. Usually drug therapy is based on one of two strategies in dosing, as follows[1]:

Target concentration: Drugs are dosed until a certain blood level is reached; therefore therapeutic effects and side effects are related to the drug concentration in the blood.
Target effect: Drugs are dosed until the desired effect is achieved or unacceptable side effects or toxicity occur.

In general, drug dosing with inhaled aerosols will need to be based on the target effect strategy: aerosol doses should be based on the desired effect, with avoidance of toxicity. Data that are now available suggest that in fact aerosol doses to neonates or children are "self-limiting" because of differences between pediatric and adult airways. Aerosol drug dose is not based on body size and blood level, but rather on amount reaching the lung.

ADVANTAGES OF AEROSOL DELIVERY IN NEONATAL AND PEDIATRIC PATIENTS

KEY POINT

Administration of inhaled aerosols to neonatal and pediatric patients limits the systemic side effects and avoids the systemic factors that can affect oral or injectable drug therapy.

The advantages of inhaled aerosol drug delivery with neonatal and pediatric patients are largely the same as in adults. Additional factors favoring the neonatal and pediatric population include the following:
• Potential for reduced systemic exposure to the drug
• Potential for use of smaller doses by inhaled aerosol compared with other routes of administration (oral, injection)
• Administration that is painless and generally safe with appropriate monitoring
• Administration that is feasible in the very young, compared with the oral route of administration with pills or tablets
• Avoidance of complicating pharmacokinetic and pharmacodynamic factors in the very young
• A rapid response such as with bronchodilators

The use of inhaled aerosols for therapeutic purposes in treating lung disease is a topical form of drug administration. As such, a drug blood level is not required and in fact is undesirable. This factor is basic to discussing the dose or amounts of inhaled drug needed with neonates or children. An aerosol drug is delivered to the airway surface where the effect is desired. For example, an inhaled β_2 agonist has its effect based on topical delivery to β_2 receptors in the airway. The therapeutic effect from an inhaled aerosol drug is a function of the amount of the drug reaching the airway surface or lung topically.[5-7] Because inhaled aerosols are topical, titrating formulas as with oral or parenteral drug administration does not work well with inhaled aerosol dosing. A major advantage in using inhaled aerosols to treat the lung is the avoidance of systemic factors that can affect oral or injectable drug therapy in neonatal and pediatric use. The effects of many drugs in neonates, infants, and children vary considerably from those in adults when given by systemic routes of administration. Some of the pharmacokinetic and pharmacodynamic factors causing these differences between adults and younger subjects are reviewed by Christensen and colleagues.[8]

FACTORS AFFECTING NEONATAL AND PEDIATRIC AEROSOL DRUG DELIVERY

KEY POINT

Although a smaller fraction of the aerosol reaches the pediatric lower airway when compared with an adult, the need for age adjustment of aerosol doses based on body weight has been clinically debated.

The same mechanisms of aerosol penetration and deposition in the lung that were outlined in Chapter 3 apply to aerosol therapy in neonatal and pediatric patients. These include inertial impaction, a function of particle size and velocity, as well as gravitational settling (sedimentation), a function of mass and residence time. However, the airway environment in neonatal and pediatric subjects differs from that of adults. Table 17-2 outlines functional and structural features of the infant lung that may affect aerosol delivery and deposition.[9]

As suggested by *in vitro* studies, the increasing upper airway geometry in adults may explain the higher amount of aerosol deposition reaching the lower airway compared with that of the neonatal and pediatric patient.[10] Therefore the impact of higher upper airway aerosol deposition in infants who are obligate nasal breathers and children wearing facemasks should always be in the mind of the clinician. A smaller fraction of the nominal dose of an aerosol reaches the lower airways with the child-size oropharynx compared with an adult-size oropharynx.[11] The smaller diameter of neonatal and pediatric lower airways, added to the effects of bronchoconstriction, inflammation, secretions, and the possible presence of an endotracheal tube, dramatically decreases aerosolized drug deposition in the lungs.[12]

TABLE 17-2

Comparison of Neonatal and Adult Respiratory Parameters

Parameter	Neonate	Adult
Tracheal diameter	~4 mm	~20 mm
Tracheal length	5-6 cm	10-12 cm
Tidal volume	6 ml/kg	6 ml/kg
Respiratory rate	30-40/min	12-14/min
Minute ventilation	200-300 ml/kg/min	6 L/min
Dead space	0.75 ml/lb	1.0 ml/lb
Inspiratory flow rate	≤100 ml/sec	~500 ml/sec

From Ruppel GL, White D: The respiratory system. In Scanlan CL, Wilkins RL, Stoller JK, editors: *Egan's fundamentals of respiratory care*, ed 8, St. Louis, Mo, 2003, Mosby.

It is also important to remember the terms and accompanying concepts used in describing aerosol drug administration at the beginning of the chapter in order to interpret study results correctly. As an example, Agertoft and associates[13] investigated delivery of inhaled budesonide in preschool children, ages 3 to 6 years, using a PARI LC Jet Plus nebulizer. Their study contained the following "doses":

Nominal dose: The 1.0 mg of budesonide solution placed in the PARI nebulizer

Inhaled or delivered dose: A mean of 25% of the nominal dose, which was measured as the amount of drug deposited on a filter placed between the mouthpiece and the nebulizer; "dose to subject"

Lung dose: Approximately 6% of the nominal dose (or 26% of the "dose to subject"), estimated indirectly from systemic drug levels

The significance of the study by Agertoft and associates is that the "inhaled dose" of 25% is not the "lung dose," which was much less (mean of 6%). In addition, the dose reaching the lungs of children was smaller than the usual 10% to 15% lung dose in adult patients.[5,14] The factors causing this reduction in lung dose are discussed subsequently. Misinterpretation of the "inhaled dose" or "dose to subject" as the "lung dose" would lead to the incorrect conclusion that the nominal dose should be reduced for pediatric subjects.

Effect of Age on the Aerosol Lung Dose

Inhaled aerosol drugs are absorbed into the body from the lung and also from the mouth and stomach if there is oropharyngeal impaction and loss. This is described by the lung/total systemic availability ratio (L/T ratio) presented in Chapter 2. If a fixed fraction of an aerosol dose, such as 10% to 15% of the nominal dose, reaches the lungs regardless of age, there would be a risk of higher drug concentrations in the circulation of neonates, infants, and children compared with adults. Systemic side effects rather than local overtreatment in the lung have been the basis for aerosol dose adjustment for age, which is usually based on body weight. An example is the dosage schedule for inhaled albuterol in the 2003 National Asthma Education and Prevention Program (NAEPP) guidelines: 0.05 mg/kg, with a minimum of 1.25 mg and a maximum of 2.5 mg.[15] With this schedule, the full 2.5 mg would be given to a 50-kg child:

$$0.05 \text{ mg}/\text{kg} \times 50 \text{ kg} = 2.5 \text{ mg}$$

The need for age adjustment of aerosol doses based on body weight has been clinically debated. The available data at this time suggest that the actual dose of an inhaled aerosol drug could be as low as <1% in neonates and infants,[16,17] and around 2.5% in young children[18] compared with the traditional 10 to 15% cited for adults. Although a smaller percentage of the aerosol deposits in the lungs, small patients may receive considerably more drug per kilogram of body weight than do adults. However, the lower deposition may provide a safety and efficacy profile comparable to that of adults.[19]

Anhøj and associates[20] found that a metered dose inhaler (MDI) of budesonide with a 250-ml steel NebuChamber having less than 2 ml of dead space delivered the *same* approximate dose to patients ranging in age from 2 to 41 years. A facemask was used for 2- to 3-year-olds and a mouthpiece for older subjects. Whereas the inhaled dose and the dose reaching the lung were not the same, the resulting plasma concentration of drug was the same in children and adults (Figure 17-1). Because the holding chamber removed oropharyngeal/stomach loss and there is high first-pass metabolism of budesonide, plasma drug levels reflect dose in the lung. If the same dose went to the lungs in adults as in 2-year-olds, higher plasma levels would be observed in younger subjects who have smaller circulating blood volumes. This report suggests that inhaled dose need not be adjusted for age to reduce systemic levels and possible toxicity.[20] When a fixed dose of 2.5 mg by nebulizer was compared with a 0.1-mg/kg body weight dose in children 4 to 12 years of age in acute asthma, there was no difference between the two dosing protocols in either clinical improvement measured by flows, oxygen saturations, and clinical score or cardiovascular and tremor side effects. The fixed dose of 2.5 mg by nebulizer was efficacious and safe.[21]

Effect of Small Tidal Volumes, Short Respiratory Cycles, and Low Flow Rates

Small pediatric patients have a low tidal volume, low vital capacity, a short respiratory cycle, and low inspiratory flow rates. Therefore, children inhale a smaller percentage of the **emitted dose** from either a small volume nebulizer (SVN) or MDI with a reservoir device (holding chamber or spacer). The aerosol deposition is reduced because of a short residence time in the airways. These factors can significantly alter the inhaled dose and the lung dose of patients less than 6 months of age.[22,23]

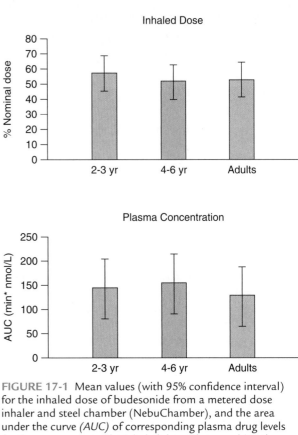

FIGURE 17-1 Mean values (with 95% confidence interval) for the inhaled dose of budesonide from a metered dose inhaler and steel chamber (NebuChamber), and the area under the curve *(AUC)* of corresponding plasma drug levels for three age ranges. The inhaled dose (dose reaching the patient) is equivalent for THE various age groups. Blood levels from lung absorption remain the same in younger subjects, indicating that the dose reaching the lung is proportionately less for younger, smaller subjects. (Data from Anhøj J, Thorsson L, Bisgaard H: Lung deposition of inhaled drugs increases with age, *Am J Respir Crit Care Med* 162:1819, 2000.)

Effect on Small Volume Nebulizer

If we assume a gas flows at 6 L/min, an adult with an inspiratory flow of 500 ml/sec (30 L/min) and a tidal volume of 500 to 1000 ml (500 ml/sec × 1 or 2 seconds) would completely inhale all of a nebulizer output. However, an **infant** with an inspiratory flow of less than 100 ml/sec (<6 L/min) and a tidal volume less than 100 ml will not completely inhale all of the nebulizer output during the inspiratory phase (Figure 17-2).

Collis and associates[24] studied the fraction of nebulizer output inspired by infants ages 1 to 12 months, children 3 to 16 years, and adults 20 to 23 years. Infants were sedated with chloral hydrate and tidal breathing was recorded by facemask and pneumotachograph. The fraction of nebulizer output inspired was lower in infants less than 6 months of age, and then reached

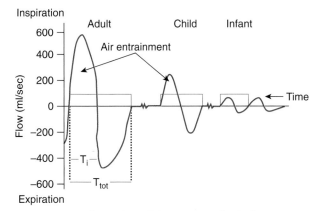

FIGURE 17-2 Illustration of the amount of nebulizer output inspired with various inspiratory patterns (volumes, flow rates, and times), indicating a smaller fraction of output inspired with low tidal volumes and flow rates in infants compared with adults. T_i, Inspiratory time; T_{tot}, total cycle time. (From Collis GG, Cole CH, Le Souëf PN: Dilution of nebulised aerosols by air entrainment in children, *Lancet* 336:341, 1990.)

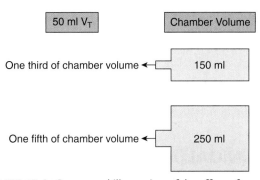

FIGURE 17-3 Conceptual illustration of the effect of small tidal volumes (V_T) on chamber evacuation with different-sized reservoir chambers.

a plateau and remained constant beyond 6 months of age. Wildhaber and colleagues[25] also found that inhaled aerosol dose from a SVN attached to a mask increased with weight in 4- to 12-month-olds and was lower in smaller infants.[26]

Effect on Reservoir Dose

The same effect of low tidal volumes would theoretically reduce the amount of volume and therefore drug mass inhaled from a reservoir chamber (Figure 17-3). The amount of reduction is proportional to the chamber volume for a given infant tidal volume. For a 50-ml tidal volume, approximately one-third of a 150-ml chamber and one-fifth (20%) of a 250-ml chamber would be inhaled. Even assuming no redistribution of aerosol in

the chamber volume, gravitational settling will further reduce available dose within seconds of MDI actuation into the chamber. The ideal volume for a spacer device is small enough to allow drug inhalation with few breaths for infants with low tidal volumes (<50 ml).

This theoretical prediction is supported by data from Everard and colleagues.[26] Delivery (not lung deposition) of MDI cromolyn sodium by reservoir and facemask with tidal volumes of 25, 50, and 150 ml was measured *in vitro*, using various sizes of chambers. Smaller tidal volumes decreased inhaled drug mass. Higher aerosol concentrations in a smaller chamber enhanced drug delivery with tidal volumes less than 150 ml. Introduction of dead space between the chamber outlet and the filter collecting inspired drug reduced the dose deposited by as much as 50% or more.[26] The results are summarized in Table 17-3.

In contrast, an *in vivo* study by Wildhaber and associates[25] that showed decreasing inhaled dose from a nebulizer with infants as small as 6 to 7 kg also found that there was no effect of size (weight) on inhaled dose for two chamber devices used with an MDI. The two reservoir devices were the Babyhaler (350-ml chamber, 40-ml dead volume) and the NebuChamber (250-ml chamber, no dead volume). The plastic reservoir device (Babyhaler, 350 ml) had the electrostatic charge removed before testing. Turpeinen and colleagues[27] compared the same reservoir devices and found that inhaled mass of budesonide from the Babyhaler did increase with increasing height, weight, and tidal volume, but not with the NebuChamber. Such variation in study results indicates that testing conditions, type of drug, and choice of reservoir device can affect inhaled dose, although not necessarily the lung dose. Box 17-2 lists factors in reservoir devices that may affect the inhaled dose to neonates, infants, and small children.

NEBULIZED DRUG DISTRIBUTION

It is hypothesized that the greater the infant's distress, the lower the lung deposition and the higher the upper respiratory tract and gastrointestinal tract deposition. Evaluation of distribution of nebulized bronchodilators in wheezy infants has shown an average of 10%-12% adherence to the patient's face, $7.8 \pm 4.9\%$ deposition in the upper respiratory and gastrointestinal tracts, and $1.5 \pm 0.7\%$ deposited in the lungs (Figure 17-4).[28,29]

The most definitive data for answering the question of how much aerosol drug reaches the lungs of neonates and pediatric patients are actual measures of

TABLE 17-3

Effect of Inspired Tidal Volumes on Mean (Range) Inhaled Aerosol Dose in Two Reservoir Devices

Device	INHALED AEROSOL DOSE (MG) AT TIDAL VOLUME OF:		
	25 ml	50 ml	150 ml
AeroChamber (150 ml)	0.33 (0.29-0.35) mg	1.15 (1.08-1.24) mg	1.41 (1.33-1.46) mg
Nebuhaler (750 ml)	0.29 (0.26-0.32) mg	0.93 (0.91-0.97) mg	1.55 (1.48-1.61) mg

Data from Everard ML, Clark AR, Milner AD: Drug delivery from holding chambers with attached facemask, *Arch Dis Child* 67:580, 1992.

Box 17-2 | **Factors That May Affect the Dose Inhaled From a Reservoir Chamber by Neonatal and Pediatric Patients**

MECHANICAL AND DESIGN FACTORS

- Chamber volume
- Electrostatic charge on plastic devices
- Shape of aerosol plume relative to chamber size
- Design of inspiratory and expiratory valves, if present
- Presence of inspiratory valve
- Amount of dead volume in mouthpiece

PATIENT FACTORS

- Breathing pattern
- Inspiratory flow rate
- Tidal volume

lung deposition for various age-groups. Such data are increasingly available and indicate that the lung dose of an aerosol drug does in fact decrease with age. This is consistent with the data of Anhøj and associates[20] discussed earlier, which found that blood levels of drug, reflecting the dose reaching the lungs, was constant in younger and older subjects, despite the smaller circulating volume of younger patients.

Figure 17-5 summarizes data on lung deposition with inhaled aerosols, compiled from four studies. All of the studies used an MDI with a reservoir device and a facemask for delivery in subjects less than 4 years of age. Values represent the percentage of total dose from the device. Fok and colleagues[30] found that 0.67% (SEM = 0.17) of the total dose of albuterol reached the lungs of infants with a mean age of 86 days (25 to 187 days).

Tal and associates[31] found 1.97% (SD = 1.4) as a lung dose of albuterol in patients with a mean age of 21 months (3 months to 5 years). Wildhaber and colleagues[32] found that 5.4% (SD = 2.1) and 9.6% (SD = 3.9) of albuterol reached the lungs of 2- to 4-year-olds and 5- to 9-year-olds, respectively. Agertoft and associates,[13]

using indirect measures of plasma levels, found that 6.1% of a budesonide dose reached the lungs of 3- to 6-year-olds. Similar data have been found for aerosol delivery with nebulizers and are listed in Chapter 3 (Table 3-4). If the amount of aerosolized albuterol reaching the lungs of infants and children in the study by Tal and colleagues[31] is used, it can be shown that the self-limiting effect of younger ages on lung dose results in the same dose per amount of body weight in children as in adults (Table 17-4). The equivalence of dose per body weight illustrated in Table 17-4 and based on lung deposition data argues strongly against the need to adjust the nominal dose of an aerosol drug for age or body size with current aerosol delivery devices. Age and size have a self-limiting effect on lung dose, producing a natural titration of dose. This conclusion may need to be revised pending more efficient aerosol delivery devices.

CLINICAL RESPONSE TO AEROSOLIZED DRUGS IN NEONATAL AND PEDIATRIC PATIENTS

KEY POINT

Aerosolized bronchodilators change respiratory mechanics in both ventilated and nonventilated infants.

The lung deposition data reviewed in the previous section argue that aerosolized drugs do reach the lungs of infants and do so in a self-regulating amount. However, the question of clinical response to aerosol drugs in infants and pediatric patients is not determined by lung deposition data. The most commonly studied drug class, and one of great interest in neonates and infants, is the adrenergic bronchodilator group. Compared with corticosteroids, the clinical response to bronchodilator

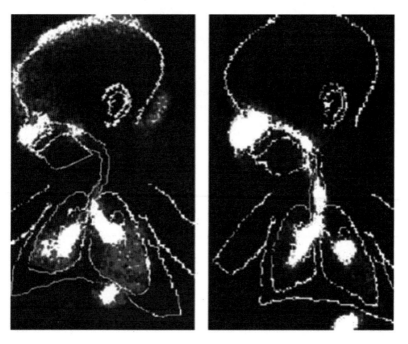

Hood   Mask

FIGURE 17-4 Scan of patient obtained during hood and mask treatments, showing deposition of aerosolized medication in the upper respiratory tract (URT) and the gastrointestinal (GI) system. Notice the considerably higher URT and GI deposition with the mask treatment. (From Amirav I, Balanov I, Gorenberg M, Groshar D, Luder AS: Nebuliser hood compared to mask in wheezy infants: aerosol therapy without tears. *Arch Dis Child* 88:719, 2003.)

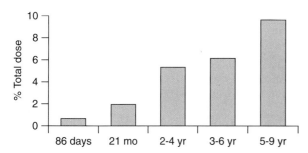

FIGURE 17-5 Data from four separate studies giving the percentage of a total aerosol dose that reaches the lungs of infants and children of various ages. In each study, the aerosol dose was delivered with a metered dose inhaler with reservoir device and a facemask to subjects less than 4 years of age. Studies are listed in the references: for 86 days: Fok and colleagues[37]; for 21 months: Tal and colleagues[32]; for 2 to 4 years and 5 to 9 years: Wildhaber and colleagues[22]; for 3 to 6 years: Agertoft and colleagues.[13]

TABLE 17-4

Calculation of Dose per Kilogram of Aerosolized Albuterol for Children and Adults, Based on Lung Deposition Data (1.97%) Showing Equivalence of Dose per Body Size

	Adult	Child
Weight	80 kg	10 kg
Lung deposition	20%*	2%
Nominal dose	200 µg	200 µg
Dose to lung	40 µg	4 µg
Per-kilogram dose	0.5 µg/kg	0.4 µg/kg

*Percentage lung deposition measured by Tal and colleagues in two adult volunteers in the same study.

Data from Tal A, Golan H, Grauer N, Aviram M, Albin D, Quastel MR: Deposition pattern of radiolabeled salbutamol inhaled from a metered-dose inhaler by means of a spacer with mask in young children with airway obstruction, *J Pediatr* 128:479, 1996.

occurs within minutes and is more feasible to study in young subjects.

Commonly cited studies from the late 1970s concluded that there was an absence of response to inhaled bronchodilators in infants and children less than 18 months of age.[22,23] These studies found no change in respiratory resistance with phenylephrine, epinephrine, or salbutamol (albuterol) in infants and children from 7 to 17 or 18 months of age, using a forced oscillation technique. The authors of the studies speculated that there was either poor development of smooth muscle at less than 18 months of age or the bronchial

TABLE 17-5

Results of Studies Examining Clinical Response to Aerosolized Albuterol in Infants

Age	Delivery	Outcome Measured	First Author	Reference No.
1-4 weeks	SVN via ETT	Improved: respiratory resistance and dynamic compliance	Rotschild, 1989	39
12 ± 8 days	MDI/spacer via ETT vs. SVN via ETT	Improved: respiratory resistance and dynamic compliance*	Sivakumar, 1999	40
8.5 ± 4.2 months	SVN	Improved: oxygen saturation, respiratory system resistance	Modl, 2005	41
14.1 ± 6.1 months	Not specified	Improved: oxygen saturation, respiratory distress	Hyvärinem, 2006	42

ETT, Endotracheal tube; MDI, metered dose inhaler; SVN, small volume nebulizer.
*MDI delivery resulted in significantly better dynamic compliance than SVN delivery, with no difference between delivery systems in respiratory resistance.

obstruction was due to secretions and airway edema rather than bronchoconstriction.

A 1993 study by Turner and associates[33] found that the level of response to a bronchodilator increases significantly with increasing age in young asthmatics between the ages of 3 and 9 years. However, studies of both ventilated and nonventilated preterm infants have shown dose-related changes in respiratory mechanics, including airway resistance, and compliance with aerosolized bronchodilators.[34-42] Table 17-5 lists several studies, and the outcomes measured, that have documented clinical efficacy of aerosolized bronchodilators in infants.

CHOICE OF DELIVERY DEVICE IN NEONATAL AND PEDIATRIC PATIENTS

Box 17-3 gives the age guidelines for use of current aerosol delivery devices in infants and children, based on the 2002 NAEPP guidelines.[15] Either a jet nebulizer or an MDI can be used with suitable auxiliary devices attached. An evidence-based review by the American College of Chest Physicians determined that for most patients with asthma, SVNs, dry powder inhalers (DPIs), and MDIs are equally effective in delivering short-acting beta agonists.[43,44] However, it is clear that children less than 5 years of age cannot effectively use, unassisted, a DPI or an MDI.[45] For both the MDI and nebulizer, a facemask is needed for the very young and a reservoir is needed additionally for the MDI. A DPI is not suitable for young children below the age of 4 or 5 years because of their limited inspiratory flow ability and more limited vital capacities.

Box 17-3 — Age Guidelines for Use of Current Aerosol Delivery Devices

Aerosol System	Age Group
SVN*	≥Neonate
MDI	>5 yr
MDI with reservoir	>4 yr
MDI with reservoir/mask	≤4 yr
MDI with ETT	≥Neonate
Breath-actuated MDI	≥5 yr
DPI	≥5 yr

DPI, Dry powder inhaler; ETT, endotracheal tube; MDI, metered dose inhaler; SVN, small volume nebulizer.
*With facemask for those unable to use a mouthpiece.
National Asthma Education and Prevention Program, National Heart, Lung, and Blood Institute, National Institutes of Health: Expert Panel Report: Guidelines for the diagnosis and management of asthma—update on selected topics 2002, NIH Publication 02-5074. Bethesda, Md, 2002, National Institutes of Health. (Available at http://www.nhlbi.nih.gov/guidelines/asthma/asthmafullrpt.pdf; accessed April 2007.)

Studies cited in Chapter 3 (Table 3-4) showing equivalent clinical response between the MDI–reservoir systems, with or without a mask as needed by age, and jet nebulizers have been confirmed in young children.[46] The MDI delivery system has the advantage of smallness and portability, plus shorter treatment time, even with an increased number of actuations, compared with gas-powered nebulizers, which require a pressurized gas source, bulky equipment, and a 10- to 15-minute treatment time, with additional preparation and cleaning time needed.

A significant disadvantage of aerosol therapy with jet nebulizers in pediatric patients is the poor tolerance often demonstrated due to noise of operation, "lengthy" treatment periods, and the need for a tight-fitting mask.[26] The absence of a tight seal between mask and patient's face results in a decrease in the amount of medication available for inhalation.[47-49] The typical pediatric patient does not tolerate a mask applied to their face, and agitation and crying are frequently observed. The efficacy of aerosol therapy administered to a combative toddler is known to be negligible.[50] Changes in respiratory patterns during nebulization have also been shown to adversely impact the delivery of aerosolized medication.[25] Often the mask is simply held near the face, a technique known as "blow-by." It has been shown that even a 1- to 2-cm gap between the mask and the face reduces the inhaled drug mass as a percentage of the nominal dose in a pediatric lung model of spontaneous breathing as much as 50%.[51] Development of more efficient, more acceptable and friendlier facemask interfaces has been evaluated as an option to improve the inhaled drug mass. Reports comparing the standard aerosol pediatric mask with other proprietary masks have shown that the newly designed masks significantly increase the inhaled drug mass.[52,53]

Amirav and colleagues compared lung deposition of salbutamol between a prototype hood and a mask attached to an SVN in wheezy infants. Because nothing touches the face, the hood provides a logical and friendly means to delivering nebulized drug to neonates, infants, and small pediatric patients. Mean total lung deposition was 2.6% with the hood and 2.4% with the mask.[29]

AEROSOL ADMINISTRATION IN INTUBATED NEONATAL AND PEDIATRIC PATIENTS

KEY POINT

An externally powered nebulizer may interfere with patient-triggered modes of ventilation, may cause increases in airway pressures and unexpected positive end-expiratory pressure (PEEP), and may result in variable F_{IO_2} (fraction of inspired oxygen) levels.

Aerosol delivery appears less efficient in intubated pediatric patients than in spontaneously breathing patients.[54] It is important to consider changes associated with the use of SVN in-line on pediatric and particularly neonatal ventilated patients, because unexpected changes in both volume and pressure may have deleterious effects. An externally powered nebulizer increases volume and pressure during volume-targeted ventilation, creates a bias flow in the ventilator circuit

that may interfere with patient-triggered modes of ventilation,[55] may result in increased airway pressure and unexpected positive end-expiratory pressure (PEEP), and may result in variable F_{IO_2} levels. Newer micropump nebulizers that require no gas flow are now available for use in ventilated patients. They do not affect airway pressures during operation as usually seen with externally gas-powered nebulizers.[56,57]

The respiratory clinician should also be aware that aerosol delivery may be less effective with manual ventilation versus mechanical ventilation.[58] Placement of the aerosol delivery device in the intubated infant requires clinician attention. Although most studies show slightly higher lung deposition with the MDI when inserted between the Y-piece and the endotracheal tube, lung deposition with an SVN placed in the inspiratory limb away from the Y-piece also averages 1% of the nominal dose.[30] In pediatric patients, an MDI–reservoir with one-way valve is associated with a significantly larger amount of inhaled drug mass.[59] No difference has been found between *in vitro* and *in vivo* studies.[60] It has been suggested that the MDI should be actuated before inspiration to improve lung deposition.[61]

Determination of doses for aerosolized drugs delivered to neonatal and pediatric patients is not completely understood. Despite the differences in drug action between adults and children, the ability to control particle size by selecting the optimal mode of aerosol delivery and placement of the delivery device, and understanding patterns of aerosol generation, are the key elements to improve efficiency of aerosol administration. Correctly gauging the ability of the patient, rather than relaying on specific age, is also essential to selecting the most appropriate device in any population.[62]

SELF-ASSESSMENT QUESTIONS

1. Can an aerosol formulation for oral inhalation be legally administered to neonates, infants and pediatric patients?
2. Can an adrenergic bronchodilator such as albuterol reduce airway resistance when used in neonates and children?
3. According to the data reviewed in this chapter, does the adult dose of an aerosol drug need to be reduced with neonatal and pediatric patients, based on weight?
4. What aerosol delivery devices could be used with a 2-year-old child?

Answers to Self-Assessment Questions are found in Appendix A.

CLINICAL SCENARIO

Case courtesy of Ruben D. Restrepo, MD, RRT, University of Texas Health Science Center at San Antonio.

A 24-month-old boy, that was born at 27 weeks, presents to the emergency room in respiratory distress. His medical history is significant for bronchopulmonary dysplasia. Vital signs are as follows: temperature (T), 37.5° C; pulse (P), 175 beats/min; respiratory rate (RR), 76 breaths/min; blood pressure (BP), 85/55 mmHg; oxygen saturation by pulse oximetry (SpO_2), 85% on room air. The physical examination reveals the presence of intercostal retractions, increased anteroposterior diameter, nasal flaring, and bilateral diffuse expiratory wheezing. The patient is administered oxygen and admitted to the pediatric intensive care unit (PICU). The attending physician orders albuterol, a 1.25-mg unit dose via a small volume nebulizer (SVN). While receiving the aerosol, the patient's pulse rate climbs to 220 beats/min and he becomes cyanotic despite the O_2 used to nebulize the drug. The patient is promptly intubated and mechanically ventilated. The patient receives albuterol throughout his hospital course and is discharged home 2 weeks later with a prescription for albuterol syrup.

What methods of aerosol delivery are appropriate and available for albuterol in this age group?

After the decision was made to use an SVN, a dose of 1.25 mg was administered, but severe tachycardia developed. Would you consider levalbuterol? What else could you recommend to the physician?

Where would you recommend placement of the SVN while administering the treatment to the ventilated patient?

Answers to Clinical Scenario Questions are found in Appendix A.

References

1. Blumer JL: Off-label uses of drugs in children, *Pediatrics* 104(suppl 3):598, 1999.
2. U.S. Food and Drug Administration: Specific requirements on content and format of labeling for human prescription drugs: revision of "pediatric use" subsection in the labeling—final rule, FDA, 21 CFR Part 201 (docket no. 92N-0165). *Fed Regist* 59:64240, 1994.
3. U.S. Food and Drug Administration: Regulations requiring manufacturers to assess the safety and effectiveness of new drugs and biological products in pediatric patients, FDA, 21 CFR Parts 201, 312, 314, and 601 (docket no. 97N-0165). *Fed Regist* 63:66631, 1998.
4. Tauer CA: Central ethical dilemmas in research involving children, *Account Res* 9:127, 2002.
5. Zainudin BM, Biddiscombe M, Tolfree SE, Short M, Spiro SG: Comparison of bronchodilator responses and deposition patterns of salbutamol inhaled from a pressurized metered dose inhaler, as a dry powder, and as a nebulised solution, *Thorax* 45:469, 1990.
6. Mestitz H, Copland JM, McDonald CF: Comparison of outpatient nebulized vs. metered dose inhaler terbutaline in chronic airflow obstruction, *Chest* 96:1237, 1989.
7. Newhouse M, Dolovich M: Aerosol therapy: nebulizer vs. metered dose inhaler, *Chest* 91:799, 1987.
8. Christensen ML, Helms RA, Chesney RW: Is pediatric labeling really necessary? *Pediatrics* 104(suppl 3):593, 1999.
9. Thompson J, Malinowski C, Wilson B: Neonatal and pediatric respiratory care. In Scanlan CL, Wilkins RL, Stoller JK, editors: *Egan's fundamentals of respiratory care*, ed 8, St. Louis, Mo, 2003, Mosby.
10. Berg E: *In vitro* properties of pressurized metered dose inhalers with and without spacer devices, *J Aerosol Med* 8(suppl):S3, 1995.
11. Olsson B: Aerosol particle generation from dry powder inhalers: can they equal pressurized metered dose inhalers? *J Aerosol Med* 8(suppl):S13, 1995.
12. Dolovich M: Aerosol delivery to children: what to use, how to choose, *Pediatr Pulmonol* 18(suppl):79, 1999.
13. Agertoft L, Andersen A, Weibull E, Pedersen S: Systemic availability and pharmacokinetics of nebulised budesonide in preschool children, *Arch Dis Child* 80:241, 1999.
14. Newman SP, Pavia D, Moren F, Sheahan NF, Clarke SW: Deposition of pressurized aerosols in the human respiratory tract, *Thorax* 36:52, 1981.
15. National Asthma Education and Prevention Program, National Heart, Lung, and Blood Institute, National Institutes of Health: Expert Panel Report: *Guidelines for the diagnosis and management of asthma—update on selected topics 2002*, NIH Publication 02-5074. Bethesda, Md, 2002, National Institutes of Health. (Available at http://www.nhlbi.nih.gov/guidelines/asthma/asthma-fullrpt.pdf; accessed April 2007.)
16. Rubin BK, Fink JB: Aerosol therapy for children, *Respir Care Clin N Am* 7:175, 2001.
17. Salmon B, Wilson NM, Silverman M: How much aerosol reaches the lungs of wheezy infants and toddlers? *Arch Dis Child* 65:401, 1990.
18. Chua HL, Collis GG, Newbury AM, Chan K, Bower GD, Sly PD, Le Souef PN: The influence of age in aerosol deposition in children with cystic fibrosis, *Eur Respir J* 7:2185, 1994.
19. Fink JB: Aerosol delivery to ventilated infant and pediatric patients, *Respir Care* 49:653, 2004.
20. Anhøj J, Thorsson L, Bisgaard H: Lung deposition of inhaled drugs increases with age, *Am J Respir Crit Care Med* 162:1819, 2000.
21. Oberklaid F, Mellis CM, Souef PN, Geelhoed GC, Maccarrone AL: A comparison of a bodyweight dose versus a fixed dose of nebulised salbutamol in acute asthma in children, *Med J Australia* 158:751, 1993.
22. Lenney W, Milner AD: At what age do bronchodilators work? *Arch Dis Child* 53:532, 1978.

23. Lenney W, Milner AD: Alpha and beta adrenergic stimulants in bronchiolitis and wheezy bronchitis in children under 18 months of age, *Arch Dis Child* 53:707, 1978.

24. Collis GG, Cole CH, Le Souëf PN: Dilution of nebulised aerosols by air entrainment in children, *Lancet* 336:341, 1990.

25. Wildhaber JH, Devadason SG, Hayden MJ, Eber E, Summers QA, LeSouef PN: Aerosol delivery to wheezy infants: a comparison between a nebulizer and two small volume spacers, *Pediatr Pulmonol* 23:212, 1997.

26. Everard ML, Clark AR, Milner AD: Drug delivery from holding chambers with attached facemask, *Arch Dis Child* 67:580, 1992.

27. Turpeinen M, Nikander K, Malmberg LP, Pelkonen A: Metered dose inhaler add-on devices: is the inhaled mass of drug dependent on the size of the infant? *J Aerosol Med* 12:171, 1999.

28. Amirav I, Balanov I, Gorenberg M, Luder AS, Newhouse MT, Groshar D: β-Agonist aerosol distribution in respiratory syncytial virus bronchiolitis in infants, *J Nucl Med* 43:487, 2002.

29. Amirav I, Balanov I, Gorenberg M, Groshar D, Luder AS: Nebuliser hood compared to mask in wheezy infants: aerosol therapy without tears, *Arch Dis Child* 88:719, 2003.

30. Fok TF, Monkman S, Dolovich M, Gray S, Coates G, Paes B, Rashid F, Newhouse M, Kirpalani H: Efficiency of aerosol medication delivery from a metered dose inhaler versus jet nebulizer in infants with bronchopulmonary dysplasia, *Pediatr Pulmonol* 21:301, 1996.

31. Tal A, Golan H, Grauer N, Aviram M, Albin D, Quastel MR: Deposition pattern of radiolabeled salbutamol inhaled from a metered-dose inhaler by means of a spacer with mask in young children with airway obstruction, *J Pediatr* 128:479, 1996.

32. Wildhaber JH, Dore ND, Wilson JM, Devadason SG, LeSouef PN: Inhalation therapy in asthma: nebulizer or pressurized metered-dose inhaler with holding chamber? *In vivo* comparison of lung deposition in children, *J Pediatr* 135:28, 1999.

33. Turner DJ, Landau LI, LeSouëf PN: The effect of age on bronchodilator responsiveness, *Pediatr Pulmonol* 15:98, 1993.

34. Holt WJ, Greenspan JS, Antunes MJ, Cullen JA, Spitzer AR, Wiswell TE: Pulmonary response to an inhaled bronchodilator in chronically ventilated preterm infants with suspected airway reactivity, *Respir Care* 40:145, 1995.

35. Denjean A, Guimaraes H, Migdal M, Miramand JL, Dehan M, Gaultier C: Dose-related bronchodilator response to aerosolized salbutamol (albuterol) in ventilator-dependent premature infants, *J Pediatr* 120:974, 1992.

36. Fok TF, Lam K, Ng PC, Leung TF, So HK, Cheung KL, Wong W: Delivery of salbutamol to nonventilated preterm infants by metered-dose inhaler, jet nebulizer, and ultrasonic nebulizer, *Eur Respir J* 12:159, 1998.

37. Gappa M, Gartner M, Poets CF, von der Hardt H: Effects of salbutamol delivery from a metered dose inhaler versus jet nebulizer on dynamic lung mechanics in very preterm infants with chronic lung disease, *Pediatr Pulmonol* 23:442, 1997.

38. Rubilar L, Castro-Rodriguez JA, Girardi G: Randomized trial of salbutamol via metered-dose inhaler with spacer versus nebulizer for acute wheezing in children less than 2 years of age, *Pediatr Pulmonol* 29:264, 2000.

39. Rotschild A, Solimano A, Puterman M, Smyth J, Sharma A, Albersheim S: Increased compliance in response to aerosolized salbutamol (albuterol) in ventilator-dependent premature infants, *J Pediatr* 115:984, 1989.

40. Sivakumar D, Bosque E, Goldman SL: Bronchodilator delivered by metered dose inhaler and spacer improves respiratory system compliance more than nebulizer-delivered bronchodilator in ventilated premature infants, *Pediatr Pulmonol* 27:208, 1999.

41. Modl M, Eber E, Malle-Scheid D, Weinhandl E, Zach MS: Does bronchodilator responsiveness in infants with bronchiolitis depend on age? *J Pediatr* 147:617, 2005.

42. Hyvarinen MK, Kotaniemi-Syrjanen A, Reijonen TM, Korhonen K, Kiviniemi V, Korppi M: Responses to inhaled bronchodilators in infancy are not linked with asthma in later childhood, *Pediatr Pulmonol* 41:420, 2006.

43. Rubin BK, Fink JB: Optimizing aerosol delivery by pressurized metered-dose inhalers, *Respir Care* 50:1191, 2005.

44. Dolovich MB, Ahrens RC, Hess DR, Anderson P, Dhand R, Rau JL, Smaldone GC, Guyatt G, American College of Chest Physicians; American College of Asthma, Allergy, and Immunology: Device selection and outcomes of aerosol therapy: evidence-based guidelines, *Chest* 127:335, 2005.

45. Ahrens RC: The role of the MDI and DPI in pediatric patients: "children are not just miniature adults," *Respir Care* 50:1323, 2005.

46. Deerojanawong J, Manuyakorn W, Prapphal N, Harnruthakorn C, Sritippayawan S, Samransamruajkit R: Randomized controlled trial of salbutamol aerosol therapy via metered dose inhaler-spacer vs. jet nebulizer in young children with wheezing, *Pediatr Pulmonol* 39:466, 2005.

47. Amirav I, Newhouse MT: Aerosol therapy with valved holding chambers in young children: importance of the facemask seal, *Pediatrics* 108:389, 2001.

48. Janssens HM, Devadason SG, Hop WC, LeSouef PN, De Jongste JC, Tiddens HA: Variability of aerosol delivery via spacer devices in young asthmatic children in daily life, *Eur Respir J* 13:787, 1999.

49. Smaldone GC, Berg E, Nikander K: Variation in pediatric aerosol delivery: importance of facemask, *J Aerosol Med* 18:354, 2005.

50. Murakami G, Igarashi T: Measurement of bronchial hyperreactivity in infants and preschool children using a new method, *Ann Allergy* 64:383, 1990.

51. Restrepo RD, Dickson SK, Rau JL, Gardenhire DS: An investigation of nebulized bronchodilator delivery using a pediatric lung model of spontaneous breathing, *Respir Care* 51:56, 2006.

52. Amirav I, Mansour Y, Mandelberg A, Bar-Ilan I, Newhouse MT: Redesigned facemask improves "real life" aerosol delivery for NebuChamber, *Pediatr Pulmonol* 37:172, 2004.

53. Lin H-L, Restrepo RD, Gardenhire DS: An *in vitro* investigation of nebulized albuterol delivery by pediatric aerosol facemasks to spontaneously breathing infants, *Respir Care* 50:1551, 2005.

54. Di Paolo ER, Pannatier A, Cotting J: *In vitro* evaluation of bronchodilator drug delivery by jet nebulization during pediatric mechanical ventilation, *Pediatr Crit Care Med* 6:462, 2005.

55. Hanhan U, Kissoon N, Payne M, Taylor C, Murphy S, DeNicola LK: Effects of in-line nebulization on preset ventilatory variables, *Respir Care* 38:474, 1993.

56. Dhand R: Basic techniques for aerosol delivery during mechanical ventilation, *Respir Care* 49:611, 2004.

57. Dhand R: New frontiers in aerosol delivery during mechanical ventilation, *Respir Care* 49:666, 2004.

58. Henry WD, Chatburn RL: Effects of manual versus mechanical ventilation on aerosol efficiency, *Respir Care* 33:914, 1988.

59. Mandhane P, Zuberbuhler P, Lange CF, Finlay WH: Albuterol aerosol delivered via metered-dose inhaler to intubated pediatric models of 3 ages, with 4 spacer designs, *Respir Care* 48:948, 2003.

60. Cameron D, Arnot R, Clay M, Silverman M: Aerosol delivery in neonatal ventilator circuits: a rabbit lung model, *Pediatr Pulmonol* 10:208, 1991.

61. Everard ML, Stammers J, Hardy JG, Milner AD: New aerosol delivery system for neonatal ventilator circuits, *Arch Dis Child* 67:826, 1992.

62. American Association of Respiratory Care (AARC): Clinical practice guideline: selection of an aerosol delivery device for neonatal and pediatric patients, *Respir Care* 40:1325, 1995.

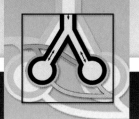

Chapter 18

Skeletal Muscle Relaxants (Neuromuscular Blocking Agents)

HINA N. PATEL

CHAPTER OBJECTIVES

After reading this chapter, the reader will be able to:
1. Define neuromuscular blocking agents (NMBAs) and their mechanism of action
2. List the classes of NMBA available and describe the differences amongst the agents
3. Explain the neuromuscular physiology of nerve conduction
4. Describe the pharmacology of NMBAs
5. Identify potential drug interactions and complications of NMBAs
6. Review indications for NMBAs and monitoring parameters

KEY TERMS AND DEFINITIONS

Acetylcholinesterase — An enzyme that breaks down the neurotransmitter acetylcholine at the synaptic cleft so that the next nerve impulse can be transmitted across the synaptic gap

Amnestic properties — Having the ability to cause total or partial loss of memory

Aspiration — Refers to the accidental inhalation of food particles, fluids, or gastric contents into the lungs

Fasciculations — Involuntary contractions or twitching of groups of muscle fibers

Myasthenia gravis — An autoimmune neuromuscular disorder characterized by chronic fatigue and exhaustion of muscles

Neuromuscular blocking agents (NMBAs) — A substance that interferes with the neural transmission between motor neurons and skeletal muscles

Neuron (nerve cell) — One of the basic functional units of the nervous system that is specialized to transmit electrical nerve impulses and carry information from one part of the body to another. A neuron consists of a cell body, axons, and dendrites

Neurotransmitter — A chemical that is released from a nerve ending to transmit an impulse from a nerve cell to another nerve, muscle, organ, or other tissue

Nosocomial pneumonia — Pneumonia that is acquired in a health care setting

Sedation — The production of a restful state of mind, particularly by the use of drugs that have a calming effect, relieving anxiety and tension

Somatic motor neurons — Part of the nervous system that controls muscles that are under voluntary control

Status asthmaticus — An exacerbation of asthma that does not respond to standard treatment

Status epilepticus — At least 30 minutes of continuous seizure activity without full recovery between seizures

---

Neuromuscular blocking agents (NMBAs), also termed "paralytics" or "muscle relaxants," are drugs that cause skeletal muscle weakness or paralysis and therefore preventing movement. These agents produce this effect at the neuromuscular junction by interfering with the action of the neurotransmitter acetylcholine. NMBAs either depolarize the pre- and postsynaptic membrane receptors or compete with acetylcholine for binding of the acetylcholine receptors at the neuromuscular junction.

KEY POINT

Neuromuscular blocking agents are used for skeletal muscle paralysis in several clinical situations, including *intubation, surgery,* and *facilitation of ventilation* in certain critically ill patients.

The NMBAs are divided into two types: depolarizing and nondepolarizing agents. The depolarizing agents bind to acetylcholine receptors and cause a sustained postsynaptic membrane depolarization. By preventing repolarization of the nerve ending, the postsynaptic ending becomes refractory and unexcitable, resulting in flaccid muscles. At present, succinylcholine is the only available agent in this class. The nondepolarizing agents produce paralysis and muscle weakness by competing

with acetylcholine for binding at the acetylcholine receptors. By preventing the binding of acetylcholine, the nondepolarizing agents block the depolarizing effects of acetylcholine, thereby preventing muscle contraction.

KEY POINT

The two types of neuromuscular blocking agents are *nondepolarizing* and *depolarizing*. Nondepolarizing agents, such as tubocurarine, *competitively block* the cholinergic nicotinic receptor on the postsynaptic muscle fiber, preventing acetylcholine from depolarizing the muscle fiber. Depolarizing agents, such as succinylcholine, act by first depolarizing the muscle fiber and then *prolonging the depolarized state* to prevent repolarization and further stimulation.

USES OF NEUROMUSCULAR BLOCKING AGENTS

The clinical uses of neuromuscular blocking agents are as follows:
- To facilitate endotracheal intubation
- For muscle relaxation during surgery, particularly of the thorax and abdomen
- To enhance patient–ventilator synchrony
- To reduce intracranial pressure in intubated patients with uncontrolled intracranial pressure

- To reduce oxygen consumption
- To terminate convulsive **status epilepticus** and *tetanus* in patients refractory to other therapies
- To facilitate procedures or diagnostic studies
- For selected patients who must remain immobile (e.g., trauma patients)

The NMBAs are usually given intravenously and exhibit a dose-related response on muscles. The primary use of NMBAs in the operating room is for anesthesia induction before endotracheal intubation. In an intensive care unit setting, NMBAs are used primarily for management of mechanical ventilation.

KEY POINT

The most common examples of *ventilated patients requiring muscle relaxation* are those with severe asthma and those requiring "uncomfortable" modes of ventilation such as pressure-controlled inverse ratio ventilation.

PHYSIOLOGY OF THE NEUROMUSCULAR JUNCTION

The autonomic nervous system consists of the central nervous system (CNS) and the peripheral nervous system (PNS). The CNS consists of the brain and the spinal cord, and the PNS includes all the nerves outside of the CNS. Moreover, the PNS is further divided into the **somatic motor neurons**, sensory afferent neurons, and the autonomic nervous system. The skeletal muscle system includes all the peripheral nerves that control "voluntary" movement. Examples of skeletal muscles include the quadriceps, biceps, and diaphragm, which are responsible for motor functions such as movement, lifting, and breathing. The autonomic nervous system includes peripheral nerves that control "involuntary" movement. These nerves stimulate visceral organs such as the heart muscles and other smooth muscles found in bronchioles, arteries, and veins. To review, refer to Chapter 5 in the text.

The basic **nerve cell**, or **neuron**, consists of a *cell body, axons*, and *dendrites* (Figure 18-1). The cell bodies of these neurons, located in the brain and spinal cord, stimulate skeletal muscles via the axons of the *peripheral nerves*. These axons are large myelinated nerve fibers extending from the peripheral nerve cell bodies to the muscle fibers. A single peripheral nerve branches and innervates many different muscle fibers as a *motor unit*. The area between the nerve and muscle, or *synapse*, is specialized into a *motor end plate*. This area between the

axon and the skeletal muscle fiber is also termed the *neuromuscular junction* (Figure 18-2).

The transmission of nerve conduction in skeletal muscle is chemically mediated by the **neurotransmitter** acetylcholine (ACh). When a nerve impulse reaches the end of the motor neuron, ACh is released from the presynaptic nerve ending into the synaptic cleft. Acetylcholine diffuses across the synaptic space and interacts with specific acetylcholine receptors on the postsynaptic muscle fiber membrane, resulting in a response by the muscle fiber. During the short period that ACh is in contact with the muscle fiber membrane, a nerve action potential, or nerve impulse, is initiated in the postsynaptic cell. Acetylcholine is then broken down and inactivated by the enzyme **acetylcholinesterase (AChE)**, allowing the muscle fiber to repolarize.

To further explain muscle stimulation, each acetylcholine receptor has two binding sites to which two acetylcholine molecules must bind to open the pore, illustrated in Figure 18-3. The generation of an action potential at the motor end plate consists of a depolarization phase and a repolarization phase. In the *depolarization phase*, the muscle membrane becomes permeable to sodium ions. As the concentration of sodium ions increases within the postsynaptic cell, a rise in membrane potential occurs. If enough receptors are activated at the same time, a critical threshold is reached and a muscle action potential occurs. As the action potential moves along the muscle fiber, intracellular release of calcium ions, which are stored in the sarcoplasmic reticulum, occurs. As calcium concentrations increase, the actin and myosin filaments of muscles interact and shorten, allowing muscle contraction to occur. In the subsequent *repolarization phase*, the membrane potential returns to a previous baseline level; sodium permeability is blocked and calcium remains inside the sarcoplasmic reticulum. The muscle fiber can be restimulated by another nerve impulse once repolarization has occurred. Until repolarization is complete, the muscle is refractory to additional depolarization and contraction.

On the basis of the neuromuscular physiology described, muscle contraction may be blocked in the following two ways:

1. Competitive inhibition: The binding and blocking of the acetylcholine receptors without depolarization; this is the action of the *nondepolarizing* agents
2. Prolonged occupation and persistent binding of the acetylcholine receptors, resulting in sustained depolarization of the neuromuscular junction; this is the action of the *depolarizing* agents

TABLE 18-1

Classification of Neuromuscular Blocking Activity

Agent	Chemical Class	Pharmacological Properties	Time of Onset (min)	Clinical Duration (min)	Mode of Elimination
Depolarizing NMBAs					
Succinylcholine (Anectine)	Dicholine ester	Ultrashort duration	1-1.5	10-15	Hydrolysis by plasma cholinesterases
Nondepolarizing NMBAs					
d-Tubocurarine	Natural alkaloid (cyclic benzylisoquinoline)	Long duration; competitive	4-6	80-120	Renal elimination; liver clearance
Atracurium (Tracrium)	Benzylisoquinoline ester	Intermediate duration; competitive	2-4	30-60	Hofmann degradation; hydrolysis by plasma esterases; renal elimination
Cisatracurium (Nimbex)	Benzylisoquinoline ester	Intermediate duration; competitive	2-3	40-60	Hofmann degradation; hydrolysis by plasma esterases; renal elimination
Doxacurium (Nuromax)	Benzylisoquinoline ester	Long duration; competitive	4-6	90-120	Renal elimination
Mivacurium (Mivacron)	Benzylisoquinoline ester	Short duration; competitive	2-4	12-18	Hydrolysis by plasma cholinesterases
Pancuronium (Pavulon)	Ammonio steroid	Long duration; competitive	4-6	120-180	Renal elimination
Pipecuronium (Arduan)	Ammonio steroid	Long duration; competitive	2-4	80-100	Renal elimination; liver metabolism and clearance
Rocuronium (Zemuron)	Ammonio steroid	Intermediate duration; competitive	1-2	30-60	Liver metabolism
Vecuronium (Norcuron)	Ammonio steroid	Intermediate duration; competitive	2-4	60-90	Liver metabolism and clearance; renal elimination

Data from *Goodman & Gilman's the pharmacological basis of therapeutics*, ed 10, New York, 2001, McGraw-Hill.

of the body. When normal conduction returns, as many as 75% of acetylcholine receptors may still be occupied by blocker. This explains why additional boluses of blocker appear more potent and have a markedly prolonged duration of action. After prolonged infusion or repeated boluses, metabolism and excretion provide the mechanism for removal of the blocking agent from the neuromuscular junction.

d-Tubocurarine and doxacurium are minimally metabolized, and approximately 60% of an injected dose is excreted by the kidneys in urine. The remainder is excreted in bile. Pancuronium is also eliminated primarily by the kidneys. However, pancuronium also undergoes some hepatic metabolism with production of an active metabolite that is eliminated by the kidneys.

Alternatively, vecuronium is an agent metabolized primarily by the liver. The metabolite of vecuronium also has activity and relies on the kidneys for excretion. All of these agents can accumulate in renal failure and cause prolonged paralysis when given in sufficient doses.

Atracurium and cisatracurium differ from other neuromuscular blocking agents regarding route of elimination. These agents are partly inactivated by a spontaneous degradation mechanism that is dependent on the pH of blood and temperature of the body. This nonenzymatic breakdown is termed *Hofmann degradation*. In addition to Hofmann degradation, these agents are also rapidly converted to less active metabolites by circulating plasma esterases that cause hydrolysis of the compounds. Because of the lack of liver and kidney elimination, atracurium and cisatracurium provide optimal choices for patients with hepatic or renal failure. Atracurium further differs from cisatracurium

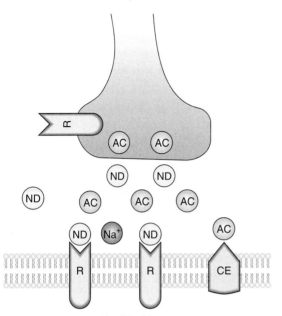

FIGURE 18-4 Competitive blocking agents, or nondepolarizers *(ND)*, occupy but do not activate acetylcholine receptors *(R)*. Acetylcholine *(AC)* is prevented from occupying receptors, and muscle contraction fails to occur. Released acetylcholine is rapidly metabolized by membrane cholinesterase *(CE)*. NDs can also bind to prejunctional acetylcholine receptors and modify AC release.

TABLE 18-2

Dose-dependent Effects of a Nondepolarizing Blocking Agent, Rocuronium, Used in Adults

Dose (mg/kg)	Time to Maximum Block (min)	Clinical Duration (min)
0.45	3	22
0.6	1.8	31
0.9	1.4	58
1.2	1	67

Data from *Drug Facts and Comparisons*, St. Louis, Mo, 2006, Facts and Comparisons, Wolters Kluwer Health.

in that it has a breakdown product of Hofmann degradation called laudanosine. Laudanosine, which is eliminated primarily by the kidneys and is slowly metabolized by the liver, has a long half-life and can cross the blood–brain barrier. Laudanosine has been associated with neurostimulatory effects. Central nervous system excitation and seizures should be considered as a possible complication, especially in patients receiving atracurium who have impaired renal function or liver failure.[2] Cisatracurium has less laudanosine production than atracurium and is considered more potent. The risk of further brain injury from seizures in patients with poor intracranial compliance (e.g., severe head injury) may make these drugs poor choices in these patients. Seizure activity might be masked by these agents, complicating assessment of the patient.

Mivacurium is one of the shortest acting NMBAs available (effect of 10 to 20 minutes in usual doses). It is unique among the nondepolarizing agents in that it is eliminated by plasma cholinesterase, just like succinylcholine, a depolarizing agent. Metabolism of mivacurium is independent of kidney or liver function.[3] However, patients with renal failure or liver dysfunction may have decreased levels of plasma cholinesterase,

therefore prolonging the duration of action of mivacurium. The effects of organ failure on NMBA duration are illustrated in Table 18-3.

Adverse Effects and Hazards
Cardiovascular Effects

It is important to understand that the nondepolarizing blocking agents also competitively block acetylcholine receptors at the autonomic ganglia, producing cardiovascular side effects on heart rate and blood pressure. They may cause a vagolytic effect, which produces tachycardia, and an increase in mean arterial pressure, by promoting an increase in norepinephrine, a potent vasoconstrictor.[3] Pancuronium has the greatest potential to cause cardiovascular side effects, especially tachycardia and hypertension. Agents such as vecuronium, doxacurium, and cisatracurium have minimal effects on heart rate and blood pressure.

Histamine Release

All of the nondepolarizing agents have a tendency to release histamine from mast cells. However, the potential for adverse cardiac effects varies among the different agents. Clinically, histamine release can cause hypotension secondary to direct vasodilation, reflex tachycardia, and bronchospasm, leading to increased airway resistance. The vasodilatory effect may also give the appearance of skin flushing. The degree of histamine release for several of the agents is demonstrated in Table 18-4. *d*-Tubocurarine is the most potent releaser of histamine and causes the most profound problems with intravenous bolus administration. Among the newer agents, mivacurium and atracurium have been reported to stimulate the most histamine release. It is recommended that these agents be given at a reduced rate or at lower doses to avoid these effects. Antihistamines may also be administered as pretreatment to avoid such effects.

TABLE 18-3

Major Metabolic Pathways of Neuromuscular Blockers and Effect on Duration of Action Caused by Organ Failure

Agent	Prolongation of Effect With Renal Failure	Prolongation of Effect With Hepatic Failure	Alternative Metabolism
d-Tubocurarine	+	+	
Doxacurium	+++	0	
Pancuronium	+++	+	
Pipecuronium	+++	0	
Atracurium	0	0	Hofmann degradation, ester hydrolysis
Cisatracurium	0	0	Hofmann degradation, ester hydrolysis
Vecuronium	++*	+	
Rocuronium	++	0	
Mivacurium	0	0	Plasma cholinesterase[†]
Succinylcholine	0	0	Plasma cholinesterase[†]

(0) None; (+) indicates degree of effect.
*Metabolic product is one-third as potent as the parent compound and is entirely removed by renal excretion.
[†]Atypical pseudocholinesterase may prolong relaxant effect dramatically.

TABLE 18-4

Comparison of Side Effects for a Variety of Neuromuscular Blocking Agents

Agent	Histamine Release	Blockade of Autonomic Ganglia	Blockade of Vagal Response	Vagal Stimulation
d-Tubocurarine	++++	+++	0	0
Doxacurium	+	0	0	0
Pancuronium	+	++	++	0
Pipecuronium	+	0	0	0
Atracurium	++	0	0	0
Cisatracurium	+	0	0	0
Vecuronium	0	0	0	0
Rocuronium	+	0	+	0
Mivacurium	++	0	0	0
Succinylcholine	+	0	0	+++

(0) None; (+) indicates degree of effect.

Inadequate Ventilation

Muscle paralysis of the diaphragm and the intercostals results in an inadequate respiratory function. Adequate airway control and ventilatory support are required until muscle recovery is adequate for spontaneous ventilation. Close patient and machine monitoring are essential in an intensive care unit setting to prevent hypoventilation and hypoxemia.

Reversal of Nondepolarizing Blockade

Muscle paralysis caused by nondepolarizing blocking agents can be reversed by use of cholinesterase inhibitors such as neostigmine. Neostigmine inhibits the cholinesterase that would normally break down acetylcholine. This allows for more acetylcholine to be available at the neuromuscular junction to compete with and displace the blocker from receptor sites. Other cholinesterase inhibitors include edrophonium and pyridostigmine. Edrophonium is rapid-acting but also has the shortest duration of action. Pyridostigmine has a slower onset and is the longest acting; it is often used to treat **myasthenia gravis** and can be given orally. Neostigmine is intermediate in onset and duration of action. Table 18-5 profiles these agents with recommended doses to reverse neuromuscular blockage produced by the nondepolarizing agents.[4]

KEY POINT

The effects of nondepolarizing agents can be reversed with an indirect-acting cholinergic agent (*cholinesterase inhibitor*) such as neostigmine. There is no reversal agent for succinylcholine.

TABLE 18-5		
Agents Used for Reversal and Antimuscarinic Effects With Nondepolarizing Blocking Agents		
Agent	**Dose**	**Time for Effect**
Reversal Agents		
Edrophonium	0.3-1.0 mg/kg	Rapid onset, short acting
Pyridostigmine	0.1-0.25 mg/kg	Slowest onset, longest acting
Neostigmine	0.01-0.035 mg/kg	Intermediate onset and duration
Antimuscarinic Agents		
Atropine	0.008-0.018 mg/kg	Rapid onset, short acting
Glycopyrrolate	0.002-0.016 mg/kg	Rapid onset, short acting

Data from Buck ML, Reed MD: Use of nondepolarizing neuromuscular blocking agents in mechanically ventilated patients, *Clin Pharm 10:32*, 1991.

KEY POINT

Myasthenia gravis is caused by an immune response to acetylcholine receptors (AChRs), which are found on nerve and muscle cells. In this disease the body produces antibodies that attack AChRs, preventing signals from reaching the muscles.

Because the reversing agents increase the levels of acetylcholine, they also increase the effects of acetylcholine at parasympathetic ganglia, producing cholinergic autonomic side effects. Major side effects of these agents include severe bradycardia and salivation. To reduce such adverse effects, agents such as atropine or glycopyrrolate are also given in conjunction with the cholinesterase inhibitors. As vagolytic and anticholinergic agents, atropine and glycopyrrolate, respectively, will prevent the bradycardia, increased salivation, and hyperperistalsis associated with excessive acetylcholine.[5]

DEPOLARIZING AGENTS

Depolarizing agents have a different mechanism of action from that of the nondepolarizing agents; they are shorter acting, and there are no agents that will reliably reverse their blockade. Succinylcholine is the only available agent in this group. An intravenous dose of 1 to 1.5 mg/kg will cause total muscle paralysis in 60 to 90 seconds that lasts from 10 to 15 minutes. Because of the quick onset and brief duration of action of succinylcholine, it is an ideal agent for patients requiring intubation.

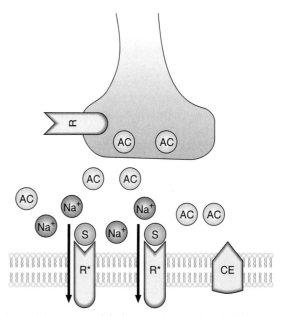

FIGURE 18-5　Succinylcholine produces a depolarizing block. Molecules of succinylcholine *(S)* occupy and activate the acetylcholine receptors *(R*)*, permitting sodium entry and an initial action potential. Continued occupancy prevents repolarization and the next action potential from released acetylcholine *(AC)*. R, Prejunctional receptor; CE, Cholinesterase. Activation of prejunctional AC receptors can modify AC release.

Mode of Action

The initial action of depolarizing neuromuscular blockers is to open sodium channels and depolarize the postsynaptic muscle membrane in the same manner as acetylcholine. The depolarizing agents are resistant to the effects of acetylcholinesterase, allowing for a persistent and longer duration at the neuromuscular junction. As depolarization lasts longer, the membrane is unable to repolarize, resulting in flaccid muscles.[5] This is illustrated in Figure 18-5, in which molecules of succinylcholine *(S)* have occupied two acetylcholine receptors, each opening a pore and allowing the local membrane to become permeable to sodium. If enough receptors are activated, depolarization occurs and is maintained until succinylcholine leaves the receptors. Further stimulation and contraction of the muscle fiber is not possible until the drug is removed by redistribution and metabolism.

Unlike any agent discussed so far, succinylcholine has a unique feature of blockade activity. On initial bolusing, succinylcholine depolarizes the membrane just like acetylcholine. The initial depolarization causes uncoordinated skeletal muscle contractions, referred to as **fasciculations**. As succinylcholine remains at the neuromuscular junction longer than acetylcholine, depolarization is prolonged and flaccid paralysis occurs. This is referred to as "phase I block." After prolonged use or large doses of succinylcholine, the type of blocking activity changes. Instead of showing depolarization characteristics, activity resembles the block produced by the nondepolarizing agents. This is referred to as "phase II block" or "desensitization block." Phase II block involves a "fading" phenomenon in which stimulation of the motor neuron is poorly sustained and paralysis is prolonged. Although cholinesterase inhibitors can reverse phase II block, they may decrease the clearance of succinylcholine and enhance further blockade. The occurrence of a desensitization block must be considered as a possibility in patients with prolonged paralysis after succinylcholine administration. The fear of this "dual" mechanism limits the use of succinylcholine in repeated doses or as a continuous infusion.

Metabolism

Succinylcholine has a very short duration of action. This is mostly due to its rapid hydrolysis by plasma cholinesterase in blood. Succinylcholine is metabolized to succinylmonocholine, which provides weak nondepolarizing activity. It is thought that succinylmonocholine accounts for some of the reason why repeated doses of succinylcholine produce prolonged blockade.

Reversal

There are no agents available for the reversal of succinylcholine. Use of cholinesterase inhibitors such as neostigmine may delay the elimination of succinylcholine, resulting in an even more prolonged depolarization and slower recovery of muscle activity.

Adverse Effects and Hazards

Succinylcholine produces many side effects. Several side effects of succinylcholine can be life threatening. The significance of these side effects may be of more concern in the intensive care unit (ICU) than during routine operating room use. Most adult patients will have a sympathomimetic response causing tachycardia and a rise in blood pressure. Repeated bolus doses of succinylcholine may produce vagal responses including bradycardia and hypotension. This is seen more often in children. Succinylcholine also provokes histamine release, resulting in bronchospasm and hypotension in susceptible individuals.[5]

Muscle pain and soreness similar to myalgias are common after the administration of succinylcholine. A relationship between the pain and muscle fasciculations has been implicated but not confirmed. Some practitioners administer a small dose of a nondepolarizing blocker (e.g., 10% of the intubating dose) before giving succinylcholine to reduce the fasciculations and pain.[6] This pretreatment is often referred to as *defasciculation*. In patients receiving a nondepolarizing agent to prevent fasciculations, higher doses of succinylcholine are needed for complete paralysis because pretreatment reduces the effectiveness of succinylcholine. This practice is considered controversial because increased doses of succinylcholine are required and pretreatment may cause partial paralysis, necessitating urgent intubation under nonideal conditions.[7] Muscle fasciculations can also cause a rise in serum potassium and creatinine phosphokinase, an effect that is also reduced but not totally eliminated by pretreatment.

Succinylcholine can cause an efflux of potassium from muscle cells, causing serum potassium to increase by 0.5 to 1.0 mEq/L in normal individuals.[6] Patients with spinal cord injury or upper motor neuron lesions, thermal injuries, and severe trauma, including closed head injury, are at a higher risk of developing life-threatening hyperkalemia if succinylcholine is administered. Effects of severe hyperkalemia include arrhythmias and cardiac arrest.

Succinylcholine-induced fasciculations can increase intraocular pressure and intragastric pressure. Patients are at risk of extrusion of intraocular contents and aspiration of gastric contents, respectively. This may be partially prevented by defasciculation.

Succinylcholine can dangerously increase intracranial pressure in patients with cerebral edema and head trauma by a mechanism that is not well understood.[6]

One of the most serious complications that can occur with succinylcholine is malignant hyperthermia. Malignant hyperthermia is caused by a genetic defect of muscle metabolism. It is a potentially fatal hypermetabolic state of skeletal muscle. An uncontrolled release of calcium from the sarcoplasmic reticulum of muscles occurs, resulting in a host of harmful effects. The clinical features can present as intractable spasm of the jaw muscles, rigidity, increased oxygen demand, severe hyperthermia, metabolic acidosis, and tachycardia. The treatment of malignant hyperthermia is dantrolene, an agent that blocks the release of intracellular calcium from the sarcoplasmic reticulum. Early recognition and treatment provide full recovery.[8]

Sensitivity to Succinylcholine

As mentioned, succinylcholine is metabolized by plasma cholinesterase, which is also called *pseudocholinesterase*. Patients with abnormal or deficient pseudocholinesterase will not metabolize succinylcholine as effectively and will experience a prolonged recovery from paralysis. In these patients, prolonged mechanical ventilation support is warranted. A family history of prolonged paralysis after surgery may suggest an abnormality in the enzyme. Laboratory tests are also available to determine the existence of abnormal cholinesterase.[9]

NEUROMUSCULAR BLOCKING AGENTS AND MECHANICAL VENTILATION

An indication for use of neuromuscular blocking agents in patients receiving mechanical ventilation is to improve ventilator–patient synchrony. Ventilator dyssynchrony can cause increased intrathoracic pressure, decreased alveolar ventilation, and increased work of breathing for the patient. The desired goal with these drugs is to improve ventilation and oxygenation and to reduce ventilation pressures. Other disease states in which neuromuscular blockade may be beneficial include the following:

- Status asthmaticus, severe bronchospasm
- Certain modes of ventilatory support (e.g., pressure-controlled inverse ratio ventilation, high-frequency oscillatory ventilation)
- Status epilepticus or other intractable convulsive activity
- Neuromuscular toxins (e.g., strychnine poisoning)
- Tetanus

Patients at highest risk of ventilator dyssynchrony include those with **status asthmaticus** and those with severe acute respiratory distress syndrome (ARDS) requiring pressure-controlled ventilation, with or without inverse ratio ventilation, to limit peak airway pressure.

Precautions and Risks

All patients receiving NMBAs should receive additional care measures in order to decrease the negative effects that can be associated with the use of these agents. For instance, proper eye care should be a standard of care for all patients receiving NMBAs. Normally, eye blinking lubricates and cleans the corneas. NMBAs cause paralysis of the eyelid muscles, which can result in corneal drying and ulceration. Appropriate eye lubrication and light taping of the eyes can prevent corneal abrasions. Eyes should be checked frequently.

With complete paralysis, the cough reflex is inhibited. Frequent suctioning along with appropriate sedation and analgesia to prevent pain and discomfort during suctioning is necessary. Retention of secretions is thought to increase the incidence of **nosocomial pneumonia** in patients receiving neuromuscular blockade for a prolonged period. Elevating the head can reduce the risk of **aspiration**.

Close monitoring of support equipment, including constant observation for extubation and ventilator malfunction, must be practiced. Alarm systems to detect hypoventilation and hypoxemia are the standard of care when NMBAs are utilized.

Those patients receiving prolonged therapy with NMBAs are at risk for developing prolonged muscle skeletal muscle weakness that persists long after the NMBA is discontinued. The myopathy, which may take months to resolve, may be more often associated with the steroid-structured agents such as vecuronium and pancuronium (see Table 18-1 for classification), especially when they are combined with corticosteroids such as prednisone. Daily physical therapy with range-of-motion exercises may lessen the potential for muscle atrophy or wasting in patients receiving prolonged blockade. Patients given an NMBA should also be turned frequently to prevent the formation of pressure sores and decubitus ulcers. The risk of developing a deep venous thrombosis (DVT) is increased in these patients because of their immobility, therefore making DVT prophylaxis imperative.

Use of Sedation and Analgesia

Of all the adjunctive therapies patients may receive, it is absolutely essential to provide adequate **sedation** and analgesia for ventilated patients receiving a blocking agent. The NMBAs cause muscle paralysis without affecting consciousness or the perception of pain. In 1947, a classic experiment that established this fact was performed by the anesthesiologist Scott M. Smith and colleagues,[10] in which Smith allowed himself to be paralyzed with *d*-tubocurarine. He reported full awareness during the paralysis, including sensations of choking while he was unable to swallow and shortness of breath even though he was being adequately ventilated. Neuromuscular blockade is unthinkable without proper sedation and pain control to prevent the nightmare of paralysis with full consciousness and sensory perception. Because clinical signs of restlessness, distress, and anxiety are lost with neuromuscular blockade continuous cardiac monitoring is necessary, and vital signs should be assessed closely. Tachycardia, hypertension, diaphoresis, and lacrimation are physiologic responses that can indicate anxiety caused by inadequate sedation or lack of pain control.

KEY POINT

Paralysis of a conscious patient is torture, and *adequate sedation* and *analgesia* are mandatory.

For short procedures including endotracheal intubation, a sedative that has **amnestic properties** should be administered. In surgery, a sedative and an analgesic agent are recommended for all patients. For patients in an ICU, a sedative should be administered on a continuous basis before initiation of neuromuscular blockade. Continuous analgesia should also be used secondary to poor assessment capabilities for pain and the discomfort associated with the constant suctioning and endotracheal tube itself. Examples of sedatives that have amnestic effects include propofol (Diprivan), lorazepam (Ativan), and midazolam (Versed). It is important to realize that these agents do not provide pain control. Analgesics commonly used for pain control include fentanyl (Sublimaze) and morphine. In many situations, deep sedation with continuously infused sedatives and analgesics may prevent the need for a blocking agent in an ICU setting. Other suggestions for sedation and analgesia are presented in Chapter 22, Drugs Affecting the Central Nervous System.

Interactions With Neuromuscular Blocking Agents

Several clinical conditions and medications may alter the effect of an administered neuromuscular blocker. Because different blocking drugs may act at different locations on the acetylcholine receptor–pore complex (e.g., external, in the pore, intercellular), combination with certain agents may be synergistic and potentiate blockade. Advantage has been taken of this potential to produce a combination of relaxant drugs that gives adequate relaxation with fewer (cardiovascular) side effects. Examples include combining inhaled anesthetics, such as halothane or isoflurane, with a nondepolarizing NMBA. The inhaled anesthetics decrease the sensitivity of the neuromuscular junction to acetylcholine, hence potentiating blockade. This allows for a reduction in the dosage of the NMBA perhaps decreasing side effects. The problem with this approach has

been the unpredictability of the duration of relaxation, which tends to be extremely prolonged, especially after repeated mixture administrations.

Some classes of drugs and other conditions have neuromuscular blocking effects themselves; these may be additive, antagonistic, or synergistic with neuromuscular blockers. The aminoglycoside antibiotics are a group of drugs often administered to critically ill patients in the ICU. Aminoglycosides produce blockade by inhibiting the release of ACh from presynaptic nerve endings and, to a lesser extent, by blocking the postsynaptic receptor. Agents such as phenytoin, azathioprine, and theophylline antagonize neuromuscular blockade.

Clinical factors such as acidosis, hypokalemia, hyponatremia, hypocalcemia, and hypermagnesemia all potentiate neuromuscular blockade. Alkalosis and hypercalcemia are known to inhibit the effects of blockade.

Factors affecting the activity of neuromuscular blocking agents are listed in Box 18-1.

Choice of Agents

The characteristics of the perfect neuromuscular blocking agent (not yet developed) are as follows:
- Nondepolarizing block
- Rapid onset of action
- Predictable and controllable duration of action
- Hemodynamic stability at all levels of block and rate of administration
- No histamine release
- Predictable kinetics independent of age, gender, and organ dysfunction
- No active metabolites or toxicity
- Inexpensive

To date, there is no NMBA that exhibits all these ideal characteristics. Selection of an appropriate NMBA is therefore situation dependent. Several factors must be taken into account when choosing an agent: duration of procedure (consider duration of action), the need for quick endotracheal intubation (consider onset of action), adverse effect profile (hemodynamic stability, histamine release), route of elimination (especially in patients with renal or hepatic insufficiency), concurrent medications/drug interactions, and cost. The depolarizing agent succinylcholine is well suited only for intubation because of its rapid onset and short duration of action. Rocuronium and mivacurium may be reasonable alternatives for succinylcholine, with a better side-effect profile. These agents have a quick onset of action but longer duration of effect than succinylcholine. For patients requiring prolonged paralysis, the nondepolarizing blocking agents are better suited. The

Box 18-1	Drugs and Conditions That Interact With Nondepolarizing Neuromuscular Blocking Agents

DRUGS

POTENTIATING FACTORS

Potent anesthetic vapors

Antibiotics
- Aminoglycosides
- Clindamycin
- Vancomycin
- Tetracycline

Local anesthetics

Antiarrhythmics
- Procainamide
- Quinidine
- Bretylium

Calcium channel blockers

β-Adrenergic blockers

Cyclosporine

Dantrolene

Cyclophosphamide

Lithium

Mineralocorticoids

Echothiophate

Tacrine

Metoclopramide

ANTAGONIZING FACTORS

Phenytoin

Carbamazepine

Theophylline

Anticholinesterase agents

Azathioprine

Ranitidine

CONDITIONS

POTENTIATING FACTORS

Acidosis

Hyponatremia

Hypocalcemia

Hypokalemia

Hypermagnesemia

Hypothermia

Renal failure

Hepatic failure

Organophosphate poisoning

ANTAGONIZING FACTORS

Alkalosis

Hypercalcemia

Demyelinating injuries

Peripheral neuropathy

DISEASES

POTENTIATING FACTORS

Myasthenia gravis

Muscular dystrophy

Amyotrophic lateral sclerosis

Poliomyelitis

Multiple sclerosis

Eaton-Lambert syndrome

ANTAGONIZING FACTORS

Diabetes mellitus

Data from Feldman S, Karalliedde L: Drug interactions with neuromuscular blockers, *Drug Safety* 15:261, 1996.

kinetics of the nondepolarizing agents allow for a longer duration of action, more gradual onset and offset of block, and fewer hemodynamic changes. They can be administered by continuous infusion and, if necessary, the blockade can be reversed with cholinesterase inhibitors.

The choice of agent for continuous paralysis involves clinical judgment and preference. The currently available nondepolarizing agents can be compared with one another regarding adverse effect profile (histamine release and cardiovascular instability), route of elimination, drug interactions, and cost effectiveness as a guide in drug choice for paralysis of ventilated patients. Tables 18-3 and 18-4 compare some of these factors for several of the NMBAs.

Most nondepolarizing agents release histamine from mast cells. As discussed earlier, *d*-tubocurarine provokes the greatest release of histamine. Pancuronium is

thought to provoke the least amount of release of histamine. Agents such as vecuronium, rocuronium, cisatracurium, and doxacurium are similar to pancuronium and have minimal histamine release relative to the other agents. Atracurium and mivacurium have also been shown to induce histamine release: more than pancuronium, but less than tubocurarine. Flushing is the most common effect of histamine release after atracurium administration. Histamine release by these drugs can be minimized by administering a bolus dose slowly over 60 seconds, administering several smaller boluses or giving the agent by slow continuous infusion.

Vecuronium, atracurium, cisatracurium, and doxacurium have minimal effects on heart rate and blood pressure. Pancuronium often produces a transient increase in blood pressure and heart rate. Pipecuronium can occasionally cause bradycardia and hypotension or hypotension alone. Rocuronium seems to cause little systemic cardiovascular effect, but an increase in pulmonary vascular resistance has been seen with this drug. Caution is recommended in using this agent with pulmonary hypertension or valvular heart disease. Bolus administration of mivacurium can cause a transient decrease in blood pressure, usually secondary to histamine release.

The method of drug elimination (e.g., renal or hepatic) is a very important factor in selecting an agent for patients with multiple-organ dysfunction syndrome requiring mechanical ventilation. Agents that depend on the liver and kidney for elimination are poorly suited for patients with disease or failure of these organs. The potential effects of organ failure on each agent are described in Table 18-3. In patients with hepatic or renal failure, atracurium, cisatracurium, and mivacurium have the advantage of plasma metabolism and do no rely on hepatic metabolism or renal excretion. The metabolite laudanosine from atracurium metabolism may be of concern in patients with kidney or liver failure. Cisatracurium results in less laudanosine than does atracurium.

Patients in the ICU have clinical conditions and are often receiving medications that can affect blockade with an NMBA. As discussed earlier, myopathy can occur in patients receiving NMBAs. The potential is increased in patients receiving concomitant corticosteroids. Agents such as vecuronium, pancuronium, and rocuronium are steroid-structured and may further prolong muscle weakness. The non-steroid-structured agents such as atracurium or cisatracurium may be better suited for patients requiring high-dose corticosteroids.

Last, cost is another important consideration in choosing an agent. Many hospitals limit the number of NMBAs available on formulary because of economic issues. The newer, shorter acting agents are very expensive, especially if used for a prolonged period in the ICU. Most hospitals restrict their use to procedures of short duration. Guidelines for blockade use in the intensive care unit have been published and suggest that cost-effective relaxation can be provided with bolus dosing or continuous infusions of pancuronium (if tachycardia is not a concern) or vecuronium in patients with ischemic cardiovascular issues.[2] For patients with hepatic and renal dysfunction, cisatracurium or atracurium provides the best option. The clinician is advised to reassess the need for continuous paralysis on a daily basis.

In summary, pancuronium provides the least expensive option for prolonged paralysis of patients who are hemodynamically stable with no organ dysfunction. For unstable patients, the nondepolarizing agents vecuronium and doxacurium produce the least amount of histamine release and fewest cardiovascular effects. Atracurium and cisatracurium offer alternative choices for ventilator management, with these agents having the advantage of alternative metabolic pathways but at a higher cost.

KEY POINT

Nondepolarizing agents are preferred for *paralysis of ventilator patients* because of the predictability, longer duration of action, and manageable side effects of these agents. Specific agents should be selected on the basis of potential for *histamine release* and *cardiovascular effects*, patient-specific *metabolic pathways*, and *cost*.

MONITORING OF NEUROMUSCULAR BLOCKADE

Patients receiving NMBAs require constant monitoring with frequent physical assessment and regularly scheduled evaluations of laboratory studies because clinical signs and symptoms of acute disease can be masked by muscle paralysis. Alarm systems to detect accidental disconnection from the ventilator are mandatory and alarms to detect hypoventilation and hypoxemia are the standard of care when neuromuscular blockade is employed.

Before initiating neuromuscular blockade of an agitated patient, ventilator malfunction must first be ruled out as the cause of agitation, or muscle paralysis could cause death in the face of inadequate machine volume or oxygen delivery.

Patients receiving paralytics can be assessed by visual, tactile, and electronic methods to evaluate muscle tone and depth of neuromuscular blockade. Direct observation of muscle activity provides the simplest means of monitoring adequacy of blockade. The sequence of paralysis of the skeletal muscles can be monitored physically: first, small, rapid moving muscles such as the eyelids; then the face, neck, extremities, abdomen, the intercostals; and finally, the diaphragm. Recovery of paralysis is in reverse order, with recovery of the diaphragm and respiratory muscles occurring first. The sensitivity of individual muscles to paralysis is related to the number of fibers innervated by each motor neuron and by regional blood flow, with areas receiving a greater blood flow having more drug delivery and therefore a quicker onset of paralysis.

TABLE 18-6

Receptor Occupancy Associated With Various Measurements of Neuromuscular Blockade

Receptors Occupied (%)	Twitch Height (%)	Train of Four	Clinical Observations
100	0	0	Total paralysis, no voluntary movement of any muscle; no PTF
98-99	0	0	Diaphragm may move; PTF present
95-98	1-5	1 or 2 twitches	Diaphragm can move minimally; PTF and fade present
90-95	10-25	2 or 3 twitches	Breathing inadequate
75-90	10-25	4 twitches, 1st > 4th	Tidal volume restored, voluntary movement apparent, can sustain head lift for 5 sec (75%-80% occupancy), NIP > 55 cmH$_2$O, vital capacity 60%-70% of normal
50-75	100	4 equal twitches	Normal strength and movement, cough strength decreased; double burst suppression abnormal
<30	100	4 equal twitches	No apparent deficits, double burst suppression normal

NIP, Negative inspiratory pressure; PTF, posttetanic facilitation.

The vast experience with neuromuscular blocking agents is in the operating room. The time course of relaxant effect and rate of recovery is not the same when these drugs are used for prolonged periods in patients in the ICU. During brief periods of paralysis, the depth of blockade or the adequacy of recovery of neuromuscular function can be assessed by simple measures of voluntary muscular functions. These include subjective assessments, such as hand-grip strength or the ability to lift the head off the bed for 5 seconds. Objective assessments include measurement of vital capacity, negative inspiratory force, and spontaneous respiratory rate. Patients requiring prolonged paralysis are not as easy to evaluate because of issues such as heavy sedation. Although clinical signs may be helpful in these patients, a more physiological and objective evaluation of neuromuscular blockade can be achieved by using electronic methods such as peripheral nerve stimulation. Examples of modes of peripheral nerve stimulation include single twitch, double burst, train of four (TOF), and tetanic and posttetanic count.

Peripheral nerve stimulation or "twitch monitoring" is used as a monitoring tool for efficacy and toxicity in both surgical and ICU patients. In peripheral nerve stimulation, a stimulator is applied to a peripheral nerve and the response of the corresponding muscle is observed. The ulnar nerve, which innervates the adductor pollicis muscle of the thumb, is the most commonly used area. Another nerve is the facial nerve, which innervates the orbicularis oculi muscle of the eye.

The nerve response to electrical stimulation depends on the current applied, the duration for which the current is applied, and placement of the electrodes. For ulnar nerve stimulation, two small conducting pads are placed on the forearm over the nerve tract, several inches apart. A single electrical stimulus is discharged from a nerve stimulator to the ulnar nerve; the responses or twitches of the thumb that occur are then measured. As the amount of paralysis increases, the strength and degree of movement of the twitch decrease.

The most commonly used technique for monitoring blockade is the train-of-four evaluation. In TOF, a supramaximal stimulus at a frequency of 2 Hz is applied to the nerve over 2 seconds. The nonpainful stimuli are delivered as four pulses, one every 0.5 second. The number of twitches that occur, ranging from 0 (100% blockade) to 4 (<75% blockade), are measured. Comparison of the strength of the fourth twitch and first twitch predicts the degree of receptor occupancy (see Table 18-6). Clinically, the degree of block can be determined by counting the number of twitches seen. Four equal twitches indicate that less than 75% of the receptors are occupied with a blocker. If only three twitches are seen, approximately 80% of receptors are blocked; if only one or two are seen, 90%-95% are blocked.

Train-of-four monitoring allows for an accurate assessment of neuromuscular blockade depth with or without baseline control. To avoid overdosing of patients, the neuromuscular blocking drug (bolus or infusion) should be titrated to produce the minimal blockade required to maintain the desired clinical response. Predefined goals such as decreased oxygen requirements, peak inspiratory pressure, and positive end-expiratory pressure (PEEP) reduction should be assessed frequently. If the response is adequate, a TOF count of at least 1-2/4 (number of twitches to stimulations) is recommended. It is possible that lesser degrees of blockade may achieve the clinical goal of ventilator synchrony or improved oxygenation. In an ICU, the depth of blockade should be assessed every 2-3 hours on initiation until a stable dose is maintained. Thereafter, TOF assessment may occur every 8-12 hours. If there is no twitch response or the clinical response is achieved at a higher twitch, the dose of the NMBA should be decreased by 10%. If three or four twitches occur without adequate response, the dose can be increased by 10%. The need for continued paralysis of the patient in the ICU should be assessed daily, and, if appropriate, should be discontinued as soon as possible.[7]

KEY POINT

Titration of drug dose and monitoring of reversal are performed with a *peripheral nerve stimulator* and train-of-four stimulation.

THE FUTURE OF NEUROMUSCULAR BLOCKING AGENTS AND REVERSAL

Research is continuing in an effort to develop an ideal NMBA. At present, gantacurium (GW280430A) has promise as a new agent. Still in the research phase, gantacurium is a nondepolarizing agent with rapid-onset and short-acting properties. Its organ-independent inactivation is ideal in patients with organ dysfunction. Histamine release has been found to occur, resulting in tachycardia and hypotension. However, the histamine release appears to be less compared with that produced by the benzylisoquinolines.[11]

At present, the method of reversing NMBAs involves the use of acetylcholinesterase inhibitors such as neostigmine, which increase the levels of acetylcholine in the synaptic cleft to compete with NMBA for receptor sites. Sugammadex, an agent currently under study, provides a newer approach to NMBA reversal. The novel mechanism of action involves the actual inactivation and removal of the NMBA from the neuromuscular junction and the body. Sugammadex functions by encapsulating the NMBA to form a complex that can no longer bind to the receptors. The stable complex that is formed is then excreted by the kidneys. Sugammadex has only been shown to effectively reverse rocuronium and vecuronium. It is much less effective for reversal of pancuronium, succinylcholine, and the benzylisoquinolines. Adverse effects are relatively mild and include nausea, dry mouth, cough, and taste perversions.[12]

Although both gantacurium and sugammadex offer promising alternatives as NMBAs, they may have drawbacks not yet discovered and require further evaluation in larger trials.

SELF-ASSESSMENT QUESTIONS

1. List four general uses of skeletal muscle relaxants.
2. What are the two classifications of neuromuscular blocking agents?
3. Identify each of the following agents by classification type: tubocurarine, vecuronium, succinylcholine, and pancuronium.
4. Which type of neuromuscular blocker can be reversed?
5. What type of drug would you use to reverse vecuronium?
6. Identify another drug that you would want to give before you reverse the vecuronium.
7. Briefly explain why you might need to paralyze a patient receiving mechanical ventilation.
8. Neuromuscular blocking agents do not block consciousness; what two types or classes of drugs would be indicated in a paralyzed patient on mechanical ventilation?
9. Identify at least two neuromuscular blocking agents that would be preferred for paralysis in a patient receiving mechanical ventilation (assume normal renal and hepatic function).
10. You are called to the recovery room to set up a ventilator for a elderly patient who has just undergone a total hip replacement and has failed to breathe after a single dose of succinylcholine. What might the problem be?
11. What would you do first to assess a ventilated patient who is restless and "fighting" the ventilator before using a paralyzing agent?

Answers to Self-Assessment Questions are found in Appendix A.

CLINICAL SCENARIO

A 64-year-old white female comes to the emergency department with a complaint of shortness of breath and congestion along with fatigue and lethargy over the last 3 days. Her problem list includes a history of diabetes mellitus, hypertension, and chronic obstructive pulmonary disease (COPD) secondary to smoking. She has had a cough productive of yellow-greenish sputum and states she has had fever and chills over the past several days. Her current medications include metformin, glyburide, lisinopril, ipratropium inhaler, albuterol inhaler as needed, and Advair inhaler.

On physical examination, her vital signs are as follows: pulse (P), 130 beats/min; blood pressure (BP), 100/72 mmHg; temperature (T), 38.5° C; and respiratory rate (RR), 30 breaths/min, with a moderate amount of respiratory distress. On auscultation, breath sounds are diminished bilaterally.

An electrocardiogram shows sinus tachycardia. Pulse oximetry showed 80% saturation on room air. Her chest radiograph shows bilateral interstitial infiltrates. Her white blood cell (WBC) count is $23.7 \times 10^3/\text{mm}^3$ with 35% bands, hemoglobin is 11.2 g/dl and hematocrit is 33.2%, and electrolytes are within normal limits, except for glucose, which is 250 mg/dl.

What additional laboratory information would be most helpful in assessing this patient and determining further treatment?

After approximately 3 hours of intense treatment with intravenous fluids, antibiotics, and albuterol/ipratropium nebulizations, the patient continues to be short of breath. She is anxious and exhibits labored breathing. Her heart rate (HR) ranges from 126 to 154 beats/min, RR is 32 to 40 breaths/min, BP is 85/60 mmHg, and her mental status has deteriorated. Arterial blood gas values on a 100% nonrebreather mask are as follows: pH, 7.24; arterial carbon dioxide pressure (Pa_{CO_2}), 38 mmHg; arterial oxygen pressure (Pa_{O_2}), 55 mmHg; and arterial oxygen saturation (Sa_{O_2}), 82%.

The decision is made to intubate and support her with mechanical ventilation.

What neuromuscular blocking agent would you consider for a rapid-sequence intubation?

After intubation and placement on the ventilator, the patient's peak airway pressures are excessive (45 cmH₂O) on 100% $F_{I_{O_2}}$ and her pulse oximetry saturation is 85%. The patient has developed acute respiratory distress with a $Pa_{O_2}/F_{I_{O_2}}$ ratio of 65. The patient is agitated and is dyssynchronous with the ventilator. You decide to provide neuromuscular blockade.

What agent would you use?

How will you monitor the effectiveness of this therapy?

If the patient were in renal or hepatic failure, what neuromuscular blocking agent would you recommend?

Answers to Clinical Scenario Questions are found in Appendix A.

References

1. Palmer T: Agents acting at the neuromuscular junction and autonomic ganglia, In Hardman JG, Limbird LE, Gilman AG, editors: *Goodman & Gilman's the pharmacological basis of therapeutics*, ed 10, New York, 2001, McGraw-Hill.
2. Society of Critical Care Medicine and American Society of Health-System Pharmacists: Clinical practice guidelines for sustained neuromuscular blockade in the adult critically ill patient, *Am J Health Syst Pharm* 59:179, 2002.
3. McManus MC: Neuromuscular blockers in surgery and intensive care, part 1, *Am J Health Syst Pharm* 58:2287, 2001.
4. *Drug Facts and Comparisons*, St. Louis, Mo, 2006, Facts and Comparisons, Wolters Kluwer Health.
5. Wheeler AP: Sedation, analgesia, and paralysis in the intensive care unit, *Chest* 104:566, 1993.
6. Fisher DM: Clinical pharmacology of neuromuscular blocking agents, *Am J Health Syst Pharm* 56(suppl):S4, 1999.
7. McManus MD: Neuromuscular blockers in surgery and intensive care, part 2, *Am J Health Syst Pharm* 58:2381, 2001.
8. Simon HB: Hyperthermia, *N Eng J Med* 329:483, 1993.
9. Davis L, Britten JJ, Morgan M: Cholinesterase: its significance in anaesthetic practice, *Anaesthesia* 52:244, 1997.
10. Smith SM, Brown HO, Toman JEP, Goodman LS: The lack of cerebral effects of *d*-tubocurarine, *Anesthesiology* 8:1, 1947.
11. Belmont MR, Lien CA, Tjan J, Bradley E, Stein B, Patel SS, Savarese JJ: Clinical pharmacology of GW280430A in humans, *Anesthesiology* 100:768, 2004.
12. Adam JM, Bennett DJ, Bom A, Clark JK, Feilden H, Hutchinson EJ, Palin R, Prosser A, Rees DC, Rosair GM, *et al.*: Cyclodextran-derived host molecules as reversal agents for the neuromuscular blocker rocuronium bromide: synthesis and structure–activity relationships, *J Med Chem* 45:1806, 2002.

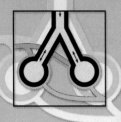

Chapter **19**

Vasopressors, Inotropes, and Antiarrhythmic Agents

HENRY COHEN, BISHOY LUKA, TERESA CHAN, NATALIE ERICHSEN

CHAPTER OBJECTIVES

After reading this chapter, the reader will be able to:
1. List the various components that make up blood pressure
2. Compare and contrast the mechanism of action of the various inotropes and vasopressors
3. Design an algorithm for the management of hypotension
4. Describe the various drug interactions that may occur with the use of vasopressors and inotropes
5. Design an algorithm that may be used in the management of ventricular fibrillation and pulseless ventricular tachycardia
6. Describe the normal conduction of the heart
7. Compare and contrast the various categories of the Vaughan Williams classification system
8. Define the mechanism of action of digoxin
9. Define the nonpharmacologic methods of treating dysrhythmias
10. List the various routes of administering medications during cardiac arrest
11. List all the dysrhythmias associated with cardiac arrest
12. Design an algorithm that may be used in the management of torsades de pointes
13. List the benefits and disadvantages of using sodium bicarbonate therapy in the setting of cardiac arrest
14. Describe the proper dosing technique of intravenous magnesium therapy in the management of torsades de pointes

KEY TERMS AND DEFINITIONS

Antiarrhythmics — A group of cardiac medications that are classified according to mechanism of action; in some instances they may pose multiple mechanisms of action. The most common classification system of antiarrhythmics is the Vaughan Williams classification system, which is divided into four distinct categories and a miscellaneous section

Atrial fibrillation — A cardiac condition in which the normal atrial contractions are replaced by rapid irregular twitchings of the muscular wall. Exceedingly rapid contractions or twitching of muscular fibrils, but not of the muscle as a whole

Atrioventricular (AV) node — Link between atrial depolarization and ventricular depolarization

Bradycardia — A slow heart rate, typically defined as less than 60 beats/min

Bohr effect — The presence of carbon dioxide aiding in the release and delivery of oxygen from hemoglobin

Cardiac output — Amount of blood that is ejected into the aorta and travels through the systemic circulation with every heartbeat

Catecholamines — Endogenous products that are secreted into the bloodstream and travel to nerve endings to stimulate an excitatory response

Chronotropic — Affecting the rate of contraction of the heart

Diastolic blood pressure (DBP) — Lowest pressure reached right before ventricular ejection

Dromotropic — Affecting the velocity of conduction at the AV node

Dysrhythmia/arrhythmia — Irregular (faster or slower) heart beat; the term *arrhythmia* is used more frequently than *dysrhythmia*

Inotrope — A drug affecting the strength of muscular contraction

Mean arterial pressure (MAP) — Pressure that drives blood into the tissues averaged over the entire cardiac cycle

Phosphodiesterase — An enzyme responsible for the breakdown of cyclic adenosine 3′,5′-monophosphate (cAMP)

Sudden cardiac death (SCD) — An episode of ventricular fibrillation, pulseless ventricular tachycardia, pulseless electrical activity, or asystole

Systolic blood pressure (SBP) — Peak pressure reached during ventricular ejection

Tachycardia — An overly rapid heart beat, usually defined as greater than 100 beats/min in adults

Vasodilator — Causing dilation of the blood vessels

Vasopressor — Causing contraction of the capillaries and arteries

Ventricular fibrillation — A cardiac condition in which normal ventricular contractions are replaced by coarse or fine, rapid movements of the ventricular muscle

OVERVIEW OF THE CARDIOVASCULAR SYSTEM

The cardiovascular system regulates blood flow to the various regions of the body. Blood flow generally travels via a pressure gradient, shifting from areas of higher pressure to lower pressure. The central nervous system relays electrical impulses through sensory receptors found systemically within the vasculature, affecting vascular tone and causing shunting of blood to and from various organ systems within the body. Vascular tone is regulated via the sympathetic nervous system and the circulation of neurotransmitters and hormones, such as epinephrine, vasopressin, and angiotensin. Several factors exert an effect on vascular tone as a response to tissue perfusion and circulatory volume.

Factors Affecting Blood Pressure

Typical measurement of blood pressure is relative to a recurring cardiac cycle of atrial and ventricular contractions and relaxations. The cycle is divided into

KEY POINT

Blood pressure is dependent on cardiac function, vascular tone, and vascular volume.

the systolic phase and the diastolic phase. The systolic phase is deemed that portion in which ventricular contraction occurs. resulting in ejection of blood through the aorta. Conversely, diastole is the period of ventricular relaxation and blood filling. On the same note, **systolic blood pressure (SBP)** is the peak pressure reached during ventricular ejection and **diastolic blood pressure (DBP)** is the lowest pressure reached right before ventricular ejection. Arterial pressure is typically recorded as SBP/DPB, for example, 120/80 mmHg. The **mean arterial pressure (MAP)** is actually of greater significance than the SBP and the DBP. The mean arterial pressure signifies the pressure that drives blood into the tissues averaged over the entire cardiac cycle. Mean arterial pressure is regulated by the

TABLE 19-1

Hemodynamic Changes in Various Shock States

Hemodynamic Parameter	Hypovolemic/Hemorrhagic	Neurogenic	Cardiogenic	Septic/Distributive
HR	↑	↔	↔/↑	↑
BP	↓	↑/↓	↑	↓
CVP (5-12 mmHg)	↓	↓	↑	↓
PCWP (10-12 mmHg)	↓	↓	↑	↓
CO (5-7 L/min)	↓	↔/↓	↓	↑
SVR (80-1440 dyn sec ·cm^{-5})	↑	↓	↑	↓

BP, Blood pressure; CO, cardiac output; CVP, central venous pressure; HR, heart rate; PCWP, pulmonary capillary wedge pressure; SVR, systemic vascular resistance.

TABLE 19-2

Inotropes and Vasopressors: Receptor Affinity

Drug	α	β$_1$	β$_2$	DA
Dopamine (Inotropin)	+ to +++*	+++*	+	0/+
Dobutamine (Dobutrex)	0 to +*	0 to +*	+	0
Epinephrine (Adrenalin)	+++*	+++	++*	0
Isoproterenol (Isuprel)	0	+++	+++	0
Norepinephrine (Levophed)	+++	++	++	0
Phenylephrine (Neo-Synephrine)	+++	0	0	0

DA, Dopamine.
*At higher doses: 0, no effect; +, slight effect; ++, moderate effect; +++, pronounced effect.

product of cardiac output (CO) and systemic vascular resistance (SVR).

$$[2(DBP)+SBP]/3$$

or

$$MAP = CO \times SVR$$

Cardiac output is the amount of blood that is ejected into the aorta and travels through the systemic circulation with every heartbeat. It is dependent on the sum of all local blood flow regulations and is demonstrated in the following equation as the product of heart rate (HR) and stroke volume (SV). Changes in either one of these components may alter the effects of the other.

$$CO = HR \times SV$$

Another component that may also affect changes in tissue perfusion is vascular volume. Intravascular volume depletion may influence SV and affect the MAP as well. This component may be indirectly measured as the pulmonary capillary wedge pressure (PCWP) or preload; in other words, the amount of fluid returning to the heart. The central venous pressure helps reflect the amount of blood returning to the heart.

Summing up all components that affect the MAP, the following equation may then better illustrate how these components relate to blood pressure:

$$MAP = HR \times SV \times SVR$$

The use of therapies such as fluids, vasopressors, and inotropes to maintain cardiovascular stability is directed toward altering each of these components, as seen in Table 19-1.

The various **vasopressors** currently on the market have different affinities for the various receptors located within the body and exert different effects on the hemodynamic parameters, as seen in Table 19-2.

To determine the cause of hypotension, such as cardiac failure or vasodilation during sepsis, the use of a monitoring device called the *pulmonary artery catheter* is necessary to evaluate patient-specific response to the use of vasoactive therapy. One should not be led to believe that vasopressors and inotropes are always first-line therapy; on the contrary, fluids are the mainstays for improving hypotensive episodes. Hence, PCWP is a viable tool to assist in measuring intravascular volume, as illustrated in Figure 19-1.

However, the use of this device is not without complications such as in the treatment of infections, trauma (placement during pneumothorax), bleeding,

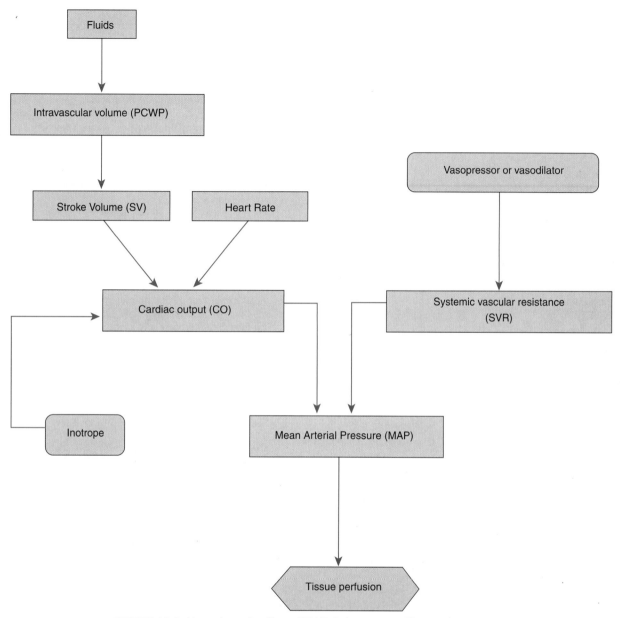

FIGURE 19-1 Hemodynamic effects. *PCWP,* Pulmonary capillary wedge pressure.

and thrombus formation. In addition, certain medications interact with various vasopressors and inotropes, leading to alterations in hemodynamic parameters as seen in Tables 19-3 and 19-4.

KEY POINT

Cardiac drugs are used to influence cardiac function and include agents to increase myocardial contractility, regulate arrhythmias, and treat cardiac arrest.

AGENTS USED IN THE MANAGEMENT OF SHOCK

KEY POINT

Cardiotonic agents stimulate the myocardium and produce a positive effect. These agents include cardiac glycosides (digitalis family), β-adrenergic stimulants, dobutamine, dopamine, isoproterenol, epinephrine, and phosphodiesterase inhibitors.

TABLE 19-3

Drug Interactions

Precipitant Drug*	Effect	Object Drug*	Comments
Dobutamine/Isoproterenol/Norepinephrine			
Bretylium	↑	Dobutamine	Concomitant use may potentiate the effects of
Halogenated hydrocarbon anesthetics		Isoproterenol Norepinephrine	vasopressors, causing arrhythmias
Guanethidine			May increase pressor response, causing severe
Oxytocic drugs			hypertension
Tricyclic antidepressants			
Phenylephrine			
Bretylium	↑	Phenylephrine	Concomitant use may potentiate the effects of
Guanethidine			vasopressors
Halogenated hydrocarbon anesthetics			
Oxytocic drugs			
Tricyclic antidepressants	↔		Tricyclic antidepressants may increase effects of phenylephrine
Dopamine			
Dopamine	↓	Guanethidine	Antihypertensive effects of guanethidine may be reversed
		Phenytoin	Concomitant use may lead to seizures, severe hypotension, and bradycardia
Tricyclic antidepressants		Dopamine	Tricyclic antidepressants may increase effects of dopamine
Halogenated hydrocarbon anesthetics	↑	Dopamine	May sensitize myocardium to actions of vasopressors, causing arrhythmia
Monoamine oxidase inhibitors (MAOIs)			Dopamine is metabolized by MAOIs. MAOIs increase (↑) pressor response to dopamine by 6- to 20-fold
Oxytocic drugs			Concomitant use may cause severe hypertension
Epinephrine			
Cardiac glycosides	↑	Epinephrine	May sensitize myocardium to actions of vasopressors, causing arrhythmia
Halogenated hydrocarbon anesthetics			
Levothyroxine antihistamines (chlorpheniramine, diphenhydramine)			
Monoamine oxidase inhibitors			Concomitant use may cause severe hypertension
Methyldopa			
Oxytocic drugs			
Reserpine			
Sympathomimetics			
Tricyclic antidepressants			
β Blockers			
α Blockers	↓	Epinephrine	Vasoconstricting and hypertensive effects of pressor may be reversed
Chlorpromazine			
Diuretics			
Epinephrine		Guanethidine	Epinephrine may antagonize effects of guanethidine, resulting in decreased (↓) antihypertensive effects

TABLE 19-3

Drug Interactions—cont'd

Precipitant Drug*	Effect	Object Drug*	Comments
Digoxin			
Amiodarone	↑	Digoxin	Amiodarone may increase (↑) digoxin blood level; reduce (↓) digoxin dose by 50%
β Blockers			Combination may cause advanced or complete heart block
Calcium channel blockers			
Calcium			Rapid administration of intravenous calcium may result in fatal arrhythmias
Succinylcholine			Succinylcholine may cause sudden extrusion of K^+ from muscle cells, leading to arrhythmias
Sympathomimetics			Combination may cause increased (↑) risk of cardiac arrhythmias
Thiazide and loop diuretics			Diuretic-induced electrolyte disturbances may predispose to digitalis toxicity
Thyroid hormones	↓	Digoxin	Thyroid hormones may reduce (↓) digoxin blood levels, hypothyroid patients may require higher dose of digoxin

↑, Object drug increased; ↓, object drug decreased; ↔, object drug unaffected.
*Precipitant drug, the drug that causes the interaction; object drug, the drug affected by the interaction.

TABLE 19-4

Cardiac Drugs: Dosing and Pharmacokinetics

Agent	Dose Range	PHARMACOKINETICS			HEMODYNAMIC EFFECTS				
		Onset (min)	Duration	Half-life	HR	MAP	PCWP	SVR	CO
Amrinone	0.75 mg/kg bolus, then 2.5-15 µg/kg/min	5-10	0.5-2 hr	4.8-8.3 hr	↓	0-↓	0-↓	0 to ↓	↓-0-↑
Dobutamine (Dobutrex)	2-20 µg/kg/min	1-2	10-15 min	2 min	0*	0-↓	↓	↓	↑
Dopamine (Inotropin)	1-5 µg/kg/min	5	<10 min	2 min	0	0	0	0	0
	5-15 µg/kg/min	5	<10 min	2 min	↑	0-↓	0-↑	↑	↑
	>15 µg/kg/min	5	<10 min	2 min	↑	0↓	0-↑	↑	↑
Epinephrine (Adrenalin)	0.01-0.1 µg/kg/min	1	3-5 min	3-5 min	↑	↑	0-↓	↓†-↑*	↑
	0.1 µg/kg/min				↑↑	↑↑	↑	↑↑	↑↑
Norepinephrine (Levophed)	0.5-30 µg/min	1-3	5-10 min	1-2 min	0-↑	↑↑↑	↑↑	↑↑↑	0-↓
Phenylephrine (Neo-Synephrine)	0.5-5 µg/kg/min	10-15	1-3 hr	2-3 hr	↓	↑	↑	↑	↓
Milrinone (Primacor)	50 µg/kg bolus, then 0.375-0.75 µg/kg/min	90	3-5 hr	2.3 hr	0-↑	↓	↓	↓	↑
Vasopressin (Pitressin)	0.04 units/min	30-60	30-60 min	10-20 min	0	↑	↑	↑	↓?

CO, Cardiac output; HR, heart rate; MAP, mean arterial pressure; PCWP, pulmonary capillary wedge pressure; SVR, systemic vascular resistance.
↑, effect increased; ↓, effect decreased; 0, effect unchanged.
*At high doses.
†At low doses.

Catecholamines

Norepinephrine (Levophed) and Epinephrine (Adrenalin)

Norepinephrine and epinephrine are endogenous **catecholamines** that are secreted by the adrenal medulla. Epinephrine is ultimately synthesized by the catalytic actions of tyrosine hydroxylase, which converts the amino acid tyrosine to L-dopa and then subsequently to dopamine, norepinephrine, and lastly to epinephrine.[2] These neurotransmitters then travel to sympathetic nerve endings, where they are released to stimulate other nerve fibers and to stimulate an excitatory response. Norepinephrine and epinephrine stimulate α receptors on the vasculature as well as β receptors, also located within the vasculature as well as in the myocardium. α Receptors within the vasculature cause vasoconstriction whereas β receptors cause vasodilation. Most vascular beds within the body contain β receptors; however, they are outnumbered by α receptors, therefore any epinephrine/norepinephrine stimulation of β receptors is negligible or of no effect, yielding a net response of vasoconstriction. In addition, β receptors densely populate the myocardium compared with the α receptors, leading to a net effect of tachycardia.[4]

Isoproterenol (Isuprel)

Isoproterenol is a synthetic catecholamine used for the treatment of symptomatic bradycardia or torsades de pointes. Isoproterenol works solely as an agonist of β receptors. By stimulating β_1-adrenergic receptors it exerts pronounced inotropic and chronotropic effects. By stimulating β_2-adrenergic receptors it leads to smooth muscle relaxation of the bronchi, skeletal muscle, vasculature, and gastrointestinal tract. Venous return to the heart is also increased by vasodilation of the venous bed. The use of isoproterenol is limited because of its pronounced stimulatory effect on the heart rate.[4]

Dopamine (Inotropin)

Dopamine (DA) is an endogenous catecholamine that is a precursor to norepinephrine. The usual vasopressor dose of dopamine is between 5 and 20 μg/kg/min; dopamine directly stimulates β receptors, producing chronotropic and inotropic effects leading to increased cardiac output, and also stimulates peripheral α receptors, causing increase systemic vascular resistance.

At one point low-dose dopamine, between 1 and 5 μg/kg/min, was thought to selectively stimulate the DA_1 and DA_2 receptors in the splanchnic and renal artery beds, causing vasodilation and increased blood flow. This belief has been nullified and is considered an antiquated form of practice. It has been suggested that dopamine's improvement of renal and splanchnic blood flow stems from its benefits on cardiac output. Cardiac output per se enhances perfusion to all major organs including blood flow to the kidney.

There is a higher likelihood of adverse effects occurring with higher doses of dopamine when used in patients with cardiac failure, because of the increase in afterload and myocardial oxygen demand. Adverse effects include tachyarrhythmias, ectopic beat, palpitations, and decreased perfusion.

Phenylephrine (Neo-Synephrine)

Unlike epinephrine, phenylephrine is purely an α agonist, yet differs from epinephrine only in that it lacks a hydroxyl group (–OH) on the benzene ring. Phenylephrine induces vasoconstriction in most vascular beds, elevating both systolic and diastolic blood pressure. Phenylephrine exerts an effect on systemic blood pressure by elevating total peripheral resistance; the direct vasoconstriction of the aortic vasculature imposes a reflex bradycardia on the heart. There are no significant adverse respiratory effects noted with phenylephrine therapy.

Vasopressin (Pitressin)

Aside from the pressor effects of vasopressin (which are discussed subsequently in the section on advanced cardiac life support), vasopressin may be used in the setting of septic shock, not only because of its pressor effect but also because of its water-retentive effects. Vasopressin is a naturally occurring hormone also known as antidiuretic hormone. Vasopressin displays affinity for V_1 and V_2 receptors located in the collecting ducts in the kidneys, which contribute to water conservation and concentration of urine. The use of vasopressin may be especially beneficial in the setting of sepsis because vasopressin is deficient in septic patients. The dose of vasopressin in the setting of septic shock is initiated at a rate of 0.04 unit/min and titrated to a dose of 0.01 unit/min. However, the 2004 practice guidelines[5] published by the Society of Critical Care Medicine do not recommend vasopressin as the initial vasopressor of choice, or as a lone agent. Precaution stems from the fact that vasopressin infusion may decrease splanchnic blood flow. Further studies are needed to evaluate the role of vasopressin in the setting of septic shock.[5] Other settings in which vasopressin may be used include diabetes insipidus at doses of 5-10 units given intramuscularly (IM) or subcutaneously (SC) and repeated two or three times per day. Vasopressin has also been used to treat esophageal bleeding at doses up to 2 units/min. Caution must also be taken when treating conditions other than shock;

myocardial ischemia may ensue as a result of the potent vasoconstrictive properties at higher doses.

Inotropic Agents
Dobutamine (Dobutrex)

Dobutamine is indicated for the short-term treatment of decompensated heart failure secondary to depressed contractility. It is a synthetic catecholamine that is chemically related to dopamine; however, unlike dopamine, it is not metabolized to norepinephrine nor does it stimulate dopamine receptors.[4] Its pharmacological actions are due to the effects of its racemic components. The (R)-isomer is responsible for its activity on the β_1 and β_2 receptors, causing predominant positive inotropic and chronotropic effects as well as vasodilatory effects, respectively. This combination of effects enhances cardiac output and stroke volume. The (S)-isomer is responsible for its activity on the α_1 receptors, causing vasoconstriction.[1,6] The vasodilatory β_2-adrenergic effect counterbalances the vasoconstrictive α_1 effects, thereby leading to minor changes in systemic vascular resistance usually seen at lower doses. However, with increasing doses, the β_2-vasodilatory actions predominate over the α_1-vasoconstrictive effect, thereby causing a fall in systemic and pulmonary vascular resistance. However, the fall in systemic and pulmonary vascular resistance may also be secondary to enhanced cardiac output.

As an inotropic agent, dobutamine has its share of adverse cardiac effects, which include arrhythmias an increase in myocardial oxygen consumption and demand, tachycardia, and hypotension. A limiting factor with the use of dobutamine is tachyphylaxis when used for more than 72 hours; this may be due to a downregulation of β_1 receptors and may be overcome by increasing the dose.

In patients with sulfite sensitivity, allergic reactions such as anaphylaxis and/or life-threatening asthmatic episodes may occur because dobutamine formulations contain sulfites.[4]

Phosphodiesterase Inhibitors: Inamrinone (Inocor) and Milrinone (Primacor)

The phosphodiesterase inhibitors (also known as inodilators), such as inamrinone (formerly known as amrinone) and milrinone, are both inotropic and vasodilator agents by increasing myocardial contractility and inducing vascular smooth muscle relaxation. These effects are mitigated by inhibition of intracellular phosphodiesterase (subclass III). **Phosphodiesterase** is an enzyme responsible for the breakdown of cyclic adenosine 3′,5′-monophosphate (cAMP). An increase in cAMP concentration mediates an increase in intracellular ionized calcium, which is responsible for its inotropic effect, and cAMP-dependent protein phosphorylation, causing relaxation of vascular muscle. Hemodynamically, phosphodiesterase inhibitors cause a decrease in systemic vascular resistance and pulmonary capillary wedge pressure and an increase in cardiac output without increasing heart rate or myocardial oxygen demand. These hemodynamic changes are related to plasma concentration. Milrinone is the phosphodiesterase inhibitor most commonly used in practice today because it has a shorter half-life than inamrinone and is less likely to cause thrombocytopenia. It undergoes renal elimination with an elimination half-life of 1 to 3 hours in patients with normal renal function; therefore steady state concentrations will be reached in 4 to 6 hours if initiated without a loading dose. The risk of hypotension occurring is higher when a loading dose is given. Milrinone may be given as an initial intravenous (IV) bolus dose of 50 μg/kg administered slowly over 10 minutes followed by continuous infusion at a rate of 0.375 to 0.75 μg/kg/min and titrated to effect. Dosage adjustment should be made in patients with severe cardiac failure or renal impairment, because of the considerable reduction in clearance.[1,4,6]

Cardiac Glycosides: Digoxin (Lanoxin)

The cardiac glycoside class consists of one medication known as digoxin (Lanoxin), which is used in the management of chronic heart failure. The implementation of digoxin in the treatment of chronic heart failure stems from its capacity to exert an inotropic effect on the myocardium. The cardiac glycosides reversibly inhibit the sodium potassium Na^+/K^+-ATPase pump located in the cardiac heart muscle, thereby leading to a net loss of potassium and a net gain in intracellular sodium concentration. This in turn results in activation of the sodium-calcium active transport system, which pumps sodium out of the cell and calcium into the cell. Elevated intracellular calcium concentrations result in further calcium secretion from the endoplasmic reticulum, ultimately stimulating the actin-myosin light chain reaction, resulting in myocardial contraction. Digoxin also has an inhibitory effect on the vagus nerve, leading to decreased heart rate and atrioventricular (AV) node prolongation. Unlike other inotropic agents such as dobutamine and milrinone, digoxin generally does not exert hypotensive effects, unless directly caused by bradycardia.

Digoxin undergoes renal elimination. In the presence of renal insufficiency, accumulation of digoxin may occur. In general, digitalis intoxication is diagnosed when the mean serum digoxin concentration exceeds 2 ng/ml; however, the clinical significance of this value depends

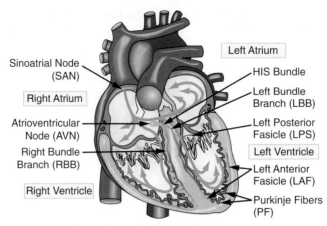

FIGURE 19-2 Cardiac conduction system.

on the time of ingestion and the time of serum sampling. Digoxin has a long distribution phase. It may take up to 4 hours after intravenous administration and up to 6 hours after oral administration for digoxin to fully distribute out of the circulatory compartment and into other regions of the body. Serum sampling of digoxin before the distribution phase may give the impression that the serum concentration is higher than it actually is. Digoxin displays a very narrow therapeutic range (0.5-2 ng/ml), particularly in the setting of hypokalemia. Hypokalemia may potentiate the adverse effects of digoxin and also render the risk of dysrhythmias and death more eminent. Adequate potassium supplementation should be used to maintain the serum potassium level within a normal range. In contrast, digitalis toxicity may cause hyperkalemia by its inhibitory actions on the Na^+/K^+-ATPase pump. Digoxin toxicity may manifest as serious life-threatening ventricular arrhythmias, including premature ventricular contractions, atrioventricular junctional rhythm, bigeminal rhythm, and second-degree atrioventricular blockade. Bradycardia may also occur early on in the setting of digoxin toxicity. The initial symptoms of digitalis toxicity are nausea, vomiting, anorexia, and abdominal pain. This may be due to a direct effect on the gastrointestinal tract or as a result of central nervous system stimulation of the chemoreceptor trigger zone. Other rare but possible neuropsychiatric effects may present as disorientation and hallucination, especially in the elderly, and also visual disturbances such as yellow-green halos. Digoxin immune Fab is the antidote used to facilitate the speedy elimination of digoxin from the body. Digoxin immune Fab is indicated in the setting of life-threatening toxicity such as ventricular arrhythmias, bradyrhythmias, ingestion of greater than 10 mg in adults or 4 mg in pediatrics, a steady state level >10 ng/ml, progressive elevation of potassium, or a potassium level >5 mEq/L.[7]

ELECTROPHYSIOLOGY OF THE MYOCARDIUM

Electrical activity is initiated by an innate pacemaker located at the sinoatrial (SA) node. Electrical potential exists across the cell membrane, and it changes in response to transmembrane movement of Na^+, K^+, Ca^{2+}, and Cl^- ions. These ions mediate the process of myocardial contraction and relaxation. Once an electrical stimulus is evoked from the SA node it generates an action potential (AP). Once generated, the AP produces a local current, which evokes further action potentials along the myocardium. An AP elicits myocardial depolarization or contraction. The link between atrial depolarization and ventricular depolarization is a portion of the conduction system called the **atrioventricular (AV) node**. The AV node slows down the electrical impulse to ensure that atrial excitation is completed before ventricular excitation. After leaving the AV node, the impulse travels to the wall between the two ventricles via the conducting system fibers known as the bundle of His. From the bundle of His, the cardiac conduction system bifurcates into three main bundle branches: the right bundle and two left bundles. These bundle branches form a conduction network, referred to as Purkinje fibers (Figure 19-2). The conduction system innervates the myocardium and causes changes in membrane polarization of the muscle fiber.[9]

An action potential (Figure 19-3) can be divided into five different phases:

Phase 0: The initial rapid depolarization of myocardial tissues, due to an abrupt transmembrane influx of sodium through "fast" sodium channels

Phase 1: The fast sodium channels are inactivated. This, coupled with the movement of K^+ and Cl^- ions, leads

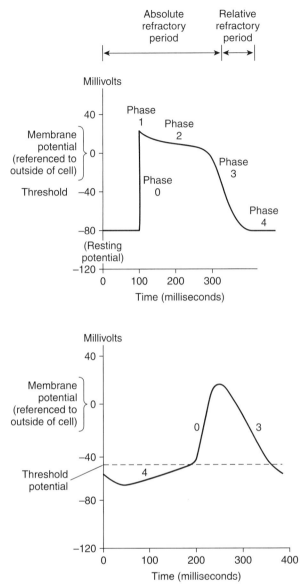

FIGURE 19-3 Action potential diagram.[13] (From Cairo JM, Pilbeam SP: Mosby's Respiratory Care Equipment, ed 7, St. Louis, 2004, Mosby/Elsevier.)

to a transient net outward current and the beginning of repolarization

Phase 2: The "plateau" phase, maintained by a balance between calcium influx and potassium efflux

Phase 3: The calcium channels close, but the membrane remains permeable to potassium, resulting in cellular repolarization

Phase 4: The cell returns to its "resting" state: the resting membrane potential is reached through

gradual depolarization related to a constant sodium influx balanced by a decreasing efflux of potassium

During the action potential, a second stimulus will not evoke a second AP; at this point the membrane is said to be in the *absolute refractory period*. The absolute refractory period does not allow the heart to undergo premature contractions or to maintain a tetanic state. Dysrhythmias are associated with abnormal impulse generation or conduction. Certain conditions that can precipitate dysrhythmias are myocardial ischemia, chronic heart failure, an oversensitivity to catecholamines, and electrolyte abnormalities.

Ablation With Radiofrequency Current

Catheter ablation is very effective when atrial fibrillation (AF) is due to a single primary circuit. The procedure involves inserting a catheter into a blood vessel in the groin or the neck, and guiding it toward the heart. When the tip of the catheter is placed against the part of the heart causing the arrhythmia, radiofrequency electrical current is applied through the catheter to produce a small burn about 6 to 8 mm in diameter. Patients should be adequately anticoagulated at least 1 month before the ablation procedure to prevent the formation of thrombi in the atria. The procedure carries a success rate in maintaining sinus rhythm over the next year of 30%-90%.[9]

Internal Cardioverter-Defibrillator

Internal cardioverter-defibrillators (ICDs) have been used since the 1980s to cardiovert, to terminate ventricular tachycardia (VT), and to provide back-up pacing for bradycardia. ICD implantation is indicated for the following conditions:

- Cardiac arrest caused by Pulseless ventricular tachycardia (VT) or ventricular fibrillation (VF) not due to a transient or reversible cause
- Spontaneous sustained VT
- Syncope of undetermined origin with clinically relevant electrophysiologically inducible sustained VT or VF when drug therapy is ineffective, not tolerated, or not preferred
- In nonsustained VT in patients with coronary artery disease, prior to a myocardial infarction, left ventricular dysfunction and lectrophysiologically inducible VT or VF not suppressed by class I antiarrhythmics

Forty to 70% of patients with ICDs require antiarrhythmic drug therapy, which puts them at risk for drug-ICD interactions.[10]

A

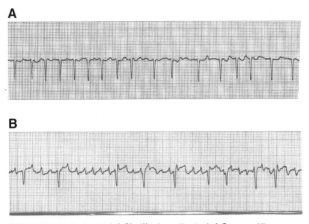

B

FIGURE 19-4 **A**, Atrial fibrillation. **B**, Atrial flutter. (From Wilkins RL, Stoller JK, Scanlan CL: Egan's Fundamentals of Respiratory Care, ed 8, St Louis, 2003, Mosby/Elsevier.)

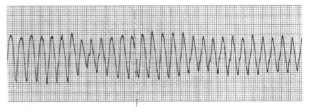

FIGURE 19-5 Ventricular tachycardia. (From Wilkins RL, Stoller JK, Scanlan CL: Egan's Fundamentals of Respiratory Care, ed 8, St Louis, 2003, Mosby/Elsevier.)

Class IB

Class IB agents are often used and have less proarrhythmic potential compared with the class IA agents. The actions of class IB agents are limited to ventricular arrhythmias.

Lidocaine (Xylocaine)

Lidocaine is used frequently to treat ventricular arrhythmia (VA) occurring during cardiac surgery or after an acute myocardial infarction. After administering IV bolus dose(s) (due to its short half-life of approximately 1.5-2 hours), continuous infusion is necessary to maintain sinus rhythm. Lidocaine is metabolized extensively in the liver to two toxic metabolites, monoethylglycinexylidide and glycinexylidide; these metabolites display antiarrhythmogenic properties but are also highly seizurogenic. Patients need to be monitored vigilantly for signs of seizure, such as tremors.[11] Other CNS side effects associated with lidocaine are as follows: insomnia, drowsiness, ataxia, agitation, and dysarthria. Caution should also be exercised in the setting of hepatic failure or chronic heart failure, because the rate of drug clearance is significantly reduced in either condition. Lidocaine infusions lasting longer than 24 hours, may prolong the half-life of lidocaine to approximately 3 hours leading to a greater risk of lidocaine accumulation and toxicity. In the setting of prolonged used of lidocaine infusion greater than 24 hours, the infusion rate should be reduced by approximately 50%. Lidocaine has also been implicated in causing respiratory depression and arrest.[4]

Mexiletine (Mexitil)

Mexiletine has a mechanism of action similar to that of lidocaine, and is available as an oral formulation. It is indicated for the treatment of life-threatening VAs. Because of its anesthetic properties it is also used at lower doses to reduce neuropathic pain associated with diabetic neuropathy. In controlled trials the most frequent adverse events were gastrointestinal disturbances (41%), tremor (12%), and lightheadedness and difficulty in coordination (>10%). Dyspnea and respiratory problems occurred in up to 5.7% of patients. With massive overdoses coma and respiratory arrest may occur.[11]

Tocainide (Tonocard)

Tocainide is the oral congener of lidocaine and is used to treat VAs, and may also be used to treat myotonic dystrophy and trigeminal neuralgia. Tocainide carries a "black box warning" (so called for the black border surrounding the warning located in the manufacturer information sheet or the package insert) for causing pulmonary disorders including pulmonary edema, fibrosing alveolitis, pneumonitis, and respiratory arrest (0.11%). These pulmonary manifestations are detectable via radiographic studies within 3-18 weeks of therapy. Another black box warning is for blood dyscrasias that are not that prevalent (0.18%) but that carry a fatality rate of up to 25%.[4]

Class IC

Class IC agents are generally not used, mainly because of their relatively higher proarrhythmic potential. Other agents from this class have been withdrawn from the market (i.e., encainide and moricizine) because of their substantially high proarrhythmic potential as demonstrated in two landmark trials: Cardiac Arrhythmia Suppression Trial I (CAST I)[18]. Class IC agents are commonly used in the management of supraventricular arrhythmias, but have activity against ventricular arrhythmias as well.

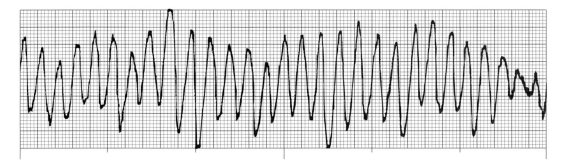

FIGURE 19-6 Torsades de pointes arrhythmia. (From Aehlert B: ECGs Made Easy, ed 3, St. Louis, St. Louis, 2006, Mosby JEMS.)

Flecainide (Tambocor)

Flecainide is indicated for the prevention of paroxysmal AF/AFL associated with disabling symptoms and PSVT, including AV nodal reentrant tachycardia, atrioventricular tachycardia, other supraventricular tachycardia in patients without structural heart disease, and sustained VT. Flecainide is efficacious in suppressing AF in 61%-92% of patients treated. Flecainide has a long half-life; therefore, the dose should not be increased more often than every 4 days. Flecainide was one of the antiarrhythmics studied in the CAST study of patients with asymptomatic non-life-threatening arrhythmias occurring 6 days to 2 years after documented myocardial infarction. Flecainide contributed to an excessive mortality or nonfatal cardiac arrest rate of 5.1 versus 2.3% for its matched placebo. Long-term oral prophylaxis with an antiarrhythmic agent poses a great risk of adverse events and relapse rates are high. It is also important to note that flecainide elimination is affected by urinary pH, leading to either toxic or subtherapeutic levels. Alkaline pH will decrease renal excretion and acidic pH will increase renal excretion of flecainide.[4]

The "pill-in-the-pocket" approach is the alternative treatment of recurrent arrhythmias, in which a pill is taken by the patient at the time of onset of palpitations. One study has assessed this approach in the conversion of AF to sinus rhythm with class IC agents, using either flecainide or propafenone, as a single oral dose to convert patients to sinus rhythm out of hospital. Flecainide was shown to be equally effective for pill-in-the-pocket treatment of recurrent AF, with a 94% efficacy rate.[12]

Propafenone (Rythmol)

Propafenone appears to be comparable to other antiarrhythmics in preventing PSVT and maintaining sinus rhythm after successful cardioversion. It is considered a first-line agent for conversion of recent-onset (<48 hours) AF, with efficacy rates of 60%-90%. Therapy is 15%-30% less effective in patients manifesting symptoms of AF for more than 48 hours. Propafenone displays nonselective β-blocking activity, hence it generally should not be used to treat patients with asthma or bronchospastic disease because β-blocking properties may inhibit bronchodilation. The highest concentrations of the drug are found in the lungs (10-fold higher than in the heart muscles or liver, and 24-fold higher than in the kidneys).[11]

Class II

Class II agents consist mainly of the β-blocking agents. These agents are used in the management of hypertension and postmyocardial infarction; metoprolol is the only agent in this class that may be used in the setting of chronic heart failure.

β Blockers

Propranolol (Inderal), metoprolol (Lopressor), atenolol (Tenormin), and nadolol (Corgard) are available as both intravenous and oral formulations, whereas esmolol (Brevibloc) is available only in the intravenous form. These agents have negative dromotropic activity but more commonly used for the negative chronotropic properties in AF/AFL and to prevent or convert SVT to normal sinus rhythm. They should not be used in settings of acute decompensated heart failure because they can exacerbate symptoms of heart failure. However, once the symptomatology of heart failure is stabilized, β blockers may be initiated at lower doses. In the setting in which patients with airway disease are overly sensitive to the bronchoconstrictive effects of β blockers, esmolol may be a convenient selection. Because of the short half-life of esmolol (~10 minutes), one may titrate the dose to meet the patient's therapeutic and safety goals.

TABLE 19-7	
Routine Laboratory Testing in Patients Receiving Amiodarone	
Type of Test	**Time When Test Is Performed**
Liver enzyme tests	Baseline and then every 6 mo
Thyroid function (T_4 and TSH)	Baseline and then every 6 mo
Serum creatinine and electrolytes	Baseline and then every 6 mo
Chest radiographic	Baseline and then yearly
Ophthalmic evaluation	Baseline and for visual impairment or symptoms, and then every 6 mo
Pulmonary function tests	Baseline and for unexplained dyspnea, especially in patients with underlying lung disease; and if there are suggestive chest radiographic abnormalities
ECG	Baseline and then yearly

T_4, Thyroxine; *TSH,* thyroid-stimulating hormone.

Class III

Class III agents are used to treat both supraventricular and ventricular arrhythmias. Bretylium, which is considered a member of this class, is no longer manufactured in the United States because of a lack of substantial efficacy data.

Amiodarone (Cordarone)

Amiodarone is effective in the management of ventricular and supraventricular arrhythmias. In the past, the life-threatening adverse effects of amiodarone have prevented it from being used as a first-line agent; it was reserved for patients with life-threatening VAs. It appears to exhibit greater efficacy and a lower incidence of proarrhythmic effects than class I or III antiarrhythmics. Today, amiodarone has become a mainstay in the management of AF, VF, and VT. Amiodarone-induced pulmonary toxicity warrants substantial concern when treating patients with arrhythmias. The main caveat associated with amiodarone is its distinctive side effect profile.[5] Baseline parameters that must be obtained before starting therapy, along with incidences of various side effects, are displayed in Table 19-7. Pulmonary toxicity is quite common, as evidenced by cough and by local or diffuse infiltrates on radiographic chest X-rays, and occurs at a rate of up to 20%. Amiodarone-induced pulmonary toxicity is managed best by discontinuation or by corticosteroid therapy; in some cases fatalities have been reported to amount to ~10%.[11] In addition, amiodarone is probably regarded as one of the most potent inhibitors of the CYP450 3A4 isoenzyme system and also inhibits CYP2C9 and CYP2C19 (hepatic drug-metabolizing enzymes), and therefore concomitant prescription medications, herbals, and over-the-counter products must be evaluated for proper detection of severe and often life-threatening interactions (see Table 19-8).

Dofetilide (Tikosyn)

Dofetilide is available as an oral formulation and is indicated for the maintenance of sinus rhythm after successful conversion, but is ineffective in paroxysmal AF. Dofetilide carries a significant risk of VAs such as torsades de pointes, associated with prolongation of the Q-T interval (duration of ventricular electrical activity). The Q-T interval can be reported as QTc, also known as the *corrected QT interval* for heart rate. This drug should be discontinued in patients with QT_c >500 msec. The risk of torsade de pointes, among patients administered dofetilide, is greatest for a subset of patients including the following:[4]

• Females
• Congenital heart disease or ischemic heart disease
• Diminished renal function
• Dofetilide doses exceeding 500 mg twice daily

This medication must be renally adjusted to avoid accumulation. Drug interactions with dofetilide pose a significant problem. Agents such as cimetidine, azole antifungals, prochlorperazine, metformin, and the trimethoprim component of Bactrim may inhibit active tubular secretion of dofetilide and increase the plasma concentration. Therapy with dofetilide must be initiated in a facility that can provide continuous ECG monitoring and the presence of personnel trained to manage severe VAs for at least 3 days. Both the prescriber and the pharmacy must be participants in a program known as the Tikosyn in Pharmacy System (T.I.P.S.) before the prescribing and dispensing of dofetilide.[13]

Sotalol (Betapace/Betapace AF)

Sotalol is available only by the oral route and works by prolonging the action potential duration as well as the relative refractory period. Sotalol can be used for both

TABLE 19-8

Clinically Significant Drug Interactions With Antiarrhythmics

Antiarrhythmic	Interacting Drug	Effect
Class IA		
Moricizine	Cimetidine	Levels ↑ 1.4-fold, ↓ clearance by 50%—initiate moricizine at lower doses (<600 mg/day)
	Digoxin	Additive PR interval prolongation (not as significant as second or third AV block)
	Propranolol	Small additive ↑ in PR interval; No change in overall ECG intervals
	Theophylline	↑Theophylline clearance by 44%-66% and half-life by 19%-33%
	Diltiazem	↑ Concentration of moricizine by diltiazem; ↓ diltiazem concentration by moricizine
Quinidine	Amiodarone	↑ Levels of quinidine → fatal dysrhythmias
	Antacids	↑ Levels of quinidine
	Barbiturates	↓ Levels and elimination half-life of quinidine
	Cholinergic drugs	Failure to terminate PSVT due to inability to antagonize vagal excitation on the atrium and the AV node
	Cimetidine	↑ Levels of quinidine
	Rifampin	↑ Metabolism and ↓ in therapeutic effect of quinidine
	Sucralfate	↓ Levels of quinidine→↓ therapeutic efficacy
	Succinylcholine	Prolonged effects of succinylcholine
	Tricyclic antidepressants	↓ Clearance of TCAs→↑ pharmacological effects or toxicity
Procainamide	Quinidine	↑ Levels of procainamide and NAPA→↑ pharmacologic effects
	Amiodarone	↑ Serum concentration of procainamide or NAPA by 33% → fatal cardiac dysrhythmias
	Anticholinergics	Additive antivagal effect on AV conduction
	Cimetidine/ranitidine	↓ Renal clearance → ↑ serum concentration of procainamide → monitor levels closely
	Quinolone antibiotics	↑ Risk of torsades de pointes
	Thioridazine/ziprasidone	Synergistic QT$_c$ prolongation→↑ risk of torsades de pointes
	Trimethoprim	↑ Procainamide and NAPA concentrations
	Neuromuscular blockers	Prolonged neuromuscular blockade → decrease dose of neuromuscular blocker
Disopyramide	Quinidine	↑ Disopyramide levels and ↓ quinidine levels
	Erythromycin	↑ Levels of disopyramide→↑ QT$_c$ interval (fatalities reported)
	Hydantoins	↓ Half-life, levels, and bioavailability of disopyramide; effects may persist for days after stopping phenytoin
Class IB		
Lidocaine	β Blockers	↑ Levels of lidocaine → possible toxicity
	Cimetidine	↓ Renal clearance → ↑ serum concentration of lidocaine (other H$_2$ blockers do not appear to interact)
	Procainamide	Additive cardiopressant action, potential for conduction abnormalities
	Tocainide	Pharmacologically similar agents → ↑ incidence of ADRs
	Neuromuscular blockers	Prolonged neuromuscular blockade
Mexiletine	Antacids/atropine/narcotics	↓ Absorption of mexiletine
	Metoclopramide	Accelerated absorption of mexiletine
	Phenytoin/rifampin	↑ Clearance of mexiletine → ↓ levels
	Theophylline	↑ Levels of theophylline → theophylline toxicity
Tocainide	Cimetidine	↓ Tocainide bioavailability and peak concentration (ranitidine does not appear to interact)
	Metoprolol	Additive effects on wedge pressure and cardiac index
	Rifampin	↓ Half-life, bioavailability, and clearance of tocainide
Phenytoin	Amiodarone	Chronic use (>2 wk) of amiodarone impairs metabolism of phenytoin → possible phenytoin toxicity↓ Amiodarone levels may be seen

Continued

TABLE 19-8

Clinically Significant Drug Interactions With Antiarrhythmics—cont'd

Antiarrhythmic	Interacting Drug	Effect
Class IC		
Flecainide	Amiodarone	↑ Levels of flecainide
	Cimetidine	↑ Bioavailability and renal excretion of flecainide
	Disopyramide	Disopyramide has (−) inotropic actions, do not use together unless risks outweigh benefits
	Propranolol	Additive (−) inotropic effects; levels of both agents may be increased
	Smoking	Smokers have greater plasma clearance than nonsmokers → use higher doses in smokers
	Digoxin	↑ Absorption, peak concentration, and bioavailability of digoxin
Propafenone	Quinidine	↑ Propafenone levels in extensive metabolizers (>90% of patients) → ↑ effect
	Cimetidine	↑ Propafenone concentration → ↑ effect
	Rifampin	↑ Clearance of mexiletine → ↓ levels, possible loss of therapeutic effect
	Anticoagulants	↑ Warfarin plasma levels; ↑ PT
	β Blockers	↑ Levels of metoprolol
	Cyclosporine	↑ Cyclosporine trough levels → ↓ renal function
	Digoxin	↑ Levels of digoxin → toxicity
Class II		
β Blockers: Propranolol Esmolol Acebutolol	Quinidine	↑ Effect of propranolol and metoprolol in extensive metabolizers
	CCBs	Pharmacologic effects of β blockers/synergistic or additive activity
	Hydralazine	↑ Levels of β blockers and hydralazine
	Warfarin	↑ Effect of warfarin by propranolol
	Ergot alkaloids	Peripheral ischemia (cold extremities, possible gangrene due to ergot alkaloid-mediated vasoconstriction) and β blocker-mediated blockade of peripheral β_2 receptors → unopposed ergot action
	Lidocaine	↑ Levels of lidocaine → toxicity
Class III		
Amiodarone	Warfarin	↑ PT, potentiation of anticoagulant response → bleeding. ↓ Warfarin dose by 30%-50%. Effect may persist for months after discontinuation of amiodarone
	Dextromethorphan	Chronic use (>2 wk) of amiodarone impairs metabolism of dextromethorphan
	Digoxin	↑ Digoxin level by ≥70% → ↓ digoxin dose by 50% and monitor levels or discontinue
	Fentanyl	↑ Fentanyl concentration → hypotension, bradycardia, ↓ cardiac output
	Gatifloxacin	↑ Risk of life-threatening arrhythmias including torsades de pointes
	Rifampin	↓ Levels of amiodarone and its active metabolite
	Ritonavir	↑ Levels of amiodarone → toxicity
Bretylium	Catecholamines	↑ Effects of catecholamines (EPI, NE, DA) → monitor BP and HR
	Digoxin	Digitalis toxicity may be aggravated by initial release of NE caused by bretylium
Dofetilide	Amiloride/triamterene/ metformin/megestrol/ prochlorperazine	Inhibit elimination of dofetilide → concurrent use is contraindicated
	Class I and III agents	Withhold class I and III antiarrhythmic agents for ≥3 plasma half-lives before dofetilide dosing
	Cimetidine	↑ Levels of dofetilide by 58% → concomitant use is contraindicated
	Digoxin	↑ Occurrence of torsades de pointes → concomitant use is not recommended
	Ketoconazole	↑ AUC and C_{max} of dofetilide by 53 and 41%, respectively, in males → concomitant use is contraindicated; ↑ AUC and C_{max} of dofetilide by 97 and 69%, respectively, in females → concomitant use is contraindicated
	Trimethoprim	↑ AUC and C_{max} of dofetilide by 103 and 93%, respectively → concomitant use is contraindicated
	Verapamil	↑ Peak plasma concentration of dofetilide by 42%, ↑ occurrence of torsades de pointes → concomitant use is contraindicated

Drug	Interacting agent	Effect/ADR
Sotalol	Thioridazine/mezoridazine/pimozide/ziprazidone/ranolazine	Concurrent use with all class III antiarrhythmics may result in an ↑ risk of Q-T prolongation, torsades de pointes, cardiac arrest → contraindicated
	Dolasetron	Concurrent use with all class III antiarrhythmics may result in an ↑ risk of Q-T prolongation, torsades de pointes, cardiac arrest
Ibutilide	None reported	
Class IV		
Calcium channel blockers (CCBs): Verapamil Diltiazem	Amiodarone	Cardiotoxicity with bradycardia and ↓ cardiac output
	β Blockers	Additive or synergistic effects; CCBs may inhibit metabolism of certain β blockers
	Cyclosporine	↑ Levels of cyclosporine
	Cimetidine/ranitidine	↑ Levels of CCBs
	Ritonavir	↑ Levels of CCBs → concomitant use (especially with bepridil) is contraindicated
	Fentanyl	CCBs may potentiate vasodilation associated with fentanyl → hypotension
	Flecainide/disopyramide	Additive effects → disopyramide should not be administered 48 hr before or 24 hr after verapamil
	Doxorubicin	↑ Levels of doxorubicin → cardiotoxicity
	Benzodiazepines	↑ Effects of midazolam and triazolam
	Digoxin	↑ Levels of digoxin → toxicity
	HMG-CoA reductase inhibitors	↑ Levels of atorvastatin → ↑ risk of rhabdomyolysis, liver enzyme elevation, neuropathies
	Lithium	With verapamil: ↓ lithium levels and toxicity/With diltiazem: neurotoxicity
	Quinidine	↑ Therapeutic and adverse effects of quinidine. Use quinidine with verapamil ONLY when no other alternative
	Theophylline	↑ Pharmacologic and toxic effects of theophylline
Class Miscellaneous		
Digoxin	Calcium (IV)	Rapid IV infusion of calcium in digitalized patients will produce cardiac dysrhythmias
	Succinylcholine	Sudden extrusion of potassium from muscle cells → cardiac dysrhythmias
	Sympathomimetics	↑ Risk of cardiac dysrhythmias
	Diuretics	Diuretic-induced electrolyte disturbances (K+, Mg2+) may predispose patients to cardiac dysrhythmias
	Thyroid hormone	Digitalized hypothyroid patient may require lower digoxin doses
	Quinidine	Marked ↑ in levels of digoxin → toxicity
	Carbamazepine	Higher degree of heart block. If possible, withhold carbamazepine for at least ~4 days before adenosine use
	Dipyridamole	Adenosine toxicity (hypotension, dyspnea, vomiting), due to inhibition of adenosine metabolism by dipyridamole. When dipyridamole is used before adenosine, ↓ adenosine dose
Adenosine	Theophylline	Effects of adenosine are antagonized by methylxanthines → use larger doses of adenosine
	Digoxin/verapamil	↑ Risk of ventricular fibrillation

ADR, Adverse drug reaction; *AV*, atrioventricular; *AUC*, area under the curve; *BP*, blood pressure; *CCB*, calcium channel blocker; C_{max}, maximal concentration; *DA*, dopamine; *EPI*, epinephrine; *HR*, heart rate; *IV*, intravenous; *NAPA*, N-acetylprocainamide; *NE*, norepinephrine; *PSVT*, paroxysmal supraventricular tachycardia; *PT*, prothrombin time; QT_c, Q-T interval (duration of ventricular electrical activity), corrected for heart rate; *TCAs*, tricyclic antidepressants.
↑, increase in; ↓, decrease in; →, leading to; therefore; (–), negative.

supraventricular as well as ventricular arrhythmias. When initiating sotalol the patient should be kept in a facility that can provide continuous ECG monitoring and the presence of personnel trained to manage severe VAs for at least 3 days.[4] As with any β-blocking agent, caution must be exercised when treating patients with restrictive airway disease.

Ibutilide (Corvert)

Ibutilide is available as an IV formulation and is an alternative to electrical cardioversion. Ibutilide is the first antiarrhythmic agent indicated for rapid conversion of AF/AFL of recent onset by the U.S. Food and Drug Administration. In clinical trials, ibutilide was more effective for the treatment of AFL than AF (>50% vs. <40%). Class I antiarrhythmics and other class III antiarrhythmics should not be given with this medication or within 4 hours of an ibutilide infusion, because of the potential to prolonged refractoriness. Since AF has potential to form clots within the atrium of the heart, patients must be adequately anticoagulated before chemical cardioversion to reduce the risk of stroke. Patients who fail electric cardioversion, will require lifelong anticoagulation.[4] There is also evidence (TIME study) to suggest that can enhance the efficacy of ibutilide and decrease the incidence of torsades de pointes by more than 30%. Before initiation all electrolytes must be maintained within normal limits and continuous ECG monitoring is required because of the high incidence of ventricular fibrillation (2.7%-4.9%).[1,14,19]

Class IV
Calcium Channel Blockers

Only two calcium channel blockers are used in the management of supraventricular arrhythmias as well as ventricular rate control for atrial fibrillation: verapamil (Isoptin) and diltiazem (Cardizem). They exert their effects by blocking calcium channels in the AV node and, hence, slowing AV nodal conduction. Unlike the β blockers, verapamil and diltiazem are not favorable agents for use in the setting of chronic heart failure; however, they are good alternatives to β blockers in the setting of airway disease.

Miscellaneous
Digoxin (Lanoxin)

Digoxin has direct AV-blocking effects and vagotonic properties, which aid in lowering the heart rate. Although digoxin prolongs the relative refractory period of the AV node and reduces the number of impulses through the AV node, it is not regarded as a first-line agent for

AF.[4,11] Digoxin does not acquire a rapid onset of effect, especially for the management of an acute condition such as AF; that is, it requires ~2 hours to achieve maximal effect. Additionally, digoxin has the potential to shorten the refractory period of atrial muscles, thereby prolonging allowing electrical impulses to be conducted throughout the myocardium and ultimately potentiating episodes of AF. It is less effective than β blockers and calcium channel blockers during states of increased sympathetic tone, such as in exercise and stress. Digoxin is not regarded as a first-line agent for the control of ventricular rate in AF except in patients with impaired left ventricular function or heart failure.[11]

Adenosine (Adenocard)

Rapid administration of adenosine is implemented to terminate SVTs. Adenosine displays an ~12-second half-life, and because of its ultrashort half-life adenosine is best administered through a central line for rapid arrival at the site of action or, if given through a brachial line, the arm should be held in the upright position followed almost instantly by a saline flush. Bronchospasms, dyspnea, hyperpnea, and cough have been reported after administration of IV adenosine in patients with asthma and chronic obstructive pulmonary disease; these symptoms are generally benign and short lasting.[15]

> **KEY POINT**
>
> Drugs used in advanced cardiac life support included antiarrhythmics, vasopressors such as epinephrine and vasopressin, the electrolyte magnesium, and atropine for bradycardia or asystole.

MANAGEMENT AND PHARMACOTHERAPY OF ADVANCED CARDIAC LIFE SUPPORT

Sudden Cardiac Death

Sudden cardiac death (SCD) is a leading cause of death in the United States and Canada and is defined as an episode of either ventricular fibrillation (VF), pulseless ventricular tachycardia (pVT), pulseless electrical activity (PEA), or asystole, all of which are life-threatening dysrhythmias.[16] Although the fatalities associated with episodes of SCD are unacceptably high, an individual may be resuscitated. Therefore, it is not uncommon for patients to be deemed as having a "history" of sudden cardiac death. The goal in treating SCD is to restore sinus rhythm, to prevent further episodes of SCD, and to prevent impairment of neurologic function. Several studies have demonstrated benefits in mortality reduction, by minimizing time to defibrillation as well as by delivery of cardiopulmonary resuscitation (CPR).[16] In the patient with VF, survival decreases by 7%-10% for every minute that passes from the time of symptom onset to defibrillation.[16] When CPR is initiated the decline in survival occurs at a more gradual rate of approximately 3%-4% for every minute between onset of symptoms and time to defibrillation.[16] Needless to say, efficient and timely delivery of defibrillation and CPR is imperative for successful management of sudden cardiac death. The 2005 American Heart Association Guidelines for Cardiopulmonary Resuscitation and Emergency Cardiovascular Care provide a discrete recommendation on the delivery of rescue breaths as follows[16]:

• Deliver each rescue breath over 1 second
• Give a sufficient tidal volume to produce visible chest rise
• Avoid rapid or forceful breaths
• When an advanced airway (i.e., endotracheal tube, Combitube, or laryngeal mask airway) is in place during two-person CPR, ventilate at a rate of 8-10 breaths per minute without attempting to synchronize breaths between compressions. There should be no pause in chest compressions for delivery of ventilations

After beginning CPR and attempting defibrillation, health care workers may begin establishing other therapeutic modalities, such as intravenous access; medication therapy should be considered, and the insertion of an advanced airway. Ventricular fibrillation and pVT are managed primarily by defibrillation/CPR and secondarily by pharmacotherapy; conversely, asystole and PEA are not managed by defibrillation and therefore are managed first by CPR only and second by pharmacotherapy as depicted in the algorithms in Figures 19-7, 19-8, and 19-9. It may be prudent to review the national consensus guidelines for further details of advanced cardiac life support algorithms.

Epinephrine

Epinephrine, an endogenous neurotransmitter, is administered in 1-mg doses as a 10-ml solution. Epinephrine stimulates β_1- and β_2-adrenergic receptors, which are found in dense proportions in the heart and lungs, respectively. However, it is the effect of epinephrine on α_1 receptors, located within the coronary and cerebral vasculature, that is more closely correlated with efficacy. Stimulation of the α_1 receptors causes vasoconstriction of the coronary and cerebral vasculature, in turn increasing blood flow to the heart's myocardium and the central nervous system. In contrast, stimulation of the β_1 receptors increases cardiac heart rate, resulting in increased oxygen demand on the heart and impairing oxygen delivery to the myocardium and the central nervous system.

One main caveat associated with epinephrine use is the occurrence of decreased receptor affinity in the setting of metabolic acidosis. Metabolic acidosis may readily ensue during SCD, due to hypoxic conditions leading to a shift in anaerobic respiration. There is at present no recommended maximal dose of epinephrine in the management of sudden cardiac death. Some side effects that may be seen postresuscitation are hypertension and tachycardia.

Vasopressin (Pitressin)

Vasopressin, also known as antidiuretic hormone, is an endogenous hormone that acts as a potent vasoconstrictor. Vasopressin is administered as a one-time dose of 40 units IV. Because the effects of vasopressin have not been shown to be exceedingly different from those of epinephrine, this dose may be administered in lieu of the first or second dose of epinephrine when treating any form of sudden cardiac death. Unlike epinephrine, vasopressin is a nonadrenergic vasoconstrictor; its vasoconstricting properties are manifested by activation of V_1 receptors (vasopressin-1), which are found in the vasculature. Once stimulated, V_1 receptors release calcium from the sarcoplasmic reticulum in vascular smooth muscle, leading to vasoconstriction and thereby increasing systemic vascular resistance as well as coronary and cerebral blood flow. In contrast to epinephrine, vasopressin receptor affinity is not compromised in the setting of metabolic acidosis. In the setting of long-term continuous infusion therapy vasopressin may cause gastrointestinal and skin ischemia; however, in the setting of SCD, these adverse events would be unlikely.

Atropine (AtroPen)

Atropine is indicated for certain forms of SCD, such as asystole or PEA usually given at the usual dose of 1 mg as intravenous push, along with epinephrine or vasopressin. Atropine acts by blocking the actions of acetylcholine, an endogenous cholinergic agent. The cholinergic system is typically involved with heart rate reduction and therefore, by blocking this effect, atropine exerts a pronounced (albeit short-lived) chronotropic effect on the heart. The recommended maximal dose of atropine used during resuscitation is 0.04 mg/kg. Because atropine affects acetylcholine globally within the body, some

**Ventricular fibrillation
"sawtooth" pattern**

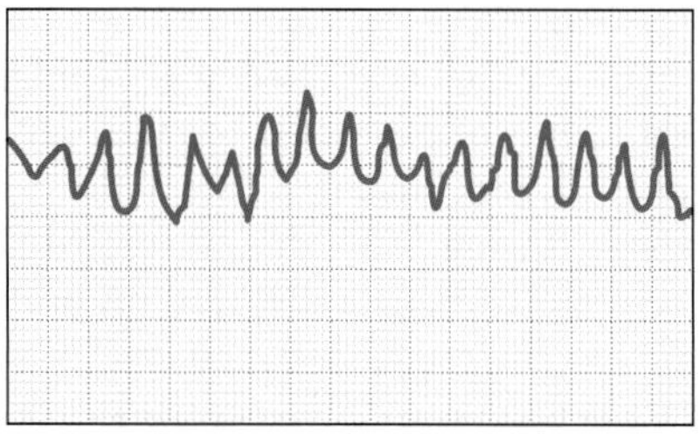

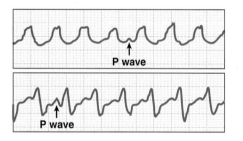

Ventricular tachycardia

P wave

P wave

**Ventricular fibrillation
pulseless ventricular tachycardia**

Defibrillation × 1 attempt

⬇

Epinephrine 1 mg q 3-5 minutes,
or vasopressin 40 units × 1 dose
(may replace 1st or 2nd dose of epinephrine)

Resume CPR
for 5 cycles

Check rhythm, if indicated
defibrillation × 1 attempt

⬇

Epinephrine 1 mg q 3-5 minutes

Resume CPR
for 5 cycles

⬇

Check rhythm, if indicated
defibrillation × 1 attempt
Consider antiarrhythmics, given
before or after shock: amiodarone, or
lidocaine

FIGURE 19-7 *Left:* Ventricular fibrillation pattern and ventricular tachycardia pattern. *Right:* Algorithm for the treatment of ventricular fibrillation and pulseless ventricular tachycardia.

**Asystole and Pulseless Electrical
Activity**

Epinephrine 1 mg IV q 3-5
minutes
or Vasopressin 40 Units × 1 dose
May replace 1st or 2nd dose of epinephrine

Resume CPR

⬇

Atropine 1 mg IV for asystole or slow
PEA rate;
(Maximum 0.04 mg/kg)

FIGURE 19-8 Algorithm for the treatment of asystole and pulseless electrical activity *(PEA)*.

Torsades de Pointes

If hemodynamically unstable: Defibrillation
Discontinue medications with QT-prolonging potential
Correct any electrolyte abnormalities

⬇

Magnesium 1-2 g (diluted in 10 ml of D5W) IV push
Or
Isoproterenol 2-10 µg/minute infusion
Or
Lidocaine 1-1.5 mg/kg IV

FIGURE 19-9 Algorithm for the treatment of torsades de pointes. *D5W,* 5% dextrose in water.

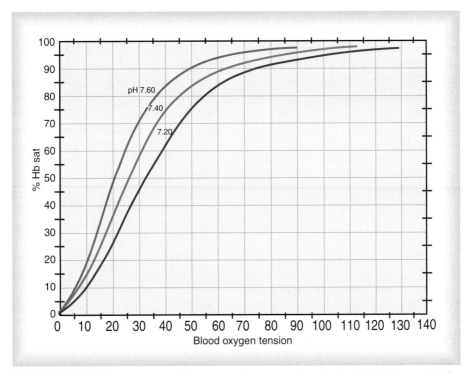

FIGURE 19-10 Bohr effect. (From Wilkins RL, Stoller JK, Scanlan CL: Egan's Fundamentals of Respiratory Care, ed 8, St Louis, 2003, Mosby/Elsevier.)

adverse effects that may be noticed are as follows: meiosis, dry mouth, urinary retention, and constipation.

Sodium Bicarbonate

Sodium bicarbonate is usually administered as 1 mEq/kg; however, its use is very limited. The use of sodium bicarbonate is limited to that setting in which a patient fails to respond to adequate ventilation, defibrillation, and cardiac compression or is refractory to vasopressor therapy. Sodium bicarbonate may be beneficial in patients with preexisting metabolic acidosis, hyperkalemia, tricyclic antidepressant overdose, or barbiturate/salicylate overdose. Nevertheless, subsequent dosing is guided by arterial blood gas analysis. The aim is to increase arterial pH to above 7.2 in order to minimize the adverse effects of systemic acidemia while at the same time avoiding the adverse effects of bicarbonate therapy. If the patient is improving without any serious negative sequelae, then waiting for renal bicarbonate regeneration and implementing heightened monitoring for clinical improvement may be a safer measure than administering bicarbonate. Most clinicians do not treat metabolic acidosis if the arterial pH is greater than 7.1.

The presence of carbon dioxide helps the release and delivery of oxygen from hemoglobin, also known as the **Bohr effect**. When comparing the oxygen dissociation curves of a serum sample with carbon dioxide and another with no carbon dioxide, we find that oxygen is able to dissociate more readily in the former state, as depicted in Figure 19-10.

In addition, sodium bicarbonate decreases hydrogen ion concentration in the serum by reacting with it, yielding carbon dioxide and water. For this reaction to continue the product (carbon dioxide) must be removed. Therefore, sodium bicarbonate therapy will aid in increasing extracellular pH only if ventilation is sufficient to remove the carbon dioxide. On the other hand, if *hypercapnia* (excess carbon dioxide in the blood) ensues, then as carbon dioxide accumulates in the serum it will eventually cross cellular membranes readily, intracellular pH may continue to decline, and further deterioration of cellular function will occur.

Magnesium Sulfate

Magnesium is often implemented in the management of torsades de pointes. Although its mechanism has not been fully elucidated, magnesium may exert its pharmacologic effect by prolonging conduction time; however, its role has been clearly delineated. Intravenous magnesium may be effective whether or not a patient is *eumagnesemic* (having a normal serum magnesium level). The typical dose consists of 1-2 g and may be repeated, separated by several minutes. No maximal dose of magnesium has been determined as yet; however, patients with normal renal function are reported to tolerate up to 16 g in a 24-hour period. A continuous infusion regimen may be initiated at a rate of 0.5-1 g/hr. Caution is warranted when treating patients with renal insufficiency. Signs and symptoms of magnesium intoxication include the following:

- Sweating
- Hypotension
- Hypothermia
- Depression of reflexes
- CNS depression

Severe hypermagnesemia may result in respiratory depression or fatal respiratory paralysis, circulatory collapse, and flaccid paralysis. Absence of patellar reflex is a clinical sign of magnesium intoxication.

ALTERNATIVE ROUTES OF MEDICATION ADMINISTRATION

Intraosseous Route

In the face of life-threatening medical emergencies, where there is a dire need for medication and fluid delivery, it becomes incumbent on the health care worker to provide vascular access in the most efficient and safest way possible. Oftentimes, intravenous access is difficult if not impossible in infants and young children or the elderly with circulatory collapse, not to mention IV drug abusers. In such situations an intraosseous (IO) needle may be inserted with relative ease, even in the most poorly perfused patients. The 2005 American Heart Association guidelines[17] for cardiopulmonary resuscitation and emergency cardiovascular care recommend the IO therapy as an alternative to direct intravenous therapy. The marrow of intraosseous bone provides a rich network of vessels that ultimately drains into the central circulation, allowing medications and fluids to gain almost instant access to the central circulation. IO access is recommended for use in children and adults. IO access may be problematic when implemented in the elderly, due to the presence of a thicker cortex of bone and smaller marrow cavity; inability to enter the marrow may increase the risk of bone fracture. Typically, an IO needle should not remain at the site of insertion for more than 3-4 hours.

Endotracheal Route

In the event that the intravenous route is not accessible, there are a few agents that are amenable to endotracheal delivery; these agents have come to be known by the acronym "LEAN," which stands for lidocaine, epinephrine, atropine, and naloxone. The following should be done when administering these agents by the endotracheal route:

- The patient should be positioned horizontally, as opposed to being in the Trendelenburg position, and chest compressions should cease.
- A catheter should be inserted into the endotracheal tube and allowed to pass the tip of the tube. The medication solution should be sprayed down the tube, followed by 5-10 rapid ventilations with a respirator bag.
- Medications should be diluted with approximately 10 ml of distilled water or normal saline. Endotracheal absorption is greater with distilled water, but distilled water has a negative impact on the partial pressure of oxygen. In general, the systemic absorption of these medications is reduced via the endotracheal route and, therefore, the dose administered should always be 2-2.5 times the usual IV dose.

Homework.

SELF-ASSESSMENT QUESTIONS

1. Mean arterial pressure is regulated by which two functions?
2. Cardiac output is regulated by which two functions?
3. Which monitoring tool reflects the presence of hypovolemia and the need in administering fluids to a patient?
4. Hypotension is first managed by what mode of therapy?
5. Which catecholamine has pronounced and selective effects on dopamine receptors in the kidney, resulting in improved urinary output?
6. What are the four categories of sudden cardiac death?
7. What are the five classes of the Vaughan Williams classification system?
8. Which category of the Vaughan Williams classification is used solely for ventricular arrhythmias?
9. Which antiarrhythmic medication should be initiated with a rate-controlling medication?
10. Which antiarrhythmic agent is highly associated with the development of lupus erythematosus?
11. Which medications constitute the class II category of the Vaughan Williams classification system?
12. Which β-blocker is included in category III within the Vaughan Williams classification system?
13. Which medication in category III within the Vaughan Williams classification system is no longer manufactured in the United States?

SELF-ASSESSMENT QUESTIONS —cont'd

14. Which medication in category III within the Vaughan Williams classification system requires continuous ECG monitoring postadministration for risk of developing ventricular arrhythmias?

15. What is the appropriate method of administering adenosine?

Answers to Self-Assessment Questions are found in Appendix A.

CLINICAL SCENARIO

R.W., a 49-year-old man, is visiting his mother, who was admitted to a nursing home for long-term rehabilitation because of a spinal cord injury. He goes to the bathroom and a few minutes later his mother hears a loud thud; she calls out to him, but there is no response. After an additional 3 minutes, the head nurse and the clinical pharmacist initiate CPR and obtain the code cart. The initial ECG reading reveals pulseless electrical activity (PEA), and they administer one dose of epinephrine and atropine given as a rapid IV push followed by a saline flush. The code team arrives to continue CPR and a subsequent ECG reading reveals ventricular fibrillation. One shock is delivered, and a dose of amiodarone 300 mg IVPB (intravenous piggyback) over 10 minutes is administered. The patient becomes conscious and hemodynamically stable.

What are the doses of epinephrine and atropine?

What alternative agent could have been given instead of epinephrine?

What is the continuous infusion rate that the patient should be maintained on, to prevent the reoccurrence of ventricular fibrillation?

What are the baseline parameters that need to be obtained prior to starting chronic amiodarone therapy?

Answers to Clinical Scenario Questions are found in Appendix A.

References

1. Barnes AD, Lee SH: Shock. In Koda-Kimble MA, Young Yee L, Kradjan WA, Gugliemo BJ, editors: *Applied therapeutics*, ed 8, Baltimore, Md, 2005, Lippincott Williams & Wilkins.
2. Guyton AC, Hall JE: *Textbook of medical physiology*, Philadelphia, Pa, 1996, W.B. Saunders.
3. Vander A, Sherman J, Luciano D: *Human physiology the mechanisms of body functions*, ed 7, New York, 1998, McGraw-Hill.
4. *Drug Facts and Comparisons* [Cardiovascular Agents], St. Louis, Mo, 2005, Facts and Comparisons, Wolters Kluwer Health.
5. Hollenberg SM, Ahrens TS, Annane D, Astiz ME, Chalfin DB, Dasta JF, Heard SO, Martin C, Napolitano LM, Susla GM, et al.: Practice parameters for hemodynamic support of sepsis in adult patients: *Crit Care Med* 1999; 27:639–60.
6. American Heart Association: The American Heart Association 2005 guidelines for cardiopulmonary resuscitation and emergency cardiovascular care, *Circulation* 112:IV-78, 2005.
7. Lewin NA: Cardiac glycosides, In Goldfrank LR, Flomenbaum NE, Lewin NA, Weisman RS, Howland MA, Hoffman RS, editors: *Toxicologic emergencies*, ed 6, New York, 1998, McGraw-Hill.
8. White MC, Song SC, Chow MS: Cardiac arrhythmias, In Koda-Kimble MA, Young Yee L, Kradjan WA, Gugliemo BJ, editors: *Applied therapeutics*, ed 8, Baltimore, Md, 2005, Lippincott Williams & Wilkins.
9. Nattel S, Opie LH: Controversies in atrial fibrillation, *Lancet* 367:262, 2006.
10. Gregoratos G, Abrams J, Epstein AE, Freedman RA, Hayes DL, Hlatky MA, Kerber RE, Naccarelli GV, Schoenfeld MH, Silka MJ, *et al.*: ACC/AHA/NASPE 2002 guideline update for implantation of cardiac pacemakers and antiarrhythmia devices: a report of the American College of Cardiology/American Heart Association Task Force on Practice Guidelines (ACC/AHA/NASPE Committee on Pacemaker Implantation). 2002. Available at http://www.acc.org/qualityandscience/clinical/guidelines/pacemaker/summary_article.pdf (accessed April 2007).
11. *AHFS Drug Information*, 24:04:04. Bethesda, Md, 2003, American Society of Health-System Pharmacists.
12. Alboni P, Botto GL, Baldi N, Luzi M, Russo V, Gianfranchi L, Marchi P, Calzolari M, Solano A, Baroffio R, Gaggioli G: Outpatient treatment of recent-onset atrial fibrillation with the "pill-in-the-pocket" approach, *N Engl J Med* 351:2384, 2004.
13. Tikosyn Product Information, Pfizer 2004. Available at http://tikosyn.com/ (accessed April 2007).
14. Corvert Product Information, Pfizer 2002. Available at http://www.pfizer.com/pfizer/download/uspi_corvert.pdf (accessed April 2007).
15. Fan MS, Mustafa J: Role of adenosine in airway inflammation in an allergic mouse model of asthma, *Int Immunopharmacol* 6:36, 2006.
16. ECC Committee, Subcommittees and Task Forces of the American Heart Association: 2005 American Heart Association guidelines for cardiopulmonary resuscitation and emergency cardiovascular care [part 2: ethical issues], *Circulation* 112:IV1, 2005.
17. ECC Committee, Subcommittees and Task Forces of the American Heart Association: 2005 American Heart Association guidelines for cardiopulmonary resuscitation and emergency cardiovascular care [see IV6-IV11], *Circulation* 112:IV1, 2005.
18. Echt D.S., Liebson P.R., Mitchell L.B., Peters R.W., Obias-Manno D., Barker A.H., Arensberg D., Baker A., Friedman L., Greene H.L.: et al. Mortality and morbidity in patients receiving encainide, flecainide, or placebo. The Cardiac Arrhythmia Suppression Trial. *N Engl J Med* 1991; 324:781–788, Mar 21, 1991.
19. Kalus JS et al. Does magnesium prophylaxis alter ibutilide's therapeutic efficacy in atrial fibrillation patients? *Circulation* 2002; 106:II-634.

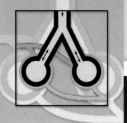

Chapter 20

Drugs Affecting Circulation: Antihypertensives, Antianginals, Antithrombotics

HENRY COHEN, ANTONIA ALAFRIS, STEVEN B. LEVY

CHAPTER OUTLINE

Epidemiology and Etiology of Hypertension
Pathophysiology of Hypertension
Hypertensive Crisis
Hypertension Pharmacotherapy
　Angiotensin-Converting Enzyme Inhibitors
　Angiotensin II Receptor Blockers
　Calcium Channel Blockers
　β Blockers
　Diuretics
　Aldosterone Antagonists
　Centrally Acting Adrenergic Agents
　α₁-Adrenergic Antagonists
　Antiadrenergic Agents
　Vasodilators

Epidemiology, Etiology, and Pathophysiology
　of Angina
Pharmacotherapy for Angina
　Nitrates
　Ranolazine
Antithrombotic Agents
　Formation and Elimination of an Acute Coronary
　　Thrombus
　Anticoagulant Agents
　Antiplatelet Agents
　Thrombolytic Agents

CHAPTER OBJECTIVES

After reading this chapter, the reader will be able to:

1. Categorize the stages of normal to high blood pressure
2. Define a hypertensive crisis
3. Design an algorithm for the pharmacotherapy of hypertension
4. Compare and contrast the clinical pharmacology among the agents used for hypertensive pharmacotherapy
5. Describe the mechanism of action of the angiotensin-converting enzyme inhibitors, calcium channel blockers, and β blockers
6. Describe the chronotherapeutic effect of blood pressure, and design a pharmacotherapy regimen based on this principle
7. Compare and contrast the clinical pharmacology of spironolactone and eplerenone

8. List antihypertensive relevant drug–drug interactions, and plausible mechanisms
9. Describe the formation and elimination of an acute coronary thrombus
10. List the agents in each of the following antithrombotic classes: anticoagulants, antiplatelets, and thrombolytics
11. Describe the mechanism of action of heparin
12. Compare and contrast the clinical pharmacology of heparin and low molecular weight heparin
13. List the laboratory parameters that may be used to monitor for the effect of heparin, low molecular weight heparin, and direct thrombin inhibitors
14. Describe the mechanism of heparin- and warfarin-induced paradoxical thrombosis

CHAPTER OBJECTIVES—cont'd

15. Compare and contrast the clinical pharmacology of aspirin, clopidogrel, ticlopidine, and dipyridamole
16. Describe the indication and mechanism of action of the glycoprotein IIb/IIIa inhibitors

17. Describe the formation and elimination of an acute coronary thrombus
18. List the indications of the thrombolytics

KEY TERMS AND DEFINITIONS

Antithrombotic — Drugs that prevent or break up blood clots in such conditions as thrombosis or embolism; include anticoagulants, antiplatelets, and thrombolytics

Arterial blood pressure (blood pressure) — Defined hemodynamically as the product of cardiac output (heart rate × stroke volume) and total peripheral resistance

Cardiovascular disease — Damage to the heart and the blood vessels or circulation, including to the brain, kidney, and the eye

Chronotropic — Influencing the rate of rhythmic movements (heartbeat)

Circadian rhythm — Human biologic variations of rhythm within a 24-hour cycle

Creatinine clearance — Measurement of the renal clearance of endogenous creatinine per unit time; considered to be an estimate of glomerular filtration rate (GFR); overestimates GFR by 10%-15%; used for drug-dosing guidelines

D-dimers — Covalently cross-linked degradation fragments of the cross-linked fibrin polymer during plasmin-mediated fibrinolysis; the level increases after the onset of fibrinolysis, and allows for identification of the presence of fibrinolysis

Dose-ceiling effect — A maximum dose of a drug, beyond which it no longer exerts a therapeutic effect; however, its toxic effect does increase

Fibrin split or fibrinogen degradation products (FDPs) — Small peptides that result following the action of plasmin on fibrinogen and fibrin in the fibrinolytic process. FDPs are anticoagulant substances that can cause bleeding if fibrinolysis becomes uncontrolled and excessive

Glomerular filtration rate (GFR) — The volume of water filtered from the plasma by the kidney via the glomerular capillary walls into Bowman capsules per unit time; considered to be 90% of creatinine clearance, and equivalent to inulin clearance

Hypertensive emergency — Blood pressures above 180/120 mmHg, when the elevation of blood pressure is accompanied by acute, chronic, or progressing target organ injury

Hypertensive urgency — Blood pressures above 180/120mmHg without signs or symptoms of acute target organ complications

Inotrope — A drug influencing the contractility of a muscle (heart)

Intrinsic sympathomimetic activity — Having the ability to activate and block adrenergic receptors, producing a net stimulatory effect on the sympathetic nervous system

Pharmacotherapy — Treatment of disease by drug therapy

Renin — An enzyme also known as angiotensinogenase, released by the kidney in response to a lack of renal blood flow, and responsible for converting angiotensinogen into angiotensin I

Substitute neurotransmitters — Neurotransmitter or hormone replacements that may be weaker or inert

---

The circulatory system comprises an integral functional part of the cardiopulmonary system. Drug therapy affecting the circulation is seen in the acute critical care, outpatient care, and home care environments. This chapter presents three classes of drug therapy, all targeted at the circulatory system. After a brief review of the epidemiology, etiology, and pathophysiology of hypertension, the multiple drug groups used as antihypertensives are described. Drugs used to treat angina pectoris are the second group of drugs described. The third group of agents affecting circulation, the antithrombotic group, is made up of several classes of drugs used to regulate clotting mechanisms.

EPIDEMIOLOGY AND ETIOLOGY OF HYPERTENSION

KEY POINT

Hypertension is defined as a blood pressure of 140/90 mmHg or greater.

More than 1 billion people worldwide and 1 in every 4 Americans has high blood pressure (≥140/90 mmHg). Hypertension adversely affects numerous body organs, including the heart, brain, kidney, and eye. Damage to these organ systems resulting from hypertension is termed **cardiovascular disease** (**CVD**). Uncontrolled hypertension increases CVD morbidity and mortality by increasing the risk of developing left ventricular hypertrophy, angina, myocardial infarction (MI), heart failure, stroke, peripheral arterial disease, retinopathy, and renal failure. One of eight deaths can be attributed to hypertension, and the World Health Organization reports that suboptimal blood pressure (systolic blood pressure above 115 mmHg) is responsible for 62% of cerebrovascular disease and 49% of ischemic heart disease. Blood pressure increases with age; thus hypertension is more prevalent in those older than 65 years of age. This is of great concern as it is estimated that by the year 2040, 25% of the American population will be more than 65 years old. Hypertension occurs more frequently in males than females and in more blacks than whites. Recent evidence suggests that individuals who are normotensive by the age of 55 have a 90% lifetime risk for developing hypertension.[1]

Hypertension is diagnosed by the mean of two or more separate seated blood pressure determinations on different days. The seventh Joint National Committee on the Prevention, Detection, Evaluation, and Treatment of High Blood Pressure (JNC VII) provides a classification of blood pressure for adults aged 18 years or older (Table 20-1).[2] Significant changes between JNC-VI[3] and JNC-VII include the development of the new blood pressure classification, in which a prehypertension category was created and stages 2 and 3 were combined. Patients with prehypertension are at increased risk for developing hypertension, and those with blood pressure in the range of 130/80 to 139/89 mmHg have a 50% greater risk of developing hypertension than those with lower values. This new classification is intended to identify those persons in whom early lifestyle modifications will reduce their blood pressure, and decrease the rate of progression to hypertension or prevent hypertension entirely.

KEY POINT

When the cause is unknown, hypertension is termed *primary* or *essential* hypertension.

In almost all cases, hypertension is caused by an unknown etiology and is termed either *primary hypertension* or *essential hypertension*. The prevalence of secondary hypertension is less than 10%, and secondary hypertension may have many disease- and drug-induced etiologies. Disease-induced causes of hypertension include renal disease, hyperthyroidism, hyperparathyroidism, Cushing's syndrome, primary aldosteronism, and pheochromocytoma. Drug-induced causes of hypertension include venlafaxine, cyclosporine, tacrolimus, erythropoietin, pseudoephedrine, amphetamines, sibutramine, nonsteroidal antiinflammatory drugs (NSAIDs) including cyclooxygenase-1 inhibitors (e.g., ibuprofen and naproxen) and cyclooxygenase-2 inhibitors (e.g., celecoxib), estrogens, corticosteroids, high-sodium-containing over-the-counter (OTC) products (e.g., Alka-Seltzer effervescent antacid tablets), and chronic alcohol ingestion.[4,5]

PATHOPHYSIOLOGY OF HYPERTENSION

KEY POINT

Arterial blood pressure is a product of cardiac output [(heart rate) × (stroke volume)] and total peripheral vascular resistance.

Arterial blood pressure, termed *blood pressure*, is generated by the interplay between blood flow and the resistance to blood flow. Arterial blood pressure reaches a peak during cardiac systole and a nadir at the end of diastole. Arterial blood pressure is defined hemodynamically as the product of cardiac output (heart rate × stroke volume) and total peripheral resistance. Venous capacitance, which affects the volume of blood *(preload)*, is a major determinant of cardiac output and systolic blood pressure. Arteriolar capacitance *(afterload)* is a major determinant of total peripheral resistance and diastolic blood pressure. Antihypertensives elicit actions on some or all of the hemodynamic parameters that define arterial blood pressure.

TABLE 20-1		
Classification of Blood Pressure for Adults Aged 18 Years and Older		
Category	Systolic (mmHg)	Diastolic (mmHg)
Normal	<120	<80
Prehypertension	120-139	80-89
Hypertension		
Stage 1	140-159	90-99
Stage 2	≥160	≥100

HYPERTENSIVE CRISIS

KEY POINT

Stage 3 hypertension, with a systolic pressure of 180 mmHg or greater and a diastolic pressure of 120 mmHg or greater, is a hypertensive crisis.

A patient with blood pressure above 180/120 mmHg is considered to be in a hypertensive crisis. A hypertensive crisis represents either a hypertensive urgency or a hypertensive emergency. **Hypertensive urgencies** usually signify high blood pressures without signs or symptoms of acute target organ complications, but may present with severe headaches, shortness of breath, nose bleeds, or severe anxiety. In these situations, reduction in blood pressure may proceed safely to a stage 1 value with oral antihypertensives over several hours to several days. Oral captopril, clonidine, and labetalol are routinely used to manage hypertensive urgencies. A **hypertensive emergency** exists when the elevation of blood pressure is accompanied by acute, chronic, or progressing target organ injury. Examples of acute target organ injury include encephalopathy, intracranial hemorrhage, severe retinopathy, renal failure, unstable angina, acute left ventricular failure with pulmonary edema, dissecting aortic aneurysm, and eclampsia. Hypertensive emergencies require admission to an intensive care unit and invasive arterial blood pressure monitoring and immediate but gradual blood pressure reduction over minutes to several hours with intravenous antihypertensives. Intravenous labetalol and nitroprusside are routinely used to manage hypertensive emergencies. Nitroprusside at high doses or when used for long durations can cause methemoglobinemia. Classic methemoglobin blood is chocolate brown and is without color change despite exposure to air.

HYPERTENSION PHARMACOTHERAPY

KEY POINT

First-line drug groups used to treat hypertension include the thiazide diuretics, β blockers, angiotensin-converting enzyme inhibitors (ACEIs), angiotensin II receptor blockers (ARBs), α-β blockers, and calcium antagonists.

KEY POINT

Second-line antihypertensives include α2 agonists, vasodilators, and antiadrenergic agents.

First-line agents for the treatment of uncomplicated hypertension are thiazide-type diuretics, or angiotensin-converting enzyme inhibitors (ACEIs), angiotensin II receptor blockers (ARBs), β blockers, and calcium channel blockers (CCBs).[2] Vasodilators, α-blocking agents, α2 agonists, and antiadrenergic agents are considered second-line antihypertensives.[2] For stage 1 hypertension, **pharmacotherapy** should be initiated for most patients with a low dose of a once-daily agent, usually a thiazide-type diuretic, and titrated upward until blood pressure control is achieved or intolerable adverse effects occur. Clinicians should be cognizant that monotherapy achieves effective blood pressure control in only 60% to 70% of patients. Thiazide diuretics profoundly decrease CVD morbidity and mortality, enhance the antihypertensive effects of the other antihypertensives, and are very useful in achieving blood pressure control. For stage 2 hypertension, because a higher response rate may be achieved by initiating low-dose *combination* antihypertensives, usually a thiazide-type agent plus an alternate first-line agent is used. The low-dose combination method may minimize adverse effects and may maximize efficacy and compliance.[6,7] An algorithm for the management of hypertension is depicted in Figure 20-1.[2]

Angiotensin-Converting Enzyme Inhibitors

ACEIs act primarily through suppression of the renin-angiotensin-aldosterone system. Because of a lack of renal blood flow, **renin** is released into the circulation, where it acts on angiotensinogen to produce angiotensin I. In the pulmonary vasculature, angiotensin I is then converted by angiotensin-converting enzyme (ACE) to angiotensin II. Angiotensin II is a highly potent endogenous vasoconstrictor that also stimulates aldosterone secretion from the zona glomerulosa cells of the adrenal cortex, contributing to sodium and water retention.[8] Angiotensin II also stimulates the release of catecholamines from the adrenergic nerve endings and mediates the release of central sympathetic outflow. ACE is abundant in the endothelial cells of blood vessels and to a lesser extent in the kidneys. ACEIs block the conversion of angiotensin I to angiotensin II by competing with the physiological substrate angiotensin I for the active site of ACE (Figure 20-2). The affinity of ACEIs for ACE is approximately 30,000 times greater than for angiotensin I. ACEIs also block the degradation of bradykinin and other vasodilating substances, including prostaglandin E_2 (PGE_2) and prostacyclin (PGI_2). Because ACEIs are potent antihypertensives in patients

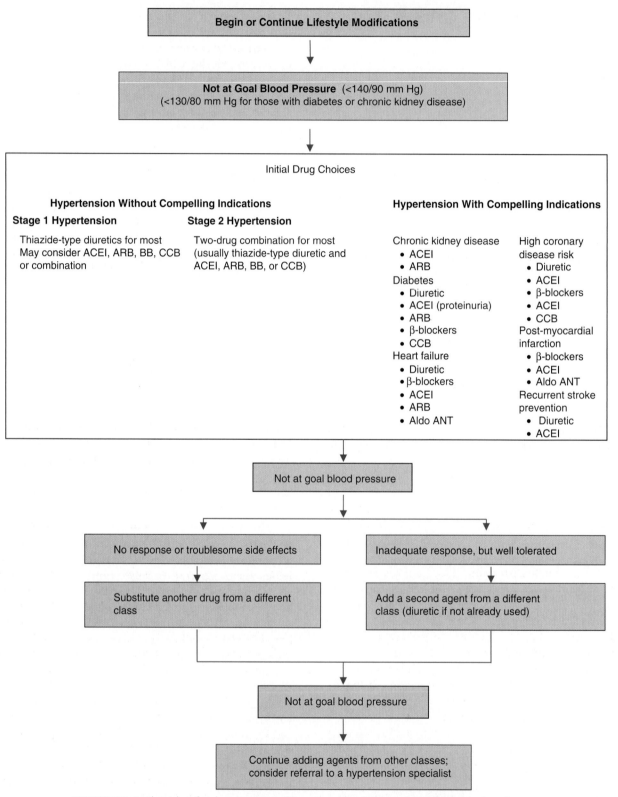

FIGURE 20-1 Algorithm for the treatment of hypertension. *ACE,* Angiotensin-converting enzyme; *ISA,* intrinsic sympathomimetic activity.

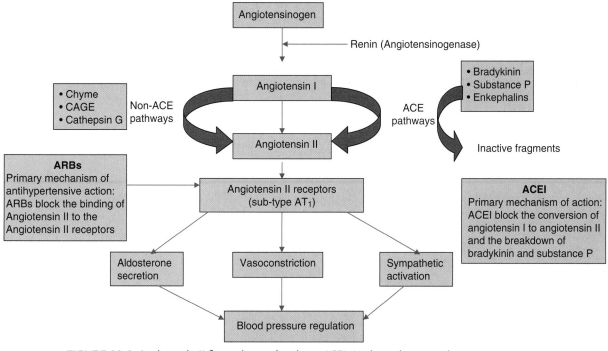

FIGURE 20-2 Angiotensin II formation and actions. *ACEI*, Angiotensin-converting enzyme inhibitors; *ARBs*, angiotensin II receptor blockers; *CAGE*, chymostatin-sensitive angiotensin II–generating enzyme.

with low-renin hypertension, the effects on bradykinin may have an integral role in the mechanism of action of these agents. The hemodynamic effects of ACEIs are a reduction of peripheral arterial resistance, an increase in cardiac output, little or no change in heart rate, an increase in renal blood flow, and unchanged **glomerular filtration rate (GFR).** ACEIs have mild antihyperlipidemic effects.

Ten ACEIs are available in the U.S. market. ACEIs are indicated for hypertension, heart failure, and systolic dysfunction, secondary prevention of MI, left ventricular dysfunction, and diabetic nephropathy. ACEIs generally decrease systolic and diastolic blood pressure by 15% to 25%. ACEIs are most effective in normal- or high-renin hypertension; however, they are also effective in low-renin hypertensives, especially when used at maximal doses. ACEIs are effective alone and in combination with other antihypertensive agents, especially thiazide-type diuretics. ACEIs rival diuretics as the most effective first-line antihypertensives to decrease CVD morbidity and mortality in various settings. With the exception of captopril, all ACEIs are generally administered once or twice daily. Enalaprilat is the only available parenteral ACEI. The pharmacokinetics and dosing guidelines for ACEIs are depicted in Table 20-2.[4,5]

The most common ACEI-induced adverse effect is a persistent nonproductive dry cough (20% to 30%). The cough may be due to ACEI-induced accumulation of kinins, prostaglandins, or substance P in the respiratory tract. The cough may develop within days to 1 year after the start of therapy. Antitussives are ineffective in relieving ACEI-induced cough. Cross-reactivity among the ACEIs is absolute; however, ARBs rarely cause cough and may be considered an alternative. ACEI-induced rash is also common; the incidence is 10%, and the reaction is usually transient. The rash often occurs in the upper extremities and is often accompanied by pruritus and erythema. A higher incidence of rash with captopril relative to other ACEIs may be due to captopril's sulfhydryl-containing structure. All other ACEIs, with the exception of fosinopril (phosphorus-containing), possess a dicarbocyl group. ACEIs are known to cause dysgeusia (6%), manifesting as a metallic or salty taste or loss of taste perception.

ACEIs may cause a slight increase in potassium that is generally inconsequential. However, the risk of hyperkalemia may be increased with concomitant use of β blockers, heparin, low molecular weight heparin (LMWH), trimethoprim, amiloride, spironolactone, elprenolone, and salt substitutes, and in patients with

TABLE 20-2

Pharmacokinetics and Dosing Guidelines for Angiotensin-converting Enzyme Inhibitors

ACEI: Generic Name (Brand Name)	Active Metabolite	Elimination Total	T$_{1/2}$ of Parent Drug (hr)*	Duration of Action (hr)	Dose Range (mg/day)	Daily Frequency	Effect of Food on Absorption
Benazepril (Lotensin)	Benazeprilat	11%-12% bile	22	24+	5-80	1	Slightly reduced
Captopril (Capoten)	None	95% urine	2	6-10	12.5-450	2-4	Reduced by 30%-40%
Enalapril (Vasotec)	Enalaprilat	94% urine and feces	11	24	2.5-40	1-2	None
Enalaprilat (Vasotec IV)	None	No data	35		1.25-5	Every 6 hr	NA
Fosinopril (Monopril)	Fosinoprilat	50% urine, 50% feces	12-15	24	10-80	1	Slightly reduced
Lisinopril (Prinivil; Zestril)	None	29% urine, 69% feces, 2% unchanged	13	24	10-40	1	None
Moexipril (Univasc)	Moexiprilat	13% urine, 53% feces	2-9	24	7.5-30	1-2	Markedly reduced
Quinapril (Accupril)	Quinaprilat	60% urine, 37% feces	2-3	24+	20-80	1-2	Reduced
Perindopril (Aceon)	Perindoprilat	96%-78% bile, 4%-12% urine	0.8-1	24	4-16	1	Reduced
Ramipril (Altace)	Ramiprilat	60% urine, 40% feces	11-17	24+	2.5-20	1-2	Slightly reduced
Trandolapril (Mavik)	Trandolaprilat	33% urine, 56% feces	24	24+	1-4	1	Reduced

ACEI, Angiotensin-converting enzyme inhibitor; *NA*, not applicable.
*Assuming normal renal function.

diabetes or renal failure. Orthostatic hypotension is common when initiating ACEI therapy, especially in patients who are in a high-renin state, such as those who are salt or volume depleted (e.g., those with heart failure, cirrhosis, diabetes, or receiving diuretics). Patients with bilateral renal artery stenosis, unilateral stenosis of a solitary functioning kidney, or in a high-renin state (especially patients with heart failure) are susceptible to developing ACEI-induced acute renal failure. Proteinuria, defined as total urinary protein exceeding 1 g/day and, rarely, accompanied by increases in blood urea nitrogen and serum creatinine, may develop in patients receiving high-dose ACEIs or with average ACEI doses and preexisting renal dysfunction. ACEI-induced blood dyscrasias such as neutropenia and agranulocytopenia occur with an incidence of less than 1% and are more common in patients with connective tissue diseases (e.g., systemic lupus erythematosus). ACEIs should be avoided in females of childbearing age because of the potential for fetal and neonatal morbidity and mortality in the second and third trimesters of pregnancy manifesting as skull hypoplasia, hypotension, anuria, and death (Pregnancy Category D).

Angioedema is rare, occurring in about 1-5 of 1000 patients, but it can be life-threatening when accompanied by dyspnea. Angioedema can occur at any time during ACEI therapy, especially when starting and stopping regimens. Angioedema generally manifests in the upper extremities, primarily the face, lips, tongue, glottis, and larynx. ACEI-induced angioedema is an absolute contraindication for the administration of alternative ACEIs and a relative contraindication for ARBs, especially in patients with a history of angioedema with dyspnea or with documented aminopeptidase P deficiency. Angioedema symptomatology may be associated with high concentrations of bradykinin. Bradykinin exerts its pharmacologic effects (vasodilation and proinflammation) on bradykinin-2 receptors, and is then metabolized primarily by ACE, to a lesser extent by aminopeptidase P, and to a minor extent by carboxypeptidase N. Delineating which patients have an aminopeptidase P plasma level deficiency may help predict which patients are predisposed to angioedema.

A significant drug interaction occurs when combining ACEIs with NSAIDs. NSAIDs increase renin release by inhibiting renal vasodilating prostaglandins (PGE$_2$

and PGI$_2$), thereby blunting or negating the antihypertensive effects of ACEIs. The NSAIDs less likely to reduce renal prostaglandins and to minimize or circumvent the interaction with ACEIs are sulindac (Clinoril), nabumetone (Relafen), etodolac (Lodine), salsalate (Disalcid), and choline magnesium trisalicylate (Trilisate). ACEIs may increase lithium concentrations and have been associated with life-threatening lithium toxicity. ACEI-induced renal sodium depletion may increase lithium renal tubule reabsorption. Patients receiving this combination should be monitored for symptoms of lithium toxicity such as nausea, vomiting, diarrhea, tremor, and mental status changes. Lithium levels should be monitored before and after initiating the ACEI. A quinapril tablet, unlike other ACEIs, contains magnesium carbonate at sufficient concentration to reduce tetracycline absorption up to 40%. The mechanism of this interaction may be chelation and plausibly may occur with fluoroquinolones. To circumvent this interaction, quinapril should be spaced 2 to 6 hours apart from tetracycline and fluoroquinolone antimicrobials.

Angiotensin II Receptor Blockers

Several nonrenin and non-ACE pathways are used for the production of angiotensin II (see Figure 20-2). Nonrenin pathways generate angiotensin II from angiotensinogen via tissue plasminogen activator, cathepsin G, and tonin. Non-ACE enzymes that generate angiotensin II from angiotensin I are cathepsin G, chymostatin-sensitive angiotensin II–generating enzyme, and chymase. Hence, ACEIs incompletely block the synthesis of angiotensin II. ARBs are angiotensin II type 1 (AT$_1$) receptor antagonists. AT$_1$ receptors are found in many tissues, such as the vascular smooth muscle, myocardial tissue, brain, kidney, liver, uterus, and adrenal glands (cortex and medulla). Many tissues also have an AT$_2$ receptor; however, it is not known to have effects on myocardial hemostasis. ARBs have thousands-fold greater affinity for AT$_1$ receptors than AT$_2$ receptors, and generally do not block the AT$_2$ receptor. Because ARBs do not inhibit ACE, they do not interfere with the concentrations of bradykinins and substance P. This kinin-sparing effect may explain why the ARBs have a low incidence of inducing cough or angioedema. However, the beneficial effects of kinins, including blood pressure–lowering potency, may be sacrificed.

Seven ARBs are available in the U.S. market. ARBs are indicated for hypertension and can be used for the treatment of heart failure. ARBs have been shown to reduce morbidity such as target organ damage (e.g., nephropathy) in patients with hypertension, and cardiovascular events in systolic heart failure patients, and progression of nephropathy in patients with type 2 diabetes. In the black population, ARBs and ACEIs may be less potent antihypertensives; however, this can be circumvented by administering maximal doses. ARBs, compared with ACEIs, are considered as potent or slightly weaker antihypertensive agents. The inhibition of bradykinin by ACEIs may account for its augmented antihypertensive effect. ARBs arguably are considered second-line agents to ACEIs for both hypertension and heart failure and are indicated when ACEI-induced cough or other adverse effects are intolerable. However, ARBs may be considered superior to ACEIs in patients with type 2 diabetic nephropathy. The ARBs are administered once or twice daily. Using the combination of an ACEI and an ARB has not been well studied; however, its beneficial effects have been observed in patients with heart failure and nephrotic syndrome. The pharmacokinetics and dosing guidelines for ARBs are depicted in Table 20-3.[4,5,8]

The side effect profile of ARBs appears to be similar to that of the ACEIs. ARBs may cause orthostatic hypotension, hyperkalemia, neutropenia, nephrotoxicity, and fetotoxicity. Similar warnings and precautions exhibited with ACEIs should be undertaken for ARBs. ARBs can cause cough; however, the incidence is significantly less than with ACEIs. ARBs cause significantly less angioedema than ACEIs; cross-reactivity has been reported. ARBs are not absolutely contraindicated in ACEI-induced angioedema; however, their use in this setting can be dangerous and should be avoided. Rash and dysgeusia are rarely reported with ARBs.

Losartan is extensively metabolized by the hepatic cytochrome P450 3A4 (CYP3A4) and CYP2C9 isoenzymes to an active carboxylic acid metabolite that is predominantly responsible for losartan's AT$_1$ blockade and antihypertensive effects. Drugs that induce these enzyme systems (e.g., phenytoin, phenobarbital, carbamazepine, oxcarbazepine, rifampin, and rifabutin) may increase the antihypertensive effects of losartan by increasing the concentration of the active metabolite. Phenobarbital has been shown to decrease the levels of losartan and its metabolite by 20%. Conversely, drugs that inhibit CYP3A4 (e.g., ketoconazole, fluconazole, erythromycin, clarithromycin, fluoxetine, and amiodarone) or CYP2C9 (e.g., amiodarone, cimetidine, and fluoxetine) or both CYP3A4 and CYP2C9 simultaneously (e.g., fluoxetine, amiodarone) may decrease the antihypertensive effects of losartan by decreasing the concentration of the active metabolite. However, a study evaluating the effects of cimetidine (CYP3A4 and CYP2C9 inhibitor) on losartan did not yield any changes in the disposition of losartan's

TABLE 20-3

Pharmacokinetics and Dosing Guidelines for Angiotensin II Receptor Blockers

ARB: Generic Name (Brand Name)	Elimination	Terminal $T_{1/2}$ (hr)	Dose Range (mg/day)	Daily Frequency	Effect of Food on Absorption
Candesartan (Atacand)	Ester hydrolysis/O-deethylation	9	8-32	1-2	No effect
Eprosartan (Teveten)	80% unchanged, 20% acyl glucuronide	5-9	400-800	1-2	No effect
Irbesartan (Avapro)	CYP2C9, CYP3A4	11-15	150-300	1	No effect
Losartan (Cozaar)	CYP2C9, CYP3A4	2	25-100	1-2	Slightly reduced
Olmesartan (Benicar)	35%-50% in urine and remainder in feces	13	20-40	1	No effect
Telmisartan (Micardis)	Conjugation to acylglucuronide	24	20-80	1	Slightly reduced
Valsartan (Diovan)	Biliary metabolism	6	80-320	1	Markedly reduced

ARB, Angiotensin II receptor blocker; *CYP*, cytochrome P450.

carboxylic acid metabolite. Telmisartan has been shown to increase digoxin peak plasma concentrations by 50%. Digoxin serum concentrations should be monitored before and after the addition of telmisartan. Several mechanistically similar drug-drug interactions that occur with ACEIs are likely to occur with ARBs, such as with NSAIDs and lithium.

Calcium Channel Blockers

Vascular smooth muscle and cardiac cell contraction is dependent on the free intracellular calcium concentration. Calcium from the extracellular fluid enters either the high-voltage–gated L-type calcium channels or the low-voltage–gated T-type calcium channels. L-channel blockade mediates coronary and peripheral vasodilation and may also cause reflex sympathetic activation or a negative inotropic effect. T-channel blockade mediates coronary and peripheral vasodilation and is devoid of a reflex sympathetic activation. The influx of calcium from extracellular fluid into cells triggers a second messenger, *inositol triphosphate*, to release stored intracellular calcium from the sarcoplasmic reticulum. The increase in cytosolic calcium results in enhanced binding to the protein *calmodulin*. A calcium-calmodulin complex activates myosin kinase, which promotes the interaction between actin and myosin, culminating in cellular contraction. Conventional calcium channel blockers inhibit only L-channels. The pharmacodynamic effects of the calcium antagonists on smooth muscle, myocardium, or specialized conduction and pacemaker tissues differ among them because of different receptor distribution and densities and the drug's inherent receptor selectivity and affinity.

Verapamil, the only diphenylalkylamine CCB, and to a lesser extent diltiazem, the only benzothiazepine

CCB, possess negative **chronotropic** effects by lowering sinoatrial (SA) node automaticity and decreasing atrioventricular (AV) node conduction; thus these agents are indicated for the treatment of angina, and arrhythmias, in addition to hypertension. Verapamil, and to a lesser extent diltiazem, are potent negative **inotropes** and may exacerbate heart failure, especially in patients with severe left ventricular dysfunction. The dihydropyridine calcium antagonists are potent vasodilators; these agents include amlodipine, felodipine, isradipine, nicardipine, nifedipine, and nisoldipine. The dihydropyridines, with the exception of nifedipine, have negligible chronotropic effects. Immediate-release nifedipine, especially when administered as a liquid (pseudo-sublingual), causes a potent reflex tachycardia that increases coronary oxygen demand and has been implicated with an increased risk of MI and stroke. Only sustained-release dosage forms of nifedipine are indicated for hypertension.[9] Amlodipine and plausibly felodipine may be used in patients with heart failure because these agents do not decrease cardiac contractility. Calcium antagonists are very effective antihypertensive agents in both elderly and black patients. The pharmacokinetics and dosing guidelines for calcium antagonists are depicted in Table 20-4.[2-5]

Verapamil (e.g., Covera HS, Verelan PM) and diltiazem (Cardizem LA) have long-acting formulations that are specifically designed to target the **circadian rhythm** of blood pressure throughout the day. Many hypertensives have a catecholamine surge with a blood pressure peak in the morning between 6 AM and 12 PM, followed by sustained high (but lower than the peak) blood pressures throughout the day, and a nadir at night. The preponderance of MIs, strokes, dysrhythmias, and venous thromboembolic events occur in the morning hours, in concert with the circadian blood pressure peaks. These

TABLE 20-4

Pharmacokinetics and Dosing Guidelines for Calcium Channel Blockers

Calcium Antagonist: Generic Name (Brand Name)	Onset of Action of Oral Dosage Forms (hr)	T$_{1/2}$ (hr)	Dose Range (mg/day)	Daily Frequency
Nondihydropyridines				
Verapamil (Calan, Isoptin)	0.5	3-7	180-480	3-4
Verapamil SR (Calan SR, Isoptin SR)	0.5	3-7	120-480	1-2
Verapamil ER (Covera HS)	4-5	2.8-7.4	180-420	Once at bedtime
Verapamil chronotherapeutic oral drug absorption (Verelan PM)	4-5	3-7	100-400	Once at bedtime
Diltiazem (Cardizem)	0.5	3.5	90-360	3-4
Diltiazem ER capsules (Cardizem CD, Cartia, Dilacor XR, Diltia XT, Tiazac, Taztia XT)	1	5	90-540	1-2
Diltiazem ER tablets (Cardizem LA)	3-4	6-9	120-540	Once daily (morning or evening)
Dihydropyridines				
Amlodipine (Norvasc)	6-12	30-50	2.5-10	1
Felodipine (Plendil)	2-5	11-16	5-20	1
Isradipine (DynaCirc)	2	8	2.5-10	2
Isradipine CR (DynaCirc)	2	8	2.5-10	1
Nicardipine (Cardene)	20 min	2-4	60-120	3
Nicardipine SR (Cardene SR)	20 min	2-4	60-120	2
*Nifedipine (Adalat, Procardia)	20 min	2-5	30-120	3-4
Nifedipine LA (Adalat CC, Procardia XL)	20 min	7	30-120	1
†Nimodipine (Nimotop)	ND	1-2	360	Every 4 hr for 21 days
Nisoldipine (Sular)	ND	7-12	20-60	1

*Nifedipine (prompt release) is not indicated for hypertension.
†Indicated for subarachnoid hemorrhage, not hypertension.
CC, Coat core; *CD,* controlled delivery; *CR,* controlled release; *ER,* extended release; *LA,* long acting; *HS, SR,* sustained release; *XL, XR,* extended release; *XT,* extended technology.

CCB dosage formulations are generally designed to be dosed at bedtime, and begin to release medication in the early morning in order to achieve a peak effect in the morning hours and a sustained effect during the day. These novel circadian dosage forms have had limited utility, because many hypertensives do not have a nadir in blood pressure in the nighttime—leaving patients unprotected with a high risk of a coronary event, and because when compared with thiazides and β blockers they have not demonstrated better effects on morbidity. Hypertensive nondippers (no nighttime nadir) are the elderly, those with renal insufficiency, and those with secondary hypertension. Both verapamil and diltiazem are available in several extended and sustained release products; the various dosage formulations of the same drug with or without circadian effects are usually not interchangeable and should not be switched on a milligram-to-milligram basis.

The incidence of verapamil-induced constipation and to a lesser extent diltiazem is high and often necessitates the use of a stimulant laxative such as bisacodyl, senna, or casanthranol. The dihydropyridines have potent peripheral vasodilating effects, and thus they have a high incidence of palpitations, orthostatic hypotension, flushing, headaches, lightheadedness, and syncope. These adverse effects are minimized with long-acting agents. All the calcium antagonists may cause peripheral edema, gingival hyperplasia, and gastroesophageal reflux (except diltiazem).

Diltiazem and verapamil inhibit CYP3A4 metabolism and plausibly the P-glycoprotein transport of alfentanil, buspirone, carbamazepine, cyclosporine, tacrolimus, methylprednisolone, lovastatin, simvastatin, digoxin, and quinidine, resulting in higher serum levels and potential toxicity. Verapamil and diltiazem inhibit the hepatic metabolism of theophylline. The dihydropyridines have negligible effects on the cytochrome P450 enzyme system or the P-glycoprotein transporter and are not expected to interact with CYP3A4 **substrates**. Grapefruit juice inhibits gut CYP3A4 and may significantly increase the levels of felodipine, nifedipine, and nisoldipine. Because many of the calcium antagonists

TABLE 20-6

Pharmacokinetics and Dosing Guidelines for Thiazides and Thiazide-like Diuretics

Thiazide/Thiazide-like Diuretic: Generic Name (Brand Name)	Bioavailability	Peak Effect (hr)	Duration of Diuresis (hr)	$T_{1/2}$ (hr)	Dose Range (mg/day)	Daily Frequency
Chlorothiazide (Diuril)	10-20	2 (PO), 0.5 (IV)	6-12 (PO), 2 (IV)	1-2	500-2000	1-2
Chlorthalidone (Hygroton)	65	2	24-72	35-55	15-200	1
Hydrochlorothiazide (Esidrix, HydroDIURIL, Oretic, Microzide)	65-75	4-6	6-12	2.5-4.5	25-100	1-3
Indapamide (Lozol)	95	2	24-36	14-18	1.25-5	1
Metolazone (Zaroxolyn)	65	2	12-24	6-20	5-20	1
Metolazone (Mykrox)		2-4	12-24	14	0.5-1 mg	1

IV, Administered intravenously; *PO*, administered orally.

possess the benzothiadiazine structure; however, they act pharmacologically like the thiazide diuretics; hence they are thiazide-like in structure and activity. Thiazide diuretics lose their antihypertensive potency in patients with a **creatinine clearance** less than 30 ml/min. Indapamide, however, retains its potency in patients with a creatinine clearance greater than 15 ml/min. Metolazone is the only thiazide-like diuretic that retains potency in patients with a creatinine clearance less than 15 ml/min. However, despite the thiazide-like structure of metolazone, its pharmacologic effects are similar to those of the loop diuretics. Metolazone is often added to a loop diuretic for refractory patients, achieving a synergistic diuretic effect. Mykrox tablets are a formulation of metolazone with a higher bioavailability than conventional metolazone, allowing it to achieve a more rapid diuretic effect; hence, Mykrox is not therapeutically equivalent to Zaroxolyn. The pharmacokinetics and dosing guidelines for the thiazide and thiazide-like diuretics are given in Table 20-6.[2,4,5]

Common thiazide side effects are hypokalemia, hypomagnesemia, hypercalcemia, hyperuricemia, hyperglycemia, hyperlipidemia, and sexual dysfunction. These abnormalities are dose related and may be minimized by using low-dose agents such as chlorthalidone, 12.5 to 25 mg daily, or hydrochlorothiazide, 12.5 mg twice daily. Less common thiazide-induced adverse effects include dyspepsia, rashes, photosensitivity, thrombocytopenia, and pancreatitis.

Loop Diuretics

Loop diuretics, which are often referred to as *high-ceiling diuretics*, act principally at the thick ascending limb of the loop of Henle, where they decrease sodium reabsorption by competing for the chloride site on the Na^+-K^+-$2Cl^-$ symporter (a transport molecule). Excretion of sodium, chloride, potassium, hydrogen ion, calcium,

magnesium, ammonium, bicarbonate, and possibly phosphate is enhanced. Diuretics such as the thiazides have a limited diuretic potency with a plateau effect, because they act primarily at sites past the ascending limb; only a small percentage of the filtered load reaches these more distal sites. Because more than 25% of the filtered load is reabsorbed in the ascending limb, loop diuretics are highly efficacious with increasing doses and hence are termed high-ceiling diuretics.

Loop diuretics are indicated for chronic heart failure, ascites, ascites of hepatic cirrhosis, renal failure, pulmonary edema, hypercalcemia, hypermagnesemia, and syndrome of inappropriate antidiuretic hormone. Loop diuretics are second-line diuretics in the management of hypertension; however, they are superior to thiazide diuretics in diuresis and decreasing blood pressure for patients with renal insufficiency. The pharmacokinetics and dosing guidelines for the oral loop diuretics are depicted in Table 20-7.[2,4,5]

Loop diuretics are very potent and as a consequence may cause severe dehydration, hypotension, hypochloremic alkalosis, and hypokalemia. Loop diuretics should not be administered at bedtime because the patient will have to urinate frequently, causing sleep disturbances. Loop diuretics may cause hyperglycemia (not reported with bumetanide), hyperuricemia, dyspepsia, photosensitivity, and ototoxicity. Ethacrynic acid is the most auditory ototoxic loop diuretic and should be considered only for patients refractory to other loop diuretics, or when there is a history of a life-threatening sulfonamide allergy.

Aldosterone Antagonists

Spironolactone (Aldactone) and eplerenone (Inspra) are aldosterone antagonists that exert their effect on the late distal tubule and collecting duct. Spironolactone, a

TABLE 20-7

Pharmacokinetics and Dosing Guidelines for Oral Loop Diuretics

Loop Diuretic: Generic Name (Brand Name)	Bioavailability (%)	Onset (hr)	Duration (hr)	$T_{1/2}$ (hr)	Dose Range (mg/day)	Daily Frequency
Bumetanide (Bumex)	70-95	0.5-1	5-6	0.8 ± 0.2	0.5-10	1
Ethacrynic acid (Edecrin)	100	0.5	6-8	2-4	50-200	1-2
Furosemide (Lasix)	60	0.5-1	6-8	0.5-1.1	40-240	1-2
Torsemide (Demadex)	80	0.5-1	1	2-4	5-200	1

TABLE 20-8

Pharmacokinetics and Dosing Guidelines for Aldosterone Antagonists

Aldosterone Antagonist: Generic Name (Brand Name)	Active Metabolite	Elimination Total	Onset of Action (hr)	Peak Response (hr)	Duration of Action (hr)	$T_{1/2}$ of Parent Drug (hr)	Dose Range (mg/day)	Daily Frequency	Effect of Food on Absorption
Spironolactone (Aldactone)	Canrenone	47%-57% renal, 35%-41% fecal	2-4	6-8 hr	16-24	1.4	25-400	1-2	Increased
Eplerenone (Inspra)	None	67% renal, 32% fecal	1-2	4 wk	24	3.5-6	50-100	1-2	No effect

weak diuretic, is used primarily for its aldosterone antagonist effects. Spironolactone is indicated for hypertension, for the management of hepatic cirrhosis (diuretic of choice), primary hyperaldosteronism, hypokalemia, and heart failure. For hypertension, spironolactone is used in combination with other antihypertensives, or to spare potassium when administered with diuretics. The chemical structure of spironolactone resembles that of the corticosteroids and may explain its sexual adverse effects such as impotence, decreased libido, gynecomastia, deepening of the voice, menstrual irregularities, and hirsutism. Other spironolactone-induced adverse effects include diarrhea, gastritis, skin rashes, drowsiness, lethargy, ataxia, headaches, and confusion. Spironolactone, similar to the other potassium-sparing diuretics, may cause hyperkalemia. The pharmacokinetics and dosing guidelines for the aldosterone antagonists are depicted in Table 20-8.[2,4,5]

Eplerenone is indicated for heart failure after MI and hypertension. Eplerenone, like spironolactone, blocks the mineralocorticoid receptor, but unlike spironolactone does not block the progesterone or androgen receptor, hence minimizing the sexual adverse effects such as gynecomastia, breast pain, impotence, and menstrual irregularities. Eplerenone has a higher incidence of severe hyperkalemia, especially in patients with reduced renal function. Because of the risk of severe hyperkalemia, eplerenone is contraindicated in all patients with a potassium values greater than 5.5 mEq/L or a creatinine clearance less than 30 ml/min; and in hypertensive patients with type 2 diabetes and microalbuminemia, or concomitant use of potassium supplements or potassium sparing diuretics, or serum creatinine greater than 1.8 mg%, or a creatinine clearance less than 50 ml/min. Vigilant monitoring of serum potassium levels is necessary when eplerenone is administered with ACEIs, ARBs, or β blockers. Eplerenone is a CYP3A4 substrate; CYP3A4 inhibitors such as verapamil, diltiazem, erythromycin, fluconazole, and saquinavir may increase eplerenone levels by 50%.

Centrally Acting Adrenergic Agents

The centrally acting adrenergic agents, or α_2 agonists, lower blood pressure by affecting both cardiac output and peripheral resistance; they are negative inotropes and chronotropes. The α_2 agonists stimulate brainstem α_2 receptors, resulting in a decrease in sympathetic outflow from the central nervous system. The α_2 agonists are very effective antihypertensives; however, they are not considered first-line therapy because of their side effect profile. They have a high incidence of anticholinergic-like side effects, such as sedation, blurred vision, dry mouth, constipation, and urinary retention, and central nervous system side effects, such as drowsiness, fatigue, headaches, depression, psychosis,

TABLE 20-9

Pharmacokinetics and Dosing Guidelines for Centrally Acting Adrenergic Agents (α_2 Agonists)

α_2 Agonist: Generic Name (Brand Name)	Onset of Action (hr)	Peak Effect (hr)	Duration of Action (hr)	$T_{1/2}$ (hr)	Elimination	Dose Range (mg/day)	Daily Frequency
Methyldopa (Aldomet)	4-6	6-9	24-48	1.25	Renal (biphasic)	500-2000	2-3
Clonidine (Catapres)	0.5-1	3-5	24	6-20	Renal (40%-60%)	0.1-2.4	2-4
Guanfacine (Tenex)	2.5	6	24	17	Renal (50%)	1-3	Once at bedtime
Guanabenz (Wytensin)	1	2-5	6-8	7-10	Renal (70%-80%)	4-32	2

and nightmares. Chronic use of these agents results in sodium and fluid retention and almost always necessitates the use of concomitant diuretics; this is especially seen with methyldopa. The α_2 agonists are not recommended for noncompliant patients and should never be withdrawn abruptly because of the risk of either rebound hypertension or overshoot hypertension.

The most effective and least toxic of the α_2 agonists is the clonidine transdermal therapeutic system (Catapres-TTS), which achieves sustained levels of clonidine for 7 days. The sustained clonidine levels avoid the peak and troughs associated with the prompt release dosage form, and hence are relatively devoid of the troublesome anticholinergic and central nervous system side effects. The clonidine patch is applied to a hairless area of intact skin on the upper torso. On the initial application, the clonidine patch will take 2-3 days to achieve target blood levels and a therapeutic effect. The most common adverse effects of the patch are local skin rashes and irritation. The pharmacokinetics and dosing guidelines for the α_2 agonists are depicted in Table 20-9.[2,4,5]

α_1-Adrenergic Antagonists

The α_1-adrenergic receptor antagonists selectively block the postsynaptic α_1 receptors. Total peripheral resistance is reduced through both arterial and venous dilation; thus these agents decrease both preload and afterload and cause a potent first-dose sympathetic reflex increase in heart rate and renin activity.[10] The α_1-adrenergic antagonists cause a first-dose phenomenon that manifests with orthostatic hypotension, tachycardia, palpitations, dizziness, headaches, and syncope. After several doses, despite persistent vasodilation, tolerance to the first-dose phenomenon develops and heart rate, renin, and cardiac output return to normal. To minimize the first-dose phenomenon, initial doses of α_1-adrenergic antagonists should be low and administered at bedtime. The α_1-adrenergic antagonists

have favorable effects on the lipoprotein profile and may decrease triglycerides and low-density lipoproteins and increase high-density lipoproteins by 5 to 10%.

The α_1-adrenergic antagonists are indicated for hypertension, benign prostatic hyperplasia, heart failure, and Raynaud's vasospasm. However, the ALLHAT (Antihypertensive and Lipid-Lowering Treatment to Prevent Heart Attack Trial) study compared doxazosin with other antihypertensives (chlorthalidone) and revealed a 25% higher incidence of combined cardiovascular morbidity in the doxazosin patients.[11] A higher incidence of doxazosin-induced stroke, heart failure, angina, and coronary revascularization was reported. On the basis of the results of this study, α_1-adrenergic antagonists are second-line antihypertensive therapy. The pharmacokinetics and dosing guidelines for the α_1-adrenergic antagonists are depicted in Table 20-10.[2,4,5]

Antiadrenergic Agents

The antiadrenergic antihypertensive agents are reserpine, guanethidine (Ismelin), and guanadrel (Hylorel). All three of these agents are second-line antihypertensives. Reserpine works by binding to storage vesicles of peripheral and central postganglionic adrenergic neurons and depleting norepinephrine. Subsequently, reserpine renders the neuronal storage vesicles dysfunctional. Reserpine may cause sedation, depression, suicidal ideation, psychosis, peptic ulcer disease, and nasal stuffiness. The side effects of reserpine can be minimized with low yet effective antihypertensive doses (0.25 mg or less). Guanethidine and guanadrel are postganglionic sympathetic inhibitors that produce a selective block of efferent peripheral sympathetic pathways. Guanethidine and guanadrel act as **substitute neurotransmitters** by replacing norepinephrine in the neuronal storage vesicle. Guanethidine and guanadrel cause

TABLE 20-10

Pharmacokinetics and Dosing Guidelines for α₁-Adrenergic Receptor Antagonists

α₁ Antagonist: Generic Name (Brand Name)	Elimination Routes	Peak (hr)	Duration (hr)	T₁/₂ (hr)	Dose Range (mg/day)	Daily Frequency
Doxazosin (Cardura)	63% feces, 9% urine	6	18-36	11	1 to 16	1
Prazosin (Minipress)	90% feces, 10% urine	1.5	8-10	2	3-40	2-3
Terazosin (Hytrin)	60% feces, 40% urine	2	24	14	120	1-2

similar adverse effects, such as orthostatic hypotension, sexual dysfunction, and diarrhea that can be occasionally explosive. The antihypertensive effects of these agents may be diminished when combined with tricyclic antidepressants, amphetamines, and ephedrine.

Vasodilators

The two common vasodilators used in the management of hypertension are hydralazine (Apresoline) and minoxidil (Rogaine, Loniten). Because of their adverse effect profile the vasodilators are second-line antihypertensive agents. Hydralazine is also indicated for heart failure and has been used for angina. These agents reduce total peripheral resistance by a direct action on vascular smooth muscle, increasing intracellular concentrations of cyclic guanosine 3′,5′-monophosphate (cGMP). These vasodilators are so potent that they cause a profound activation of baroreceptors, leading to reflex tachycardia, renin release, and an increase in cardiac output. To minimize tachycardia and fluid retention, these agents are often administered concomitantly with a β blocker and a loop diuretic, respectively. Hydralazine has been associated with peripheral neuropathy and drug-induced systemic lupus erythematosus–like syndrome. When hydralazine is administered with food its bioavailability may double and may cause cardiac toxicity. Hydralazine should be administered consistently with or without food. Minoxidil-induced adverse effects include hirsutism, nausea and vomiting, and pericardial effusions.

EPIDEMIOLOGY, ETIOLOGY, AND PATHOPHYSIOLOGY OF ANGINA

KEY POINT

Angina pectoris is a marker for myocardial ischemia.

Ischemic heart disease can present as many clinical variants such as stable exertional angina; unstable (rest, preinfarction, crescendo) angina; coronary vasomotion; vasospasm associated with atypical, variant, or Prinzmetal's angina; silent myocardial ischemia; or an MI. Angina pectoris (chest pain) is a symptom or marker of myocardial ischemia. Ischemia is defined as a lack of oxygen and decreased or no blood flow to the myocardium. The annual incidence of angina pectoris is about 5 per 1000. Women often initially present with angina, whereas men will present with an MI. Angina pectoris can present with a heavy weight or pressure on the chest, a burning sensation, or shortness of breath. The chest tightness or pressure can occur over the sternum, left shoulder, and lower jaw. Chest pain can be precipitated by exercise, cold environment, physical exercise, or emotional stress (anger). The duration of pain intensity may range from a few minutes to half an hour. During angina an imbalance of myocardial oxygen supply and myocardial oxygen demand occurs. Factors that increase myocardial oxygen demand include increased heart rate, increased systolic wall force or tension, or increased contractility. Factors that decrease myocardial oxygen supply include a decrease in the concentration of oxygen (e.g., anemia), a decrease in coronary blood flow (e.g., thrombus), or the myocardium's inability to extract oxygen from the blood.

PHARMACOTHERAPY FOR ANGINA

KEY POINT

Pharmacotherapy for angina includes the nitrates (e.g., nitroglycerin), β blockers, and calcium antagonists.

Pharmacotherapy for angina pectoris includes the nitrates, β blockers, calcium antagonists, and ranolazine (Ranexa). Ranolazine was approved by the U.S.

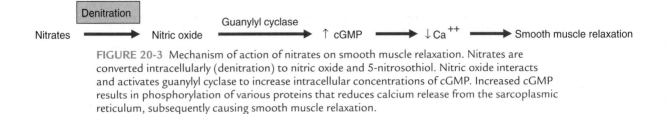

FIGURE 20-3 Mechanism of action of nitrates on smooth muscle relaxation. Nitrates are converted intracellularly (denitration) to nitric oxide and 5-nitrosothiol. Nitric oxide interacts and activates guanylyl cyclase to increase intracellular concentrations of cGMP. Increased cGMP results in phosphorylation of various proteins that reduces calcium release from the sarcoplasmic reticulum, subsequently causing smooth muscle relaxation.

Food and Drug Administration (FDA) in 2006 for the treatment of chronic stable angina in combination with amlodipine, β blockers, or nitrates.[12] For the management of vasospastic and chronic stable angina, diltiazem, verapamil, amlodipine, and nifedipine are indicated. For the management of angina, β blockers are usually dosed to achieve a resting heart rate of 50 to 60 beats/min and a maximal exercise heart rate of 100 beats/min. All patients with angina should receive daily aspirin to prevent an MI.[13,14]

Nitrates

Nitroglycerin reduces myocardial oxygen demand by causing venodilation of coronary arteries and collaterals, resulting in decreased end-diastolic pressures. Venous effects predominate; however, nitroglycerin can affect arteries at high doses. The cellular mechanism of action of nitrates is depicted in Figure 20-3. Nitrates are indicated for acute treatment or prophylaxis of angina, acute MI, acute heart failure, low-output syndromes, and hypertension (intravenous). Nitrates may be administered by various routes and are readily available in multiple preparations, including oral, intravenous, ointment, transdermal, translingual, and sublingual tablets. Sublingual nitroglycerin is indicated for acute anginal relief. Sublingual nitroglycerin has an onset of action of minutes and duration of action of 30 minutes. Sublingual nitroglycerin should be administered every 5 minutes until relief is obtained. If pain relief is not achieved after three doses in 15 minutes, emergency care should be sought. Sublingual tablets must always be stored in their original container or they may lose potency. In addition, unused tablets should be discarded 6 months after the original container is opened, because a loss of potency may have occurred. Other forms of nitroglycerin are isosorbide dinitrate (Isordil) and isosorbide mononitrate (Imdur, ISMO, and Monoket). The pharmacokinetics and dosing guidelines of the nitrates is depicted in Table 20-11.

Serious adverse reactions to nitrates are uncommon and involve mainly the cardiovascular system. The most frequent adverse effects include tachycardia, palpitations, postural hypotension, dizziness, flushing, and headache. Case reports of clinically significant methemoglobinemia are rare at conventional doses. Methemoglobinemia formation is dose related and occurs by the nitrite ion reacting with the ferrous hemoglobin. Tolerance to the vascular and antianginal effects may occur with prolonged use. Because most evidence supports the central role of cGMP stimulation in nitrate-induced vasodilation, it has been suggested that the tolerance results from sulfhydryl depletion at the nitrate receptor. Sulfhydryl depletion leads to reduced S-nitrosothiol production and therefore a decreased production of cGMP. Theoretically, administration of a sulfhydryl donor, such as N-acetylcysteine or captopril, may restore vascular response to nitrates. Increasing doses of nitroglycerin overcome tolerance, but this is short-lived. To circumvent nitrate tolerance, a nitrate-free interval of 10 to 14 hours is suggested. Nitrates are contraindicated in patients concomitantly taking phosphodiesterase type 5 inhibitors for erectile dysfunction, such as sildenafil (Viagra), vardenafil (Levitra), and tadalafil (Cialis), because of pronounced potentiation of nitric oxide resulting in significant decreases in blood pressure that may be fatal.

Ranolazine

Ranolazine is indicated for the treatment of chronic angina patients who have not achieved an adequate response with other antianginal drugs. Ranolazine provides antiischemic effects that complement the benefits of CCBs, β blockers, and nitrates. Ranolazine is believed to reduce fatty acid oxidation, shifting myocardial energy production from fatty acid oxidation to glucose oxidation. The oxygen demands required for glucose oxidation are less than for fatty acid oxidation, allowing the myocardium to maintain its normal function at times of ischemia. Ranolazine increase exercise tolerance, which reduces angina frequency, and the need for emergent nitroglycerin interventions. Unlike the standard antianginal medications, ranolazine does not alter blood pressure or heart rate. The initial adult dose of ranolazine extended release tablets is 500 mg twice daily, with a maximal dose of 1 g twice daily.

TABLE 20-11

Pharmacokinetics and Dosing Guidelines for Nitrates

Name	Dosage Forms	Onset of Action (min)	Duration of Action (hr)	Initial Dose
Nitroglycerin	Buccal tablet, ER Oral capsule, ER Oral tablet, ER Sublingual spray Sublingual tablet Intravenous solution Topical ointment Transdermal patch	Angina pectoris • Oral ER: 20-45 • Sublingual: 1-3 • Topical ointment: 30-60 • Transdermal patch: 30-60 • Translingual spray: 2 Perioperative hypertension • IV: 1-5	Oral ER: 3-8 Sublingual: up to 1 Topical ointment: 7 Transdermal patch: 8-10 Transdermal spray: up to 1	Angina pectoris • IV: 5-25 µg/min to response • Oral capsule, ER: 2.5-9 mg every 12 hr; may increase to every 8 hr if needed and if tolerated • Topical ointment: 7.5-30 mg applied twice daily to a 36-square-inch area of truncal skin • Transdermal patch: 0.2-0.4 mg/hr • Sublingual tablet: 0.3-0.6 mg every 5 min, 3 times • Sublingual spray: 1-2 metered sprays onto or under the tongue; may repeat in 3-5 min, with no more than 3 metered sprays in 15 min Chronic heart failure • IV: non-PVC tubing, 5 µg/min, initial titration should be in 5-µg/min increments at intervals of 3-5 min guided by patient response Perioperative hypertension • IV: 5 µg/min, initial titration should be in 5-µg/min increments at intervals of 3 to 5 min, guided by patient response
Isosorbide dinitrate	Oral capsule, ER Oral tablet Oral tablet, chewable Oral tablet, ER Sublingual tablet	Oral: 60 Oral tablet, chewable: 2-3 Sublingual tablet: 2-10	Oral: 8 Oral tablet, chewable: 2 Sublingual tablet: 1-2	Angina pectoris • Oral tablet (immediate release): 5-20 mg bid-tid • Oral tablet/capsule, ER: 40 mg once daily to bid • Oral tablet, chewable: 5-10 mg every 2-3 hr or as needed; titrate to effect Chronic heart failure • Sublingual tablet: 5-15 mg every 2-3 hr • Oral: 30-160 mg/day in divided doses
Isosorbide mononitrate	Oral tablet Oral tablet, ER	45-60	6-12	Angina pectoris • Oral tablet (immediate release): 5-20 mg bid-tid • Oral tablet: 20 mg every morning, then 20 mg 7 hr later • Oral tablet, ER: 30-60 mg once daily Myocardial infarction Oral tablet: 20 mg once daily to tid

ER, Extended release; *IV*, intravenous.

Adverse reactions observed with ranolazine include dizziness, palpitations, headache, constipation, nausea, abdominal pain, and peripheral edema. Small, reversible increases in serum creatinine and blood urea nitrogen (BUN) have also been observed without the incidence of renal toxicity. Ranolazine is excreted primarily in the urine (75%) and to a lesser extent via the feces (25%); however, the manufacturer suggests that no dose adjustments are needed in renally impaired patients. Nevertheless, ranolazine patients who are renally impaired were observed

Box 20-1	List of Antithrombotic Agents

ANTICOAGULANT AGENTS

PARENTERAL ANTICOAGULANTS

High molecular weight heparin
- Unfractionated heparin

Low molecular weight heparins
- Dalteparin (Fragmin)
- Enoxaparin (Lovenox)
- Tinzaparin (Innohep)

Selective factor Xa inhibitor
- Fondaparinux (Arixtra)

Direct thrombin inhibitor
- Argatroban
- Bivalirudin (Angiomax)
- Desirudin (Iprivask)
- Lepirudin (Refludan)

Oral anticoagulants
- Warfarin sodium (Coumadin)

ANTIPLATELET AGENTS

Aspirin
Clopidogrel (Plavix)
Cilostazol (Pletal)
Dipyridamole (Persantine)
Aspirin and extended release dipyridamole (Aggrenox)
Ticlopidine HCl (Ticlid)
Glycoprotein IIb/IIIa inhibitors
- Abciximab (ReoPro)
- Eptifibatide (Integrilin)
- Tirofiban (Aggrastat)

THROMBOLYTIC AGENTS

Alteplase (Activase)
Reteplase (Retavase)
Streptokinase (Streptase)
Tenecteplase (TNKase)

to have a 15-mmHg increase in blood pressure—frequent blood pressure monitoring is prudent in such patients. Ranolazine can dose dependently prolong the cardiac QT_c interval (Q-T interval [duration of ventricular electrical activity], corrected for heart rate) and place patients at risk of torsades de pointes. A dose of 1 g twice daily prolongs the QT_c by 6 milliseconds (msec), and is more pronounced with hepatic dysfunction. Ranolazine is contraindicated in patients with any degree of hepatic dysfunction, or who are receiving other QT_c-prolonging agents. Baseline and follow-up electrocardiograms (ECGs) should be completed during ranolazine therapy.

Ranolazine is extensively metabolized in the gut and liver by CYP3A4 and to a lesser extent by CYP2D6. CYP3A4 inhibitors such as ketoconazole, fluconazole, macrolides, diltiazem, and verapamil can significantly increase the plasma levels of ranolazine—and are contraindicated. Moreover, ranolazine is a substrate of P-glycoprotein and it should not be taken with verapamil,

a known inhibitor of P-glycoprotein. Ranolazine is a P-glycoprotein inhibitor, and has been shown to increase the plasma concentration of digoxin by 1.5-fold. Ranolazine is also an inhibitor of CYP3A4 and CYP2D6, plausibly increasing the plasma levels of drugs that are substrates of these enzymes such as statins, tricyclic antidepressants, and antipsychotics.

ANTITHROMBOTIC AGENTS

KEY POINT

Antithrombotic agents include anticoagulants (heparin and coumarins), antiplatelet agents (aspirin, dipyridamole, cilostazol, pentoxifylline, ticlopidine, clopidogrel, and glycoprotein IIb/IIIa inhibitors), and thrombolytic agents (agents that lyse clots, e.g., streptokinase, alteplase).

Antithrombotics may be defined as agents that prevent or break up blood clots in such conditions as thrombosis or embolism. Three categories of antithrombotic agents are currently available in the United States and include the anticoagulants, antiplatelets, and thrombolytics. The anticoagulant agents work by preventing the formation of the fibrin clot and preventing further clot formation in already existing thrombi. Antiplatelet agents inhibit the action of platelets in the initial stage of the clotting process. Thrombolytics break up thrombi by degrading fibrin. Box 20-1 lists the currently available antithrombotic agents.[15]

Formation and Elimination of an Acute Coronary Thrombus

Under normal conditions, the body maintains an equilibrium state between clot formation (thrombosis) and clot breakdown (fibrinolysis).[16] Thromboses are initiated by an injury to the endothelial wall of a coronary vessel. When injury occurs, the anticoagulated endothelial surface is disrupted and the highly procoagulant subendothelial surface is exposed. Instantaneously, platelets will aggregate in response to the release of chemotactic substances, such as thromboxane A_2, followed by platelet adhesion to the subendothelial vessel surface, representing the initial step in clot formation. Platelet adhesion is mediated mainly by von Willebrand factor. von Willebrand factor is present in the subendothelium and is actively recruited when the subendothelium is injured. Adhered platelets are exposed to many subendothelial proteins, such as collagen and thrombin. Collagen and thrombin also promote platelet activation. Activated platelets release platelet agonists such

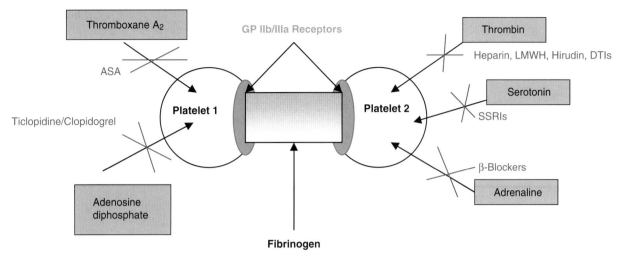

FIGURE 20-4 Triggers affecting platelet aggregation and their antagonists. Numerous agonists can mitigate platelet activation, which can be inhibited by drugs with corresponding mechanisms of action. However, expression of the platelet receptor GP IIb/IIIa on the platelet surface causes fibrinogen to bind to the platelet and subsequent linking of the two platelets (aggregation). This is the final common pathway to platelet aggregation. *ASA*, Aspirin; *DTIs*, direct thrombin inhibitors; *LMWH*, low molecular weight heparin; *GP*, glycoprotein; *SSRIs*, selective serotonin reuptake inhibitors.

as adenosine diphosphate, norepinephrine, serotonin, and arachidonic metabolites, mitigating and amplifying platelet aggregation and forming an unstable thrombus or platelet plug. The most important consequence of platelet activation is the expression of platelet receptor glycoprotein (GP) IIb/IIIa on the platelet's surface, allowing binding to fibrinogen. Fibrinogen then binds to the two GP IIb/IIIa molecules, causing a cross-linking of receptors on adjacent platelets and initiating platelet aggregation. Triggers affecting platelet aggregation and their antagonists are depicted in Figure 20-4. Fibrinogen is then converted into fibrin monomers by the action of thrombin; this is the final step in clot formation. Homeostasis is complete when the fibrin clot becomes insoluble within the vessel. This stable fibrin clot is the end result of the coagulation cascade. Under normal conditions, multiple inhibitors and control mechanisms keep these reactions localized to the site of the injury.

The fibrin clot ultimately must be removed for hemostasis to be maintained. Activation of the fibrinolytic system by tissue plasminogen activators (t-PA), which are present in most body fluids and tissues, results in the conversion of plasminogen to plasmin, initiating the dissolution of fibrin and fibrinogen. The breakdown of fibrinogen and fibrin results in polypeptides termed **fibrin split** or **fibrinogen degradation products** (**FDPs**). FDPs are anticoagulant substances that can cause bleeding if fibrinolysis becomes uncontrolled

and excessive. The **D-dimers** are fragments of plasmin-digested, cross-linked fibrin that rise in concentration after the onset of fibrinolysis. Blood testing for D-dimer fragments may assist in the diagnosis of pathogenic venous thromboembolism. The extrinsic and intrinsic pathways of the coagulation system are depicted and described in Figure 20-5.[2,3,14]

Anticoagulant Agents
Heparins: Unfractionated Heparin and Low Molecular Weight Heparin
Heparin is a nonionic sulfated glycosaminoglycan anticoagulant naturally present in the secretory granules of human mast cells. When heparin is released from mast cells it is ingested and destroyed by macrophages. Heparin is not detectable in plasma, except in pathologic circumstances (e.g., mastocytosis). Commercially available unfractionated heparin (UFH), or simply *heparin*, is indicated for the prevention and treatment of venous thromboembolism, the prevention and treatment of pulmonary embolism, the treatment of atrial fibrillation with embolization, the diagnosis and treatment of disseminated intravascular coagulation, and the prophylaxis and treatment of peripheral arterial embolism.

Heparin is extracted from porcine intestinal mucosa or bovine lungs; however, because of the high propensity of thrombocytopenia with the bovine lung derivative, only the porcine derivative is routinely employed

Intrinsic Pathway   **Extrinsic Pathway**

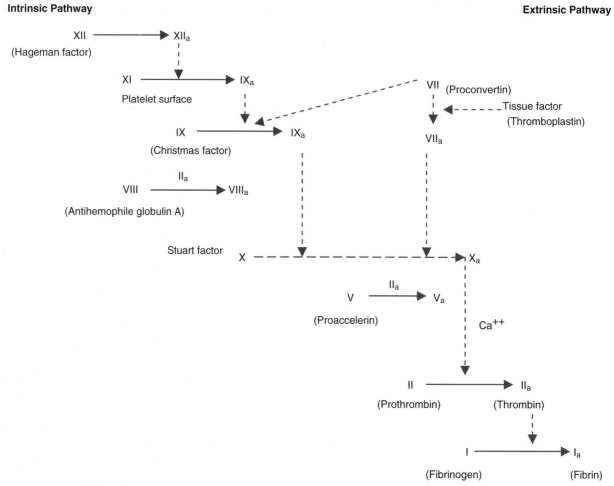

FIGURE 20-5 Extrinsic and intrinsic pathways of the coagulation system. The coagulation system is divided into the intrinsic pathway and extrinsic pathway. The intrinsic or contact activation pathway is activated by trauma or infection, which causes inflammatory proteins to be released in the circulation. The main role of the extrinsic pathway is to initiate coagulation during hemostasis. The activated forms of factors X and V catalyze, in the presence of calcium, the conversion of prothrombin to thrombin.

in practice. Heparin serves as a catalyst that accelerates the rate of the thrombin-to-antithrombin III reaction by at least 1000-fold by serving as a catalytic template to which both bind, resulting in a ternary complex (heparin, thrombin, and antithrombin). Antithrombin III is a large protein (58,000 daltons) that is synthesized in the liver and is known as a *suicide substrate*. Heparin is a high molecular weight complex mucopolysaccharide containing specific pentasaccharide units and approximately 45 monosaccharide side chains with a mean molecular mass of 12,000 daltons (range, 5000-30,000 daltons).[17] Most of the monosaccharide side chains of UFH are more than 18 monosaccharides long, and are necessary to form the ternary complex. Heparin molecules that possess fewer than

18 monosaccharide units (<5400 daltons) do not catalyze the thrombin-to-antithrombin III reaction. However, the heparin molecules that include fewer than 18 monosaccharides catalyze a conformational change on antithrombin III that inhibits the effects of factor Xa (Stuart factor), and does not require a ternary complex. Low molecular weight heparin (LMWH) is generally about 4500 daltons (range, 1000-10,000 daltons) in size and contains 15 monosaccharide units, and hence do not form a ternary complex. Their anticoagulant activity is exhibited via factor Xa inhibition. Because factor Xa occurs earlier in the coagulation cascade, the inhibition of a single molecule of Xa prevents thousands of thrombin molecules from forming. The anti-factor Xa to anti-factor IIa ratio of

UFH is 1:1 compared with that of LMWH, which ranges from 2:1 (tinzaparin) to 3.8:1 (enoxaparin). Heparin also inhibits the conversion of fibrinogen to fibrin and inhibits the activation of factor XIII, thereby preventing the formation of a stable fibrin clot. LMWH is postulated to suppress von Willebrand factor, which increases platelet aggregation, and to stimulate the release of tissue factor pathway inhibitor, which inhibits factor Xa.

LMWHs include dalteparin (Fragmin), enoxaparin (Lovenox), and tinzaparin (Innohep). UFH, unlike LMWH, binds extensively to plasma proteins such as glycoproteins, vitronectin, lipoproteins, fibrinogen, platelet proteins such as platelet factor-4, acute-phase reactant proteins, and endothelial cells, yielding poor UFH bioavailability and an unpredictable effect. The predictable bioavailability of LMWH allows for subcutaneous administration for all indications. UFH is administered subcutaneously for venous thromboembolism prophylaxis, but must be administered as a continuous infusion for serious indications such as an MI and to minimize the risk of hemorrhage. High molecular weight heparin (UFH) is cleared faster and requires more frequent dosing or an intravenous continuous infusion. The half-life of UFH is approximately 30 to 60 minutes whereas the half-life of LMWH is 4-5 hours, allowing for once or twice daily LMWH administration. The onset of action of heparin is within 6 hours of initiation of a continuous infusion. The LMWH time to peak anti-factor Xa activity is 2-5 hours. Each commercially available LMWH is synthesized by different mechanisms, possesses moderately different pharmacokinetic and pharmacodynamic characteristics, and has different FDA-approved indications and dosing regimens, and hence these agents are not interchangeable.

The activated partial thromboplastin time (aPTT) is used to monitor the effects of heparin because it is sensitive to the inhibitory effects of thrombin, factor Xa, and factor IXa and correlates with heparin levels. When the concentration of plasma heparin is 0.1-1 U/ml, the aPTT and thrombin time are prolonged. The goal of heparin therapy is to achieve the prevention of unwanted clotting without an increased risk of hemorrhage. This may be accomplished by maintaining the aPTT between 2 and 2.5 times the upper limit of the control value. The aPTT should not be used to monitor LMWH. The effect of LMWH may be monitored on the basis of anti-factor Xa levels; however, because the relationship between anti-factor Xa levels and clinical outcomes is tenuous, routine measurement is not indicated, and should be reserved for special populations such as renal patients, the obese, and the underweight.

UFH- and LMWH-induced adverse effects include bleeding, hematoma, early thrombocytopenia, delayed thrombocytopenia with or without the white clot syndrome, hyperkalemia, osteoporosis, and an increase in liver enzyme tests (LETs). An increase in LETs may occur in up to 10%-30% of patients receiving low or high molecular weight heparins. However, the increase in LETs appears to be benign and has not been associated with any cases of hepatic sequelae. Early-onset heparin-induced thrombocytopenia type 1 (HIT-1) manifests with a decrease in platelets of approximately 50,000/mm^3. The decrease in platelets is transient and inconsequential. Delayed-onset heparin-induced thrombocytopenia type 2 (HIT-2) is due to the formation of anti-platelet antibodies between days 6 and 12. HIT-2 is dependent on platelet factor-4 binding. These platelet antibodies aggregate and form the basis for the paradoxical heparin-induced white clot syndrome. The white clot syndrome may manifest as pulmonary embolism, MI, stroke, renal or hepatic thrombosis, or skin necrosis and gangrene. The diagnosis of HIT-2 is clinical and may be confirmed by several laboratory tests. Clinical diagnosis of HIT-2 includes a significant reduction in the platelet count of greater than 50% and/or a decrease in the platelet count to less than 100,000/mm^3. Ostensibly, the risk of thrombocytopenia is greatest with unfractionated heparin and lowest with LMWH; however, LMWH cannot be administered as an alternative to heparin because of greater than 95% cross-reactivity. However, Fondaparinux (Arixtra), a pentasaccharide-selective anti-Xa inhibitor agent, does not possess a risk of cross-reactivity and is currently being studied in clinical trials as a treatment modality for HIT-2 and the white clot syndrome. Current treatment options for HIT-2 include the direct thrombin inhibitors (DTIs) Argatroban and Lepirudin (Refludan), which are structurally and pharmacologically unrelated to the heparins.

The antidote for heparin is protamine sulfate. Protamine sulfate is derived from the sperm of mature testes of salmon and related species. Protamine is electropositive and will rapidly bind to the electronegative heparin to form salts that have no anticoagulant effect. In addition, protamine will also cause a dissociation of heparin-antithrombin III complexes in favor of a heparin-protamine complex. The recommended neutralizing dose of protamine is 1 mg for every 100 units of heparin, up to a total of protamine 50 mg per dose. Protamine should be administered by slow intravenous infusion over at least 1 to 3 minutes to prevent hypotension, bradycardia, or dyspnea. Patients who have previously received protamine-containing insulin, have undergone a vasectomy, or have a known sensitivity to fish or medications derived from fish (calcitonin-salmon, cold water fish oils containing omega-3 fatty acids, and oyster shell-derived calcium supplements) are at an increased risk for experiencing allergic reactions such as anaphylaxis and developing anti-protamine antibodies.[17] Excessive protamine may act as an anticoagulant, resulting in bleeding complications; therefore a careful underdosing strategy is suggested. There is no proven method for neutralizing LMWH. Protamine appears to neutralize approximately 60% of the anti-factor Xa activity of LMWH. Therefore, UFH may be the preferred parenteral anticoagulant in patients who are at risk for clinically significant bleeding, for example, those with end-stage renal disease receiving hemodialysis treatments.

Direct Thrombin Inhibitors

There are four commercially available highly specific DTIs. Desirudin (Iprivask) is indicated for deep vein thrombosis prophylaxis, and Bivalirudin (Angiomax) is indicated for unstable angina. Argatroban and Lepirudin (Refludan) are indicated for prophylaxis or treatment of thrombosis in patients with HIT-2 and are used for anticoagulation against thromboembolic conditions in patients with or at risk for HIT-2. The DTIs exert their anticoagulant effects by directly inhibiting the effects of thrombin on a sustained fibrin clot. One molecule of a DTI binds to one molecule of thrombin. DTIs are independent of antithrombin III reactions and are not inhibited by platelet factor IV. The aPTT is used to monitor the effects of DTIs, and is generally maintained at about 1.5 to 2.5 times the upper limit of the control.

The most common adverse effect of the DTIs is minor and major hemorrhage. DTIs may cause allergic skin reactions, and anaphylactic reactions manifesting with bronchospasm, stridor, and dyspnea. There are no proven antidotes for DTIs. However, there may be a role for recombinant human factor VIIa (rFVIIa) (NovoSeven) in DTI bleeding toxicities. rFVIIa is cloned from hamster kidney cells; it is a vitamin K–dependent glycoprotein (molecular mass, 50 daltons) structurally similar to human plasma–derived factor VIIa. rFVIIa can activate factor IX to IXa, and factor X to Xa, converting prothrombin to thrombin, and fibrinogen to fibrin, forming a hemostatic plug.

Natural hirudin is produced in trace amounts by the salivary glands of the leech *Hirudo medicinalis*. Lepirudin is a recombinant hirudin derived from yeast cells. The recommended initial dosing regimen is 0.4 mg/kg body weight as an intravenous bolus injection followed by

0.15 mg/kg/hr continuous infusion. Lepirudin has a half-life of 1.3 hours. The aPTT value should be obtained about 4 hours after the start of the infusion. Lepirudin is almost exclusively renally eliminated, requiring careful dosing adjustments in mild to moderate renal dysfunction, and it is contraindicated in severe renal impairment. The anticoagulant effects may be enhanced in patients with hepatic disease, and thus close monitoring in this population is recommended. The formation of lepirudin–anti-hirudin antibody complexes has been observed in 40% of lepirudin patients, and may enhance the effect of lepirudin by delaying its renal elimination. An advantage of lepirudin is its lack of effect on the international normalized ratio (INR) value, facilitating accurate warfarin monitoring and dosing (see the next section for more details on the INR).

Argatroban is a synthetic agent, derived from L-arginine, that reversibly binds to the thrombin active site. Dosing is accomplished through continuous intravenous infusion. The half-life of argatroban is 30-50 minutes. The route of elimination is primarily via the hepatic CYP3A4/5 isoenzyme system and, therefore, the potential for drug interactions exists with CYP3A4/5 inhibitors and inducers. There are four argatroban hepatic metabolites; only M1 is active. It is about 3- to 5-fold weaker than the parent, and is present at 0 to 20% relative to the parent. The recommended initial dose of argatroban is 2 μg/kg/min. An aPTT value should be attained 1 to 3 hours after initiation. In patients with hepatic dysfunction, the initial dose of argatroban should be reduced to 0.5 μg/kg/min. The effects of argatroban are not significantly influenced by renal impairment, and hence dosage adjustments are not necessary in this setting. When used in combination with warfarin, argatroban, especially at doses exceeding 2 μg/kg/min, has the potential to prolong the INR beyond that of warfarin alone. However, argatroban exerts no additional effects on vitamin K–dependent factor Xa activity. Therefore, special warfarin dosing considerations are required when concomitantly using argatroban and warfarin.

Warfarin (Coumadin)

Warfarin (Coumadin) is an oral anticoagulant indicated for the prophylaxis and treatment of venous thrombosis, pulmonary embolism, and thromboembolic complications associated with atrial fibrillation, cardiac valve replacement, and as an adjunct in the treatment of coronary occlusion. Warfarin is also used to reduce the risk of death, reinfarction, and thromboembolic events such as stroke or systemic embolization after MI. Warfarin is a racemic mixture; the (S)-isomer has a half-life of 2 days, and the less potent (R)-isomer has a half-life of 1.3 days and thus is dosed once daily. The full anticoagulant effect of warfarin has a delayed onset of 3-5 days, necessitating overlap with a parenteral heparin agent when rapid anticoagulation is preferred. The initial dose of warfarin should be the expected maintenance dose. Loading doses of warfarin are no longer recommended. A study found that when hospitalized patients were given an average warfarin maintenance dose of 5 mg, the INR was usually ≥2 within 4 or 5 days and was associated with less excessive anticoagulation compared with a 10-mg dose.[18] Warfarin starting doses of less than 5 mg may be most appropriate in elderly patients. Warfarin interferes with the hepatic synthesis of vitamin K–dependent clotting factors II, VII, IX, and X and endogenous anticoagulant proteins C and S. The time to complete anticoagulation with warfarin is not immediate. Inhibition of coagulation factors begins 12 to 24 hours after administration; however, the complete antithrombotic effects of warfarin may not occur until 5 to 7 days after initiation of therapy.

The international normalized ratio (INR) is the standard for monitoring warfarin therapy. The prothrombin time (PT) as a tool for monitoring warfarin therapy is problematic because thromboplastin reagents vary in their responsiveness to warfarin-induced reduction in clotting factors, a variability that is dependent on their method of preparation. The INR is a *mathematical correction* of the results of the one-stage PT time that standardizes the reporting of PT determinations worldwide. The INR takes into account the sensitivity of the thromboplastin used in each specific laboratory to determine the PT. The target INR range for warfarin in most clinical scenarios is 2 to 3. The INR should be used exclusively to dose warfarin clinically; however, the PT should be reviewed in conjunction with the INR to aid in detecting laboratory errors in calculation or assay methodology.

Hemorrhage is the most common adverse effect associated with warfarin and ranges from minor to life-threatening major bleeding. Bleeding manifestations may include ecchymoses, petechiae, purpura, melena, hematochezia, hematuria, hemoptysis, hematemesis, epistaxis, or gingival bleeding. Because warfarin inhibits protein C (half-life, 8 hours) and protein S (half-life, 30 hours), which have shorter half-lives than factors II (half-life, 60 hours), IX (half-life, 24 hours), and X (half-life, 72 hours), there is a risk of a paradoxical hypercoagulability, thrombus formation, and skin necrosis with gangrene. The procoagulant effect of warfarin can be enhanced in patients who are protein C and protein S deficient. To minimize the immediate procoagulant effect of warfarin,

an overlap of 3 to 5 days with a parenteral anticoagulant is warranted. Purple toe syndrome, caused by the release of atheromatous plaque emboli and cholesterol-rich microembolization, occurs approximately 3 to 10 weeks after initiation of coumarin therapy. The purple toe syndrome is reversible, and is typically characterized by a purplish or mottled discoloration of the plantar surfaces and sides of the toes that blanches on moderate pressure and fades with elevation of the legs. Oral or parenteral vitamin K_1 (phytonadione) may be administered to reverse the anticoagulation effects of warfarin.

Many factors such as diet, disease states, and drugs can alter the pharmacologic characteristics and effects of warfarin.[18] Patients should be counseled to eat a healthy and consistent diet. An increased intake of vitamin K–containing supplements and foods, such as green leafy vegetables, may result in a reduced anticoagulant response, decreased INR, and subsequently treatment failure such as an embolism. Conversely, abrupt decreases in vitamin K dietary intake may result in an increased anticoagulant response with an increased INR and subsequent risk of hemorrhage. Hepatic disease and to a lesser extent renal disease may decrease warfarin's elimination and increase the effects of warfarin. A plethora of drugs can increase or decrease the effects of warfarin. It is prudent to measure the INR frequently when factors that interact with warfarin are added to a patient's regimen. Table 20-12 lists selected significant warfarin drug interactions. Because warfarin is a high-risk medication that can significantly interact with many medications, requires frequent INR monitoring, and is pharmacokinetically challenging to dose, pharmacist-based warfarin clinics with physician supervision and collaboration have become a standard of best practice—more than 1500 such clinics are active in the United States today.

Antiplatelet Agents
Aspirin

In platelets, the prostaglandin derivative thromboxane A_2 is a major inducer of platelet aggregation and vasoconstriction. Aspirin is hydrolyzed to salicylic acid and inhibits prostaglandin production by acetylating cyclooxygenase, the initial enzyme in the prostaglandin biosynthesis pathway. This inhibition of platelet aggregation lasts for the life of the platelet, which is approximately 7 to 10 days. By inhibiting platelet aggregation, aspirin will increase bleeding times. Low doses of aspirin inhibit platelet aggregation, whereas larger doses inhibit cyclooxygenase in arterial walls, which interferes with prostacyclin production. Prostacyclin is a potent vasodilator and inhibitor of platelet aggregation. Lower

TABLE 20-12	
Selected Significant Drug Interactions With Warfarin	
Precipitant Drug	**Mechanism**
Amiodarone Cimetidine Lovastatin Metronidazole Omeprazole Quinidine SMZ-TMP	These agents may increase the anticoagulant effect of warfarin by inhibiting the hepatic cytochrome P450 isozymes (CYP2C9, CYP3A4, or CYP1A2) involved in its metabolism. The risk of bleeding may be increased
Chloral hydrate Loop diuretics Nalidixic acid NSAIDs	These agents may increase the anticoagulant effect of warfarin by displacement from protein-binding sites (albumin). The risk of bleeding may be increased
Antimicrobials NSAIDs Salicylates	These agents may increase the anticoagulant effect of warfarin either by inhibition of gastrointestinal vitamin K or by inhibiting platelet aggregation. The risk of bleeding may be increased
Barbiturates Carbamazepine Oxcarbazepine Etretinate Glutethimide Rifampin Rifabutin	These agents may decrease the anticoagulant effect of warfarin by the induction of those hepatic cytochrome P450 isozymes (CYP2C9, CYP3A4, or CYP1A2) involved in its metabolism. A lack of warfarin efficacy and thrombosis may occur
Cholestyramine Estrogens Oral contraceptives Spironolactone Sucralfate Thiazide diuretics Vitamin K	These agents may decrease the anticoagulant effect of warfarin by various mechanisms. A lack of warfarin efficacy and thrombosis may occur

NSAIDs, Nonsteroidal antiinflammatory drugs; *SMZ-TMP*, sulfamethoxazole-trimethoprim.

doses therefore plausibly may be more effective than higher doses in preventing coronary heart disease; however, this has not been proven clinically.

Aspirin has many indications including fever and pain associated with headaches, neuralgias, myalgias, and arthralgias. Antithrombotic indications for aspirin include reducing the risk of thrombosis, such as in the primary and secondary prevention of nonfatal or fatal MI in patients with/or without a previous MI or unstable angina; and preventing recurrent transient ischemic attacks (TIAs) or stroke. The dose of aspirin for its analgesic, antiinflammatory, and antipyretic effects is considered high dose and may be 325 to 650 mg up to every 4 hours daily as needed. The dose of aspirin for its antithrombotic indications is considered low dose; the range for prevention of MI is 81 to 325 mg daily, and for TIA/stroke it is 50 to 325 mg daily. Up to 25% of patients taking aspirin as an antithrombotic may be genetically prone to aspirin resistance, and higher doses may be necessary to overcome resistance (e.g., 500 mg-1.5 g daily). Aspirin resistance is best detected by means of bleeding time tests; however, these tests are not yet validated, standardized, nor are they routinely employed in clinical practice.

Aspirin-induced adverse effects are dose dependent and include peptic ulcer disease, renal dysfunction, increased blood pressure, tinnitus, pulmonary dysfunction, and bleeding. The risk of clinically significant hemorrhage with aspirin, for example, gastrointestinal bleeds, is dose dependent. However, any dose of aspirin carries a risk of major bleeding when compared with placebo controls. Therefore, patients should be counseled on the signs and symptoms of bleeding, which may include anemia, abnormal bruising, epistaxis, or bleeding of the gums, and dizziness and lightheadedness associated with low blood pressure and rapid heart rate. Aspirin, especially at high doses, can induce or exacerbate asthma by inhibiting bronchodilatory prostaglandins (PGE_2 and PGI_2), and can exacerbate dyspnea in patients with chronic obstructive pulmonary disease. Aspirin is contraindicated in patients who have a history of allergy, especially anaphylaxis to NSAIDs. Patients with rhinorrhea, nasal polyps, and aspirin- or NSAID-induced dyspnea are at greatest risk of aspirin- or NSAID-induced anaphylaxis. Aspirin should not be administered to children or teenagers with viral infections, because of the risk of Reye's syndrome.

An important drug-drug interaction between ibuprofen and aspirin has been identified. Ibuprofen interferes with aspirin access to the platelet serine-binding site, and inhibits the pharmacologic effect of aspirin. This drug interaction occurs during single ingestion when ibuprofen is administered before aspirin, or with chronic use of ibuprofen and aspirin irrespective of whether ibuprofen is administered before or after aspirin. Diclofenac (Voltaren), celecoxib (Celebrex), and rofecoxib (Vioxx) do not seem to interact with aspirin; other NSAIDs have not been studied. The combination of aspirin and NSAIDs may lead to a high risk of life-threatening gastropathy, especially in the elderly population or among patients using concomitant antithrombotic agents. Aspirin and NSAIDs inhibit gastrointestinal vasodilatory prostaglandins (PGE_2 and PGI_2), increasing the accumulation of aggressive factors (acid) and decreasing the supply of defensive factors (sodium bicarbonate). Such patients should be immediately placed on gastropathy prophylaxis with proton pump inhibitors (omeprazole) or misoprostol (Cytotec).

Dipyridamole

Dipyridamole is a vasodilator and platelet adhesion inhibitor. It has been postulated that patients with prosthetic heart valves have abnormally shortened platelet survival time. Dipyridamole lengthens the abnormally shortened platelet survival time in a dose-dependent manner. The primary effect of dipyridamole is to inhibit cyclic guanosine 3',5'-monophosphate (cGMP)-specific phosphodiesterase, increasing cGMP levels and augmenting the effects of nitric oxide. Dipyridamole weakly inhibits red blood cell, endothelial cell, and platelet uptake of the platelet activity inhibitor adenosine, and inhibits the formation of thromboxane A_2; this effect occurs in a dose-dependent manner (0.5-1.9 µg/ml). This uptake inhibition results in dipyridamole inhibiting platelet function by inhibiting cyclic adenosine 3',5'-monophosphate (cAMP)-specific phosphodiesterase, which leads to increased cellular concentrations of cAMP within platelets, in turn preventing platelet aggregation by stimuli such as collagen and adenosine diphosphate. Dipyridamole does not alter prothrombin time levels, but can increase the platelet bleeding time.

Dipyridamole (Persantine) is only indicated as an adjunct to warfarin in the prevention of postoperative thromboembolic complications of cardiac valve replacement. Intravenous dipyridamole, occasionally used for cardiac exercise stress testing, may decrease blood pressure, and increase heart rate and cardiac output; this effect is generally not seen with the oral dosage form. Dipyridamole is eliminated via hepatic conjugation and glucuronidation; hence it does not undergo hepatic cytochrome P450 elimination. Dipyridamole has a weak metabolite and undergoes negligible renal elimination. The half-life of dipyridamole is 13 hours. Adverse reactions to dipyridamole are transient and include headache, dizziness, hypotension, and abdominal distress. Rarely, dipyridamole has aggravated angina symptoms; the intravenous form has precipitated acute myocardial ischemia. Dipyridamole can potentiate the effects of intravenous adenosine, causing fatal asystole or sustained ventricular tachycardia; a decreased dose of adenosine should be used when treating paroxysmal supraventricular tachycardias.

Aggrenox is a combination gelatin capsule containing 200 mg of extended-release dipyridamole with 25 mg of aspirin and is indicated to reduce the risk of stroke for patients who have had transient ischemic attacks or completed ischemic strokes. The steady state dipyridamole peak and trough plasma levels are 2 and 0.5 µg/ml, respectively, allowing for dipyridamole to achieve its effects on cAMP and cGMP throughout the dosing interval; this is not likely to occur with prompt-release dipyridamole. Dipyridamole requires an acidic environment for gut absorption; the Aggrenox product contains tartaric acid, allowing for maximal bioavailability in patients who have gut hypochlorhydria or achlorhydria (e.g., the elderly). The second European Stroke Prevention Study (ESPS-2) has shown that dipyridamole modified-release formulation, 200 mg given twice daily, is effective in the secondary prevention of stroke and transient ischemic attack compared with placebo and that coadministration with aspirin, 25 mg twice daily, provides additional benefit.[19] ESPS-2 showed that the relative risk reduction for stroke with aspirin administration was 18.1% ($P=0.013$); for modified-release dipyridamole, the relative risk reduction was 16.3% ($P=0.039$); and with the combination, it was 37% ($P<0.001$), when compared with placebo. Aggrenox must not be substituted by prompt-release dipyridamole and aspirin.

Clopidogrel

Clopidogrel (Plavix) is a prodrug thienopyridine derivative platelet aggregation inhibitor that interferes with platelet membrane function by inhibiting adenosine

TABLE 20-13

Characteristics of Glycoprotein IIb/IIIa Inhibitors

	Abciximab (ReoPro)	Tirofiban (Aggrastat)	Eptifibatide (Integrilin)
Common uses	Adjunct to PCI	Management of ACS, medically or with PCI	Management of ACS, medically or with PCI; adjunct to PCI
Pharmacology	Chimeric human–murine monoclonal antibody Fab fragment GP IIb/IIIa inhibitor	Non-peptide GP IIb/IIIa inhibitor	Cyclic heptapeptide GP IIb/IIIa inhibitor
Origin	Antibodies from immunized mice	Chemically derived	Active component of snake venom peptides
Binding to platelets	Irreversible	Reversible	Reversible
Elimination half-life	30 min	2 hr	2.5 hr
Platelet function recovery	~48 hr	~4 hr	~4 hr
Elimination	Renal, lymphatic system	65% renal, 25% biliary	50% renal, 30% metabolized in plasma into amino acids

ACS, Acute coronary syndrome; *GP*, glycoprotein; *PCI*, percutaneous coronary intervention.

TABLE 20-14

Pharmacologic Properties of Thrombolytic Agents

	Streptokinase	Alteplase (rtPA)	Reteplase (rPA)	Tenecteplase (TNK-tPA)
Brand name	Streptase	Activase	Retavase	TNKase
Source	Streptococcal culture	Recombinant DNA technology using heterologous mammalian tissue culture	Recombinant DNA technology using *Escherichia coli*	Recombinant DNA technology using Chinese hamster ovary cells
Common uses	Pulmonary embolism, deep vein thrombosis, peripheral arterial occlusion, clearance of occluded central venous access devices, ST segment elevation	Pulmonary embolism, stroke, clearance of occluded central venous access device, ST segment elevation	Infarction, myocaradial, ST segment elevation	Infarction, myocaradial, ST segment elevation
Type of agent	Bacterial proactivator	Tissue plasminogen activator	Tissue plasminogen activator	Tissue plasminogen activator
Plasma half-life (min)	12-18	2-6	13-16	90-130
Fibrinolytic activation	Systemic	Systemic	Systemic	Systemic
Antigenic	Yes	No	No	No
Fibrin specific	+	+++	++	++++
Systemic bleeding risk	+++	++	++	+
ICH risk	+	++	++	++

ICH, Intracranial hemorrhage; *rPA*, recombinant plasminogen activator; *rrPA*, recombinant tissue-type plasminogen activator; *TNK*, tenecteplase; *tPA*, tissue-type plasminogen activator.

of stroke within the last 3 months, active internal bleeding, suspected aortic dissection, closed head or facial trauma within 3 months, uncontrolled blood pressure, and current use of anticoagulants.

The most common adverse effect associated with these agents is major and minor bleeding. Sites of major bleeding include gastrointestinal, genitourinary, respiratory tract, retroperitoneal, and intracranial hemorrhage.

Minor bleeding often manifests as superficial or surface bleeding as a result of arterial punctures and surgical intervention. Thrombolytic-induced hemorrhagic stroke in those greater than 75 years of age occurs more often with alteplase than streptokinase. Patients greater than 75 years of age should receive streptokinase rather than alteplase. Alteplase and tenecteplase are known to be fibrin specific because they promote the conversion of plasminogen into plasmin in the presence of clot-bound fibrin only, with limited systemic proteolysis. The increased fibrin specificity is believed to induce less extensive systemic depletion of clotting factors such as fibrinogen and plasminogen. The clinical relevance of thrombolytic fibrin specificity has not been elucidated. The thrombolytics have rarely been associated with cholesterol embolization manifesting as purple toe syndrome, livedo reticularis, acute renal failure, gangrene, MI, bowel infarction, stroke, and rhabdomyolysis. When thrombolytics are used for ACS they can cause reperfusion arrhythmias manifesting as bradycardia or ventricular tachyarrhythmias. The pharmacological properties of the thrombolytic agents are depicted in Table 20-14.[25]

SELF-ASSESSMENT QUESTIONS

1. List the adverse effects associated with angiotensin-converting enzyme inhibitors (ACEIs).
2. Which of the β blockers possess intrinsic sympathomimetic activity (ISA)?
3. Which of the β blockers possess selective β₁-blocker activity?
4. List the adverse effects associated with α₁-adrenergic antagonists.
5. What are the most common side effects of nitrates?
6. List the metabolic effects associated with thiazide diuretics.
7. List five medications that may cause drug-induced increases in blood pressure.
8. Which calcium channel blocker is most likely to cause constipation?
9. What is the best parameter available to monitor the effects of warfarin?
10. What is the antidote for heparin?
11. What is the mechanism of action of warfarin?
12. Name the pharmacological class responsible for inhibiting the final pathway in platelet aggregation.
13. Which thrombolytic is recommended for patients greater than 75 years of age who present with ST segment elevation myocardial infarction?
14. Name the only ACEI that is available in a parenteral dosage form.
15. What is the best parameter available to monitor the effects of heparin?
16. Is clopidogrel or ticlopidine superior to aspirin for stroke prevention?

Answers to Self-Assessment Questions are found in Appendix A.

CLINICAL SCENARIO

A 75-year-old male presents to the emergency department complaining of chest pain of 1 hour in duration. He has had intermittent chest pain for the past week. He describes experiencing substernal pain that radiates down his left arm. The pain is associated with diaphoresis and is not relieved by change in body position. He has had a history of hypertension for the past 10 years. He has no history or family history for coronary artery disease. He is currently taking labetalol, 200 mg twice daily, and an enteric-coated aspirin, 81 mg daily. He has no known allergies.

On physical examination, he appears anxious and is complaining of chest pain. His vital signs are as follows: blood pressure (BP), 140/70 mmHg; pulse (P), 74 beats/min; and respiratory rate (RR), 20 breaths/min. His heart sounds are normal, with no murmurs or gallops present. His lungs are clear on auscultation, and his abdomen, extremities, and funduscopic examination are unremarkable. His skin is cool and clammy.

Electrocardiography displays evidence of sinus bradycardia with a heart rate of 49 beats/min. His cardiac enzymes all were elevated (creatine kinase [CK], 200 U/L; CK-MB [CK isoenzymes found in muscle and brain fractions], 20 U/L; and troponin I, 2 mcg/ml).

In summary, this 75-year-old male, based on his history, physical examination, and ECG, is diagnosed with a non-ST segment elevation myocardial infarction (MI).

Is this patient a candidate for immediate administration of a glycoprotein IIb/IIIa inhibitor?

Is this patient a candidate for immediate administration of thrombolytic therapy?

Answers to Clinical Scenario Questions are found in Appendix A.

References

1. Vasan RS, Beiser A, Seshadri S, Larson MG, Kannel WB, D'Agostino RB, Levy D: Residual lifetime risk for developing hypertension in middle-aged women and men: the Framingham Heart Study, *JAMA* 287:1003, 2002.
2. Chobanian AV, Bakris GL, Black HR, Cushman WC, Green LA, Izzo JL Jr, Jones DW, Materson BJ, Oparil S, Wright JT Jr, *et al.*; Joint National Committee on Prevention, Detection, Evaluation, and Treatment of High Blood Pressure National Heart, Lung, and Blood Institute, National High Blood Pressure Education Program Coordinating Committee: Seventh Report of the Joint Committee on detection, evaluation and treatment of high blood pressure [JNC-VII], *Hypertension* 42:1206, 2003.

3. Joint National Committee on Prevention, Detection, Evaluation, and Treatment of High Blood Pressure: The Sixth Report of the Joint Committee on detection, evaluation and treatment of high blood pressure [JNC-VI], *Arch Intern Med* 157:2413, 1997.

4. *Drugs facts and comparisons*, St. Louis, Mo, 2000, Facts and Comparisons, Wolters Kluwer Health.

5. Oates J: Antihypertensive agents and the drug therapy of hypertension, In Hardman J, Limbrid L, editors: *Goodman & Gilman's the pharmacological basis of therapeutics*, ed 9, New York, 1995, McGraw-Hill.

6. Weir M: When antihypertensive monotherapy fails: fixed-dose combination therapy, *South Med J* 93:548, 2000.

7. Psaty BM, Smith NL, Siscovick DS, Koepsell TD, Weiss NS, Heckbert SR, Lemaitre RN, Wagner EH, Furberg CD: Health outcomes associated with antihypertensive therapies used as first-line agents, *JAMA* 277:739, 1997.

8. Weber M, Messerli F, Bruner H: Angiotensin II receptor inhibition, *Arch Intern Med* 156:1957, 1996.

9. Grossman E, Messerli FH, Grodzicki T, Kowey P: Should a moratorium be placed on sublingual nifedipine capsules given for hypertensive emergencies and pseudoemergencies, *JAMA* 276:1328, 1996.

10. Veelken R, Schimieder R: Overview of α_1-adrenegic antagonism and recent advances in hypertensive therapy, *Am J Hypertens* 9:139S, 1996.

11. Furberg C, Wright J, Davis B, Cutler J, Alderman M, Black H, Cushman W, Francis C, Grimm R, Haywood L, *et al.*; ALLHAT Officers and Coordinators for the ALLHAT Collaborative Research Group: Major cardiovascular events in hypertensive patients randomized to doxazosin vs chlorthalidone: the Antihypertensive and Lipid Lowering Treatment to Prevent Heart Attack Trial (ALLHAT), *JAMA* 283:1967, 2000.

12. Chaitman BR, Pepine CJ, Parker JO, Skopal J, Chumakova G, Kuch J, Wang W, Skettino SL, Wolff AA; Combination Assessment of Ranolazine In Stable Angina (CARISA) Investigators: Effects of ranolazine with atenolol, amlodipine, or diltiazem on exercise tolerance and angina frequency in patients with severe chronic angina: a randomized controlled trial, *JAMA* 291:309, 2004.

13. Thandani U: Treatment of stable angina, *Curr Opin Cardiol* 14:349, 1999.

14. Williams G: Hypertensive vascular disease. In Fauci AS, Braunwald E, Isselbacher KJ, Wilson JD, Martin JB, Kasper D, Hauser SL, Longo DL, editors: *Harrison's principles of internal medicine*, ed 14, New York, 1998, McGraw-Hill.

15. Mathis AS: Newer antithrombotic strategies in the initial management of non-ST-segment elevation acute coronary syndromes, *Ann Pharmacother* 34:208, 2000.

16. Heesen M, Winking M, Kemkes-Matthes B, Deinsberger W, Dietrich GV, Matthes KJ, Hempelmann G: What the neurosurgeon needs to know about the coagulation system, *Surg Neurol* 47:32, 1997.

17. Hirsh J, Raschke R: Heparin and low-molecular-weight heparin: the Seventh ACCP Conference on Antithrombotic and Thrombolytic Therapy, *Chest* 126:188S, 2004.

18. Ansell J, Hirsh J, Poller L, Bussey H, Jacobson A, Hylek E: The pharmacology and management of the vitamin K antagonists: the Seventh ACCP Conference on Antithrombotic and Thrombolytic Therapy, *Chest* 126:204S, 2004.

19. Diener HC, Cunha L, Forbes C, Sivenius J, Smets P, Lowenthal A: European Stroke Prevention Study. 2. Dipyridamole and acetylsalicylic acid in the secondary prevention of stroke, *J Neurol Sci* 143:1, 1996.

20. CAPRIE Steering Committee: A randomized, blinded, trial of clopidogrel versus aspirin in patients at risk of ischaemic events (CAPRIE), *Lancet* 348:1329, 1996.

21. Gent M, Blakely JA, Easton JD, Ellis DJ, Hachinski VC, Harbison JW, Panak E, Roberts RS, Sicurella J, Turpie AG: The Canadian-American Ticlopidine Study (CATS) in thromboembolic stroke, *Lancet* 1:1215, 1989.

22. Hass WK, Easton JD, Adams HP Jr, Pryse-Phillips W, Molony BA, Anderson S, Kamm B: A randomized trial comparing ticlopidine hydrochloride with aspirin for the prevention of stroke in high-risk patients (TASS), *N Engl J Med* 321:501, 1989.

23. Latour-Perez J: Risk and benefits of glycoprotein IIb/IIIa antagonists in acute coronary syndrome, *Ann Pharmacother* 35:472, 2001.

24. Albers GW, Amarenco P, Easton JD, Sacco RL, Teal P: Antithrombotic and thrombolytic therapy for ischemic stroke, *Chest* 119:300S, 2001.

25. Ohman EM, Harrington RA, Cannon CP, Agnelli G, Cairns JA, Kennedy JW: Intravenous thrombolysis in acute MI, *Chest* 119:253S, 2001.

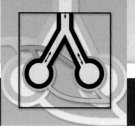

Chapter 21

Diuretic Agents

RUBEN D. RESTREPO, LORENA M. FERNANDEZ-RESTREPO

CHAPTER OUTLINE

CHAPTER OBJECTIVES

After reading this chapter, the reader will be able to:

1. Define *diuretics*
2. Describe renal function, filtration, reabsorption, and acid–base balance
3. List and describe the various groups of diuretics
4. List some of the indications for diuretic therapy
5. List the most common adverse reactions associated with the use of diuretics
6. Describe special situations related to diuretic therapy

KEY TERMS AND DEFINITIONS

Congestive heart failure (CHF) — Failure of the heart to pump the blood adequately, resulting in lung congestion and tissular edema

Diuretic — A drug that increases urine output

Edema — Swelling due to an abnormal accumulation of fluid in intercellular spaces of the body

Glomerular filtration — Mechanism by which hydrostatic pressure forces fluid out of the glomerular capillaries and into the renal ducts

Hypovolemia — Abnormally decreased volume of blood circulating in the body

Nephrocalcinosis — Renal lithiasis in which calcium deposits form in the renal parenchyma, resulting in reduced kidney function and the presence of blood in the urine

Nephron — The microscopic functional unit of the kidney, responsible for filtering and maintaining fluid balance. Each kidney has approximately 2 million nephrons

Ototoxicity — Damage to the ear, specifically the cochlea or auditory nerve and sometimes the vestibulum, by a toxin

Reabsorption — The return to the blood of most of the water, sodium, amino acids, and sugar that were removed during filtration; occurs mainly in the proximal tubule of the nephron

Synergistic effect — When the effect of two chemicals on an organism is greater than the effect of either chemical individually

Urine output — Amount of urine produced in 24 hours. Normal urine output averages 30 to 60 ml/hr

KEY POINT

Diuretics increase urine output.

KEY POINT

The kidney is a highly specialized organ responsible for maintaining homeostasis between the internal volume and electrolyte status.

The main purpose of **diuretics**, or agents that increase **urine output**, is to eliminate excess fluid from the body. Diuretics were introduced into medicine in 1958. They are drugs that increase the excretion of solutes and water by directly increasing urine output. The preceding definition excludes agents, such as digitalis, that promote urine output without a *direct* action on the kidney. In general, the primary goal of diuretic therapy is to reduce extracellular fluid volume in order to lower blood pressure or to rid the body of excess interstitial fluid. The following is a summary of the essentials of the clinical pharmacology of diuretics that briefly reviews renal function with an emphasis on acid–base balance. The major groups of diuretics, their modes of action, and common interactions and side effects are each summarized. These groups include osmotic diuretics, carbonic anhydrase inhibitors, thiazides, loop diuretics, and potassium-sparing agents.

RENAL STRUCTURE AND FUNCTION

The kidneys are paired retroperitoneal organs found on either side of the spinal cord at the level of the umbilicus. In the adult, each kidney weighs approximately 160 to 175 g and is 10 to 12 cm long. The renal artery provides perfusion to the kidneys. Kidneys receive the highest blood flow per gram of organ weight in the body. Approximately 22% of the cardiac output, or about 1.1 liters/min in a normal 70-kg adult, flows through the kidneys. Like the heart and brain, the kidney is an active organ (not a passive filter) with high oxygen consumption. For this reason, impaired circulation can cause renal failure or damage.

Figure 21-1 illustrates the kidney and a **nephron**, which like the alveolus in the lung, is the functional unit of the kidney. The nephron is composed of the glomerulus, proximal tubule, loop of Henle, distal tubule, and collecting duct. Although each kidney contains as many as a million nephrons, 75% of them may be compromised before renal disease is apparent.

The renal artery branches into the afferent arteriole, which enters and forms the capillary tuft of the glomerulus. This blood flow then leaves in the efferent arteriole, which then forms the capillary network around the tubules and loop of Henle. This capillary network rejoins to form the renal vein.

The glomerulus is supported and surrounded by an epithelial-lined capsule named Bowman's capsule. The glomerular capsule is actually the beginning of the proximal tubule, and filtration of fluid from the blood to the tubule occurs in the glomerulus. This fluid is the glomerular filtrate, which empties into the proximal tubule, goes through the descending and ascending loops of Henle, into the distal tubule, and later into the collecting duct. Each of

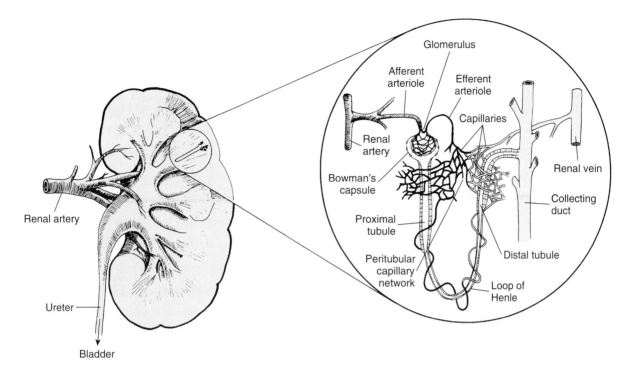

FIGURE 21-1 Basic structure of the kidney, with a detailed view of the nephron.

the nearly 250 collecting ducts collects urine from about 4000 nephrons. The collecting ducts merge to form larger ducts that eventually empty into the renal papillae, and finally empty into the ureter to be stored in the bladder.

The principal function of the nephron is to maintain homeostasis or equilibrium between the internal volume and electrolyte status and that of the environment's influences, diet and intake. This mission is accomplished by almost 2 million nephrons through the processes of glomerular ultrafiltration, tubular reabsorption, and tubular secretion. The kidney cannot regenerate new nephrons. Therefore, renal injury, disease, and aging are associated with a gradual decrease in nephron number. The body maintains blood pressure at the expense of extracellular fluid volume (ECFV). Its control is achieved by adjusting sodium chloride (NaCl) and water (H_2O) excretion.

Glomerular Filtration

Beginning in the glomerulus, the nephron forms a cell-free ultrafiltrate, with a relatively small amount of protein, which has the same ionic concentration (Na^+, Cl^-, HCO_3^-, etc.) as plasma. Twenty percent of the total blood flow that goes through the nephron, or about 130 ml/min, is filtered through the glomerulus. More than 99% of this **glomerular filtrate** is reabsorbed in the tubules, and less than 1% of the fluid is excreted as urine.

KEY POINT

Urine output less than 0.5 to 1 ml/min or less than 30 to 60 ml/hr is known as *oliguria*. The presence of oliguria and *anuria* (no urine output) are commonly associated with renal failure of any etiology. Greater than normal urine output is known as *polyuria*.

Therefore, the total urine output for an adult is approximately 0.5 to 1 ml/min or about 30 to 60 ml/hour. Because diuretics interfere with the **reabsorption** of water in the tubules of the nephron, they increase the urine output.

Electrolyte Filtration and Reabsorption

The ions listed in Box 21-1 are filtered and exchanged in the tubules.

Sodium: About 70% of the sodium in the filtrate is reabsorbed in the proximal tubules, 20% in the loops of Henle, and about 10% in the distal tubules. There is an exchange of Na^+ for H^+ or K^+ in the distal tubules.

Potassium: Most filtered K^+ is reabsorbed in the proximal tubules. The K^+ found in the urine is that secreted by the distal tubule.

Chloride and bicarbonate: These are passively reabsorbed in the proximal and distal tubules.

Box 21-1	Common Electrolytes

- Sodium (Na^+)
- Potassium (K^+)
- Chloride (Cl^-)
- Bicarbonate (HCO_3^-)
- Hydrogen (H^+)
- Calcium (Ca^{2+})
- Magnesium (Mg^{2+})

Water is also passively reabsorbed or excreted, depending on the concentration of electrolyte, primarily Na^+, in the filtrate. By inhibiting sodium reabsorption, diuretics cause less water to be retained and more is excreted in the filtrate.

Aldosterone, a mineralocorticoid secreted by the adrenal cortex, increases sodium and water reabsorption in the distal tubule. A diuretic such as spironolactone can increase sodium and water loss by inhibiting aldosterone.

Acid–Base Balance

Because a fundamental function of the kidney is the control of buffering substances, especially HCO_3^-, diuretics may cause acid–base imbalances to occur as they increase water loss. Figure 21-2 illustrates the hydrogen and bicarbonate pathways that regulate pH. The filtration and reabsorption of Na^+, Cl^-, and HCO_3^-, described previously, can be seen in Figure 21-2.

The important exchange for acid–base balance is that of Na^+. Sodium is reabsorbed in the tubules by several means, as follows:

- Reabsorption with *chloride* to preserve electrical neutrality
- Exchange of Na^+ for H^+ or K^+, again preserving neutrality

Either *low chloride* (hypochloremia) or *low potassium* (hypokalemia) will force Na^+ to exchange for H^+, producing a loss of H^+ and metabolic alkalosis:

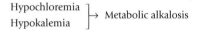

$$\left.\begin{array}{c}\text{Hypochloremia}\\\text{Hypokalemia}\end{array}\right\} \rightarrow \text{Metabolic alkalosis}$$

Finally, preventing the HCO_3^- in the *filtrate* from forming CO_2 and water will lead to a loss of bicarbonate buffer in the urine and metabolic acidosis.

DIURETIC GROUPS

The primary therapeutic goal of diuretic use is to reduce the ECFV. Therefore, NaCl output *must* exceed NaCl intake. Diuretics primarily prevent Na^+ entry into the tubule cell. Diuretics need to access the tubule fluid to

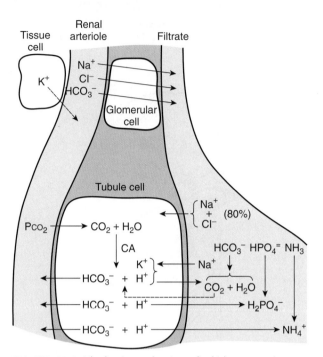

FIGURE 21-2 The basic mechanisms for kidney retention of bicarbonate with hydrogen ion buffering. Sodium exchange with chloride and for hydrogen is also indicated. *CA*, Carbonic anhydrase.

KEY POINT

Diuretic agents are important in reducing the morbidity and mortality of cardiovascular patients with fluid retention.

exert their action. Once in the tubule fluid, the nephron site at which the diuretic acts determines its effect. In addition, the site of action also determines which electrolytes, other than Na^+, will be affected. All diuretics except spironolactone exert their effects from the lumenal side of the nephron.[1]

There are five major groups of diuretics described in this chapter. Figure 21-3 illustrates the site of action, and Table 21-1 summarizes the mechanism of action, and the indications for use of each of the five major groups of diuretics.[2-5]

Because hypertension affects one-third of adults in the United States,[6] the diuretics of most immediate relevance to respiratory and critical care clinicians are those used to treat hypertension and **congestive heart failure** (**CHF**). There is evidence that diuretic-based therapy is effective in reducing morbidity and mortality among elderly hypertensive patients.[7-10] Diuretics are also used to aid in the treatment of other conditions associated

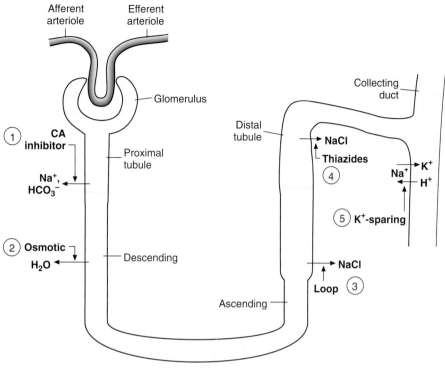

FIGURE 21-3 Illustration of the nephron, from glomerulus to collecting duct, showing the various sites of action for the diuretic groups. *CA,* Carbonic anhydrase. *1-5,* points at which the five major groups of diuretics exert their effects.

with fluid retention such as corticosteroid therapy, and certain renal and liver diseases.

Osmotic Diuretics

KEY POINT

Osmotic diuretics are often used in the management of head trauma with cerebral edema.

Osmotic diuretics (Table 21-2) are freely filtered at the glomerulus but are not reabsorbed. These agents remain in the tubule lumen and impair the ability of the proximal tubule and thick ascending limb of Henle to reabsorb NaCl. The net result is that osmotic substances are potent diuretics that lead to increased excretion of water and NaCl. However, the resultant increased delivery of sodium and chloride to the distal tubule results in increased exchange of Na^+ for K^+, producing a net potassium loss in urine.

Of the four currently available osmotic diuretics (glycerin, isosorbide, mannitol, and urea), mannitol is

the typically selected agent because of its lower toxicity. Mannitol has a relatively short half-life and therefore manifests with a rapid onset and quick offset of action. To maintain a continued diuretic action, the drug is frequently administered via continuous infusion. Osmotic diuretics are often used in the management of cerebral **edema**.

Carbonic Anhydrase Inhibitors

KEY POINT

Although carbonic anhydrase inhibitors (CAIs) are considered very weak diuretics, they are commonly used in glaucoma, metabolic alkalosis, and altitude sickness.

The primary site of action of carbonic anhydrase inhibitors (CAIs) is within the proximal tubule. Carbonic anhydrases are enzymes that catalyze the hydration of carbon dioxide and the dehydration of bicarbonate: $CO_2 + H_2O \leftrightarrow HCO_3^- + H^+$. CAIs prevent the normal breakdown of carbonic acid and, therefore, decrease bicarbonate reabsorption. The CAIs also inhibit NaCl reabsorption at the proximal tubule. The decreased osmotic gradient for water reabsorption results in increased delivery of

TABLE 21-1		
Diuretics: Site and Mechanism of Action, Main Indications, and Other Uses		
Diuretic Class (Mechanism of Action)	**Main Indications**	**Other Uses**
Osmotic Diuretics		
Freely filtered, nonreabsorbable osmotic agents such as mannitol, glycerol, and urea: Reduction of the reabsorption of H_2O and solutes, including NaCl, primarily in the proximal tubule and descending loop of Henle	To treat or prevent acute renal failure (ARF)	To reduce intracranial or intraocular pressure
Carbonic Anhydrase Inhibitors		
Acetazolamide, methazolamide, and dichlorphenamide: Inhibition of CA in lumenal membrane of proximal tubule, reducing proximal sodium and bicarbonate reabsorption	To reduce intraocular pressure in glaucoma; to lower $[HCO_3^-]_p$ in "mountain sickness"; to raise urine pH in cystinuria	Periodic paralysis; adjunctive therapy in epilepsy
Loop Diuretics		
Furosemide, bumetanide, torsemide, and ethacrynic acid: Inhibition of $Na^+/K^+/Cl^-$ reabsorption in the thick ascending limb of Henle	Hypertension, congestive heart failure (CHF) (in the presence of renal insufficiency or for immediate effect); ARF; chronic renal failure (CRF), ascites, and nephrotic syndrome	Acute pulmonary edema; to enhance urinary excretion of chemical toxins; hypercalcemia
Thiazide Diuretics		
Chlorothiazide, hydrochlorothiazide, etc.: Inhibition of NaCl reabsorption in early distal tubule (DT)	Hypertension; CHF; idiopathic hypercalciuria (renal calculi)	Nephrogenic diabetes insipidus (prevent further urine dilution from taking place in the DT); CRF
K⁺-Sparing Diuretics		
Spironolactone: Competitively blocks the actions of aldosterone on the cortical collecting ducts (CCDs) Amiloride and triamterene: Inhibition of the Na/K pump by reducing Na entry across the lumenal membrane of the CCDs	Chronic liver disease: To treat secondary hyperaldosteronism due to hepatic cirrhosis complicated by ascites CHF: To counteract the hypokalemic effect of other diuretics	Primary hyperaldosteronism (Conn's syndrome)

$[HCO_3^-]_p$, Plasma bicarbonate concentration.

$NaHCO_3$, NaCl, and water from the proximal tubule. (Figure 21-4). However, much of the NaCl will be reabsorbed in the thick ascending loop of Henle. The net result is a moderate increase in sodium and bicarbonate in the urine along with increased water excretion.

The potential for metabolic acidosis coupled with their weak diuretic properties limit the use of CAIs as the first-line treatment for patients who require more aggressive management of their hypervolemic status.

Other, more common uses of CAIs include the treatment of glaucoma, metabolic alkalosis, and altitude sickness. CA is an important enzyme in the formation of intraocular fluid. Therefore CAIs effectively decrease intraocular pressure and are used to treat glaucoma. Short-term CAIs may also correct metabolic alkalosis, as a result of the acidosis they produce. Finally, CAIs have been shown to be useful against altitude sickness, although the exact mechanism of action is not known. The most common adverse effect of CAIs is hypokalemia resulting from the increased amount of sodium presented to the collecting duct, which is then reabsorbed in exchange for potassium excretion.

Loop Diuretics

KEY POINT

Loop diuretics produce a hemodynamic effect characterized by acute vasodilation and manifested by a decrease in pulmonary capillary wedge pressure, blood pressure, and systemic vascular resistance.

TABLE 21-2

Characteristics of Diuretics

Drug	Route	Onset (min)*	Peak (hr)	Duration (hr)	Half-life (hr)	Oral Bio-availability (%)	Typical Dose
Osmotic							
Glycerin	PO	10-30	1-1.5	4-5	0.5-0.75	N/D	1-2 g/kg
Isosorbide	PO	10-30	1-1.5	5-6	5-9.5	N/D	1-3 g/kg
Mannitol	IV	30-60	1	6-8	0.25-1.5	N/A	50-100 g
Urea	IV	30-45	1	5-6	N/A	N/A	1-1.5 g/kg
Thiazide							
Bendroflumethiazide	PO	120	4	12-16	3-4	100	5 mg
Benzthiazide	PO	120	4-6	16-18	N/D	N/D	50-100 mg/day
Chlorothiazide	PO	120	4	12-16	0.75-2	10-21	0.5-2.0 g/day
	IV	15	0.5	12-16	0.75-2	10-21	0.5-2.0 g/day
Chlorthalidone	PO	120-180	2-6	24-72	40	64	50-100 mg/day
Hydrochlorothiazide	PO	120	4-6	12-16	50.6-14.8	65-75	50-200 mg/day
Hydroflumethiazide	PO	120	4	12-16	17	50	25-200 mg/day
Indapamide	PO	60-120	<2	36	14	93	1.25-5 mg/day
Methylclothiazide	PO	120	6	24	N/D	N/D	5 mg
Metolazone	PO	60	2	12-24	N/D	65	5-20 mg/day
Polythiazide	PO	120	6	24-48	25-37	N/D	2-4 mg/day
Quinethazone	PO	120	6	18-24	N/D	N/D	50-100 mg/day
Trichlormethiazide	PO	120	6	24	2.3-7.3	N/D	2-4 mg/day
Loop							
Bumetanide	PO	30-60	1-2	4-6	1-1.5	72-96	0.5-2.0 mg
	IV	5	0.25-0.5	0.5-1	1-1.5	72-96	0.5-2.0 mg
Ethacrynic acid	PO	30	2	6-8	1	100	50-100 mg
	IV	5	0.25-0.5	2	1	100	50-100 mg
Furosemide	PO	60	1-2	6-8	2	60-64	20-80 mg
	IV	5	0.5	2	2	60-64	20-80 mg
Torsemide	PO	60	1-2	6-8	3.5	80	5-20 mg
	IV	10	<1	6-8	3.5	80	5-20 mg
Potassium Sparing							
Amiloride	PO	2 hr	6-10	24	6-9	30-90	5-20 mg/day
Spironolactone	PO	24-48 hr	48-72	48-72	20	73	25-400 mg/day
Triamterene	PO	2-4 hr	6-8	12-16	3	30-70	200-300 mg/day

IV, Intravenous; *N/A*, not applicable; *N/D*, no data; *PO*, oral.
*Unless otherwise indicated.

Loop diuretics (see Table 21-2) are often called "high ceiling" diuretics because they can cause up to 20% of the filtered load of sodium chloride and water to be excreted in the urine. They inhibit the reabsorption of NaCl at the thick ascending limb of Henle, where about 20% of filtered NaCl is usually reabsorbed.[11] They lead to increased Na^+, K^+, Cl^-, and water excretion.

When administered intravenously, loop diuretics produce an acute hemodynamic effect independent of their diuretic properties.[12] Within 5 minutes of the administration of intravenous loop diuretics to cardiac patients, an acute vasodilatory effect is observed. This effect is manifested by a decrease in pulmonary capillary wedge pressure, blood pressure, and systemic vascular resistance. The effect seems to be derived from the renal release of vasodilating prostaglandins.[13,14]

Because the diuretic effect of intravenous loop diuretics is typically not seen for 15 to 20 minutes after administration, patients with acute pulmonary edema may derive a clinical benefit from intravenous loop diuretics before the onset of diuresis. The hemodynamic effect is short lived, with all measurements returning to baseline once diuresis has begun. The acute hemodynamic effect

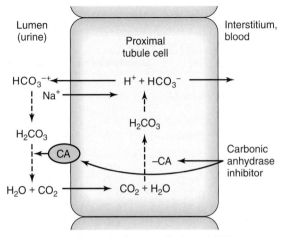

Lumen
(urine)

Proximal
tubule cell

Interstitium,
blood

FIGURE 21-4 Effect of carbonic anhydrase inhibitor diuretics, such as acetazolamide, which block the availability of hydrogen to exchange for sodium in the proximal tubule, causing a loss of sodium, bicarbonate, and water, along with reduced bicarbonate reabsorption into the cell and the blood. *CA,* Carbonic anhydrase.

has also been reported to activate the sympathetic nervous system, resulting in an adverse hemodynamic profile characterized by increased afterload and diminished cardiac function before the onset of diuresis.[15] This effect is also short lived and dissipates with the onset of diuresis. Because the diuretic effect may last several hours, several doses per day may be required to maintain a net diuretic effect for 24 hours. Patients requiring frequent bolus doses may benefit from continuous infusion.

Administration of loop diuretics to patients with renal dysfunction results in less total drug reaching the site of action within the nephron; therefore the administration of larger doses is required to achieve a therapeutic effect.[16-18] In these patients, differences exist among the effects of furosemide, bumetanide, and torsemide. Furosemide may have a more prolonged effect in patients with renal dysfunction. However, patients may be resistant to furosemide compared with bumetanide. Because loop diuretics are the most potent diuretics, they are effective at very low creatinine clearance levels (a low creatinine clearance level indicates kidney disease). Loop diuretics as single agents should be considered as first-line therapy in patients with creatinine clearance values below 40 ml/min. If this dose is inadequate to produce diuresis within 20 minutes, the dose can be doubled every 20 minutes until a response occurs or until a maximum dose is reached. Various studies have reported a ceiling effect to furosemide of approximately 250 mg.[19,20]

Therefore, increasing the dose above this ceiling dose may not produce an increased response.

Although patients with renal dysfunction require larger doses to deliver diuretics into the urine, the remaining nephrons in these patients continue to function normally. Overall, sodium excretion may be limited as a result of diminished sodium filtration. To overcome this relative resistance, an effective response may occur by administering a large enough effective dose several times a day. Certain disease states result in a diminished response that does not improve by administering larger doses. Although the mechanism for this effect is unknown, it has been reported in patients with congestive heart failure, cirrhosis, or nephrotic syndrome.[21] In these patients, multiple doses should be given rather than larger single doses. This finding implies a modest ceiling dose of loop diuretics in patients with congestive heart failure and cirrhosis.

Thiazide Diuretics

KEY POINT

Thiazide diuretics are considered the first line of therapy for mild hypertension.

Thiazide diuretics (see Table 21-2) block NaCl reabsorption at the distal tubule.[21,22] Thiazide diuretics are of moderate potency because only about 5% to 10% of filtered NaCl is reabsorbed in the distal tubule. However, they are considered the first line of therapy for mild hypertension. Thiazide diuretics are effective to a creatinine clearance of approximately 30 ml/min. Thiazide diuretics have a limited dose–response curve when compared with loop diuretics. This results in a narrow difference between maximal and minimal effective doses. Doses above 50 mg may not produce greater diuresis, but they may predispose the patient to increased toxicity.

Doses above 50 mg may, however, be useful in the treatment of hypertension. The use of thiazide diuretics in the treatment of hypertension produces an effect initially as a result of diuresis-induced decreases in blood volume.[2,21]

Long-term benefits of thiazide diuretics in hypertension are most likely not due to a diuretic response. One proposed mechanism is decreased peripheral vascular resistance.[23] Although the exact mechanism of action is unknown, hypertensive patients may respond to thiazide diuretic doses above 50 mg/day.

Potassium-Sparing Diuretics

The potassium-sparing diuretics include spironolactone, amiloride, and triamterene (see Table 21-2). They are weak diuretics that block sodium reabsorption by slightly different mechanisms of action. Whereas *amiloride* and *triamterene* block the Na^+ channels in the lumenal membrane of the principal cells of the cortical collecting ducts, *spironolactone* is a competitive aldosterone antagonist at the cytosolic receptor level. On the basis of its mechanism of action, spironolactone is specifically used for conditions known to have elevated aldosterone concentrations, such as hyperaldosteronism (primary and secondary), cirrhosis and ascites, adrenal hyperplasia, and renal artery stenosis. The most common use is in patients with cirrhosis and ascites. Because the duration of effect of spironolactone is one or more days, the dose should be increased every 3 or 4 days until the desired level of diuresis is attained.[24]

In the distal tubule, sodium is typically exchanged for potassium and hydrogen. Blocking this exchange is what makes these agents *potassium-sparing diuretics*. Although frequently used in combination with thiazide diuretics to produce better diuresis and to diminish potassium loss, the rationale is controversial. Only about 5% of patients receiving thiazide diuretics become potassium depleted.[21] In addition, the potassium-sparing agents may produce hyperkalemia, which is a more life-threatening situation than potassium depletion.

Triamterene is a short-acting agent requiring multiple doses per day. Triamterene must be converted to an active metabolite by the liver; therefore this agent may be a poor choice in patients with liver dysfunction.[25]

Amiloride has a moderately long half-life and does not require metabolic activation. Coadministration of potassium supplements, angiotensin-converting enzyme inhibitors, and nonsteroidal antiinflammatory agents, along with renal dysfunction may predispose patients receiving potassium-sparing diuretics to develop hyperkalemia.

DIURETIC COMBINATIONS

Various diuretic combinations may be used in an attempt to obtain additive or synergistic effects in patients who respond poorly to one agent. By using agents with different sites of action within the nephron, the diuretic response may be enhanced. The most common combination is of a loop diuretic and a thiazide.[26] Although not consistently effective, combinations occasionally may result in pronounced diuresis.[27]

TABLE 21-3	
Drug Interactions and Their Potential Side Effects Associated With Use of Diuretics	
Interacting Drug	**Potential Side Effect**
Angiotensin-converting enzyme inhibitors **AND** K⁺-sparing diuretics	Hyperkalemia and cardiac irritability
Aminoglycosides **AND** loop diuretics	Ototoxicity and nephrotoxicity
Digoxin **AND** thiazide and loop diuretics	Hypokalemia
β Blockers **AND** thiazide diuretics	Hyperglycemia, hyperlipidemia, hyperuricemia
Steroids **AND** thiazide and loop diuretics	Increased risk of hypokalemia
Carbamazepine or chlorpropamide **AND** thiazide diuretics	Increased risk of hyponatremia

DRUG INTERACTIONS

Because diuretics are commonly prescribed in combination with other medications, a knowledge of drug interaction plays an important role in the selection of the diuretic agent. Clinicians responsible for prescription of diuretics need to be informed of associated comorbidity such as the presence of diabetes, renal disease, hepatic disease, or gout. Table 21-3 summarizes some of the most common drug interaction side effects associated with diuretic agents.

ADVERSE EFFECTS

KEY POINT

Hypovolemia and acid–base abnormalities are the most common side effects of diuretic therapy.

Although diuretics have been used successfully for more than 40 years, they have the potential to cause adverse effects (Table 21-4). Most complications associated with diuretic use can be anticipated as an extension of their pharmacological activity, with *hypovolemia*, and *electrolyte* and *acid–base abnormalities*, being the most common.

Some of the rare side effects that need immediate medical attention include black, tarry stools; blood in the urine or stools; cough or hoarseness; fever or chills; joint pain; lower back or side pain; painful or difficult urination; pinpoint red spots on the skin; ringing

TABLE 21-4

Common Side Effects of Diuretic Therapy

Drug	Effect
Osmotic diuretics	Acute expansion of ECFV and increased risk of pulmonary edema Acute hyperkalemia Nausea and vomiting; headache
Loop diuretics	*Depletions:* Hypokalemia; hypomagnesemia; hyponatremia; hypovolemia *Retention:* Hyperuricemia Metabolic: Hyperglycemia (insulin resistance) Metabolic alkalosis (partly due to ECFV reduction) Ototoxicity and diarrhea (mainly with ethacrynic acid)
Thiazide diuretics	*Depletions:* Hypokalemia, hyponatremia, hypovolemia *Retentions:* Hyperuricemia due to enhanced urate reabsorption; hypercalcemia due to enhanced Ca^{2+} reabsorption Metabolic alkalosis (hypochloremia) Metabolic: Hyperglycemia (insulin resistance), hyperlipidemia Hypersensitivity (fever, rash, purpura, anaphylaxis) Interstitial nephritis
K⁺-sparing diuretics	*Spironolactone:* Hyperkalemia, gynecomastia, hirsutism, menstrual irregularities, testicular atrophy (with prolonged use) *Amiloride:* Hyperkalemia, glucose intolerance in diabetic patients *Triamterene:* Hyperkalemia; megaloblastic anemia in patients with liver cirrhosis
Carbonic anhydrase inhibitors	Metabolic acidosis (due to HCO_3^- depletion) Drowsiness, fatigue, CNS depression, paresthesia

ECFV, Extracellular fluid volume.

Box 21-2 Causes of Volume Depletion With Diuretics

- Initiation of treatment or increased dose
- Improved compliance
- Reduced dietary sodium intake
- Development of diarrhea
- Ingestion of drugs that impair diuretic administration
- Improved underlying disease state not requiring diuretics

Hypovolemia

Because diuretics promote sodium and fluid excretion, elimination may exceed intake, resulting in **hypovolemia**. Hypovolemia should be suspected if dizziness, extreme thirst, excessive dryness of the mouth, decreased urine output, dark-colored urine, or constipation is observed.

Certain situations may predispose a patient to hypovolemia (Box 21-2). Diuretic-induced hypovolemia should be treated by discontinuation of the diuretic. Mild cases of hypovolemia may respond to liberalization of sodium intake, whereas more severe cases will require intravenous volume replacement.

Hypokalemia

Preserving potassium balance has emerged as one of the most important factors in the management of hypertension.[29] Potassium is exchanged for sodium in the distal convoluted tubule and collecting duct. Any diuretic that increases sodium delivery to those regions may potentially induce hypokalemia. In addition to a direct potassium loss, diuretic-induced volume depletion produces reabsorption of sodium via release of aldosterone in the distal tubule in an effort to bolster intravascular volume. This additional sodium reabsorption also contributes to potassium excretion. Dietary sodium intake and chloride depletion may also influence potassium excretion.

Diuretic-induced hypokalemia appears to be dose related, with loop diuretics having a lower incidence than thiazide diuretics.[30] Although studies have tried to identify the incidence of diuretic-induced hypokalemia, it is impossible to predict whether a particular patient will develop hypokalemia.[31-33] The issue of potassium supplementation is also controversial. Who to treat, when to treat, and how to treat hypokalemia are all unresolved questions. At the center of this unresolved issue is whether hypokalemia poses a risk for arrhythmias or sudden cardiac death. Supplemental potassium should be considered in patients with a history of cardiac disease, patients with symptoms indicating hypokalemia,

or buzzing in the ears or any loss of hearing; skin rash or hives; severe stomach pain with nausea and vomiting; unusual bleeding or bruising; yellow eyes or skin, and yellow vision. Other adverse effects are even more rare or idiosyncratic and cannot be anticipated or prevented. There is a particular concern with the suggested association between long-term diuretic therapy and the risk of developing renal cell carcinoma.[28]

TABLE 21-5

Pediatric Dosages of Commonly Prescribed Diuretics

Drug	Age of Patient	Route	Typical Dose
Furosemide	Neonates	PO	1-4 mg/kg/dose, 1-2 times daily
		IV/IM	1-2 mg/kg/dose, q 12-24 hr
	Children	PO/IV/IM	1-2 mg/kg/dose, q 6-12 hr
Bumetanide	<6 mo	PO/IV/IM	N/D
	>6 mo	PO/IV/IM	0.015 mg/kg/dose, qd or qod; maximum, 0.1 mg/kg/dose
Hydrochlorothiazide	<6 mo	PO	2-3.3 mg/kg/day, divided bid
	>6 mo	PO	2 mg/kg/day, divided bid
Chlorthiazide	<6 mo	PO	20-40 mg/kg/day, divided bid
		IV	2-8 mg/kg/day, divided bid
	>6 mo	PO	20 mg/kg/day, divided bid
		IV	4 mg/kg/day
Metolazone	Children	PO	0.2-0.4 mg/kg/day, divided q 12-24 hr
Spironolactone	Children	PO	1.5-3.5 mg/kg/day, divided q 6-24 hr

IM, Intramuscular; *IV*, intravenous; *N/D*, no data; *PO*, oral.
Modified from Bestic M, Reed M: Pharmacology review: common diuretics used in the preterm and term infant, *Neoreviews* 6: 392, 2005.

patients with a serum potassium level less than 3.0 mEq/L, and patients receiving digitalis therapy.[34]

Potassium-sparing diuretics may induce a hyperkalemic state in up to 8.6% of patients receiving spironolactone and in up to 23% of patients receiving a potassium-sparing diuretic and potassium supplementation.[33,35]

Acid–Base Disorders

With diuresis and volume depletion, hypokalemia and hypochloremia may result. This state may then cause metabolic alkalosis, which is responsive to potassium and chloride replacement therapy. The exceptions are carbonic anhydrase inhibitors, the use of which may result in metabolic acidosis.

Glucose Changes

Loop and thiazide diuretics have been associated with hyperglycemia. The average rise in serum glucose is between 6.5 and 9.6 mg/dl, although cases of diabetic ketoacidosis have also been reported.[36,37] The severity of glucose elevation in these reports was related to the dose of diuretic used, as well as to the drop in potassium levels. Although the cause of hyperglycemia is not completely understood, several possible etiologies have been postulated. These include decreased pancreatic insulin release and insulin resistance with impaired uptake of glucose in response to insulin.

Ototoxicity

The loop diuretics may cause a dose-related **ototoxicity** consisting of tinnitus and clinical or subclinical hearing loss. The ototoxicity results from anatomical and chemical abnormalities produced within the inner ear.[34] Ototoxicity is related to the blood level of these agents. Therefore rapid infusion and drug accumulation with large parenteral doses in renal failure both predispose patients to ototoxicity. Reducing the infusion rate or administering the drug orally may alleviate the hearing loss.[38,39] The majority of ototoxicity is reversible; however, cases of irreversible hearing loss have occurred. Ethacrynic acid has a higher likelihood of causing irreversible hearing loss.[39,40] Limited data on bumetanide indicate that it may have a lower incidence of ototoxicity than furosemide and ethacrynic acid.

To minimize diuretic-induced ototoxicity, ethacrynic acid should be avoided. In addition, chronic doses greater than 500 mg in patients with advanced renal disease and repetitive dosing in patients with acute renal failure and rapid infusions should be avoided.

OTHER CONSIDERATIONS

Diuretics are not recommended for pregnant women because the effects of the drug on the fetus are unknown. As many diuretics pass into breast milk, diuretics are not recommended to breastfeeding women, because of the risk of dehydration in the baby.

Children can safely take diuretics because the side effects are similar to those in adults. However, they may require smaller doses of the drug (Table 21-5). Furosemide is one of the most effective and least toxic diuretics used in pediatric practice. However, long-term use of loop diuretics in children should be carefully evaluated because of the risk of **nephrocalcinosis** and potential decrease in bone mass density.[41,42]

SELF-ASSESSMENT QUESTIONS

1. What is a diuretic?
2. Identify the five major groups of diuretics used clinically.
3. If an agent such as one of the loop diuretics causes a loss of potassium, how will this lead to a metabolic alkalosis?
4. Which diuretics would preserve potassium?
5. What is the potential effect of a carbonic anhydrase inhibitor on acid–base balance?
6. Explain how a diuretic such as furosemide can be helpful in acute congestive heart failure with pulmonary and vascular edema.
7. Which diuretic agent has a vasodilatory effect when used chronically?
8. In an otherwise healthy adult with mild hypertension, what diuretic agent should be considered as the first line of treatment?
9. Match each set of drugs on the left with the most likely interaction on the right.

Gentamicin **PLUS** furosemide	Hyperglycemia
Hydrochlorothiazide **PLUS** prednisone	Ototoxicity and nephrotoxicity
Spironolactone **PLUS** enalapril	Hyperkalemia
Hydrochlorothiazide **PLUS** carbamazepine	Hyponatremia

10. Which of the following drugs is indicated specifically for the treatment of primary hyperaldosteronism?

Answers to Self-Assessment Questions are found in Appendix A.

CLINICAL SCENARIO

Case courtesy **Douglas J. Pearce, MD, cardiologist.**

A 73-year-old white male presents to the emergency department with a chief complaint of severe dyspnea that began about 8 hours before presentation. The patient's history is significant for long-standing hypertension and coronary artery disease. In 1985, he had an inferior myocardial infarction and then in 1989 had another myocardial infarction of unknown location. After this, he underwent a coronary artery bypass graft procedure. His left internal mammary artery was used to bypass the left anterior descending artery, a saphenous vein graft was placed to the posterior descending artery, and a sequential saphenous vein graft was placed to the first and second obtuse marginal arteries.

Cardiac catheterization before bypass grafting revealed inferior wall akinesis with global hypokinesis of the remaining walls. His left ventricular ejection fraction was estimated to be 40%. Since his bypass surgery, he has not had any further angina or infarctions, but he has had two admissions for acute pulmonary edema. Both episodes were felt to have been precipitated by medical noncompliance, but this could not be confirmed. At this presentation, the patient again denies chest pain. He states that he began feeling dyspneic the night before presentation and then awoke about 5 AM severely dyspneic and coughing up white, foamy phlegm. When queried about his compliance with his medicines, he admits that he sometimes forgets to take his clonidine.

The patient has chronic renal insufficiency and has had right inguinal hernia repair. He denies any allergies.

The patient is taking the following medications: clonidine 0.1 mg PO bid; atenolol 50 mg PO hs each night; aspirin 325 mg PO qd; transdermal nitroglycerin 0.4 mg qh (he places a patch on in the morning and takes it off at bedtime); and furosemide 40 mg PO q AM.

Physical examination reveals an elderly white male in obvious respiratory distress. His vital signs are as follows: pulse (P), 120 beats/min and regular; respiratory rate(RR), 32 beats/min; blood pressure (BP), 230/140 mmHg, and he is afebrile. His neck shows positive jugular venous distention. Heart auscultation reveals a regular rate, with an I/VI systolic ejection murmur, negative S_3, and positive S_4. His lungs demonstrate bibasilar rales half of the way up the thorax. His abdomen is flat and bowel sounds are present; no masses or tenderness are identified. His extremities are slightly cool, and pulses are felt in all extremities, but are somewhat thready.

The patient's laboratory results are as follows: Na, 138 mEq/L; K, 3.6 mEq/L; blood urea nitrogen (BUN), 40 mg/dl; and creatinine, 2.8 mg/dl. His ECG shows sinus tachycardia, with inferior Q waves and lateral Q waves of questionable significance. A chest radiograph shows mild cardiomegaly with bilateral infiltrates consistent with pulmonary edema.

This is a 73-year-old white male with ischemic heart disease, hypertension, and chronic renal insufficiency. His history, physical examination, and diagnostic data are consistent with acute pulmonary edema. His blood pressure is markedly elevated. There is a history of possible medical noncompliance, which would make one suspicious that he has not taken his clonidine. Acute hypertension in the face of already impaired left ventricular systolic function is a common cause of acute pulmonary edema. Of note, the patient does have some evidence of renal insufficiency with an elevated creatinine level. His potassium is at the lower end of normal, probably secondary to his furosemide.

True or False: In addition to oxygen and morphine sulfate 2 mg intravenously, a thiazide-type diuretic should be administered immediately.

If the patient fails to respond to furosemide 80 mg intravenously, should another loop diuretic be tried?

True or False: When the patient begins to diurese, close observation of the potassium level will be needed.

Answers to Clinical Scenario Questions are found in Appendix A.

References

1. Dirks JH, Sutton RL: *Diuretics: physiology, pharmacology, and clinical use*, Philadelphia, Pa, 1986, W.B. Saunders.
2. Hardman JG, Gilman AG, Limbird LE: *The pharmacological basis of therapeutics*, New York, 1995, McGraw-Hill.
3. Katzung BG: *Basic and clinical pharmacology*, Norwalk, Ct, 2001, Appleton & Lange.
4. Melmon KL: *Clinical pharmacology: basic principles in therapeutics*, New York, 1992, McGraw-Hill.
5. Messerli D: *Diuretics in cardiovascular drug therapy*, Philadelphia, Pa, 1996, W.B. Saunders.
6. Ferdinand KC, Saunders E: Hypertension-related morbidity and mortality in African-Americans: why we need to do better, *J Clin Hypertens* 8:21, 2006.
7. Messerli FH, Grossman E, Goldbourt U: Are β-blockers efficacious as first-line therapy for hypertension in the elderly? A systematic review, *JAMA* 279:1903, 1998.
8. Messerli FH: Antihypertensive therapy: β-Blockers and diuretics—why do physicians not always follow guidelines?, *Proc (Bayl Univ Med Cent)* 13:128, 2000.
9. Joint National Committee on Prevention, Detection, Evaluation, and Treatment of High Blood Pressure: The Sixth Report of the Joint Committee on detection, evaluation and treatment of high blood pressure, *Arch Intern Med* 157:2413, 1997.
10. Guidelines Subcommittee: 1999 World Health Organization–International Society of Hypertension guidelines for the management of hypertension, *J Hypertens* 17:151, 1999.
11. Chennavasin P, Seiwell R, Brater DC, Liang WM: Pharmacodynamic analysis of the furosemide-probenecid interaction in man, *Kidney Int* 16:187, 1979.
12. Martin S: Continuous infusion of loop diuretics: pharmacodynamic concepts and clinical applications, *Clin Trends Pharm Pract* 8:10, 1994.
13. Dikshit K, Vyden JK, Forrester JS, Chatterjee K, Prakash R, Swan HJ: Renal and extrarenal hemodynamic effects of furosemide in congestive heart failure after myocardial infarction, *N Engl J Med* 288:1087, 1973.
14. Bourland WA, Day DK, Williamson HE: The role of the kidney in the early nondiuretic action of furosemide to reduce elevated left atrial pressure in the hypervolemic dog, *J Pharmacol Exp Ther* 202:221, 1977.
15. Francis GS, Siegel RM, Goldsmith SR, Olivari MT, Levine TB, Cohn JN: Acute vasoconstrictor response to intravenous furosemide in patients with chronic heart failure, *Ann Intern Med* 103:1, 1985.
16. Hammarlund-Udenaes M, Benet LZ: Furosemide pharmacokinetics and pharmacodynamics in health and disease: an update, *J Pharmacokinet Biopharm* 17:1, 1988.
17. Beerman B, Leinfelder J, Anderson SA: Clinical pharmacology of torsemide, a new loop diuretic, *Clin Pharmacol Ther* 42:187, 1987.
18. Brater DC: Diuretics: In Williams RL, Brater DC, Mordenti J, editors: *Rational therapeutics: a clinical pharmacologic guide for the health professional*, New York, 1989, Marcel Dekker.
19. Voelker JR, Cartwright-Brown D, Anderson S, Leinfelder J, Sica DA, Kokko JP, Brater DC: Comparison of loop diuretics in patients with chronic renal insufficiency: mechanism of difference in response, *Kidney Int* 32:572, 1987.
20. Rudy DW, Gehr TW, Matzke GR, Kramer WG, Sica DA, Brater DC: The pharmacodynamics of intravenous and oral torsemide in patients with chronic renal insufficiency, *Clin Pharmacol Ther* 56:39, 1994.
21. Brater DC: Pharmacology of diuretics, *Am J Med Sci* 319:38, 2000.
22. Seely JF, Dirks JH: Site of action of diuretic drugs, *Kidney Int* 11:1, 1977.
23. Van Brummelen P, Man in't Veld AJ, Schalekamp MADH: Hemodynamic changes during long-term thiazide treatment of essential hypertension in responders and non-responders, *Clin Pharmacol Ther* 27:328, 1980.
24. Ochs HR, Greenblatt DJ, Bodem G, Smith TW: Spironolactone, *Am Heart J* 96:389, 1978.
25. Villenuve JP, Rocheleau F, Raymond G: Triamterene kinetics and dynamics in cirrhosis, *Clin Pharmacol Ther* 35:831, 1984.
26. Sica DA, Gehr TWB: Diuretic combinations in refractory oedema states, *Clin Pharmacokinet* 30:229, 1996.
27. Ellison DH: The physiologic basis of diuretic synergism: its role in treating diuretic resistance, *Ann Intern Med* 14:886, 1991.
28. Grossman E, Messerli FH, Goldbourt U: Does diuretic therapy increase the risk of renal cell carcinoma?, *Am J Cardiol* 83:1090, 1999.
29. Sica DA: Antihypertensive therapy and its effects on potassium homeostasis, *J Clin Hypertens* 8:67, 2006.
30. Carlsen JE, Kober L, Torp-Pedersen C, Johansen P: Relation between dose of bendrofluazide, antihypertensive effect, and adverse biochemical effects, *BMJ* 300:975, 1990.
31. Schnaper HW, Freis ED, Friedman RG, Garland WT, Hall WD, Hollifield J, Jain AK, Jenkins P, Marks A, McMahon FG, *et al.*: Potassium restoration in hypertensive patients made hypokalemic by hydrochlorothiazide, *Arch Intern Med* 149:2677, 1989.

32. Toner JM, Ramsay LE: Thiazide-induced hypokalemia: prevalence higher in women, *Br J Clin Pharmacol* 18:449, 1984.

33. Widmer P, Maibach R, Kunzi UP, Capaul R, Mueller U, Galeazzi R, Hoigne R: Diuretic-related hypokalemia: the role of diuretics, potassium supplements, glucocorticoids and β_2-adrenoceptor agonists: results from the Comprehensive Hospital Drug Monitoring Programme, Berne (CHDM), *Eur J Clin Pharmacol* 49:31, 1995.

34. Greenberg A: Diuretic complications, *Am J Med Sci* 319:10, 2000.

35. Greenblatt DJ, Koch-Weser J: Adverse reactions to spironolactone: a report from the Boston Collaborative Drug Surveillance Program, *J Am Med Assoc* 225:40, 1973.

36. Amery A, Berthaux P, Bulpitt C, Deruyttere M, de Schaepdryver A, Dollery C, Fagard R, Forette F, Hellemans J, Lund-Johansen P, *et al.*: Glucose intolerance during diuretic therapy: results of trial by the European Working Party on Hypertension in the Elderly, *Lancet* 1(8066):681, 1978.

37. Savage PJ, Pressel SL, Curb JD, Schron EB, Applegate WB, Black HR, Cohen J, Davis BR, Frost P, Smith W, *et al.*: Influence of long-term, low-dose, diuretic-based, antihypertensive therapy on glucose, lipid, uric acid, and potassium levels in older men and women with isolated systolic hypertension, *Arch Intern Med* 158:741, 1998.

38. Dormans TP, Gerlag PG: Combination of high-dose furosemide and hydrochlorothiazide in the treatment of refractory congestive heart failure, *Eur Heart J* 17:1867, 1996.

39. Rybak LP: Ototoxicity of loop diuretics, *Otolaryngol Clin North Am* 26:829, 1993.

40. Seligmann H, Podoshin L, Ben-David J, Fradis M, Goldsher M: Drug-induced tinnitus and other hearing disorders, *Drug Saf* 14:198, 1996.

41. Auron A, Alon US: Resolution of medullary nephrocalcinosis in children with metabolic bone disorders, *Pediatr Nephrol* 20:1143, 2005.

42. Bestic M, Reed M: Pharmacology review: common diuretics used in the preterm and term infant, *Neoreviews* 6:392, 2005.

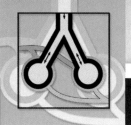

Chapter 22

Drugs Affecting the Central Nervous System

LOUIS LOVETT

CHAPTER OBJECTIVES

After reading this chapter, the reader will be able to:

1. Describe the multiple functions of the central nervous system
2. Recognize various effects of medications on the central nervous system and their ability to modulate neurotransmitters
3. Comprehend psychiatric medications, including their classification, use, and side effect profiles
4. Recognize the effects of alcohol on the central nervous system during acute intoxication, chronic use, and after abrupt withdrawal
5. Distinguish physiological and psychological bases of pain and the classes of analgesics used to treat it
6. Recognize indications for the use of both local and general anesthesia
7. Describe the concept of conscious sedation, and its indications and guidelines for use
8. Distinguish drugs that stimulate the central nervous and respiratory systems and describe the indications for application

KEY TERMS AND DEFINITIONS

Analgesics — Analgesics are drugs that provide pain relief. They can be subdivided into narcotic and nonnarcotic medications. The narcotic drugs are derivatives of opium, such as morphine and codeine. The non-narcotic medications are useful in treating pain and inflammation. They also have antipyretic activity

Anesthetics — Anesthetics are drugs that depress the nervous system. They can be divided into local and general anesthetics. General anesthesia causes total loss of consciousness and reflexes, which results in the absence of pain perception. Local anesthetics are applied to a specific site and decrease pain perception at the specific site and do not affect level of consciousness. Both types of anesthetics are often used during surgical procedures

Antidepressants — Antidepressants are drugs that can alter levels of certain neurotransmitters, in particular norepinephrine and serotonin, within the brain. Depending on the class of antidepressant, they can either inhibit the reuptake of neurotransmitters or decrease their degradation, ultimately allowing for increased levels of neurotransmitter at the nerve terminal

Antipsychotics — Antipsychotics are drugs used to treat psychotic disorders, such as schizophrenia. These drugs affect primarily the neurotransmitter dopamine

Anxiolytics — Anxiolytics are known as minor tranquilizers. They are drugs used to treat several conditions, including anxiety disorders and insomnia. The most common class of anxiolytics is the benzodiazepines. They bind to the γ-aminobutyric acid (GABA) receptor to increase the inhibitory actions of this neurotransmitter

Central nervous system — The brain and spinal cord make up the functional components of the central nervous system. The spinal cord provides nerve fibers that transport signals to and from the brain. The brain is largely made up of three components: the cortex, midbrain, and brainstem. These together provide for all conscious and subconscious functions of the body

Cholinesterase inhibitors — Cholinesterase inhibitors are drugs that block the activity of cholinesterase, an enzyme that inactivates the neurotransmitter acetylcholine. Acetylcholine is found at nerve terminals in both the central and peripheral nervous systems. Cholinesterase inhibitors are used in the treatment of dementia to slow the progression of cognitive decline

Conscious sedation — Conscious sedation is a method used during certain invasive procedures. The goal of conscious sedation is to decrease the level of consciousness, relieve anxiety and pain, while allowing the patient to follow verbal commands. Conscious sedation is achieved through the use of several classes of drugs, including benzodiazepines and narcotic analgesics

Mood stabilizers — Mood stabilizers are drugs used primarily to treat bipolar disorders

Neurotransmitter — A neurotransmitter is a chemical substance that allows neurons to transmit electrical impulses throughout the central and peripheral nervous systems. The action of the electrical impulse is determined by the chemical structure of the neurotransmitter and the receptor to which it binds

Stimulants — Stimulants are drugs that increase activity of the brain. They can be divided into two classes: the amphetamines, and respiratory stimulants. Amphetamines cause increased wakefulness, improved concentration, and appetite suppression. Respiratory stimulants include doxapram, xanthines, carbonic anhydrase inhibitors, salicylates, and progesterone

---

The most widely used drugs, both therapeutic and recreational, are those affecting the central nervous system. Humans are intrinsically concerned with and perhaps even defined by the processes of thinking and feeling. These processes originate within the brain. Thoughts and feelings, although poorly understood, reside primarily with neurochemical interactions and balance in the brain. Drugs that affect the **central nervous system (CNS)** are used to affect perception and mood. Whereas the gross anatomy of the brain has been elegantly described, the complex interaction of various brain areas and individual neurons is less well understood.

In general, the cortex, or outer covering, of the brain is considered to be the location of thought, memory, self-awareness, and personality. Perception of sensation and control of body movement, including speech, are also represented in specific areas of the cortex. The midbrain functions as a relay station for information traveling to and from the cortex. It also integrates and modulates autonomic functions; this function occurs primarily in the hypothalamus. The brainstem, or medulla, contains the control areas for autonomic functions such as breathing and cardiovascular control, as well as the areas responsible for alertness, the reticular activating system. The spinal cord enters the brain at the brainstem, and the cerebellum, immediately behind the brainstem, affects fine motor control and coordinates movement. Much of our understanding of brain organization and function comes from removing areas of brain and identifying resulting deficits in animals. Some information has been acquired by studying humans who have had strokes or destructive brain surgery. These observations have led to a general understanding of functional neuroanatomy and recognizing that the brain can recover significant function after damage to important areas.

More complicated than the gross anatomy would suggest, individual neurons have a wide array of connections with many different neurons in diverse areas of the brain. These patterns are different in different individuals and also change with time in the same individual. It is apparent that many functions are represented in multiple ways, making them resistant to damage. Although the number of individual neurons does not increase after adulthood is reached, the brain is able to change and increase the number of connections and complexity of the neuronal circuitry throughout life. Although each neuron releases only a single **neurotransmitter** and occasionally a coneurotransmitter, the actual effect of these neurotransmitters on the next neuron is modified by additional presynaptic and postsynaptic neurons, which may inhibit or augment the primary neurotransmitter effect

Several diseases appear related to loss of particular neurons with specific neurotransmitters. For example, Parkinson disease is caused by a loss of dopamine-containing neurons in the *substantia nigra* area of the midbrain. It is characterized by resting tremor; rigidity; bradykinesia, or slowness in effecting movement; gait disturbances; and postural instability. Treatment of the disease involves increasing the amount of dopamine contained in and released from the remaining neurons.[1,2] Some forms of depression are believed to be caused by reduced activity of norepinephrine neurons in the brain, particularly those in the *locus ceruleus*.[3] There appears to be a decrease in both the preganglionic augmentation effects of serotonin and direct stimulatory effects of norepinephrine. Treatment is to restore more normal activity of the norepinephrine neurons by inhibiting the reuptake of serotonin by modulating neurons, enhancing the amount of norepinephrine released, and increasing the duration of its effects in the synapse.

It is clear from the diversity of neuronal connections and the plasticity of the central nervous system that drugs used for central nervous system therapy will have widespread and varying effects. This functional and chemical complexity of the brain and peripheral nervous system explains why side effects and toxicities are common with central nervous system drug therapy.

KEY POINT

Drugs that affect the *central nervous system* are *commonly prescribed*. They exert their effects by interacting with *neurotransmission;* by affecting neurotransmitter *release, metabolism*, or *uptake;* or by acting at primary or modifying receptors or *transport proteins*.

NEUROTRANSMITTERS

KEY POINT

The clinical effects of central nervous system drugs depend on the localization of specific neurotransmitters in specific brain areas.

KEY POINT

Because the organization of the central nervous system is complex, the main cause of side effects of this class of drugs is their interaction in diffuse brain areas.

KEY POINT

Central nervous system drugs may increase or decrease individual neuronal activity. The balance of activity of different types of neurons seems to affect brain function and mood. Restoration of this balance is the goal of treatment of mood disorders.

Each neuron releases predominantly one type of neurotransmitter from its axon to synapse with the next neuron. If enough receptors are activated on the postsynaptic membrane, electrical depolarization occurs and a signal is passed to the next neuron. The functional anatomy and components of neurotransmission are illustrated in Figures 22-1 and 22-2. Released neurotransmitters are bound to and transported by proteins in the synapse, taken back up by the releasing nerve terminal, repackaged into vesicles, and recycled. Bound neurotransmitters are not available for receptor interactions, and alterations in the transport proteins in amount or affinity affect the signal propagation potential. Some of the released neurotransmitter is metabolized by membrane-bound enzymes on the postsynaptic cell membrane. The resulting constituent components are taken up presynaptically and used as precursors for neurotransmitter synthesis. Receptors on both the presynaptic membrane and the postsynaptic membrane specific for the released

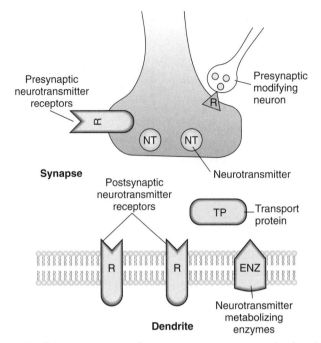

FIGURE 22-1 Schematic of the components of neuron-to-neuron communication. Neurotransmitter is synthesized in the nerve and transported and stored in the nerve terminal. Other components of neurotransmission include transport proteins *(TP)* in the synapse, receptors *(R)* on the postjunctional membrane, receptors *(R)* on the prejunctional membrane, membrane-bound enzymes *(ENZ)*, and modifying neurons.

chemicals, as well as for other chemicals from modulating and neighboring neurons, affect the activity of the neuron.

Examples of chemicals that behave as neurotransmitters are listed in Table 22-1. The effect of the neurotransmitter released is determined by many factors, including the amount of neurotransmitter released, type and quantity of transport proteins, previous release of neurotransmitters, presence of modifying substances, efficiency of reuptake processes, and activities of modulating interneurons. Specifics of this transmission modulation system differ for various brain areas, mental functions, and neurotransmitters. Central nervous system–active drugs may have effects on specific parts of a neurotransmitter system or have generalized effects on brain function. Augmentation or inhibition of neurotransmission can result from drug interaction at any of the sites illustrated in Figures 22-1 and 22-2.

PSYCHIATRIC MEDICATIONS

Antidepressants

Depression is one of the most common psychiatric disorders and a major cause of worldwide disability. In the United States the 1-month prevalence of a major depressive episode has been estimated to involve more than 2%

> **KEY POINT**
>
> *Depression* is a common *mood disorder*. Several classes of drugs, including the *tricyclic antidepressants (TCAs)*, *monoamine oxidase inhibitors (MAOIs)*, and *selective serotonin reuptake inhibitors (SSRIs)*, are used for this disorder and exhibit a wide range of side effects.

> **KEY POINT**
>
> Other *psychotherapeutic* drugs include the *major tranquilizers* and *sedative-hypnotic* drugs.

of the population.[4] The Global Burden of Disease Study found unipolar depression to be the fourth leading cause of worldwide disability, even after excluding deaths from suicide.[5] The prevalence of major depressive disorder may be on the increase, and it is predicted that by 2020, unipolar major depression will be the second leading cause of disability worldwide.[6]

Depressive disorder has multiple etiologies, including biological, psychological, and social factors. Serotonin and norepinephrine have been shown to be important neurotransmitters, and their relative deficiency has been linked to depression. For more than a decade,

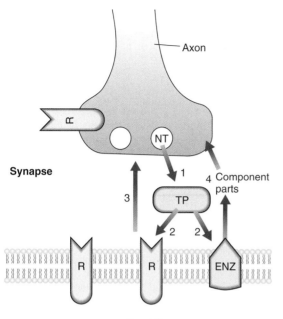

FIGURE 22-2 Schematic for the pathways that neurotransmitters follow after release into the synapse. After axonal depolarization, the stored neurotransmitter *(NT)* is released into the synapse *(1)*, where it is bound to the transport or carrier protein *(TP)*. NT is transported to and binds with postjunctional receptors *(2)*, is metabolized by membrane-bound enzymes *(2)*, is actively taken up by the releasing neuron *(3)*, or is released and binds to prejunctional receptors. NT substance that is degraded to its component parts is taken up by the releasing neuron to be resynthesized and reused *(4)*.

TABLE 22-1	
Central Nervous System Chemicals That Function as Neurotransmitters	
Chemical Class	**Neurotransmitter**
Biogenic amines	Norepinephrine
	Epinephrine
	Dopamine
	Acetylcholine
	Histamine
	Serotonin (5-hydroxytryptamine)
Amino acids	γ-Aminobutyric acid (GABA)
	Glutamate
	Glycine
	Aspartate
Nucleotides and nucleosides	Adenosine triphosphate
	Adenosine
Peptides	Thyrotropin-releasing hormone
	Enkephalins
	Angiotensin II
	Oxytocin
	Vasopressin
	Bradykinin
	Dynorphin
	Substance P
	Substance K
	Neuropeptide Y
	β-Endorphin
	Luteinizing hormone–releasing factor
	Corticotropin-releasing factor
	Somatostatin
	Secretin
	Melanocyte-stimulating hormone

the first line of medical treatment for major depressive disorder has been the *selective serotonin reuptake inhibitors (SSRIs)*. These drugs are preferred because they are safer and more tolerable than the older medications, such as tricyclic antidepressants and monamine oxidase inhibitors. In addition, newer drugs target both norepinephrine and serotonin. They are called *serotonin norepinephrine reuptake inhibitors*. These drugs and their side effects are listed in Tables 22-2 and 22-3.

Mood Stabilizers

Mood stabilizers are used primarily for bipolar disorder. This affective disorder involves alternating episodes of depression and mania or hypomania. Mania is characterized by at least a week of elevated or irritable mood, and at least three of the following: inflated self-esteem or grandiosity, decreased need for sleep, being more talkative than usual, rapid thoughts, or the subjective experience that one's thoughts are racing, distractibility, an

increase in goal-directed behavior, or excessive involvement in pleasurable activities that have a high potential for painful consequences.[7] Hypomania is similar to mania, but less intense and of shorter duration.[7]

Medical treatment of any degree of bipolar disorder must begin with a mood stabilizer. These drugs include lithium, anticonvulsants such as valproic acid, carbamazepine, gabapentin, lamotrigine, and **antipsychotics**, which are discussed subsequently. The main side effect of these drugs, except for lithium, is sedation. Lithium has a narrow therapeutic window, and consequently must be used judiciously. Lithium can cause tremor, cognitive slowing, hypothyroid, renal insufficiency, leukocytosis, polyuria, and polydipsia. Lithium toxicity can result in coma.[8] A list of common mood stabilizers is found in Table 22-4.

TABLE 22-2

Drugs Used to Treat Depression

Class	Generic Drug	U.S. Brand Name(s)
Selective serotonin reuptake inhibitors (SSRIs)	Citalopram	Celexa
	Fluoxetine	Prozac
	Paroxetine	Paxil, Paxil CR, Pexeva
	Sertraline	Zoloft
	Escitalopram oxalate	Lexapro
Serotonin and norepinephrine reuptake inhibitors	Venlafaxine	Effexor, Effexor XR
	Duloxetine	Cymbalta
Serotonin receptor antagonist	Nefazodone	Nefazodone
Dopamine reuptake inhibitor	Bupropion	Wellbutrin, Zyban
Tricyclic antidepressants (TCAs)	Amitriptyline	Amitriptyline
	Clomipramine	Anafranil
	Desipramine	Norpramin
	Doxepin	Sinequan
	Imipramine	Tofranil
	Nortriptyline	Aventul, Pamelor
	Protriptyline	Vivactil
	Trimipramine	Surmontil
Tetracyclic antidepressants	Maprotiline	Maprotiline
	Mirtazapine	Remeron
Monoamine oxidase inhibitors (MAOIs)	Phenelzine	Nardil
	Tranylcypromine	Parnate
	Isocarboxazid	Marplan
Herbal remedy	Hypericum	St. John's wort
Miscellaneous drugs	Trazodone	Desyrel

CR, controlled release; *XR,* extended release.

Antipsychotics

Psychotic disorders are characterized by impaired reality testing. They include schizophrenia spectrum disorders as well as psychosis associated with depression or mania. Pharmacotherapy is generally used to increase dopamine in the brain. These drugs are most efficacious for the active psychotic symptoms, such as hallucinations and abnormal thought processes. Older drugs such as thorazine, thioridazine, and haloperidol had numerous side effects, which affected compliance. These include extrapyramidal symptoms such as cogwheel rigidity, acute dystonia, oculogyric crisis, as well as cholinergic side effects. Newer agents, such as risperidone, olanzapine, and quetiapine, are more tolerable. A list of some of the common antipsychotics is found in Table 22-5.

Drugs for Alzheimer's Dementia: Cholinesterase Inhibitors

Alzheimer's dementia is associated with cognitive deficits secondary to decreased acetylcholine levels within the brain. The **cholinesterase inhibitors** improve cognition and function in patients with Alzheimer's disease. These drugs include donepezil, tacrine, galantamine, and rivastigmine. The use of these drugs is sometimes limited by gastrointestinal side effects, which include nausea, vomiting, diarrhea, and hepatotoxicity, especially with tacrine.[9] These drugs are listed in Table 22-6.

Anxiolytics

KEY POINT

Hypnotic drugs primarily *activate the γ-aminobutyric acid (GABA) receptor*–mediated chloride channel, hyperpolarizing the cell and decreasing consciousness, anxiety, and recall.

KEY POINT

GABA channel activation may also be important in the production of general anesthesia and sleep. Sleep is a complex activity and induction of sleep can be pharmacologically influenced by sedative drugs; however, the quality of the sleep so induced is poor.

TABLE 22-3

Incidence of Various Side Effects of Commonly Used Antidepressants

Medication	Sedation	Agitation	Anticholinergic Effects*	Postural Hypotension	Gastrointestinal Upset	Sexual Dysfunction	Weight Gain	Weight Loss
Serotonin and Norepinephrine Reuptake Inhibitors								
Tricyclics (Tertiary Amines)								
Amitriptyline	++++	0	++++	+++	+	+	++	0
Doxepin	++++	0	++++	+++	+	+	+	0
Imipramine	++++	0	++++	+++	+	+	+	0
Tricyclics (Secondary Amines)								
Desipramine	+++	0	+++	++	+	+	+	0
Nortriptyline	+++	0	+++	++	+	+	+	0
Bicyclic								
Venlafaxine†	++	+	++	0	+++	++	0	+
Selective Serotonin Reuptake Inhibitors								
Citalopram	0	0	+	0	++	+	+	+
Fluoxetine	+	++	+	0	++	++	+	+
Paroxetine	++	0	+	0	++	++	+	+
Sertraline	+	+	+	0	++	++	+	+
Serotonin norepinephrine reuptake inhibitor								
Duloxetine	++	+	++	+	++	+	+	+
Norepinephrine Reuptake Inhibitor, Dopamine Reuptake Inhibitor								
Bupropion	+	++	++	0	++	0	+	++
Serotonin Antagonists and Reuptake Inhibitors								
Nefazodone	++	0	++	+	+	0	0	0
Trazodone	++++	0	++	+	+	0	+	+

From Whooley MA, Simon GE: Managing depression in medical outpatients, *N Engl J Med* 343:1947, 2000.
0, None; +, minimal (<5% of patients); ++, low frequency (5% to 20%); +++, moderate frequency (21% to 40%); ++++, high frequency (>40%).
*Side effects may include dry mouth, dry eyes, blurred vision, constipation, urinary retention, tachycardia, or confusion.
†Venlafaxine may cause a dose-related elevation in diastolic blood pressure; monitoring of blood pressure is recommended.

TABLE 22-4

Drugs Used as Mood Stabilizers

Generic Drug	Brand Name(s)
Carbamazepine	Tegretol, Epitol, Carbatrol, Equetro
Lamotrigine	Lamictal
Lithium	Lithobid, Eskalith
Valproic acid	Depakene, Depakote, Depakote ER

ER, Extended release.

KEY POINT

Antagonism of the *benzodiazepine* receptor site can be accomplished with *flumazenil*, which binds to the receptor site, but does not activate the receptor.

TABLE 22-5

Drugs Used in the Management of Psychotic Disorders

Class	Generic Drug	Brand Name
Phenothiazines	Chlorpromazine	Thorazine
	Fluphenazine	Prolixin
	Perphenazine	Trilafon
	Trifluoperazine	Stelazine
Thioxanthene	Thiothixene	Navane
Butyrophenones	Droperidol	Inapsine
	Haloperidol	Haldol
Miscellaneous agents	Clozapine	Clozaril
	Lithium	Lithobid, Eskalith
	Olanzapine	Zyprexa
	Pimozide	Orap
	Quetiapine	Seroquel
	Risperidone	Risperdal
	Ziprasidone	Geodon

The benzodiazepines are a group of agents that have been used to reduce anxiety under a variety of circumstances. **Anxiolytics** are also used as amnestics, preventing conversion of short-term experience into permanent memory. By themselves, they cause no change in respiration; however, they may augment the depression induced by opioids. They have little effect on cardiac function and are very safe agents from this standpoint. Benzodiazepines are excellent induction agents when providing general anesthesia and are useful

TABLE 22-6

Drugs Used in the Treatment of Dementia

Class	Generic Drug	Brand Name
Cholinesterase inhibitors	Donepezil	Aricept
	Galantamine	Reminyl
	Rivastigmine	Exelon
	Tacrine	Cognex

TABLE 22-7

Drugs Used to Treat Anxiety and Insomnia

Class	Generic Drug	U.S. Brand Name(s)
Benzodiazepines	Alprazolam	Xanax
	Clorazepate dipotassium	Tranxene
	Chlordiazepoxide	Librium
	Diazepam	Valium
	Estazolam	ProSom
	Flurazepam	Dalmane
	Lorazepam	Ativan
	Midazolam	Versed
	Oxazepam	Oxazepam
	Temazepam	Restoril
	Triazolam	Halcion
Benzodiazepine antagonist	Flumazenil	Romazicon
Other anxiolytics	Buspirone HCl	BuSpar
	Doxepin HCl	Sinequan
	Hydroxyzine	Vistaril
	Meprobamate	Equanil, Miltown

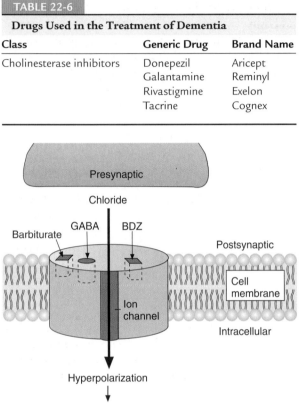

FIGURE 22-3 Mode of action by which barbiturates and benzodiazepines *(BDZ)* depress central nervous system function; stimulation of receptors on the chloride ion channel facilitates γ-aminobutyric acid *(GABA)*–induced inhibition of neuronal function.

in preventing unpleasant recall during uncomfortable interventions. They may be used as somnifics. These agents are used to terminate seizures and will elevate seizure threshold. Benzodiazepines exert their effects by binding to benzodiazepine receptors in the γ-aminobutyric acid (GABA) receptor complex on neurons, increasing the GABA chloride channel permeability, which hyperpolarizes the neuron, making depolarization less likely (Figure 22-3). A specific antagonist, flumazenil (Romazicon), can reverse the sedative effects of the benzodiazepines.

Several other drugs are used to treat anxiety and insomnia. Some of these are listed with the benzodiazepines in Table 22-7. Their mechanisms of action are not related to interactions with the benzodiazepine receptor or the GABA system. Some of the drugs in Table 22-7 are used to promote sleep; these and other nonrelated sleep-inducing agents are listed in Table 22-8. Although they induce sleep, benzodiazepines and other drug classes interfere with the normal sleep cycles by reducing the amount of time spent in rapid eye movement (REM) sleep.

Barbiturates

One of the oldest group of sedative drugs, the barbiturates, is a derivative of barbituric acid. Because of their toxic potential and rapid development of tolerance, they have largely been replaced by the benzodiazepines, except for a few specialized uses. Several ultrashort-acting barbiturates are used for anesthetic induction (thiopental, thiamylal, and methohexital), as hypnotics (pentobarbital and secobarbital), and for seizure control and prophylaxis (phenobarbital). Use of barbiturates as hypnotics is limited by rapid development of tolerance and reduction in the quality of sleep (decreased amount of REM sleep). They are potent inducers of the CYP450 drug-metabolizing system that can alter the levels of many other drugs. Although many of the therapeutic effects of barbiturates are mediated by a specific receptor at the GABA-mediated inhibitory receptor, they have widespread depressive effects on neuron activity. Intentional or accidental overdose results in respiratory arrest and cardiovascular collapse because of brain control center depression. This drug class also carries a high risk of addiction and abuse. Severe withdrawal symptoms, including seizures, occur after abruptly stopping chronic barbiturates.

TABLE 22-8

Medications Used to Induce Sleep

Class	Generic Drug	Brand Name
Benzodiazepines	Estazolam	ProSom
	Flurazepam HCl	Dalmane
	Quazepam	Doral
	Temazepam	Restoril
	Triazolam	Halcion
Barbiturates	Secobarbital	Seconal
	Pentobarbital	Nembutal
	Butabarbital	Butisol
Antihistamines	Cyproheptadine	Cyproheptadine
	Diphenhydramine	Benadryl
	Hydroxyzine	Vistaril
Miscellaneous	Chloral hydrate	Somnote
	Ethanol	Alcohol
	Eszopiclone	Lunesta
	Paraldehyde	Paral
	Ramelteon	Rozerem
	Zaleplon	Sonata
	Zolpidem	Ambien

Other Hypnotics

Difficulty sleeping is a common clinical complaint that frequently results in the prescription of a hypnotic. In addition to the short-acting benzodiazepines and barbiturates mentioned above, several other sedatives are used for inducing sleep. Unfortunately, all disrupt sleep patterns and may not improve overall well-being. Hypnotics to induce sleep are generally recommended for brief periods (1 or 2 weeks). However, some patients continue to take these medications for years. A new drug, eszopiclone, is approved for long-term use. Medications used for sleep enhancement are listed in Table 22-8.

ETHYL ALCOHOL

Alcohol is a by-product of sugar fermentation. It is used as a socially acceptable nonprescription, sedative-hypnotic agent. Ingested to excess, it behaves like a general anesthetic, depressing all brain areas, resulting in loss of voluntary muscle control and consciousness. At toxic levels (400 to 600 mg/dl, blood alcohol level) the respiratory center is affected and death as a result of respiratory arrest is likely. The disinhibiting effects of modest alcohol intoxication result from depression of higher cortical behavior control centers, probably by decreasing the GABA receptor effects of endogenous mediators. At higher levels, diffuse membrane-disruptive effects occur, causing generalized neurological depression. When combined with other sedative-hypnotic drugs, the degree of intoxication is additive. Chronic alcohol ingestion results in upregulation of GABA receptors and other brain functions, with the development of tolerance to the intoxicating and toxic depression caused by alcohol. Abrupt withdrawal after prolonged use may result in the syndrome of *delirium tremens (DTs)*, characterized by central nervous system hyperactivity, including hyperthermia, increased blood pressure, muscle twitching, hallucinosis, and seizures. The mortality from DTs is high, ranging from 5% to 10% if seizures occur. The withdrawal syndrome can be prevented or treated with any of the sedative-hypnotic drugs, and usually a benzodiazepine is chosen because of its relative safety.

Because alcohol is a carbohydrate, if ingested in large quantities, it replaces many of the dietary calories and decreases appetite. Protein, fat, and vitamin malnutrition are often seen with chronic alcohol abuse. Alcohol is metabolized to CO_2 and H_2O, producing acetaldehyde in the process. Because it is a food, ethyl alcohol saturates the metabolic enzyme system and undergoes first-order elimination kinetics. This means that a constant amount of alcohol is removed per unit time, rather than a fixed percentage of the blood concentration as with most other drugs. In the average person, this results in about 10 to 12 g of alcohol removed per hour.

PAIN TREATMENT

Pain is a common human problem. Because pain is a subjective, unpleasant experience, it is difficult objectively to observe and quantitate. Recognition of the physiological and psychological consequences of inadequate pain treatment has led to increased attention to pain control in patients. In hospitalized patients, estimation of pain has been raised to the level of a vital sign, on par with blood pressure, heart rate, respiratory rate, and temperature. Pain is now often referred to as the fifth vital sign. Besides the difficulty of estimating the amount of pain, it is well known that many factors alter patient responses to a given degree of discomfort. Physiological, social, and psychological factors profoundly alter patient perception and tolerance of pain.[10,11] The meaning of pain to the individual can affect the reported pain and the response of the pain to treatment. It is helpful to view the pain experience as composed of at least two components: the sensation of *pain* as mediated by the central nervous system receiving nociceptive input from peripheral pain receptors; and *suffering*, the negative, personal emotional response to the pain experience. The integration and expression of these two components produce the pain behavior, which influences the patient's analgesic requirements.

Medications may be directed at the origin, integration, or interpretation of the pain experience. Often combinations of medications are more effective than a single approach to this common problem.

Nonanalgesic drugs also affect perception and tolerance of pain. Sedative drugs such as the barbiturates and benzodiazepines appear to reduce pain tolerance, actually increasing the amount of pain perceived and reported by patients receiving them. This probably occurs by reducing cortical modulation of the pain perception, thereby increasing pain behaviors. These agents, when combined with **analgesics**, however, seem to decrease the painful experience and enhance analgesia. When interviewed after resolution of the pain episode, patients do not usually report having experienced pain of the extreme magnitude that was perceived by caregivers.

Another factor that must be taken into account when assessing pain is that patients have poor pain memories. With time, the ability to recall the severity and characteristics of pain diminishes. This applies to the effects of treatment as well. Patients asked whether past pain treatment was effective almost always report improvement in pain, even if objective evaluation at the time documents no change or even worsening pain.[12] **Antidepressants** combined with analgesics are used to treat chronic pain states. They may be effective by modifying the depressed mood that accompanies chronic discomfort.

Although there are external clues to the presence and magnitude of a person's pain, personal reports are the only way to judge the presence and magnitude of pain. Visual or numerical analog pain scales (VAS) are the most commonly employed methods for estimating the magnitude of pain. The simplest and most common pain scale employed is an 11-point scale, with 10 being the worst imaginable pain and 0 being totally without pain. Patients are asked to rate their pain from the worst imaginable pain (10) to no pain at all (0). These scales appear to have internal and external validity.[13-15] The numerical rating is convenient and recognizable, and it lends itself to frequent repetition and consistent reporting. In children, a series of smiling and frowning faces, such as the Wong/Baker Rating Scale, may be used to allow the child to report the degree of pain.[16] These scales help in assessing the adequacy of analgesia and also create a shorthand way for patients to communicate their need for additional analgesia to the bedside caregiver.

Caregivers must integrate VAS reports, patient pain behaviors, and vital signs with their own biases[17] as to the degree of pain that should be present to decide whether to administer additional analgesic drugs.[18] It appears that caregivers often deliver inadequate amounts of analgesics.[19] Inappropriate expectations of the degree of pain in both the patient and caregiver contribute to this reluctance to administer potent analgesics. Acute pain remains undertreated in many patients.

Nonsteroidal Antiinflammatory Drugs

> **KEY POINT**
>
> Pain may be relieved by *local anesthetics* blocking sensory transmission, by *nonsteroidal antiinflammatory drugs (NSAIDs)* modifying peripheral inflammation and central integration, and *opiates* modifying the spinal cord transmission, brainstem processing, and cortical perception of pain.

One of the frequently used analgesic classes, nonsteroidal antiinflammatory drugs (NSAIDs), is employed to treat moderate pain (Table 22-9). NSAIDs work by affecting the hypothalamus and by inhibiting the production of inflammatory mediators, primarily prostaglandins, at the peripheral site of the painful stimulus. The salicylates are the oldest member of this class and have been known for more than 100 years for their effects as antipyretics. Aspirin is a common component of over-the-counter (OTC) analgesics and cold remedies. Aspirin decreases the synthesis of prostaglandin by irreversibly inhibiting two enzymes: cyclooxygenase-1 and cyclooxygenase-2 (COX-1 and COX-2). COX-1 is located primarily on tissues, including blood vessels, kidney, and gastric mucosa, and COX-2 is associated primarily with inflammation. Unlike aspirin, others in this group reversibly inhibit these enzymes. Although selective COX-2 inhibitors are thought to cause fewer gastrointestinal side effects, there are no clinical trials clearly demonstrating this profile.[20]

Gastric irritation and ulceration are major problems with administering NSAIDs. Renal injury can result from prolonged use and high dosage of these medications. They also inhibit platelet aggregation and this compounds the problem of gastrointestinal bleeding. The antiplatelet effects are used therapeutically either after or to prevent cardiac thrombosis. Aspirin use in childhood febrile illness has been associated with an increased incidence of Reye syndrome, an often fatal rise in intracranial pressure associated with massive hepatic dysfunction.[21,22] Allergic reactions to this class of drugs are common. Rashes, urticaria, angioneurotic edema, asthma, and anaphylaxis have been seen.

TABLE 22-9		
Nonsteroidal Antiinflammatory Drugs		
Class	**Generic Drug**	**Brand Name(s)**
Nonspecific cyclooxygenase inhibitors		
Salicylates	Aspirin	
	Choline salicylate	Arthropan
	Diflunisal	Dolobid
	Magnesium salicylate	
	Salsalate	Amigesic, Disalcid
	Sodium salicylate	
	Sodium thiosalicylate	
Aniline derivative	Acetaminophen	Tylenol, Tempra
Indoles	Etodolac	Lodine
	Indomethacin	Indocin
	Sulindac	Clinoril
Propionic acid derivatives	Ibuprofen	Advil, Motrin
	Fenoprofen	Nalfon
	Flurbiprofen	Ansaid
	Ketoprofen	Orudis
	Naproxen	Aleve, Anaprox, Naprelan, Naprosyn
	Oxaprozin	Daypro
Piroxicam derivative	Piroxicam	Feldene
Miscellaneous	Diclofenac	Voltaren, Cataflam
	Ketorolac	Toradol
	Meclofenamate	Meclofenamate
	Mefenamic acid	Ponstel
	Nabumetone	Relafen
	Tolmetin	Tolectin
COX-2 inhibitors		
	Celecoxib	Celebrex
	Meloxicam	Mobic
	Rofecoxib	Vioxx*
	Valdecoxib	Bextra[†]

COX-2, Cyclooxygenase-2.
*Manufacturer voluntarily withdrew agent from the market.
[†]U.S. Food and Drug Administration removed April 7, 2005.

Acetaminophen (Tylenol), although a weak inhibitor of the cyclooxygenase system, has no significant antiinflammatory effects but is effective in relieving mild to moderate pain. It does not inhibit platelets or cause gastric ulcers. In large doses, it can cause lethal hepatic necrosis. Because it is used in many nonprescription cold preparations, accidental overdose from combined dosing during self-medication occasionally occurs.

Recently, COX-2 inhibitors have been reevaluated for their potential to cause adverse cardiovascular events. Rofecoxib (Vioxx) and valdecoxib (Bextra) have been withdrawn from the market. Other COX-2 inhibitors are currently undergoing trials to assess their potential to increase cardiovascular risk.

Opioid Analgesics

KEY POINT

Depression of respiratory drive is an important *side effect* of several classes of central nervous system drugs, including the general anesthetics and *opioid analgesics.*

KEY POINT

Opiate effects can be antagonized with *naloxone* or *naltrexone.*

Opioids or narcotic analgesics are derivatives of the naturally occurring drug mixture opium, derived from the poppy, *Papaver somniferum.* These agents are used for the treatment of moderate to severe pain. They act by binding to opioid receptors in the brain and spinal cord. They modify pain pathways at the spinal level, as well as profoundly influence the subjective response to pain at the cortical level. Endogenously occurring opioids, the endorphins and enkephalins, are neuromodulators affecting pain perception and mood. Opioids exert their effects and side effects by binding to receptors for these naturally occurring agents. There are at least three distinct opioid receptors, *mu (μ), kappa (κ),* and *delta (δ),* and several subtypes. Agonist drugs may bind at one or more of these receptors, accounting for some of the differences seen in their effects. Besides pain relief, high enough doses of opioids can result in loss of consciousness and, because of a profound dose-dependent depression of respiratory drive, respiratory arrest. The opioids produce a euphoric effect on mood, making them popular drugs of abuse. Tolerance develops rapidly and withdrawal is very painful and unpleasant. These factors contribute to the highly addictive potential of the opioids.

The μ-receptor is responsible for the analgesic effects in the central nervous system and spinal cord. It also accounts for respiratory depression, constipation, nausea and vomiting (from the chemotactic trigger zone receptors), and antitussive effects. κ-Receptors located in the spinal cord and, to a lesser extent, in the central nervous system, mediate analgesia. They may be the receptors responsible for the analgesic effects of the mixed agonist-antagonist drugs. The δ-receptor is the receptor for the naturally occurring mediator enkephalin; its role in analgesia is not clear. It may be important in the spinal mediation of pain perception. This is just the outline of the opioid receptor system; there are other types and subtypes of receptors. Their actual function in human health is not understood. The effect of various opioids can be explained by their actions at one or more of these receptors.

Opioids are listed in Table 22-10. Some have pure agonist effects, acting as the endogenous mediators at the receptors, and others antagonize the endogenous mediators but have a small agonist effect (mixed drugs or agonist-antagonist drugs). There are several strictly antagonist agents. These drugs are used to reverse the analgesic and respiratory depressive effects of the opioids. The most serious side effect of the opioid antagonists is respiratory depression, which is mediated by decreased sensitivity of the respiratory center to elevations in arterial carbon dioxide pressure (Pa_{CO_2}). Miosis (small pupils) is pathognomonic for opioid drug administration and is a consequence of effects on the sympathetic nervous system. Constipation results from opioid depression of motility of the stomach and intestines. Nausea and vomiting are a direct effect on the brainstem effectors. Cough suppression results from a direct central effect of the opioid.

Because of their effects on pain perception, narcotics are often used as part of a balanced anesthetic. Doses that cause profound depression of respiration have minimal or no effect on cardiac function. Because of this safety, opioids are the basis for anesthesia for the seriously cardiovascular-compromised patients. By themselves, opioids have no effect on consciousness or memory. Combined with small doses of benzodiazepines or gaseous **anesthetics**, they can be used to provide surgical anesthesia.

Strong opioid drugs are often referred to as *narcotics*, from the Greek word for stupor. The word *narcotic* has significant legal overtones. For this reason, its use has been avoided in this section. *Opiates* are compounds derived from opium and represent a small number of the drugs discussed above. *Opioids*, as used in this section, implies simply that the agents interact with one or more of the opioid receptors.

Routes of Opioid Administration

KEY POINT

Inadequate pain relief has been identified as a serious problem. Many pain control options are available to hospitalized patients.

TABLE 22-10		
Opioid Drugs		
Effect at the Opioid Receptor	**Generic Drug**	**Brand Name(s)**
Agonist	Morphine	MSIR, MS Contin
	Opium	Paregoric
	Codeine	Codeine
	Alfentanil	Alfenta
	Dihydrocodeine	Synalgos, Compal
	Fentanyl	Sublimaze, Actiq, Duragesic
	Heroin	None
	Hydrocodone	Only available in combination with other agents
	Hydromorphone	Dilaudid
	Levomethadyl	ORLAAM
	Levorphanol	Levo-Dromoran
	Meperidine	Demerol
	Methadone	Dolophine, Methadose
	Oxycodone	Roxicodone, OxyContin
	Oxymorphone	Numorphan
	Propoxyphene	Darvon
	Remifentanil	Ultiva
	Sufentanil	Sufenta
	Tramadol	Ultram
Mixed agonist-antagonist	Buprenorphine	Buprenex, Subutex
	Butorphanol	Stadol
	Nalbuphine	Nubain
	Pentazocine	Talwin
Antagonist	Nalmefene	Revex
	Naloxone	Narcan
	Naltrexone	ReVia

MS, Morphine sulfate; *MSIR*, morphine sulfate immediate release.

KEY POINT

Patient-controlled (opioid) analgesia (PCA), epidural analgesia with local anesthetics and opioids, and combinations of analgesic classes can result in excellent postoperative pain relief.

As discussed previously, pain is a subjective experience. Inadequate analgesia is a common complaint voiced by patients. This is especially true after surgery. Fear of respiratory depression is often given as the reason caregivers are reluctant to administer more opioids. Novel ways of treating pain have been developed to improve treatment of pain. Patient-controlled analgesia (PCA) is a method by which patients can self-administer a predetermined intravenous bolus of an opioid at a set interval. This avoids the delay in getting a dose requested from and later delivered by a nurse. More total analgesia drug is needed if pain is allowed to intensify between drug doses. It is more effective to keep control of pain than to regain control of it. Continuous administration of a background opioid rate also may help with this problem. Patients using PCA for postoperative pain use less total opioid and report subjectively less pain than patients receiving scheduled or as-needed opioids delivered by nurses.

Opioid Inhalation

Opioids are occasionally administered by inhalation. This route has been suggested to be more effective than systemic opioids for decreasing the sensation of dyspnea in patients with advanced respiratory failure. Opioid receptors have been found in lung tissue, but their exact function in modifying the sensation of dyspnea has not been determined. Inhaled (nebulized) opioids may affect dyspnea by a central mechanism because these drugs are rapidly absorbed from the lung. No controlled studies have demonstrated improved effectiveness of opioids when administered by inhalation; however, this route may be an alternative when intravenous access is not available.[23] Terminal cancer patients without lung disease have been given their systemic doses of analgesics through this route with good clinical effect.

Local Anesthetics

KEY POINT

Local anesthetics consist of a *hydrophilic end* connected to an active *amino end* connected by an *amine* or *ester* linkage.

KEY POINT

Local anesthetics block *sodium channels* in axons and abolish neural transmission.

Pain treatment can be achieved by blocking transmission of the pain impulse from the damaged area. Local anesthetics are used to interrupt these nervous signals. Local anesthetics produce nerve conduction block by blocking sodium channels. These are located all along the cell, including the axon. When depolarization occurs, the impulse is propagated down the axon by an abrupt increase in the membrane sodium permeability. When the drug binds to and occludes the channel pore, sodium is unable to enter the cell

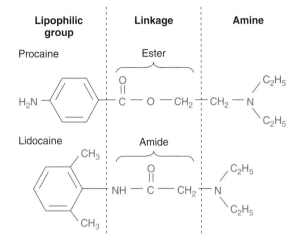

FIGURE 22-4 Chemical structures of the local anesthetics procaine and lidocaine, showing their respective ester and amide linkages, location of the lipophilic group, and the ionizable amine group.

and propagation of the electrical impulse is stopped. All local anesthetics consist of a lipophilic part and a hydrophilic, amine part connected by either an amide or ester linkage. This is illustrated in Figure 22-4. Several of the common agents are listed in Table 22-11. Sodium channel blockade makes some of these drugs useful in terminating cardiac conduction abnormalities, as well as providing analgesia. Some evidence suggests that systemic administration or inhalation may also enhance bronchodilation in asthma, as well as suppress irritant tracheal cough responses. At toxic levels, central nervous system excitation occurs and frank seizures may result. Epinephrine is often added to a local anesthetic for vasoconstriction to delay its absorption, thus prolonging its effect and decreasing blood levels and potential toxicity. Bupivacaine is very cardiotoxic, and a toxic dose may result in profound and prolonged cardiac depression or arrest.

Epidural Analgesia

Continuing epidural infusions for analgesia have improved postoperative pain therapy. There is evidence that patient outcome may also be improved with epidural infusions of local anesthetics, opioids, or both.[24,25] This is especially true for the very ill.[26-29] The quality of the analgesia and the ability to eliminate pain in many body areas are superior with local anesthetic infusion compared with systemic analgesics. Minimal effects on normal sensory and motor function

TABLE 22-11

Examples of Local Anesthetics

Class	Generic Drug	Brand Name(s)
Esters	Benzocaine	Hurricane, Solarcaine
	Chloroprocaine	Nesacaine
	Procaine	Novocain
	Tetracaine	Pontocaine
Amides	Articaine	Septocaine
	Bupivacaine	Marcaine, Sensorcaine
	Levobupivacaine	Chirocaine
	Lidocaine	Xylocaine
	Mepivacaine	Carbocaine, Polocaine
	Prilocaine	Citanest
	Ropivacaine	Naropin

Box 22-1   Side Effects of Agents Used for Epidural Analgesia

LOCAL ANESTHETICS
- Motor weakness
- Numbness
- Hypotension
- Difficulty diagnosing epidural hematoma

OPIOIDS
- Respiratory depression (equal to or less than with systemic opioids)
- Reduced gastrointestinal motility (greater than with systemic opioids)
- Nausea and vomiting (equal to that with systemic opioids)
- Difficult micturition (greater than with systemic opioids)
- Pruritus (much greater than with systemic opioids)

TABLE 22-12

Some Examples of Combinations of NSAIDs and Opioid Analgesics

NSAID		OPIOID		
Agent	Dose	Agent	Dose	Brand Name
Acetaminophen	650 mg	Propoxyphene	100 mg	Darvocet N100
Acetaminophen	650 mg	Propoxyphene	50 mg	Darvocet 50
Aspirin	325 mg	Codeine	30 mg	Empirin #3
Aspirin	325 mg	Codeine	60 mg	Empirin #4
Acetaminophen	500 mg	Hydrocodone	5 mg	Duocet
Acetaminophen	650 mg	Hydrocodone	10 mg	Lorcet 10/650
Acetaminophen	650 mg	Hydrocodone	7.5 mg	Lorcet Plus
Acetaminophen	500 mg	Hydrocodone	2.5 mg	Lortab 2.5/500
Acetaminophen	500 mg	Hydrocodone	5 mg	Lortab 5/500
Aspirin	325 mg	Oxycodone	4.5 mg	Percodan
Aspirin	325 mg	Oxycodone	2.25 mg	Percodan-Demi
Acetaminophen	325 mg	Oxycodone	5 mg	Roxicet, Percocet
Acetaminophen	300 mg	Codeine	15 mg	Tylenol #2
Acetaminophen	300 mg	Codeine	30 mg	Tylenol #3
Acetaminophen	300 mg	Codeine	60 mg	Tylenol #4
Acetaminophen	500 mg	Oxycodone	5 mg	Tylox
Acetaminophen	500 mg	Hydrocodone	5 mg	Vicodin
Ibuprofen	200 mg	Hydrocodone	7.5 mg	Vicoprofen
Acetaminophen	650 mg	Propoxyphene	65 mg	Wygesic

NSAID, Nonsteroidal antiinflammatory drug.

can be achieved with very dilute local anesthetics. Addition of opioids to the mixture permits even less local anesthetic to be infused. If sympathetic blockade produces unacceptable hypotension, local anesthetics can be eliminated completely, with significant analgesia obtained with narcotic infusion alone. Pain modulation from epidural opioids occurs at receptors at the spinal cord segmental level. The major side effects of epidural analgesia using local and/or opioid infusions are listed in Box 22-1.

Combinations of Analgesic Classes

Another strategy to improve analgesia and to reduce the likelihood of opioid overdose is to combine several different classes of analgesics. Prescription combinations of NSAIDs and opioids are widely available. Some of these are listed in Table 22-12. The concept of attacking pain at several places is useful, but the fixed combinations of drugs with different effects, toxicities, and half-lives make titration to an individual patient's needs difficult with these agents. Use of the separate agents, independently titrated, may improve this problem but makes the taking of many medications more difficult for patients.

CHRONIC PAIN SYNDROMES

Surgery or trauma causing acute pain can lead to central sensitization and persistence of pain after the peripheral lesion has resolved. It is not known how frequently this problem leads to a chronic pain syndrome, but information is accumulating suggesting that specific treatment in the acute period may reduce the likelihood of a neuropathic problem later.

Neuropathic pain may start with nerve injury, which results in axon degeneration and regeneration. Associated with this process in animal models are abnormal discharges at the spinal cord level, leading to sensitization, abnormal sensation, phantom pain, and rapid changes in the functional architecture of the pain pathways at the level of the spinal cord and lower brain. *Hyperesthesia* (increased and unpleasant sensitivity to all sensory modalities), *hyperpathia* (increased unpleasant abnormal feeling from mildly uncomfortable stimuli), and *allodynia* (painful feeling from gentle stimuli) can be demonstrated to occur soon after acute painful trauma in some patients, especially after surgery on or near major nerve trunks. In some patients, this process may persist and advance to result in a chronic pain syndrome. The characteristics of neuropathic pain include evidence of a primary injury; pain involving (but not confined to) a body area with a sensory deficit; burning, electric, or shooting character to the pain; dysesthesias in the area; pain spreading beyond the cutaneous nerve distribution; sympathetic hyperactivity; and allodynia, hyperpathia, and hyperalgesia. In some complex regional pain syndromes, the autonomic deregulation results in skin changes, edema, and nail and hair loss. This syndrome may lead to severe suffering and incapacitation. Once established, neuropathic pain is poorly responsive to analgesic treatment, but may respond to sympathetic interruption or α-receptor blockade.[30] It is possible that modification of the initial pain input may decrease the incidence or reduce the severity of the syndrome that develops over time.

Preemptive analgesia is the delivery of adequate and appropriate analgesia before initiation of nociceptive input from the surgical incision. By totally abolishing the painful stimulus, the potential for chronic pain syndromes should be reduced. Although general anesthetics and opioids do modify the central sensitization to some extent, regional analgesia, antiinflammatory agents, central α-receptor blockers, and *N*-methyl-*d*-(+)-aspartate (NMDA) receptor antagonists, alone or in combination, offer hope of actually preempting pain and eliminating postoperative pain syndromes.

ANESTHESIA

The state of general anesthesia is a drug-induced absence of perception. Stronger stimuli may require deeper anesthesia. Anesthetics are usually administered by inhalation or intravenously because of the more predictable time course of drug actions. Often, combinations of drugs are used to achieve the state of anesthesia. The ideal anesthetic would include the following:

- A pleasant and rapid induction and emergence
- Rapid changes of depth of anesthesia to match surgical demands
- Skeletal muscle relaxation to facilitate surgical exposure
- A wide margin of safety
- No toxic or adverse effects

The first and most common anesthetic agents are the gases and volatile liquids. These are listed in Table 22-13. Dosage and potency are compared by using the concept of minimal alveolar concentration (MAC), which is the amount necessary to achieve the anesthetic state. This is a statistical concept, much like the ED_{50} (effective dose for 50% of subjects to respond), based on the measured agent concentration in exhaled gas (which is in equilibration

TABLE 22-13

Gases and Volatile Liquids Used to Produce General Anesthesia

Class	Agent	Common or Brand Name
Gases	Cyclopropane	
	Ethylene	
	Nitrous oxide	Laughing gas
Liquids	Halothane	Fluothane
	Isoflurane	Forane
	Enflurane	Ethrane
	Sevoflurane	Ultane
	Desflurane	Suprane
	Methoxyflurane	Penthrane

with the blood) sufficient to prevent movement on surgical incision in half of the subjects. The mechanisms by which anesthetic gases and vapors exert their effects are poorly understood but may be receptor mediated (the GABA receptor being a top candidate) or may be more diffuse, temporary disruption of nerve cell communication. The facts that anesthetic vapor potency is linearly related to fat solubility and that anesthetics can be reversed by high pressures (50 to 100 atmospheres) suggest that cell wall swelling from the agent dissolving in the lipid membrane is an important contributor to the anesthetic state.

Volatile anesthetics by themselves achieve some of the characteristics of the ideal anesthetic in that depth of anesthesia can be changed rapidly, induction and emergence are rapid (with some agents), and there are few toxic concerns. These agents do not reliably provide muscle relaxation. Neuromuscular blockers and other adjuvant drugs are often titrated to create the desired anesthetic state and to prevent potent agent overdose. Neuromuscular blockers are discussed in Chapter 18. Their use in anesthesia includes facilitation of tracheal intubation (often a short-acting agent) and surgical relaxation, necessary for intrathoracic, intraabdominal, and other procedures. Pharmacological reversal of the long-acting neuromuscular blocking agents is also discussed in Chapter 18. Because volatile anesthetics provide little analgesia, narcotic and nonnarcotic analgesics are often a part of the anesthetic mixture. Analgesics may reduce the amount of volatile agent necessary to achieve anesthesia. The use of a mixture of agents to achieve the anesthetic state is often referred to as *balanced anesthesia*, in which each element is provided in balance and by a different drug. Induction of general anesthesia is usually facilitated by a rapidly effective, sedative-hypnotic agent, although inhalation induction with a newer volatile agent (sevoflurane) is rapid and not unpleasant. Intravenous induction agents commonly used are listed in Table 22-14.

Depth of anesthesia is determined by patient response to painful stimuli and is often judged by the sympathetic response, that is, a change in heart rate or blood pressure. Because other factors may influence these signs, determination of anesthetic depth is much more of an art than a science. Monitors are available that are based on the processed electroencephalogram, and that are touted to predict depth of anesthesia (bispectral index [BIS] monitor), but these devices are subject to other influences as well. During the course of surgery and anesthesia, the degree of surgical stimulus and the depth of anesthesia vary, and one function of the anesthesiologist is to match these two. Analgesia may be needed intraoperatively, as well as being part of pain management in the postoperative period. In medically compromised patients, the main activity of the anesthesiologist is to obtain and maintain stability and prevent death; the anesthetic may simply consist of preventing pain and abolishing recall of interoperative events. The entire cardiovascular armamentarium may be used as part of anesthetic management for these critically ill, unstable patients.

Conscious Sedation

KEY POINT

Conscious sedation is a technique using sedatives and analgesics to prevent patient discomfort during invasive procedures. To prevent catastrophe, a *dedicated individual* must *monitor* the progress of sedation and be prepared to correct airway and cardiovascular problems.

Fear and pain are frequent side effects of many clinical interventions. The pain experience, which includes the physical and emotional components, associated with clinical interventions is unnecessary and may increase morbidity and mortality. For these reasons, minimizing fear and pain is an important part of clinical care.

Besides general anesthesia, many approaches are available to modify the unpleasant experience of diagnostic and therapeutic procedures. Patient preparation, education, relaxation exercises, hypnosis, and drugs may be useful. *Conscious sedation* is the term applied to the pharmacological modification of painful and frightening experiences during medical procedures. As implied in the name, sedated patients should remain conscious and able to communicate, protect their own airway, and breathe adequately. Improved patient comfort and outcome are the goal of sedation. However, because of variations in patient responses, consciousness as well as the patient's ability to maintain an unobstructed airway may be lost during sedation.

TABLE 22-14		
Anesthetic Induction Agents		
Class	**Generic Drug**	**Brand Name**
Barbiturates	Methohexital	Brevital
	Thiopental	Pentothal
Benzodiazepines	Diazepam	Valium
	Lorazepam	Ativan
	Midazolam	Versed
Miscellaneous agents	Etomidate	Amidate
	Ketamine	Ketalar
	Propofol	Diprivan

Institutional standards for safe and effective provision of **conscious sedation** are required by the Joint Commission on Accreditation of Healthcare Organizations and other regulatory agencies. These standards must be adhered to throughout the institution, whether sedation is provided by a nurse, respiratory therapist (RT), anesthesiologist, or other healthcare provider. Many concerned groups have developed guidelines for providing safe conscious sedation. RTs should understand sedative and analgesic pharmacology and may actively participate in provision of conscious sedation.[31,32] Because most of the serious complications of conscious sedation relate to airway compromise, RTs are uniquely qualified to safeguard patients and improve outcomes during conscious sedation.

Standards for Providing Conscious Sedation

Most conscious sedation guidelines and many clinical reports differentiate several levels of sedation. Often a clear distinction is drawn between conscious and deep sedation.[33] However, the progression from conscious sedation to deep sedation to general anesthesia is difficult to control clinically and each deeper level implies increased risks and mandates more intensive monitoring and an increased level of support. The definitions of

these states and suggested requirements for monitoring are given in Table 22-15.

All published conscious sedation standards insist on the presence of *more than one* person during the period of sedation (at least the operator and a monitoring assistant). Several guidelines suggest that deep sedation and general anesthesia are *indistinguishable* and that at least three qualified people must be continually present during the sedation period.[34] The standards also suggest that one person must have, *as sole responsibility*, continual monitoring of the patient and recording of vital signs. When providing conscious sedation, it is necessary to continuously assess and ensure oxygenation, ventilation, and temperature maintenance. Although some conscious sedation guidelines suggest how to monitor these vital functions, the decision to use a particular device and frequency of repeated observations is left to the responsible clinician.[35] What is not left to the discretion of the clinician is the number of personnel necessary and that they must be specially qualified and assigned *only* to monitor one patient's vital functions and the progress of sedation. There must be resuscitation equipment immediately available and individuals trained to use it. To be competent at providing conscious sedation requires a didactic understanding of the pharmacology of the drugs discussed in this chapter and a

---

TABLE 22-15

Levels of Sedation and Recommendations for Monitoring

Level of Sedation	Definition	Suggested Monitors
Conscious sedation	Minimally depressed level of consciousness, retaining the patient's ability to maintain the airway independently and continuously and to respond to physical stimulation and verbal commands	Dedicated monitoring assistant Pulse oximetry IV access Blood pressure measurement every 15 min
Deep sedation	Depressed consciousness accompanied by partial loss of protective reflexes and inability to respond purposefully to verbal command	Skilled airway person Monitoring and recording person IV access Pulse oximetry Continuous ECG monitoring Blood pressure measurement every 5 min
General anesthesia	Unconsciousness accompanied by partial or complete loss of protective reflexes and inability to maintain an airway independently	Anesthesia personnel Anesthesia assistant IV access Pulse oximetry Carbon dioxide measurement device Continuous ECG monitoring Blood pressure measurement every 5 min Other requirements dictated by the patient's physiological condition

ECG, Electroencephalogram; *IV*, intravenous.

performance-based competency including intravenous therapy, monitor use, and supervised clinical practice.[36]

CENTRAL NERVOUS SYSTEM AND RESPIRATORY STIMULANTS

KEY POINT

Central nervous system–stimulating drugs include the *methylxanthines* (caffeine and aminophylline) and doxapram. These agents have little clinical usefulness in treating respiratory failure or drug-induced respiratory depression.

KEY POINT

Specific antagonists for benzodiazepine sedative drugs and opioids are more useful for reversing drug-induced hypoventilation.

In contrast to most of the sedative drugs discussed in this chapter, some drugs can *increase* activity of the brain rather than depress it. Such drugs are termed *analeptic* drugs. If the effects are primarily on the respiratory center, the agent may be a respiratory or ventilatory stimulant. Stimulant drugs are used for treatment of narcolepsy, attention-deficit hyperactivity disorder (ADHD), obesity, and, to a lesser extent, respiratory failure. Some of these drugs are listed in Table 22-16. Most of the stimulant drugs are sympathomimetics, acting directly on α and β receptors. Their abuse potential is great and their side effects are predictable. They interfere with sleep and are used (and abused) to promote wakefulness and weight loss.

Some drugs can increase ventilation. Doxapram has been used in the past as a treatment for acute and chronic respiratory failure. It was given intravenously and would cause a transient increase in rate and depth of ventilation. It is rarely used as no sustained improvement of respiratory failure has been demonstrated. Methylxanthines, used to promote bronchodilation, also increase catecholamines and increase ventilation. Caffeine, a common component in popular beverages, is used therapeutically in apnea-bradycardia syndromes of premature births. Agents causing metabolic acidosis such as salicylate toxicity, including carbonic anhydrase inhibitor diuretics, can increase ventilation in response to the systemic acidosis that develops. This increase in minute ventilation is not, however, considered therapeutic. Progesterone can cause a sustained increase in ventilation and fall in $Paco_2$ and is occasionally used to treat chronic elevations in CO_2 from advanced obstructive lung disease. Hormonal effects on mood and breast development limit its usefulness.

Respiratory failure resulting from sedative or opioid drug overdose should be treated with specific antagonists, flumazenil and naloxone, rather than with nonspecific analeptic drugs. Respiratory **stimulants** have little or no clinical role in treating respiratory failure.

TABLE 22-16

Central and Peripheral Nervous System–Stimulating Drugs

Class	Use	Generic Drug	Brand Name(s)
Sympathomimetics	Diet	Benzphetamine	Didrex
		Diethylpropion	Tenuate
		Phendimetrazine	Adipost, Bontril
		Phentermine	Pro-Fast, Ionamin
		Sibutramine	Meridia
	Diet and CNS stimulant	Amphetamine	Adderall
	Diet and CNS stimulant	Methamphetamine	Desoxyn
	CNS stimulant	Dextroamphetamine	Dexedrine, Dextrostat
Xanthines	CNS stimulant	Aminophylline	
		Caffeine	
Progestational agent	CNS stimulant	Medroxyprogesterone acetate	Provera
Respiratory stimulant	Peripheral chemoreceptor stimulant	Doxapram	Dopram
Miscellaneous	ADHD	Dexmethylphenidate	Focalin
		Methylphenidate	Ritalin, Methylin, Concerta, Daytrana

ADHD, Attention-deficit hyperactivity disorder; *CNS,* central nervous system.

Elevated Pa_{CO_2} caused by muscle fatigue from increased work of breathing as a result of chronic obstructive pulmonary disease (COPD), acute respiratory distress syndrome (ARDS), or severe bronchospasm would not be expected to improve with catecholamine-stimulating agents. Mechanical ventilation, muscle rest, and bronchodilators are more appropriate approaches.

SELF-ASSESSMENT QUESTIONS

1. What is the difference between sedation and analgesia?
2. Identify the general class of each of the following agents (sedative-hypnotic, analgesic, tranquilizer, anesthetic, antipsychotic): lorazepam, phenobarbital, doxapram, chloral hydrate, thiopental, midazolam, nitrous oxide, chlorpromazine, halothane, morphine, ibuprofen.
3. You are planning to extubate and remove a patent from the ventilator. However, the nurse administers a large dose of lorazepam (Ativan) for anxiety. What problem may occur if you proceed?
4. What is the most serious side effect of tranquilizers, sedatives, or analgesics (especially opioids)?
5. You have two patients, both of whom have overdosed on central nervous system depressants
   • Patient 1: Comatose, cyanotic, dilated pupils
   • Patient 2: Comatose, cyanotic, pinpoint pupils
   Which patient may have taken a barbiturate and which a narcotic analgesic?
6. Identify your initial priorities as a respiratory therapist in caring for a subject with an overdose of tranquilizers.
7. What is the mode of action of the benzodiazepines?
8. Identify an agent that can reverse the effects of benzodiazepines such as midazolam and triazolam.
9. Will barbiturates be helpful in managing pain in a ventilator patient?
10. Would meperidine be helpful to prevent or lessen perception of pain?
11. For a patient with a bleeding disorder, such as hemophilia, or one who is taking anticoagulants such as warfarin, suggest an analgesic for minor pain.
12. Are there any serious side effects to use of a ventilatory stimulant such as doxapram?

Answers to Self-Assessment Questions are found in Appendix A.

CLINICAL SCENARIO

Case courtesy **Robert Aranson, MD, Pulmonologist/ Intensivist, formerly of Emory University School of Medicine, Grady Memorial Hospital, Atlanta, Ga.**

A 35-year-old black male was admitted to the hospital with lethargy, after being found in his apartment by a friend. An empty bottle of amitriptyline pills was lying next to the man. In the emergency room, the patient became more lethargic to the point of unresponsiveness and developed hypopnea and bradypnea. He was subsequently intubated and mechanically ventilated with a volume-cycled ventilator. The patient had a history of depression, but had been in good physical health. He was taking amitriptyline, which was prescribed by his psychiatrist for his depression. In an act of despair, he had taken an overdose of his medication. The man had no allergies, and his past medical history and family history were unremarkable.

Physical examination revealed a mesomorphic male appearing his stated age, markedly sedated, intubated, and mechanically ventilated. His vital signs were as follows: temperature (T), 39° C rectally; pulse (P), 140 beats/ min; respiratory rate (RR), 12 breaths/min on an assist/ control (A/C) rate of 12 breaths/min; blood pressure (BP), 110/60 mmHg, right arm, supine. Head, eyes, ears, nose, and throat (HEENT) were unremarkable except for oral endotracheal tube (ETT) in place. His chest was normoresonant to percussion and his lungs had clear breath sounds bilaterally. Cardiovascular examination revealed that on palpation, the point of maximal impulse was located normally in the fifth intercostal space in the midclavicular line. Auscultation revealed normal S_1 and S_2 without murmurs, gallops, or rubs. He had normal jugular venous pressure, and his pulses were 2+ throughout. The man's abdomen was mildly distended with absent bowel sounds. No masses or organomegaly were present. His extremities were unremarkable, and his skin was very warm and dry. He was unresponsive to visual, auditory, or tactile stimuli, and his pupils were equally dilated and sluggishly responsive to light. All of his extremities were flaccid, and his reflexes were 1+ throughout. His plantar reflexes were downgoing.

Laboratory results revealed normal hemogram, electrolytes, blood urea nitrogen (BUN), creatinine, and liver function test results. The tricyclic antidepressant (TCA) level was in the toxic range. His chest radiograph was normal. The ETT was approximately 2 cm above the carina. The ECG showed sinus tachycardia at 140 beats/ min, with prolonged PR and QRS intervals. Arterial blood gas (ABG) on A/C ventilation at 12 breaths/min, with a tidal volume (V_T) of 800 ml and a fraction of inspired

Continued

oxygen (F_{IO_2}) of 1.0, resulted in the following: pH, 7.44; arterial carbon dioxide pressure (Pa_{CO_2}), 38 torr; arterial oxygen pressure (Pa_{O_2}), 550 torr.

The patient was diagnosed with a TCA overdose, and admitted to the medical intensive care unit (MICU), where he was treated with activated charcoal 30 g via nasogastric tube q6h, along with normal saline hydration intravenously. After the first dose of charcoal, his heart rate dropped to approximately 120 beats/min, and his F_{IO_2} was eventually tapered to 0.35, with the resulting ABG results: pH, 7.43; Pa_{CO_2}, 40 torr; and Pa_{O_2}, 175 torr. Several hours after the second charcoal dose, he awoke and was able to write notes to the MICU staff, stating that he was anxious to be extubated. The staff wanted to oblige and placed him on a T-piece with 35% O_2 from a large-reservoir nebulizer. About 2 hours later, the patient fell asleep while on the T-piece, and an ABG at that time revealed pH, 7.36; Pa_{CO_2}, 48 torr; and Pa_{O_2}, 165 torr. An astute respiratory therapist noticed the marked change in the ABG parameters, and placed the patient back on the ventilator. The patient was eventually able to be extubated uneventfully several hours after the fourth dose of charcoal. He was transferred in stable medical condition to the psychiatry service the day after extubation.

What are the toxic side effects of TCAs, and what class of drugs (and what drug in particular) do they mimic in this regard?

How is TCA overdose typically treated?

Why did the patient awaken and then fall back asleep in between doses of activated charcoal?

What implications does this phenomenon have for respiratory therapists in freeing TCA-overdosed patients from the ventilator? When would it have been deemed safe to extubate this patient?

What did the ABG on T-piece imply regarding the patient ventilatory status? Could the patient have been extubated with this particular ABG? Why or why not?

Was supplemental oxygen ever needed for this patient? Why or why not?

Answers to Clinical Scenario Questions are found in Appendix A.

References

1. Olanow CW, Hauser RA, Gauger L, Malapira T, Koller W, Hubble J, Bushenbark K, Lilienfeld D, Esterlitz J: The effect of deprenyl and levodopa on the progression of Parkinson disease, *Ann N eurol* 38:771, 1995.
2. Lozano AM, Lang AE, Hutchison WD, Dostrovsky JO: New developments in understanding the etiology of Parkinson disease and in its treatment, *Curr Opin Neurobiol* 8:783, 1998.
3. Ressler KJ, Nemeroff CB: Role of norepinephrine in the pathophysiology and treatment of mood disorders, *Biol Psychiatry* 46:1219, 1999.
4. Regier DA, Boyd JH, Burke JD Jr, Rae DS, Myers JK, Kramer M, Robins LN, George LK, Karno M, Locke BZ: One month prevalence of mental disorders in the United States, *Arch Gen Psychiatry* 45:977, 1988.
5. Murray C, Lopez A: Global mortality, disability, and the contribution of risk factors: Global Burden of Disease Study, *Lancet* 349:1436, 1997.
6. Murray C, Lopez A: Alternative projections of mortality and disability by cause 1990-2020, *Lancet* 349:1498, 1997.
7. American Psychiatric Association: *Diagnostic and statistical manual of mental disorders*, ed 4, Washington, DC, 2000, American Psychiatric Association.
8. American College of Physicians: *ACP Medicine*, ch 13, section II, pp. 1-12. New York, 2006, WebMD Professional Publishing.
9. Abramowicz M, editor: Tacrine for Alzheimer's disease, *Med Lett Drugs Ther* 35:87, 1993.
10. Chen AC, Dworkin SF, Haug J, Gehrig J: Human pain responsivity in a tonic pain model: psychological determinants, *Pain* 37:143, 1989.
11. Carragee EJ, Vittum D, Truong TP, Burton D: Pain control and cultural norms and expectations after closed femoral shaft fractures, *Am J Orthop* 28:97, 1999.
12. Feine JS, Lavigne GJ, Dao TT, Morin C, Lund JP: Memories of chronic pain and perceptions of relief, *Pain* 77:137, 1998.
13. Chambers CT, Reid GJ, McGrath PJ, Finley GA: Development and preliminary validation of a postoperative pain measure for parents, *Pain* 68:307, 1996.
14. McGrath PA, Seifert CE, Speechley KN, Booth JC, Stitt L, Gibson MC: A new analogue scale for assessing children pain: an initial validation study, *Pain* 64:435, 1996.
15. Colwell C, Clark L, Perkins R: Postoperative use of pediatric pain scales: children self-report versus nurse assessment of pain intensity and affect, *J Pediatr Nurs* 11:375, 1996.
16. Wong DL, Baker CM: Pain in children: comparison of assessment scales, *Pediatr Nurs* 14:9, 1988.
17. Todd KH, Samaroo N, Hoffman JR: Ethnicity as a risk factor for inadequate emergency department analgesia, *JAMA* 269:1537, 1993.
18. Sjostrom B, Haljamae H, Dahlgren LO, Lindstrom B: Assessment of postoperative pain: impact of clinical experience and professional role, *Acta Anaesth Scand* 41:339, 1997.
19. Beauregard L, Pomp A, Choiniere M: Severity and impact of pain after day-surgery, *Can J Anaesth* 45:304, 1998.
20. Abramowicz M: *COX2 alternatives and GI protection*, *Med Lett Drugs Ther*, 46: 91, 2004.
21. Hurwitz ES, Barrett MJ, Bregman D, Gunn WJ, Pinsky P, Schonberger LB, Drage JS, Kaslow RA, Burlington DB, Quinnan GV, *et al.*: Public Health Service study of Reye syndrome and medications: report of the main study, *JAMA* 257:1905, 1987.

22. Forsyth BW, Horwitz RI, Acampora D, Shapiro ED, Viscoli CM, Feinstein AR, Henner R, Holabird NB, Jones BA, Karabelas AD, *et al.*: New epidemiologic evidence confirming that bias does not explain the aspirin/Reye syndrome association, *JAMA* 261:2517, 1989.

23. Manning HL: Dyspnea treatment, *Respir Care* 45:1342, 2000.

24. Ballantyne JC, Carr DB, deFerranti S, Suarez T, Lau J, Chalmers TC, Angelillo IF, Mosteller F: The comparative effects of postoperative analgesic therapies on pulmonary outcome: cumulative meta-analyses of randomized, controlled trials, *Anesth Analg* 86:598, 1998.

25. McNeely JK, Farber NE, Rusy LM, Hoffman GM: Epidural analgesia improves outcome following pediatric fundoplication: a retrospective analysis, *Reg Anesth* 22:16, 1997.

26. Yeager MP, Glass DD, Neff RK, Brinck-Johnsen T: Epidural anesthesia and analgesia in high-risk surgical patients, *Anesthesiology* 66:729, 1987.

27. Pelton JJ, Fish DJ, Keller SM: Epidural narcotic analgesia after thoracotomy, *South Med J* 86:1106, 1993.

28. Ackerman III, WE Molnar JM, Juneja MM: Beneficial effect of epidural anesthesia on oxygen consumption in a parturient with adult respiratory distress syndrome, *South Med J* 86:361, 1993.

29. Kirsch JR, Diringer MN, Borel CO, Hanley DF, Merritt WT, Bulkley GB: Preoperative lumbar epidural morphine improves postoperative analgesia and ventilatory function after transsternal thymectomy in patients with myasthenia gravis, *Crit Care Med* 19:1474, 1991.

30. Hayes C, Malloy AR: Neuropathic pain in the postoperative period, *Int Anesthesiol Clin* 35:67, 1997.

31. Anonymous: Administration of sedative and analgesic medications by respiratory care practitioners: a position statement from the American Association for Respiratory Care, *Respir Care* 43:655, 1998.

32. Durbin CG Jr.: Respiratory therapists and conscious sedation, *Respir Care* 44:909, 1999.

33. Phero JC: Pharmacologic management of pain, anxiety, and behavior: conscious sedation, deep sedation, and general anesthesia, *Pediatr Dent* 15:429, 1993.

34. Rosenberg MB, Campbell RL: Guidelines for intraoperative monitoring of dental patients undergoing conscious sedation, deep sedation, and general anesthesia, *Oral Surg Oral Med Oral Pathol* 71:2, 1991.

35. Matthews RW, Malkawi Z, Griffiths MJ, Scully C: Pulse oximetry during minor oral surgery with and without intravenous sedation, *Oral Surg Oral Med Oral Pathol* 74:537, 1992.

36. Glassman P, Garrison R: A suggested curriculum for teaching conscious sedation in advanced general practice programs: GPR and AEGD, *Special Care Dent* 13:27, 1993.

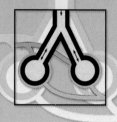

Answers to Self-Assessment Questions and Clinical Scenarios

CHAPTER 1

Self-Assessment Questions

1. What is the definition of the term *drug*?

   Answer: A *drug* may be defined as any chemical that alters an organism's function.

2. What is the difference between the generic name and the trade (or brand) name of a drug?

   Answer: The generic name of a drug is nonproprietary, whereas the brand name is the name given by a particular manufacturer of the drug. If a physician prescribes a particular brand of the drug, the pharmacist must sell that brand unless generic substitution is indicated on the prescription.

3. What part of a prescription contains the name and amount of the drug being prescribed?

   Answer: The inscription.

4. A physician's order reads as follows: "gtts iv of racemic epinephrine, 3 cc of normal saline, q4h, while awake." What has been ordered?

   Answer: Four drops of racemic epinephrine with 3 cc of normal saline, to be given every 4 hours while the patient is awake.

5. The drug salmeterol was released for general clinical use in the United States in 1994. Where would you look to find information about this drug, such as the available dosage forms, doses, properties, side effects, and action?

   Answer: Several sources of information would be available on a new drug, in addition to research reports in the journal literature: the package insert with the drug, the *Physician's Desk Reference* (PDR), and the United States Pharmacopeia–National Formulary USP–NF). Usually a new drug release is accompanied by marketing literature, from the manufacturer, that is available from drug representatives or at conferences.

Clinical Scenario

Where could you find information on the drug, Primatene Mist, that he was taking?

Answer: Primatene Mist is a good example of the need for problem-solving in seeking drug information. A first reference to check would be the PDR; however, you will not find Primatene Mist listed there because this is an old agent in long use. If you cannot find a drug listed in the PDR, other sources would be the package insert for the agent, obtained from a pharmacy, or a current compendium of agents available in the United States, such as *Drug Facts and Comparisons.* This will provide information about the drug, including its pharmacokinetics (onset, duration) and side effects. Finally, textbooks featuring respiratory care drugs, such as this one, provide the same information in the appropriate chapter.

In general, what is the fundamental error this person displayed?

Answer: Failure to seek medical help while self-treating with an over-the-counter (OTC) drug product. He probably did not realize that (1) Primatene Mist is epinephrine, which is short-acting (1 to 2 hours in duration) and will not control the full development of an asthma exacerbation, termed the *late-phase* reaction; and (2) a progressive asthma episode can cause serious obstruction of the airway and often worsens in the evening or night. Given his continued symptoms, he required more aggressive therapy than Primatene Mist.

CHAPTER 2

Self-Assessment Questions

1. If a drug is in liquid solution, what routes of administration are available for its delivery, considering only its dosage form?

   Answer: Oral, injection, inhalation (nebulization), topical (possibly). The type of drug, pharmacokinetics, and intended effect will further narrow the choice of route of administration.

2. Although generic drug equivalents all have the same amount of active drug, will formulations of the same drug from different manufacturers all have the same ingredients?

Answer: No, not necessarily. Ingredients other than the active drug may differ. For example, in a tablet preparation, the substances used to form the active drug into a molded tablet may vary.

3. If 200 mg of a drug results in a plasma concentration of 10 mg/L, what is the calculated volume of distribution (V_D)?

Answer: $V_D = 200$ mg/(10 mg/L) = 20 L.

4. If the V_D of a drug such as phenobarbital is 38 L/70 kg and an effective concentration is 10 mg/L, what loading dose would be needed for an average adult (assuming total bioavailability)?

Answer: Dose = V_D × concentration = 38 L × 10 mg/L = 380 mg.

5. If an inhaled aerosol has zero gastrointestinal absorption of active drug, and only lung absorption, what is the L/T ratio?

Answer: 1.0; L/T = lung availability/(lung + stomach availability); and stomach = 0.

6. True or False: A patient uses a reservoir device with an inhaled aerosol and there is no swallowed portion of the drug; therefore there will be no systemic side effects.

Answer: False. Systemic drug levels are due to *total* drug absorbed, from the gastrointestinal tract and lungs. Sufficient lung absorption of active drug could produce extrapulmonary side effects.

7. Which receptor system signal mechanism is responsible for the effects caused by β-receptor activation, such as those seen with adrenergic bronchodilators (e.g., albuterol)?

Answer: G protein–linked receptors.

Clinical Scenario

What may be a likely cause of the patient's respiratory symptoms?

Answer: The pharmacokinetics of the drug are not suitable for a qid schedule. Assuming there is no other complication developing (and that should be ruled out by assessing the patient), the duration of the drug's effect is too short. The improvement in airway resistance has declined, and the patient is working harder to breathe again.

What solutions could you offer?

Answer: You could administer the isoetharine more frequently, on a q3h schedule instead of the qid schedule. However, a better choice might be to identify a longer-acting bronchodilator with a duration of 4 to 6 hours, such as one of the noncatecholamine agents (see Chapter 6) if the qid schedule is maintained. Less-frequent dosing is more cost effective for an in-hospital patient as well.

CHAPTER 3
Self-Assessment Questions

1. What are the three most common aerosol-generating devices used to deliver inhaled drugs?

Answer: Small volume nebulizer (SVN), metered dose inhaler (MDI) with or without a reservoir device, and dry powder inhaler (DPI).

2. Describe the inspiratory pattern you would instruct a patient to use with an MDI.

Answer: Exhale to end-tidal volume; begin to inhale slowly through the mouth and simultaneously actuate the MDI; continue to inhale to total lung capacity, and hold the breath for 5 to 10 seconds.

3. What are three advantages offered by a reservoir device used with an MDI?

Answer: Reservoir devices can modify the aerosol plume from an MDI in three ways: (1) allow time/distance between actuation and inhalation for particle evaporation and reduced particle size; (2) allow distance for the high initial particle velocity to slow; and (3) somewhat simplify the hand-breathing coordination required with MDI use. The net effect of the first two influences reduces oropharyngeal impaction and loss.

4. Would a dry powder inhaler be appropriate for a 3-year-old child with asthma?

Answer: No. These devices require an inspiratory flow rate of 60 L/min or more for optimal use. This probably exceeds the capability of most 3-year-old children. DPIs are not recommended for children younger than 5 years.

5. What is meant by the term *dead volume* in an SVN?

Answer: The dead volume is the residual amount of solution left in a nebulizer when the nebulizer "sputters" and is no longer able to generate aerosol. This is usually around 0.5 to 1.0 ml in most disposable nebulizers.

6. What is the optimal filling volume and power gas flow rate to use with an SVN?

Answer: For most disposable nebulizers, the optimal filling volume is 3 to 5 ml and the power gas flow rate is 8 to 10 L/min. A flow rate of 8 L/min probably gives the maximal particle size penetrating the lower respiratory tract and therefore the maximal drug mass able to reach the airway. However, a flow rate of 10 L/min will reduce particle size further and decrease the treatment time.

7. How does the electrostatic charge affect an MDI when used with a holding chamber?

   Answer: The electrostatic charge pulls the particles out of suspension, thereby decreasing the amount of drug available to the patient. At present, some manufacturers produce "antistatic" chambers; however, it has been found that washing a standard holding chamber with household detergent will decrease the static. Decreasing static increases available drug to the patient.

8. Which device would be better to deliver a β agonist to an adult patient in the emergency department: an SVN, MDI, or DPI?

   Answer: It really depends on a number of factors, including drug availability, patient or clinical preference, practicality, and convenience. The best choice would be an SVN or MDI with a holding chamber. An MDI without a holding chamber, or a DPI, would not be a good selection because of the patient not being able to coordinate and decreased inspiratory flow.

Clinical Scenario

What would you do to analyze this situation and ensure that the MDI is functioning properly?

Answer: First, check to be sure there are in fact no obstructions in the mouthpiece of the actuator. After shaking well, discharge a dose to room air (away from everyone) to see whether there is a visible plume. If possible, you might compare the aerosol plume from his canister with another MDI, to see whether they appear comparable. If you have a laboratory (e.g., in the hospital) try to have the canister weighed to ensure adequate fullness. Short of analyzing the aerosol, you cannot guarantee a correct dose of albuterol, but you can measure the person's peak expiratory flow with a peak flow meter or his FEV_1 with a portable spirometry screening unit before and after use. If he exhibits his usual amount of reversibility, this is indirect evidence of drug delivery. Also, ask him if he obtains relief when he uses the MDI during wheezing or chest tightness.

Assuming the MDI appears functional based on the preceding check, how would you explain the situation with hydrofluoroalkane (HFA) albuterol to the patient?

Answer: The HFA formulation of albuterol has a higher plume temperature and a lower plume force on actuation. It is a softer and gentler spray. Patients who may have used a chlorofluorocarbon (CFC) formulation of albuterol by MDI often think they are not getting the usual dose because they cannot feel the colder, forceful blast they experienced with the CFC formulation.

CHAPTER 4

Self-Assessment Questions
Prepared-Strength Dosage Calculations

1. A bottle is labeled Demerol (meperidine), 50 mg/cc. How many cubic centimeters are needed to give a 125-mg dose?

   Answer: 50 mg/1 cc = 125 mg/x cc; x = 2.5 cc.

2. Promazine HCl comes as 500 mg/10 ml. How many milliliters are needed to give a 150-mg dose?

   Answer: 500 mg/10 ml = 150 mg/x ml; x = 3 ml.

3. Hyaluronidase comes as 150 U/cc. How many cubic centimeters are needed for a 30-U dose?

   Answer: 150 U/cc = 30 U/x cc; x = 0.2 cc.

4. Morphine sulfate 4 mg is ordered. You have a vial with 10 mg/ml. How much do you need?

   Answer: 10 mg/ml = 4 mg/x ml; x = 0.4 ml.

5. A dosage schedule for the surfactant poractant calls for 2.5 ml/kg birth weight. How much drug will you need for an 800-g baby?

   Answer: 800 g × 1 kg/1000 g = 0.8 kg; 2.5 ml/kg × 0.8 kg = 2 ml.

6. Diphenhydramine (Benadryl) elixir contains 12.5 mg of diphenhydramine HCl in each 5 ml of elixir. How many milligrams are there in a one-half teaspoonful dose (1 tsp = 5 ml)?

   Answer: 1/2 teaspoon = 2.5 ml.
   12.5 mg/5 ml = x mg/2.5 ml; x = 6.25 mg.

7. A pediatric dose of oxytetracycline 100 mg is ordered. The dosage form is an oral suspension containing 125 mg/5 cc. How much of the suspension contains a 100-mg dose?

   Answer: 125 mg/5 cc = 100 mg/x cc; x = 4 cc.

8. How many units (U) of heparin are found in 0.2 ml, if you have 1000 U/ml?

   Answer: 1000 U/ml = x units/0.2 ml; x = 200 U.

9. Albuterol syrup is available as 2 mg/5 ml. If a dose schedule of 0.1 mg/kg is used, how much syrup is needed for a 30-kg child? How many teaspoons is this?

   Answer: 30 kg × 0.1 mg/kg = 3 mg
   2 mg/5 ml = 3 mg/x ml; x = 7.5 ml
   7.5 ml × 1 tsp/5 ml = 1.5 tsp

10. Terbutaline is available as 2.5-mg tablets. How many tablets do you need for a 5-mg dose?

    Answer: 2.5 mg/1 tab = 5 mg/x tab; x = 2 tablets.

11. If Tempra is available as 120 mg/5 ml, how much dose is there in 1/2 tsp?
Answer: 1/2 tsp = 2.5 ml; 120 mg/5 ml = x mg/2.5 ml; x = 60 mg.

12. Theophylline is available as 250 mg/10 ml and is given intravenously at 6 mg/kg body weight. How much solution do you give for a 60-kg woman?
Answer: 60 kg × 6 mg/kg = 360 mg; 250 mg/10 ml = 360 mg/x ml; x = 14.4 ml.

13. Terbutaline sulfate is available as 1 mg/ml in an ampoule. How many milliliters are needed for a 0.25-mg dose?
Answer: 1 mg/ml = 0.25 mg/x ml; x = 0.25 ml.

14. A patient is told to take 4 mg of albuterol four times daily. The medication comes in 2-mg tablets. How many tablets are needed for one 4-mg dose?
Answer: 2 mg/tab = 4 mg/x tab; x = 2 tablets.

15. Metaproterenol is available as a syrup with 10 mg/5 ml. How many teaspoons should be taken for a 20-mg dose?
Answer: 1 tsp = 5 ml.
10 mg/5 ml = 20 mg/x ml; x = 10 ml.
10 ml × 1 tsp/5 ml = 2 tsp.

16. If you have *d*-(+)-tubocurarine at 3 mg/ml, how many milliliters are needed for a dose of 9 mg?
Answer: 3 mg/ml = 9 mg/x ml; x = 3 ml.

17. If a dosage schedule requires 0.25 mg/kg of body weight, what dose is needed for an 88-kg person?
Answer: 0.25 mg/kg × 88 kg = 22 mg.

18. If theophylline is available as 80 mg/15 ml, how much is needed for a 100-mg dose?
Answer: 80 mg/15 ml = 100 mg/x ml; x = 18.75 ml.

19. How much drug is needed for a 65-kg adult, using 0.5 mg/kg?
Answer: 0.5 mg/kg × 65 kg = 32.5 mg.

20. The pediatric dosage of an antibiotic is 0.5 g/20 lb of body weight, not to exceed 75 mg/kg/24 hr.
a. What is the dose for a 40-lb child?
Answer: 0.5 g/20 lb × 40 lb = 1.0 g.
b. If this dose is given twice in 1 day, has the maximal dose been exceeded?
Answer: 2 doses = 2 × 1.0 g = 2.0 g = 2000 mg.
40 lb × 1 kg/2.2 lb = 18 kg.
2000 mg/18 kg = 111.1 mg/kg.
Yes, the maximal dose has been exceeded: two doses give 2000 mg/40 lb, which is 2000 mg/18 kg, or 111.1 mg/kg/day.

Percentage-Strength Problems

1. How many grams of calamine are needed to prepare 120 g of an ointment containing 8% calamine?
Answer: 0.08 = x g/120 g; x = 9.6 g.

2. One milliliter of active enzyme is found in 147 ml of solution. What is the percentage strength of active enzyme in the solution?
Answer: x = 1 ml/147 ml; x = 0.0068 = 0.68%.

3. If theophylline is available in a 250-mg/10 ml solution, what percentage strength is this?
Answer: x = 0.25 g/10 ml; x = 0.025 = 2.5%.

4. You have epinephrine 1:100. How many milliliters of epinephrine would be needed to contain 30 mg of active ingredient?
Answer: 0.01 = 0.03 g/x ml; x = 3 ml.

5. A dose of 0.4 ml of epinephrine HCl 1:100 is ordered. This dose contains how many milligrams of epinephrine HCl (the active ingredient)?
Answer: 0.01 = x g/0.4 ml; x = 0.004 g = 4 mg.

6. If you administer 3 ml of a 0.1% strength solution, how many milligrams of active ingredient have you given?
Answer: 0.001 = x g/3 ml; x = 0.003 g = 3 mg.

7. A drug is available as a 1:200 solution and the maximal dose that may be given by aerosol for a particular patient is 3 mg. What is the maximal amount of solution (in milliliters) that may be used?
Answer: 1:200 = 0.5% = 0.005; 3 mg = 0.003 g; 0.005 = 0.003 g/x ml; x = 0.6 ml.

8. Epinephrine 1:1000 contains how many milligrams per milliliter?
Answer: 1:1000 = 0.1% = 0.001; 0.001 = x g/1 ml; x = 0.001 g = 1 mg.

9. How many milligrams per milliliter are there in 0.3 ml of 5% strength metaproterenol?
Answer: 0.05 = x g/0.3 ml; x = 0.015 g = 15 mg.

10. How many milligrams of sodium chloride are needed for 10 ml of a 0.9% solution?
Answer: 0.009 = x g/10 ml; x = 0.09 g = 90 mg.

11. If you have lidocaine (Xylocaine) at 5 mg/ml, what percentage strength is this?
Answer: x = 0.005 g/ml; x = 0.005 = 0.5%.

12. A 0.5% strength solution contains how many milligrams in 1 ml?
Answer: 0.005 = x g/ml; x = 0.005 g = 5 mg.

13. Cromolyn sodium contains 20 mg in 2 ml of water. What is the percentage strength?
Answer: x = 0.02 g/2 ml; x = 0.01 = 1%.

14. How much active ingredient of acetylcysteine (Mucomyst) have you given with 4 cc of a 20% solution?
Answer: 0.2 = x g/4 cc; x = 0.8 g = 800 mg.

15. You have 20% acetylcysteine; how many milliliters do you need of this to form 4 ml of an 8% solution?
Answer: 0.08 = 0.2(x) ml/4 ml; 0.2(x) = 0.32; x = 1.6 ml, and saline qs for 4 ml.

16. The recommended dose of metaproterenol 5% is 0.3 cc. How many milligrams of solute are there in this amount?
    Answer: $0.05 = x$ g/0.3 cc; $x = 0.015$ g $= 15$ mg.

17. The Mucomyst brand of acetylcysteine was marketed as 10% acetylcysteine with 0.05% isoproterenol. How many milligrams of each ingredient were in a 4-cc dose of solution?
    Answer: Acetylcysteine: $0.10 = x$ g/4 cc; $x = 0.4$ g $= 400$ mg.
    Isoproterenol: $0.0005 = x$ cc/4 cc; $x = 0.002$ g $= 2$ mg.

18. Which contains more drug: 1/2 cc of a 1% drug solution with 2 ml of saline, or 1/2 cc of a 1% drug solution with 5 ml of saline?
    Answer: They each contain the same amount of drug: 5 mg ($0.01 = x$ g/0.5 cc; $x = 0.005$ g $= 5$ mg). The different amounts of diluent (2 ml, 5 ml) will change the resulting percentage strength and the total amount of new solution, but not the amount of drug.

19. How many milligrams per milliliter are in a 20% solution?
    Answer: $0.20 = x$ g/ml; $x = 0.2$ g $= 200$ mg.

Intravenous Infusion Rates

1. You wish to give a solution of 500 mg/L of dobutamine at a rate of 10 µg/kg/min, to a 50-kg woman. What drip rate will you need?
   Answer: Dose $= 10$ µg/kg/min $\times 50$ kg $= 500$ µg/min.
   Concentration $= 500$ mg/L $= 0.5$ mg/ml $= 500$ µg/ml.
   Flow rate (drops/min) $= 500$ µg/min $\times 1$ ml/500 µg $\times 15$ drops/ml $= 15$ drops/min.

2. If you have 2 mg of isoproterenol in 500 ml of solution, and you wish to deliver 5 µg/min intravenously, what drip rate is needed?
   Answer: Concentration $= 2$ mg/500 ml $= 0.004$ mg/ml $= 4$ µg/ml.
   Flow rate (drops/min) $= 5$ µg/min $\times 1$ ml/4 µg $\times 15$ drops/ml $= 18.75$ drops/min.

3. You have 250 mg of dobutamine in 1 L of solution. You want to deliver 5 µg/kg/min to a 60-kg man. What infusion rate in milliliters per minute, and in drops per minute, is needed?
   Answer: Concentration $= 250$ mg/1000 ml $= 0.25$ mg/ml $= 250$ µg/ml.
   Dose $= 5$ µg/kg/min $\times 60$ kg $= 300$ µg/min.
   Flow rate (ml/min) $= 300$ µg/min $\times 1$ ml/250 µg $= 1.2$ ml/min.
   Flow rate (drops/min) $= 1.2$ ml/min $\times 15$ drops/ml $= 18$ drops/min.

4. You have 250 ml of D_5W and a drip rate of 15 drops/min. How long will the bag of solution last?

Answer: Flow rate (ml/min) $= 15$ drops/min $\times 1$ ml/15 drops $= 1$ ml/min.
Time (min) $= 250$ ml $\times 1$ min/ml $= 250$ min.

5. You have an epinephrine solution, 1 mg/250 ml. What drip rate is needed to deliver 4 µg/min?
   Answer: Concentration $= 1$ mg/250 ml $= 0.004$ mg/ml $= 4$ µg/ml.
   Flow rate (drops/min) $= 4$ µg/min $\times 1$ ml/4 µg $\times 15$ drops/ml $= 15$ drops/min.

6. If you wish to deliver 500 ml of a solution in 1 hour and 40 minutes, what drip rate should you set?
   Answer: 1 hour and 40 minutes $= 100$ minutes.
   Flow rate (ml/min) $= 500$ ml/100 min $= 5$ ml/min.
   Flow rate (drops/min) $= 15$ drops/ml $\times 5$ ml/min $= 75$ drops/min.

7. A recommended dose of intravenous epinephrine is 15 ml/hr, using a solution of 4 µg/ml. What drip rate is needed to achieve the recommended infusion rate?
   Answer: Flow rate (ml/min) $= 15$ ml/hr $\times 1$ hr/60 min $= 15$ ml/60 min $= 0.25$ ml/min.
   Flow rate (drops/min) $= 0.25$ ml/min $\times 15$ drops/ml $= 3.75$ drops/min.

Clinical Scenario

Can you use the 1 N solution as diluent, unchanged?
Answer: A 1 normal (N) solution contains 1 g equivalent weight (GEW) of solute per liter of solution. If we calculate the percentage strength of a 1 N solution of NaCl, we can compare this with 0.9% to determine equivalence or lack of equivalence. The molecular weights of sodium (Na) and chlorine (Cl) are 23.0 and 35.5, respectively. A GEW is the molecular weight divided by the valence of the elements. So,

$$1 \text{ GEW, NaCl} = 23.0 \text{ g} + 35.5 \text{ g} = 58.5 \text{ g.}$$
$$1 \text{ N solution} = 1 \text{ GEW/L} = 58.5 \text{ g/L } or$$
$$5.85 \text{ g/100 ml} = 5.85\%.$$

Therefore a 1 N solution of NaCl is 5.85% strength and is not the same concentration as normal saline, which is 0.9% strength. A 0.9% solution would be 0.9 g/100 ml, not 5.85 g/100 ml. Use of the more concentrated 1 N solution, which is hypertonic relative to body fluid, may cause bronchial irritation in a nebulizer solution for inhalation.

CHAPTER 5
Self-Assessment Questions

1. Which portion of the nervous system is under voluntary control: the autonomic or the skeletal muscle motor nerve portion?
   Answer: The skeletal muscle motor nerve portion.

2. What is the neurotransmitter at each of the following sites: neuromuscular junction, autonomic ganglia, most sympathetic end sites?

Answer: Neuromuscular junction—acetylcholine. Autonomic ganglia—acetylcholine. Most sympathetic end sites—norepinephrine.

3. Where are muscarinic receptors found?

Answer: At parasympathetic nerve terminal sites.

4. What is the effect of cholinergic stimulation of airway smooth muscle?

Answer: Bronchoconstriction.

5. What is the effect of adrenergic stimulation on the heart?

Answer: Increased rate and force of contraction.

6. Classify the drugs pilocarpine, physostigmine, propranolol, and epinephrine.

Answer: Pilocarpine—direct-acting cholinergic. Physostigmine—indirect-acting cholinergic. Propranolol—adrenergic-blocking agent (β_1 and β_2). Epinephrine—adrenergic agonist (stimulates α and β receptors).

7. How do indirect-acting cholinergic agonists (parasympathomimetics) produce their action?

Answer: Indirect-acting parasympathomimetics, such as neostigmine, inhibit the enzyme cholinesterase, which increases the amount of acetylcholine available to stimulate postsynaptic sites at the nerve terminal.

8. What effect would the drug atropine have on the eye and on airway smooth muscle?

Answer: Atropine is a competitive blocking agent for muscarinic receptors. The drug would block the eye circular iris muscle to dilate the pupil (mydriasis), paralyze the ciliary muscle to flatten the lens (cycloplegia), and antagonize cholinergically induced bronchoconstriction in the airway.

9. What is the general difference between α and β receptors in the sympathetic nervous system?

Answer: The α receptors generally cause an excitatory effect (e.g., vasoconstriction), and β receptors generally produce inhibition (e.g., airway smooth muscle relaxation).

10. What is the primary mechanism for terminating the neurotransmitters acetylcholine and norepinephrine?

Answer: Acetylcholine is metabolized by cholinesterase enzymes; norepinephrine is reabsorbed back into the presynaptic neuron.

11. What is the predominant sympathetic receptor type found on airway smooth muscle?

Answer: The β_2 receptor.

12. Identify the adrenergic receptor preference for phenylephrine, norepinephrine, epinephrine, and isoproterenol.

Answer: Phenylephrine—α receptors (α_1 specifically). Norepinephrine—$\alpha > \beta$ receptors. Epinephrine—α and β receptors equally. Isoproterenol—β (β_1 and β_2 receptors).

13. What is the autoregulatory receptor on the sympathetic presynaptic neuron?

Answer: α_2 Receptors.

14. Classify the following drugs by autonomic class and receptor preference: dopamine, ephedrine, albuterol, phentolamine, propranolol, and prazosin.

Answer: Dopamine—sympathomimetic (dopamine receptors, α, β). Ephedrine—sympathomimetic (α and β). Albuterol—sympathomimetic (β_2 preferential). Phentolamine—α sympatholytic (α_1 and α_2). Propranolol—β sympatholytic (β_1 and β_2). Prazosin—α_1 sympatholytic.

15. What is the autoregulatory receptor on the parasympathetic presynaptic neuron at the terminal nerve site?

Answer: The muscarinic receptor subtype M_2.

16. Contrast α_1 and α_2 receptor effects, in general.

Answer: α_1-Receptor effects are generally excitatory (e.g., vasoconstriction of peripheral blood vessels). α_2-Receptor effects are generally inhibitory (e.g., inhibition of norepinephrine release from nerve terminals).

17. What substance may be the neurotransmitter in the NANC (nonadrenergic, noncholinergic) inhibitory nervous system in the lung?

Answer: Vasoactive intestinal peptide (VIP) or possibly nitric oxide (NO).

18. What substance is the neurotransmitter in the NANC excitatory nervous system in the lung?

Answer: Substance P.

Clinical Scenario

What may have led to the wheezing and dyspnea of the patient?

Answer: This is an example of altering the balance of autonomic control in the lung. Propranolol (Inderal) is a nonspecific β blocker (β_1 and β_2). As a β_1-blocking agent, the drug will slow the heart rate. However, the blockade of β_2 receptors in the airway prevents endogenous epinephrine and exogenous adrenergic agents from stimulating those receptors. The intravenous dose directly antagonizes the effect of the β-receptor stimulation in the airways with the adrenergic bronchodilator albuterol, and it inhibits the degree of bronchodilation achieved in this asthmatic, whose airways tend to react to stimuli and constrict. The balance between adrenergic relaxation of the airway and cholinergic constriction is tipped in favor of unbalanced cholinergic activity. She begins to exhibit symptoms of bronchoconstriction (wheezing, dyspnea).

What changes in the therapeutic approach would you suggest in a case such as this?

Answer: Prevention is the best approach. In a patient such as an asthmatic, β-receptor stimulation is an important property to preserve. The use of a drug other than a β-blocking agent would be indicated for the supraventricular tachycardia (SVT), to avoid the undesirable side effect of β blockade in the lung. Alternative drugs for tachycardia are discussed in subsequent chapters; these would include a calcium channel–blocking agent such as verapamil or an agent such as adenosine. Her use of the β-adrenergic bronchodilator albuterol, which is a β_2 agonist, should also be reviewed, to ensure proper dosage and frequency of use. Although β_2 specific, an adrenergic agonist can stimulate the heart.

CHAPTER 6

Self-Assessment Questions

1. Identify three adrenergic bronchodilators used clinically that are catecholamines.
   Answer: Epinephrine, isoproterenol, isoetharine.
2. Which of the catecholamine bronchodilators given by aerosol is β_2 specific?
   Answer: Isoetharine.
3. What is the duration of action of the catecholamine bronchodilators?
   Answer: Approximately 1.5 hours; up to 3 hours at most.
4. Identify two advantages introduced with the modifications of the catecholamine structure in adrenergic bronchodilators.
   Answer: Increased β_2 specificity and longer duration of action.
5. Identify the usual dose by aerosol for an SVN for levalbuterol and albuterol.
   Answer: Levalbuterol—0.63 to 1.25 mg.
   Albuterol—0.5 cc of a 0.5% concentration.
6. What is an extremely common side effect with β_2-adrenergic bronchodilators?
   Answer: Muscle tremor.
7. Identify the approximate duration of action for isoetharine, pirbuterol and salmeterol.
   Answer: Isoetharine—1 to 3 hours.
   Pirbuterol—4 to 6 hours.
   Salmeterol—12 hours.
8. Identify the generic drug for each of the following brand names: Alupent, Tornalate, Maxair, Serevent, Ventolin.
   Answer: Alupent—metaproterenol.
   Tornalate—bitolterol.
   Maxair—pirbuterol.
   Serevent—salmeterol.
   Ventolin—albuterol.
9. Which route of administration is more likely to have greater severity of side effects with a β agonist, oral or inhaled aerosol?
   Answer: Oral (tremor is more severe).
10. You notice a pinkish tinge to aerosol rainout in the large-bore tubing connecting a patient's mouthpiece to a nebulizer after a treatment with racemic epinephrine; what has caused this?
    Answer: The catecholamine epinephrine will be broken down by light and air to the adrenochrome form, producing a pinkish, or pinkish-brown residue in tubing.
11. A patient exhibits paradoxical bronchoconstriction from the Freon propellant when using his albuterol by MDI. Suggest an alternative for the patient.
    Answer: Consider trying the HFA formulation or an alternative delivery form such as a nebulizer solution. If the albuterol is effective with the patient, this will allow him to continue use of the drug.
12. If you are working with an asthmatic with occasional symptoms of wheezing and chest tightness, which respond well to an inhaled β agonist, would you suggest using salmeterol?
    Answer: No; salmeterol is indicated for maintenance therapy of asthmatics needing regular use of a β agonist or step 2 therapy (regular β agonist and inhaled corticosteroid or other agents).
13. Suggest a β agonist that would be appropriate for the patient in question 12.
    Answer: Any of the following: albuterol, pirbuterol, levalbuterol, metaproterenol.

Clinical Scenario

How could you assess the presence of airflow obstruction in this patient?

Answer: A peak expiratory flow measure, which indicates approximately 80% of his predicted value. Alternatively, office spirometry would provide more complete information on his FEV_1 and mid-maximal flow rates. A "before and after" bronchodilator study would further determine if he has *reversible* obstruction; however, his history and symptoms suggest this.

Given his symptoms, your physical findings, and a reduced peak flow, would you recommend a β agonist?

Answer: Yes. He exhibits measures of airflow obstruction, and it is reasonable to treat him with a bronchodilator.

If you recommend a bronchodilator, suggest an appropriate agent.

Answer: A $β_2$-selective, short-acting inhaled drug would be appropriate for relief now. This could include levalbuterol, albuterol, pirbuterol, or metaproterenol. A long-acting agent such as salmeterol is not appropriate because of its time course.

How could you assess his response to a β-agonist bronchodilator?

Answer: The simplest approach is to wait about 15 minutes after he inhales the β agonist and test his peak flow again or his FEV_1. Improvement in his flow rate indicates reversibility.

At this point, suggest a β agonist to prescribe for his use at home or work when he leaves the clinic.

Answer: At the least, he needs a rescue β-agonist bronchodilator. A short-acting agent such as albuterol, pirbuterol, or levalbuterol in an MDI would be appropriate.

What type of instructions and follow-up would you suggest for this patient?

Answer: First, be sure to demonstrate correct use of the MDI, with a return demonstration using a placebo inhaler. If he has difficulty, a holding chamber should be prescribed. Second, he should be given a basic action plan to deal with recurrences of bronchospasm, which includes how much and often to use his β-agonist inhaler and when to seek help. Third, follow-up testing for allergies and to establish a diagnosis of asthma requires an immediate referral to a pulmonologist or an allergist, for more complete assessment, ongoing monitoring, and management.

CHAPTER 7

Self-Assessment Questions

1. What was the first U.S. Food and Drug Administration (FDA)–approved anticholinergic bronchodilator for aerosol inhalation?
   Answer: Ipratropium (Atrovent).
2. What is the usual recommended dose of ipratropium by MDI and by SVN?
   Answer: MDI: 36 μg, two actuations, each 18 μg (from the mouthpiece). SVN: 500 μg, 2.5 ml of a 0.02% solution.

3. Identify a long-acting anticholinergic bronchodilator and give its duration of action.
   Answer: Tiotropium (Spiriva); duration of effect up to 24 hours.
4. What is the usual clinical indication for use of an anticholinergic bronchodilator such as ipratropium?
   Answer: Maintenance treatment of chronic obstructive pulmonary disease (COPD).
5. Which disease state, asthma or COPD, may show greater response to an anticholinergic bronchodilator than a β agonist?
   Answer: COPD patients are likely to have a greater response to an anticholinergic agent rather than a β agonist in reversibility of airflow obstruction.
6. With which type of anticholinergic agent are you more likely to observe systemic side effects: the tertiary ammonium or quaternary ammonium compounds?
   Answer: Tertiary; these are less ionized and are better absorbed and distributed through body tissues.
7. What are the most common side effects seen with inhaled ipratropium?
   Answer: Dry mouth and cough.
8. Can ipratropium be used with subjects who have glaucoma?
   Answer: Yes. However, use with caution, have patient notify the ophthalmologist, and monitor intraocular pressures.
9. Can ipratropium be alternated with or combined with a β agonist in the treatment of COPD and asthma?
   Answer: Yes. The two types of agents may have additive effects in reversing airflow obstruction. In addition, they have complementary sites and mechanisms of action, and the time to peak effect is later for ipratropium compared with that of a β agonist, resulting in more sustained peak bronchodilation.
10. What precautions should you observe if administering ipratropium by SVN?
    Answer: Protect the eyes from exposure to nebulized drug, using a mouthpiece instead of a mask whenever possible or covering the eyes if a facemask is used for administration. This is done to avoid ocular effects of mydriasis and cycloplegia.
11. What is the clinical indication for the use of an anticholinergic intranasal spray?
    Answer: Rhinorrhea associated with nonallergic perennial rhinitis, colds, and allergic rhinitis if unresponsive to intranasal corticosteroids.

Clinical Scenario

Would you recommend a bronchodilator for Mr. C.?

Answer: A bronchodilator should be considered after assessing the degree of reversibility of his airflow obstruction by spirometry after bronchodilator administration. In fact, Mr. C.'s forced expiratory volume in 1 second (FEV_1) and FEV_1/forced vital capacity (FVC) improved by approximately 20% with a β agonist.

What type of bronchodilator would you think best to start for Mr. C.?

Answer: An anticholinergic bronchodilator, specifically ipratropium or tiotropium, is indicated for maintenance treatment of COPD with reversible airflow obstruction. The most convenient formulation of Atrovent is an MDI and a starting dose of 2 puffs (inhalations) qid could be prescribed. Tiotropium is available only as a DPI and is prescribed once daily.

If Mr. C. has trouble with MDI use, what actions could you take?

Answer: First, review instructions for correct use of the MDI with Mr. C. and have him practice with a placebo inhaler. Second, consider using a reservoir device with the MDI.

Third, if he is unable or unwilling to use the MDI, you could change to the nebulizer solution.

What lifestyle change(s) would you emphasize to Mr. C.?

Answer: First and foremost, quit smoking. Give smoking cessation material and program information to him. Second, consider a rehabilitation or disease management educational program, to incorporate knowledge of the disease, its treatment options, exercise, and nutrition.

CHAPTER 8

Self-Assessment Questions

1. What drug in the xanthine group is used most often therapeutically?

   Answer: Theophylline (aminophylline).

2. What is the difference between aminophylline and theophylline?

   Answer: Aminophylline is a salt of theophylline, designed to increase aqueous solubility for intravenous administration.

3. What is the recommended therapeutic plasma level for theophylline in asthma?

   Answer: 5 to 15 µg/ml.

4. How do you know whether a given dose of theophylline will produce a satisfactory treatment effect in an asthmatic?

Answer: The most exact method is to monitor the plasma level of theophylline and adjust the dose to maintain a therapeutic plasma level. Alternatively, and less precisely, the dose can be adjusted to control symptoms and side effects.

5. Identify at least three adverse side effects seen with theophylline.

   Answer: Gastric irritation, insomnia, anxiety/shakiness, tachycardia, nausea, loss of appetite, headache.

6. What is meant by a "narrow therapeutic margin"?

   Answer: For a drug with a narrow therapeutic margin, the dose required to produce a therapeutic effect is close to the dose that begins to produce toxic side effects.

7. Although theophylline is a weak bronchodilator, what other effects make it useful in treating chronic airflow obstruction?

   Answer: (1) Stimulation of ventilatory drive in the central nervous system and (2) strengthening of diaphragmatic contractile force.

8. True or False: Theophylline causes bronchodilation and improved airflow by inhibiting phosphodiesterase, which breaks down cyclic adenosine 3′,5′-monophosphate (cAMP).

   Answer: False. The mode of action of theophylline is unclear.

Clinical Scenario

What is the first drug that is indicated by this individual's blood sample values?

Answer: Oxygen. Although a Po_2 of 64 mmHg on room air, with a saturation of 90%, appears to be satisfactory, this is achieved by a labored pattern of respiration, with tachypnea (respiratory rate [RR], 22 breaths/min), and is accompanied by increased blood pressure (170/112 mmHg) and tachycardia (120 beats/min). In addition, he is mildly anemic. Relieving his hypoxemia, and thereby reducing his work of breathing and myocardial work, may prevent the need for ventilatory support.

Would you continue use of ipratropium bromide; if so, what dose would you suggest?

Answer: Yes; ipratropium is a drug of choice in COPD, including an acute exacerbation. However, a dose of 2 inhalations from the MDI may well be insufficient and the dose should be titrated to 6 or 8 actuations for inhalation, given immediately with a reservoir device, because he is tachypneic and may have trouble coordinating breathing and actuation. A larger dose of ipratropium can be administered if the SVN solution of 500 µg is administered instead.

What additional bronchodilator therapy could you recommend?

Answer: A β_2 agonist, such as albuterol, pirbuterol, levalbuterol, or metaproterenol, should be administered by MDI with a reservoir preferably or, if available, as an SVN solution, by that mode. This should be administered at the same time as the ipratropium. In addition, this patient may benefit from theophylline.

What is the rationale for use of theophylline in this patient?

Answer: Theophylline has a weak bronchodilating effect in the airways, which may help reverse his airflow obstruction. In addition, the drug can strengthen diaphragmatic contractile force, improving his ability to ventilate, and the drug is a ventilatory stimulant. Finally, theophylline has been shown to reduce dyspnea, even in the absence of improvement in objective measures of airflow.

What would you check before initiating therapy with theophylline?

Answer: Question the patient on use of theophylline before his admission to the hospital. Although he did not state use of theophylline in his initial assessment, this should be checked before administering the drug, because there is a narrow therapeutic margin. If he does recall regular use of the drug, or any use before admission, a theophylline blood level should be checked as soon as possible.

What serum theophylline level would you target, if the patient is started on theophylline?

Answer: Optimal results with minimal side effects will be obtained with a blood level of 10 to 12 µg/ml in most patients.

CHAPTER 9

Self-Assessment Questions

1. Identify the two mucolytic agents approved for inhalation as an aerosol in the United States—give the generic and brand names.
   Answer: Dornase alfa (Pulmozyme), given 2.5 mg daily by jet nebulization; and *N*-acetylcysteine (NAC; or Mucomyst), 4 ml of a 10% solution by jet nebulization (however, the latter is not of proven benefit for airway disease).
2. What is the mode of action for dornase alfa?
   Answer: Depolymerizes extracellular DNA, decreasing sputum tenacity.
3. What is the clinical indication for use of dornase alfa?
   Answer: To promote secretion clearance in persons with cystic fibrosis.
4. What are contraindications to the use of mucolytic medications?
   Answer: Poor or absent cough reflex, weakness, inability to protect the airway, allergy or documented sensitivity to the medication used.
5. How do macrolide antibiotics affect mucus and what are their indications for use?
   Answer: Low-dose macrolide and azalide antibiotics are mucoregulatory medications that decrease mucus hypersecretion due to inflammation while preserving the normal or constitutive secretion.
6. How should dornase alfa be administered when high-frequency oscillation is used?
   Answer: It seems to be at least as effective, and probably easier to administer, when given concomitant with high-frequency chest wall compression (HFCWC).
7. What is a common side effect seen with NAC by aerosol?
   Answer: Bronchospasm, airway inflammation, and decreased pulmonary function.
8. What are the indications for the use of acetylcysteine?
   Answer: Acetylcysteine is approved for systemic use in treating acetaminophen overdose. There are no indications for giving this as an aerosol.
9. How and when should bicarbonate aerosol or instillation be used?
   Answer: Never.

Clinical Scenario

What aerosol medications would be indicated for her?

Answer: Her pulmonary function tests indicate mild to moderate airway obstruction, accompanied by the usual problematic secretions seen in cystic fibrosis. Her recent history also suggests recurrent pulmonary infections, with purulent sputum production and a need for intravenous antibiotic therapy and hospitalizations. She may benefit from dornase alfa (Pulmozyme), 2.5 mg daily by nebulizer. She may also find continued use of a β agonist such as albuterol helpful to improve or maintain lung function and secretion clearance. Finally, continued use of aerosolized antibiotic such as tobramycin should be considered to reduce the bacterial burden of her respiratory secretions.

What outcomes would you assess to determine the effectiveness of dornase alfa in her case?

Answer: (1) The use of parenteral antibiotics over the coming year; (2) the use of oral quinolones such as ciprofloxacin over the next year; (3) the need for hospitalizations for acute exacerbations; and (4) maintenance or hopefully even improvement in her pulmonary function.

CHAPTER 10

Self-Assessment Questions

1. What is the definition of a *surface-active substance*?
   Answer: An agent that can change surface tension at liquid-air interfaces.
2. In general, what is the clinical indication for use of exogenous surfactants?
   Answer: Prevention (prophylaxis) of respiratory distress syndrome (RDS) in premature newborns with immature lungs or newborns with evidence of immature lung development, and treatment (rescue) of infants who have developed RDS.
3. What type (category) of exogenous surfactant is each of the following: colfosceril palmitate, beractant, calfactant, and poractant alfa?
   Answer:
   Beractant (Survanta)—modified natural bovine extract.
   Calfactant (Infasurf)—natural bovine extract.
   Poractant alfa (Curosurf)—natural porcine extract.
4. What are the major ingredients of natural pulmonary surfactant?
   Answer: Lipids (about 90%), including dipalmitoyl-phosphatidylcholine (DPPC); proteins, 10%.
5. Give the dosage schedule of each of the current exogenous surfactants.
   Answer: Exosurf—5 ml/kg.
   Survanta—100 mg/kg, or 4 ml/kg.
   Infasurf—3 ml/kg.
   Curosurf—2.5 ml/kg.
6. What is the difference between "rescue" and "prophylaxis" treatment with these agents?
   Answer: Rescue—drug given in the presence of RDS. Prophylaxis—drug given *before* the onset of RDS.
7. Identify at least three possible adverse effects with use of exogenous surfactant treatment.
   Answer: Apnea, overventilation, overoxygenation, airway occlusion, desaturation, and bradycardia.
8. Why does the improvement in lung compliance last, after only one or two administrations of exogenous surfactant?
   Answer: Apparently, exogenous surfactant enters the recycling pool in alveolar cells.
9. How would you assess the effectiveness of exogenous surfactant treatment in a premature newborn with respiratory distress?
   Answer: Monitor vital signs, including color and activity, for evidence of airway occlusion, desaturation,

and bradycardia. Be prepared to manually ventilate and suction the airway. Assess changes in level of ventilation: chest rise, arterial oxygen saturation (Sa_{O_2}) or tcP_{O_2} transcutaneous oxygen pressure, and exhaled volumes or peak inspiratory pressures. Modify ventilator settings and fraction of inspired oxygen ($F_{I_{O_2}}$) on the basis of changes.

Clinical Scenario

Is there an indication for administration of an exogenous surfactant in this case? Support your decision with the available data.
Answer: Yes. The gestational age and low birth weight indicate prematurity, which is associated with lung immaturity and lack of endogenous surfactant. The chest radiograph confirms the presence of neonatal RDS. Beractant (Survanta) was chosen for administration, and arterial blood gas (ABG) values after treatment were as follows: pH, 7.38; Pa_{CO_2}, 48 mmHg; and Pa_{O_2}, 62 mmHg. There was good chest rise, and exhaled tidal volume averaged 5 to 6 ml/kg body weight. Pulse oximetry readings stabilized in the range of 93% to 96%. Over the next few hours, the $F_{I_{O_2}}$ was lowered to 0.60, and the peak inspiratory pressure (PIP) decreased to 17 cmH_2O.

Would this administration of surfactant be a rescue or prophylactic treatment, if given immediately after placement on ventilatory support?
Answer: Although RDS is present on the radiograph, immediate treatment with surfactant is considered prophylactic rather than rescue; the infant has not yet developed full-blown respiratory failure (note Apgar score at 5 minutes). However, this is likely to occur without treatment.

What pharmacological treatment is now indicated?
Answer: A second dose of surfactant should be administered in an attempt to reverse the subsequent decline in lung function indicated by the decrease in compliance, deteriorating vital signs, and oxygenation. Ventilation and oxygenation should be monitored after a repeat dose, and adjustments made to avoid overventilation and overoxygenation.

CHAPTER 11

Self-Assessment Questions

1. Identify all corticosteroids approved for clinical use by oral inhalation in the United States, using generic names.
   Answer: Beclomethasone dipropionate, triamcinolone acetonide, flunisolide, fluticasone, budesonide, and mometasone furoate.

2. What is the major therapeutic effect of corticosteroids?

Answer: Their antiinflammatory effect.

3. Identify two common respiratory diseases in which inhaled corticosteroids are prescribed.

Answer: Asthma, and (less frequently) chronic obstructive pulmonary disease (COPD).

4. What is the rationale for administering corticosteroids by the inhalation route, rather than by the oral route, in asthma?

Answer: By targeting the lung directly with corticosteroids that have high topical potency, systemic levels can be minimized and systemic side effects decreased or avoided.

5. Contrast the effects of β agonists with those of corticosteroids on the early phase and late phase of asthma.

Answer: β Agonists may relieve the early phase of bronchoconstriction, whereas corticosteroids can reduce airway inflammation, preventing both the early and late phases of asthma.

6. What is the effect of orally administered corticosteroids on growth, bone density, and adrenal function?

Answer: Growth is decreased in children; bone density is decreased, causing osteoporosis; normal adrenal steroid secretion is suppressed, and in general the hypothalamic-pituitary-adrenal (HPA) axis activity is suppressed.

7. What is the purpose of alternate-day steroid therapy?

Answer: To reduce exposure of the body to exogenous corticosteroids and thereby reduce systemic side effects, such as adrenal suppression.

8. Can you transfer an asthmatic patient from oral steroid use to inhaled steroid use? Explain the precautions or reasons, as appropriate.

Answer: Transfer can be accomplished; however, the patient should be weaned from the oral dose, using tapering doses while initiating inhaled steroids, to allow adequate recovery of adrenal function, because inhaled steroids will not maintain significant plasma levels at the recommended doses.

9. Identify a common side effect with inhaled steroids.

Answer: Oral thrush (candidiasis), dysphonia.

10. Identify two methods of minimizing the side effect identified in question 9.

Answer: (1) Use of a reservoir device with MDI orally inhaled corticosteroids; (2) rinsing of the throat with gargling after inhaling a corticosteroid.

11. Have inhaled corticosteroids traditionally been used with an asthmatic during an acute episode?

Answer: No; there is no acute bronchodilating effect, and the dose of inhaled steroids is too low for acute management of airway inflammation. However, inhaled corticosteroids have been investigated for emergency department treatment of acute severe asthma, along with aggressive bronchodilator therapy (see discussion in Chapter 11).

Clinical Scenario

What inhaled aerosol agents would you recommend as appropriate at this time for discharge?

Answer: A bronchodilator as a reliever and a corticosteroid as a controller would seem to benefit this individual, given her history. An inhaled steroid by either MDI or DPI, depending on drug choice, should be recommended. A shorter, more rapid-acting β agonist, such as albuterol by MDI, should also be prescribed for as-needed use in acute symptoms. Salmeterol by MDI twice daily can be added as an additional controller agent if symptoms persist and may prevent the need for increasing the inhaled corticosteroid dose. The combination products, fluticasone/salmeterol in a DPI formulation and budesonide/formoterol or fluticasone/salmeterol in an MDI, are available for convenient dosing.

What precautions and recommendations would you make with this patient?

Answer: Check to see whether she has been taking oral or intravenous steroids during her hospital stay; if so, taper the dose with oral prednisone while she begins using an inhaled steroid. This is intended to prevent adrenal suppression and exacerbation of symptoms. Instruct her to use a reservoir device with her inhaled steroid if an MDI formulation is prescribed, unless an integral spacing tube is supplied with the drug (e.g., triamcinolone acetonide, Azmacort). Instruct her to rinse her throat with water after inhalation to avoid oropharyngeal side effects such as dysphonia or oral thrush. Explain that poor compliance with the inhaled steroid will prevent a full therapeutic effect and that regular use is needed for control of airway inflammation, even though she may not "feel" an immediate effect. Clarify the use of the long-acting agent salmeterol versus the shorter-acting agent albuterol. Salmeterol is not helpful for acute symptoms, and overuse may lead to toxic accumulation. Albuterol has favorable pharmacokinetics for treating acute symptoms. Review the correct use of an MDI and reservoir device, with a return demonstration from the individual. Finally, she should be instructed in self-assessment with a peak flow–measuring device and told to contact her physician if her symptoms return and are not controlled by this regimen.

CHAPTER 12

Self-Assessment Questions

1. Identify five nonsteroidal antiasthmatic drugs used in the management of chronic asthma (give both generic and brand names).

   Answer: Cromolyn sodium (Intal), nedocromil sodium (Tilade), montelukast (Singulair), zafirlukast (Accolate), and zileuton (Zyflo).

2. Which immunoglobulin is implicated in allergy and is termed *cytophilic*?

   Answer: Immunoglobulin E (IgE).

3. Which type of asthma involves allergic reaction to an antigenic stimulus?

   Answer: Extrinsic, or atopic.

4. Which type of helper T cell, Th1 or Th2, is involved primarily in the atopic allergic response?

   Answer: Th2 cells (helper type 2 lymphocytes).

5. A resident wishes to order nebulized cromolyn sodium for a young asthmatic patient in the emergency department who is wheezing and in moderate distress. Would you agree?

   Answer: No. Cromolyn sodium, as a mediator antagonist, is a prophylactic agent to *prevent* mast cell degranulation and mediator release; the drug has no bronchodilating properties.

6. Which of the following could be recommended as possible choices for the asthmatic patient in question 5: inhaled albuterol, inhaled salmeterol, inhaled ipratropium, theophylline either orally or intravenously?

   Answer: All the agents listed could be used in an acute asthma episode, except for salmeterol, because its pharmacokinetics are not useful for an acute attack.

7. What is the usual dose of nedocromil sodium by inhalation in adults?

   Answer: By MDI, 2 actuations with 1.75 mg per actuation, four times daily.

8. An asthmatic patient has been taking 40 mg of oral prednisone for 1 week after an acute asthma attack and an emergency department visit. His physician now wants to switch him to inhaled nedocromil and discontinue the oral prednisone. What is the risk in doing this and what would you recommend?

   Answer: There is a risk of adrenal insufficiency caused by the steroid therapy and HPA suppression, and by the fact that nedocromil is not a steroid. A tapered dose regimen of the oral prednisone while the nedocromil is started should be recommended.

9. Briefly compare and distinguish the mode of action of nedocromil sodium versus cromolyn sodium.

   Answer: Nedocromil sodium has a broader effect, with inhibition of multiple inflammatory cells, including mast cell degranulation, eosinophil protein release, cytokine release from airway epithelial cells, suppression of adhesion molecules from epithelial cells (e.g., intercellular adhesion molecule-1 [ICAM-1]), and inhibition of sensory nerve activation; cromolyn sodium has a more specific action inhibiting IgE-mediated mast cell degranulation and mediator release.

10. How does the mode of action of zafirlukast and montelukast differ from that of zileuton?

    Answer: Zafirlukast and montelukast act by competitive antagonism of leukotriene receptors (CysLT$_1$ receptors), whereas zileuton acts by inhibition of the 5-lipoxygenase enzyme.

11. What are the recommended dose and route of administration for zafirlukast, montelukast, and zileuton?

    Answer: Zafirlukast—20 mg twice daily, by the oral route.

    Montelukast—10 mg once daily, orally.

    Zileuton—600 mg four times daily, orally.

12. Which of the three antileukotriene agents in question 11 offers the most convenient dosing and fewest drug interactions?

    Answer: Montelukast (Singulair), with once-daily dosing, and no significant drug interactions such as can occur with zileuton or zafirlukast.

13. When would you recommend using omalizumab?

    Answer: In a patient with uncontrolled moderate to severe asthma, especially uncontrolled by corticosteroids.

14. A 17-year-old asthmatic has been treated for symptoms for the last 12 months. His symptoms have not improved despite the use of the highest inhaled corticosteroid dose and regular use of salmeterol; in addition, trials on montelukast, cromolyn sodium, and oral theophylline have been unsuccessful. What would you recommend for this patient?

    Answer: Omalizumab would be a great recommendation. The use of omalizumab may be able to decrease the use of corticosteroids being administered.

Clinical Scenario

How would you treat her asthma attack at this point?

Answer: She was placed on oxygen at 2 L/min by nasal cannula and given albuterol, 4 actuations using an MDI with holding chamber, every 20 minutes. A plasma theophylline level showed 12.8 μg/ml. After approximately 1 hour (three albuterol treatments), her respiratory rate had decreased to 14 breaths/min, she appeared comfortable, and her wheezing had diminished, with breath sounds heard over both lung fields. She stated her chest felt "much more open." She was given a prescription for 1 week of oral prednisone, tapered dose, and asked to see her physician within a week.

What medications would you consider for maintenance of her asthma, given her recent history and prior medications?

Answer: Her increasing use of the inhaled β agonist on most days of the week indicates the need for an antiinflammatory agent. A trial of either cromolyn sodium or nedocromil sodium could be considered to target her inflammation. Given her recent cough symptoms, aspirin sensitivity, and history of nasal polyps, she may be a good candidate for use of an antileukotriene agent. Alternatively, the broad inhibitory effect of nedocromil sodium on the inflammatory process may prove beneficial. Either type of agent is an alternative to use of inhaled steroids. The inhaled β agonist should be continued. The theophylline could be discontinued in light of her headaches, gastrointestinal symptoms, and insomnia and replaced with either nedocromil or an antileukotriene while monitoring for any deterioration of her asthma symptoms. She was started on nedocromil sodium, 2 inhalations by MDI four times daily, together with pirbuterol, 2 to 4 inhalations as needed. She was also instructed in the use of a peak flow meter, to evaluate control of her symptoms. Because she had occasional mornings with chest tightness and a need for use of the pirbuterol, and because of more convenient dosing, she subsequently changed to oral montelukast, 10 mg each evening. She has done well on this combination of rescue β agonist and an antileukotriene.

CHAPTER 13

Self-Assessment Questions

1. Identify the disease states for each of these drugs is used when inhaled as an aerosol: pentamidine, ribavirin, tobramycin, and zanamivir.

   Answer: Pentamidine—Pneumocystis carinii pneumonia (PCP) prophylaxis in acquired immunodeficiency syndrome (AIDS) (last option).

   Ribavirin—respiratory syncytial virus (RSV) treatment with risk of severe or complicated infection. Tobramycin—management of *Pseudomonas aeruginosa* in cystic fibrosis.

   Zanamivir—treatment of acute influenza infection.

2. Briefly, what is the rationale for aerosolizing an antibiotic such as tobramycin in cystic fibrosis?

   Answer: The oral route gives inadequate lung levels; inhaled and intravenous routes give higher lung tissue levels.

3. What is the brand name of aerosolized pentamidine?

   Answer: NebuPent.

4. What is the dose and frequency for aerosolized pentamidine?

   Answer: 300 mg q4wk.

5. What device is approved for aerosolization of pentamidine?

   Answer: Respirgard II.

6. Identify the common airway effects with aerosolized pentamidine, and suggest a method for preventing or lessening these effects.

   Answer: Cough, bronchoconstriction; pretreat with a β agonist.

7. What is a major risk to the caregiver when aerosolizing pentamidine to a patient with AIDS?

   Answer: Contraction of tuberculosis (TB) infection.

8. What is the current Centers for Disease Control and Prevention (CDC)-recommended prophylactic treatment for PCP in AIDS patients?

   Answer: Use trimethoprim-sulfamethoxazole (TMP-SMX) orally as long as side effects are tolerated and acceptable. If side effects are too severe, switch to parenteral pentamidine. The use of inhaled pentamidine can be used; however, it not recommended by the CDC.

9. What is the brand name and dose for aerosol ribavirin?

   Answer: Virazole 6 g/300 ml (2%), 12 to 18 hr/day for 3 to 7 days.

10. What is the mode of action of ribavirin?

    Answer: Virostatic. As a nucleoside analog, ribavirin interferes with viral transcription and replication.

11. Identify two serious hazards when ribavirin is given to a patient undergoing mechanical ventilation.

    Answer: (1) Occlusion of endotracheal tube; (2) expiratory valve and sensor occlusion.

12. How, in general, can you prevent environmental contamination when delivering ribavirin to an oxygen hood?

    Answer: A containment/scavenging system around the hood.

13. What is the recommended dosage for inhaled tobramycin?

    Answer: 300 mg by PARI LC Plus SVN twice daily, alternating 28 days on/28 days off.

14. What common side effects have been observed with aerosolized tobramycin?

    Answer: Tinnitus and voice changes.

15. Identify two potential hazards to family members with aerosolized tobramycin at home.

    Answer: Exposure to aerosolized drug in ambient air may lead to (1) allergic reactions in those sensitive to the drug and (2) fetal harm in a pregnant female.

16. Give the brand name and dosage for zanamivir.

    Answer: Relenza 2 inhalations (10 mg) twice daily 12 hours apart, for 5 days.

17. In one sentence, describe the mode of action of zanamivir.

    Answer: Zanamivir inhibits the viral enzyme neuraminidase, causing viral aggregation and clumping, hence preventing viral release and spreading.

18. What are common hazards in the use of inhaled zanamivir?

    Answer: Pulmonary function deterioration, including bronchospasm in those with reactive airway disease, and inappropriate treatment or undertreatment of nonviral bacterial infections.

19. What factors cause debate over the use of zanamivir in treating influenza?

    Answer: Essentially cost versus efficacy—small reduction in symptoms; no inexpensive, easily available test to confirm influenza infection; increased possible risk in airway disease.

Clinical Scenario

What would you suggest as key elements of his respiratory care plan?

Answer: Continue with his usual cystic fibrosis medications (vitamins, iron supplement, Pancrease enzymes). *Oxygen* is indicated by his Sp_{O_2} (oxygen saturation by pulse oximetry) value. *Antibiotic therapy* will be needed to reduce his bacterial burden, as indicated by his temperature and WBC count. An aggressive program of bronchial hygiene is usual to clear his secretions, and would include *chest physiotherapy* with postural drainage and percussion as tolerated for mobilization of secretions; β_2 *agonist* by aerosol to maintain airway patency; possible administration of the anticholinergic bronchodilator *ipratropium* by either SVN or MDI; and, finally, adequate fluid intake and balanced nutrition.

What is the risk of using ciprofloxacin as an antibiotic to treat his symptoms of infection?

Answer: Because he has completed a course of ciprofloxacin and symptoms are now recurring, there is the possibility of resistance to the ciprofloxacin. A different, or at the least an additional, antibiotic may be needed.

His physician decides to institute a course of tobramycin rather than repeating the ciprofloxacin. Can this antibiotic be given orally as an effective antibacterial agent for Mr. P.'s respiratory infection?

Answer: No. Oral administration of aminoglycosides, antibiotics that are very effective in treating the gram-negative infections typical in cystic fibrosis, do not give suitably high lung levels.

Identify two alternative routes of administration for tobramycin in this case.

Answer: Either intravenously or by aerosol. Aerosol administration would directly target the lung.

Mr. P.'s physician orders intravenous tobramycin, as well as by aerosol, 300 mg bid, and he asks you to make a detailed suggestion on administration by nebulizer. What would you suggest?

Answer: The nebulizer used in clinical trials of aerosolized tobramycin was the PARI LC Plus. Other nebulizers may give suitable drug output and particle size. The PARI should be operated either by a suitable powerful compressor, such as the Pulmo-Aide, or used with 6 to 8 L/min of air powered by 50 psi. Administer the β_2 agonist by MDI before the antibiotic treatment. A nebulizer system with one-way intake and expiratory valves and a scavenging filter on the expiratory side is strongly recommended, to reduce personnel exposure to ambient aerosol of the antibiotic.

How would you evaluate (1) the aerosolized antibiotic therapy and (2) the treatment plan for Mr. P.?

Answer: (1) The aerosol antibiotic therapy can be evaluated during and after a treatment by monitoring respiratory rate and pattern, pulse, and breath sounds. (2) Over the course of his therapy, vital signs, including temperature, chest radiograph, WBC count, sputum production characteristics (color, amount, consistency), sputum cultures, and bedside spirometry (especially FEV_1) will provide information about his progress. The treatment plan described in the question above on key elements, including intravenous and aerosol tobramycin, was in fact successfully implemented, and Mr. P. steadily improved. On his eighth day postadmission, intravenous antibiotic therapy was discontinued, and on the eleventh day, Mr. P. was discharged, with no wheezing and some rales on auscultation of his lung fields.

CHAPTER 14

Self-Assessment Questions

1. What is the difference between bacteriostatic and bactericidal antimicrobial agents?

   Answer: Bacteriostatic agents inhibit the growth of bacteria, whereas bactericidal agents kill bacteria.

2. Describe the difference between antimicrobial agents that act in a concentration-dependent manner and agents that act in a time-dependent manner.

   Answer: Concentration-dependent antimicrobials have a proportional increase in their rate of microbial kill when their concentrations are increased. Time-dependent (or concentration-independent) antimicrobials do not have proportional increases in microbial kill with increasing concentrations of the agent. Time-dependent agents require maintenance of drug concentration above the minimal inhibitory concentration (MIC) (or some factor of the MIC) for optimal activity.

3. Describe at least three parameters that may indicate antibiotic failure in a patient.

   Answer: Continued fever spikes, elevated WBC count, repeated positive cultures, and nonresolution or worsening of symptoms (such as hypotension or mental status change) may indicate antibiotic failure.

4. Why is it useful to use combination antimicrobial therapy? (Be specific.)

   Answer: Antimicrobial combinations can provide broad-spectrum activity as part of an empiric regimen. Certain infections are polymicrobial and so require a combination of antimicrobials to be therapeutically effective. Antimicrobial combinations can be used for their synergistic effect and reduce the emergence of resistance.

5. Describe the mechanism of action of penicillin antibiotics. Name at least two additional antibiotic classes with similar mechanisms of action.

   Answer: Penicillins bind to cell wall proteins to inhibit the cross-linkage of peptidoglycan, which reduces the structural integrity of the cell wall, resulting in lysis. Cephalosporins, carbepenems, and monobactams have a similar mechanism of action.

6. Which β-lactam antibiotic is least likely to cause an allergic reaction in a patient with a penicillin allergy?

   Answer: Aztreonam.

7. Name three antimicrobial agents that would be useful in the treatment of community-acquired pneumonia.

   Answer: Azithromycin, clarithromycin, levofloxacin, gatifloxacin, moxifloxacin, cefuroxime, or erythromycin.

8. What is the antimicrobial agent of choice for the treatment of PCP?

   Answer: Trimethoprim-sulfamethoxazole.

9. What agents are considered first-line therapy for the treatment of pulmonary tuberculosis?

   Answer: Isoniazid, rifampin or rifabutin, pyrazinamide, and ethambutol.

10. Which antimicrobial agents are useful for the treatment of nosocomial pneumonia caused by *Pseudomonas aeruginosa*?

    Answer: Imipenem or meropenem or cefepime or ceftazidime or piperacillin/tazobactam plus an aminoglycoside (gentamicin, tobramycin, or amikacin) or ciprofloxacin.

Clinical Scenario

What signs and symptoms of infection in this patient are consistent with the diagnosis of community-acquired pneumonia?

Answer: The symptoms consistent with this diagnosis include productive cough, fever, chills, and shortness of breath. The signs of infection include his elevated temperature, heart and respiratory rates, decreased oxygen saturation, bilateral respiratory crackles, elevated WBC count, many WBCs in his sputum, and left lower lobe infiltrate on chest X-ray film.

What is the most likely pathogen responsible for community-acquired pneumonia in this patient?

Answer: The Gram stain reveals gram-positive cocci in pairs and chains, which is consistent with the most likely pathogen, *Streptococcus pneumoniae*.

Name two antibiotics that can be used to treat this patient's community-acquired pneumonia.

Answer: Numerous antibiotics may be used, including azithromycin, clarithromycin, levofloxacin, gatifloxacin, or moxifloxacin. A β-lactam (e.g., a penicillin or cephalosporin) must be avoided because of the patient's allergy history.

If the sputum stains are acid-fast positive, what precautions should be taken and what drug therapy should be initiated?

Answer: The patient must be placed in respiratory isolation, using a negative-pressure room. Health care personnel should wear fitted respiratory masks when tending to this patient. The patient should be initiated on isoniazid, rifampin, pyrazinamide, ethambutol, and pyridoxine for treatment of tuberculosis.

CHAPTER 15

Self-Assessment Questions

1. Identify the four classes of ingredients found in cold medications.

   Answer: Adrenergic decongestants, antihistamines (H_1 blockers), expectorants, antitussives. *Note:* An analgesic may be added.

2. For each of the following agents, identify the category (e.g., adrenergic, antitussive, etc.): codeine, chlorpheniramine, phenylephrine, dextromethorphan, pseudoephedrine.

   Answer: Codeine—antitussive.
   Chlorpheniramine—antihistamine.
   Phenylephrine—adrenergic.
   Dextromethorphan—antitussive.
   Pseudoephedrine—adrenergic.

3. What is the intended purpose of α-adrenergic agents in cold medications?

   Answer: Topical vasoconstriction, to open upper (nasal) airway.

4. What is the intended effect of antihistamines (H_1 blockers) in cold medications?

   Answer: To dry secretions (rhinitis) produced by histamine release and stimulation of H_1 receptors.

5. Are antihistamines in cold remedies H_1 or H_2 blockers?

   Answer: H_1 blockers. (H_2 blockers, e.g., ranitidine [Zantac], are antiulcer drugs.)

6. You drink several beers at a friend's house after taking a dose of Chlor-Trimeton. Should you drive home, and why or why not?

   Answer: No. Antihistamines cause drowsiness, and alcohol produces an additive effect on this—reflexes are decreased.

7. Identify the most common expectorant in over-the-counter (OTC) cold remedies.

   Answer: Guaifenesin (glyceryl guaiacolate).

8. Briefly explain how guaifenesin stimulates mucus production.

   Answer: Probably through stimulation of vagal receptors in the stomach.

9. List some specific fluids you would recommend to someone with a cold.

   Answer: Water, juices, milk.

10. Differentiate a "cold" from the "flu."

    Answer: Cold—nonbacterial upper respiratory infection with mild malaise and runny, stuffy nose (more localized than the flu).
    Flu—systemic viral infection with fever, chills, headache, muscle ache, extreme fatigue.

Clinical Scenario

What other symptoms would you ask about to differentiate his complaint as a cold versus the flu?

Answer: Temperature, headache, muscle ache, degree of malaise, and rapidity of onset. In response to questioning, he denies headache or muscle ache, describes the malaise as a very mild fatigue, and states that he noticed a gradually increasing rhinitis over a period of hours, with sneezing beginning during the first 6 hours of these symptoms. He has no fever. You could also ask if he has any ache in the area of his sinuses. A general question about history of any upper respiratory problems would be helpful.

What is your conclusion, at this point?

Answer: His symptoms indicate a cold rather than the flu.

Based on your information, what would you suggest to him for self-treatment?

Answer: Point out that there is no "cure" if this is a rhinovirus infection. He should treat his symptoms, however. An adrenergic *decongestant* may be helpful in opening his nasal passages and reducing some of the rhinitis. The use of a topical agent will give fewer systemic effects, such as a feeling of shakiness, and central nervous system stimulation than an oral agent. Caution him to use the decongestant sparingly to avoid rebound nasal congestion; treating the rebound congestion with additional sprays can produce a self-sustaining congestion. An antitussive agent, such as dextromethorphan, can be helpful if he has a nonproductive, dry, irritating cough, particularly if this prevents adequate rest at night. The use of an antihistamine should be avoided if possible, to prevent impaction of secretions and subsequent sinus problems. However, if an antihistamine is used, it should be taken only at night or when alert activity (including driving) is not needed. Rest and good nutrition, including juices, will assist his own immune response to recover from the infection.

What is your assessment now?

Answer: Based on his symptoms, there is a secondary infection, probably bacterial, causing an acute bronchitis. Identification of a causative organism would be desirable, but in its absence treatment with a broad-spectrum antibiotic should be considered. This could be with penicillin, tetracycline, or a third-generation cephalosporin to cover gram-negative bacteria.

CHAPTER 16

Self-Assessment Questions

1. What is the disease state in which an α_1-proteinase inhibitor (API) is indicated?

   Answer: Congenital α_1-antitrypsin deficiency.

2. What is the route of administration for α_1-proteinase inhibitor?

Answer: Intravenous.

3. What is the mode of action of α_1-proteinase inhibitor in treating emphysema associated with inadequate API levels?

Answer: Intravenous administration of exogenous α_1-proteinase inhibitor increases blood levels and diffuses into the lung tissue to increase epithelial fluid levels, where the API inactivates the enzyme neutrophil elastase (NE), which can destroy lung tissue.

4. Is treatment with API indicated for age-related emphysema or in general for those who smoke and have emphysema later in life?

Answer: No. Use of API is recommended only for those who have congenital α_1-antitrypsin (α_1-AT) deficiency and severe COPD. Such individuals often are smokers, which is a risk factor for development of COPD in α_1-AT deficiency, usually at an early age (third or fourth decade).

5. Identify three pharmaceutical formulations of nicotine that are used as smoking cessation aids.

Answer: The transdermal patch, chewing gum, lozenge, nasal spray, inhaler.

6. What is the usual effect of nicotine, whether in a smoking cessation aid or in cigarettes, on blood pressure?

Answer: Nicotine acts at the ganglionic synapses to increase blood pressure, with peripheral vasoconstriction; epinephrine is released from the adrenal medulla, contributing to hypertension, tachycardia, and vasoconstriction.

7. Name two nonnicotine agents used in the treatment of smoking cessation.

Answer: Varenicline (CHANTIX), bupropion (Zyban, Wellbutrin)

8. What is the effect of inhaled nitric oxide?

Answer: Relaxation of the pulmonary vascular endothelium and reduction of pulmonary hypertension.

9. Identify two potentially toxic by-products of inhaled nitric oxide.

Answer: Methemoglobin and nitrogen dioxide.

10. What is the usual dose of inhaled nitric oxide?

Answer: The recommended dose is 20 ppm, maintained up to 14 days or until the underlying oxygen desaturation has resolved and weaning from inhaled nitric oxide can be accomplished.

11. Identify two disease states in which nitric oxide has been used to reverse pulmonary hypertension.

Answer: Persistent pulmonary hypertension of the newborn and acute respiratory distress syndrome.

12. Can insulin be inhaled? Explain.

Answer: Exubera is available in 1- and 3-mg blisters of powdered insulin for inhalation. However, it should not be used in patients with uncontrolled lung disorders.

Clinical Scenario

Given this presenting scenario, what laboratory tests would you recommend Dr. G. obtain to further evaluate her respiratory status?

Answer: Important laboratory tests to evaluate her respiratory status would be a complete blood count (CBC) and differential, electrolytes, sputum sample, chest radiograph (anteroposterior and lateral), ABGs, and pulmonary function test. These tests were performed, and the results showed a mild elevation of her WBC count (13.1×10^3/mm^3), normal hemoglobin and hematocrit, normal electrolytes, and *Pseudomonas* and normal flora in her sputum. Her chest radiograph showed some hyperlucency; hyperinflation with moderately lowered, somewhat flattened hemidiaphragms on full inspiration; and an infiltrate in the right lower lobe. ABG values on room air were as follows: pH, 7.35; Pa$_{CO_2}$, 54 mmHg; Pa$_{O_2}$, 66 mmHg; HCO$_3^-$, 30 mEq/L; and Sa$_{O_2}$, 92%. Pulmonary function tests revealed an FEV$_1$ that was 60% of predicted, with an elevated residual volume (RV) and RV/total lung capacity (TLC) ratio, an increased TLC above predicted, and a decreased D$_{L_{CO}}$ (diffusing capacity of the lung for CO).

Based on her clinical picture and the laboratory results, what further test would Dr. G. want now?

Answer: Her clinical and laboratory findings support a diagnosis of chronic obstructive pulmonary disease (COPD). However, her smoking history is not sufficient to produce the degree of severity seen, and her age is incompatible with the usual presentation of COPD. You may want to obtain an α_1-proteinase inhibitor blood level. This was obtained, in fact, and her value was found to be approximately 5 µM, by the purified laboratory standard.

With these results, would the use of α_1-proteinase inhibitor therapy be indicated?

Answer: Yes. She was subsequently started on Prolastin, 60 mg/kg intravenously once a week, with a diagnosis of moderately severe emphysema secondary to α_1-proteinase inhibitor deficiency.

CHAPTER 17

Self-Assessment Questions

1. Can an aerosol formulation for oral inhalation be legally administered to neonates, infants, and pediatric patients?

Answer: Yes, using appropriate devices and techniques and with a duly licensed physician's order.

2. Can an adrenergic bronchodilator such as albuterol reduce airway resistance when used in neonates and children?

Answer: Yes. Multiple studies have found improved airway mechanics with aerosolized albuterol delivered by either MDI/reservoir system or nebulizer.

3. According to the data reviewed in this chapter, does the adult dose of an aerosol drug need to be reduced with neonatal and pediatric subjects, based on weight?

Answer: No. Because of multiple factors in neonatal and pediatric patients, the actual dose of an inhaled aerosol reaching the lungs is proportionately less than an adult lung dose and increases/decreases with increasing/decreasing age.

4. What aerosol delivery devices could be used with a 2-year-old child?

Answer: A nebulizer (with mask if necessary) or an MDI with a reservoir and mask.

Clinical Scenario

What methods of aerosol delivery are appropriate and available for albuterol in this age group?

Answer: Either an MDI or an SVN could be used, based on the age and patient interface (endotracheal tube, ETT).

After the decision was made to use an SVN, a dose of 1.25 mg was administered, but severe tachycardia developed. Would you consider levalbuterol?

Answer: You could utilize levalbuterol, a dose of 1.25 mg of levalbuterol is the maximal recommended dose. The use of lower doses may be appropriate.

What would you recommend to the physician?

Answer: A dose of 2.5 mg of albuterol is the maximal recommended dose. Because the side effect of sinus tachycardia is noted with this dose, it would be appropriate to reduce the dose. The dose schedule of 0.05 mg/kg would result in an ineffectively low dose of only 0.04 mg, which is less than 0.01 ml of a 0.5% solution. The minimal recommended dose of 1.25 mg would be reasonable and, in fact, was then delivered after allowing the heart rate to return to baseline. The heart rate remained at 164 to 176 beats/min throughout the subsequent treatment, and improved volume exchange was noted.

Where would you recommend placement of the SVN while administering the treatment to the ventilated patient?

Answer: Placement of the aerosol delivery device in the intubated infant requires clinician attention. Lung deposition with an SVN should be placed in the inspiratory limb away from the Y-piece.

CHAPTER 18
Self-Assessment Questions

1. List four general uses of skeletal muscle relaxants.
Answer: To facilitate endotracheal intubation
   - For muscle relaxation during surgery, particularly of the thorax and abdomen
   - To enhance patient-ventilator synchrony
   - To reduce intracranial pressure in intubated patients with uncontrolled intracranial pressure
   - To reduce oxygen consumption
   - To terminate convulsive *status epilepticus* and *tetanus* in patients refractory to other therapies
   - To facilitate procedures or diagnostic studies
   - For selected patients who must remain immobile (e.g., trauma patients)

2. What are the two classifications of neuromuscular blocking agents?
Answer: Nondepolarizing and depolarizing.

3. Identify each of the following agents by classification type: tubocurarine, vecuronium, succinylcholine, and pancuronium.
Answer: Tubocurarine—nondepolarizing. Vecuronium—nondepolarizing. Succinylcholine—depolarizing. Pancuronium—nondepolarizing.

4. Which type of neuromuscular blocker can be reversed?
Answer: Nondepolarizing.

5. What type of drug would you use to reverse vecuronium?
Answer: Cholinesterase inhibitor (e.g., neostigmine).

6. Identify another drug that you would want to give before you reverse the vecuronium.
Answer: Atropine or glycopyrrolate (antimuscarinic agents).

7. Briefly explain why you might need to paralyze a patient receiving mechanical ventilation.
Answer: To relax the chest wall and prevent spontaneous breathing efforts that are out of phase with the ventilator, causing increased intrathoracic pressure and decreased alveolar ventilation.

8. Neuromuscular blocking agents do not block consciousness; what two types or classes of drugs would be indicated in a paralyzed patient on mechanical ventilation?
Answer: Analgesics and sedatives.

9. Identify at least two neuromuscular blocking agents that would be preferred for paralysis in a patient receiving mechanical ventilation (assume normal renal and hepatic function).

   Answer: Doxacurium and vecuronium have minimal histamine release and cardiovascular effects; mivacurium, atracurium, and rocuronium are also alternatives.

10. You are called to the recovery room to set up a ventilator for a elderly patient who has just undergone a total hip replacement and has failed to breathe after a single dose of succinylcholine. What might the problem be?

    Answer: Atypical plasma cholinesterase.

11. What would you do first to assess a ventilated patient who is restless, and "fighting" the ventilator, before using a paralyzing agent?

    Answer: Assess ventilator function and patient status. Ventilator—possible malfunction; inappropriate settings (flow, F_{IO_2}, volume, inspiratory:expiratory [I:E] ratio, etc.)

    Patient-airway patency, Sao_2 or Spo_2, possible pain or anxiety requiring analgesia and sedation rather than paralysis.

Clinical Scenario

What additional laboratory information would be most helpful in assessing this patient and determining further treatment?

Answer: An arterial blood gas. Her low oxygen saturation indicates hypoxia and pulse oximetry does not give her pH or carbon dioxide level.

What neuromuscular blocking agent would you consider for a rapid-sequence intubation?

Answer: Either a nondepolarizing or a depolarizing agent could be used. However, succinylcholine has the advantage of rapid onset and short duration. This will avoid the need to manually ventilate the patient for several minutes, because of the slower onset of action when using a nondepolarizing agent. After sedation, succinylcholine was administered and the patient was nasally intubated.

What agent would you use?

Answer: A nondepolarizing agent is indicated in this situation, because a longer duration of action is needed for a patient requiring continuous paralysis. Options include pancuronium, vecuronium, cisatracurium, atracurium, pipecuronium, and doxacurium. An agent should be chosen based on side effect profile, route of elimination, potential drug interactions, and cost and formulary issues.

How will you monitor the effectiveness of this therapy?

Answer: Using peripheral (ulnar) nerve stimulation, the neuromuscular blocking drug should be titrated to maintain at least one twitch during train-of-four (TOF) evaluation. This will minimize the amount of blocking agent and prevent overdosage. TOF peripheral nerve stimulation should be monitored at 15- to 30-minute intervals while the neuromuscular blocking infusion continues. The goals of neuromuscular blockade in this patient should also be assessed. Ventilatory pressures with an adequate respiratory rate and I:E ratio should be seen. The improvement noted in arterial blood gases reflects improved gas exchange with the level of ventilatory support.

If the patient were in renal or hepatic failure, what neuromuscular blocking agent would you recommend?

Answer: This additional factor leads to consideration of atracurium or cisatracurium, neither of which is eliminated in the liver or kidneys. However, monitoring for cerebral toxicity and excitation caused by the metabolite, laudanosine, is needed. Alternatively, mivacurium provides a blocking agent not dependent on significant liver or kidney elimination. Mivacurium has a relatively short duration of action, which can be prolonged in end-stage liver or kidney disease. All three agents can cause more histamine release than vecuronium or pancuronium.

CHAPTER 19
Self-Assessment Questions

1. Mean arterial pressure is regulated by which two functions?

   Answer: Cardiac output and systemic vascular resistance.

2. Cardiac output is regulated by which two functions?

   Answer: Heart rate and stroke volume.

3. Which monitoring tool reflects the presence of hypovolemia and the need to administer fluids to a patient?

   Answer: Central venous pressure and pulmonary capillary wedge pressure.

4. Hypotension is first managed by what mode of therapy?

   Answer: Fluid administration.

5. Which catecholamine has pronounced and selective effects on dopamine receptors in the kidney, resulting in improved urinary output?

   Answer: None of the catecholamine agents has significant effects on the kidney; any effect of improved urinary output stems mainly from the improvement of cardiac output, which enhances perfusion to the kidney.

6. What are the four categories of sudden cardiac death?
   Answer: Ventricular fibrillation, pulseless ventricular tachycardia, pulseless electrical activity, and asystole.

7. What are the five classes of the Vaughan Williams classification system?
   Answer: Class IA, IB, IC, II, III, IV, and miscellaneous.

8. Which category of the Vaughan Williams classification is used solely for ventricular arrhythmias?
   Answer: Class 1B.

9. Which antiarrhythmic medication should be initiated with a rate-controlling medication?
   Answer: Quinidine.

10. Which antiarrhythmic agent is highly associated with the development of lupus erythematosus?
    Answer: Procainamide.

11. Which medications constitute the class II category of the Vaughan Williams classification system?
    Answer: Esmolol, propranolol, metoprolol, nadolol, and atenolol.

12. Which β blocker is included in category III within the Vaughan Williams classification system?
    Answer: Sotalol.

13. Which medication in category III within the Vaughan Williams classification system is no longer manufactured in the United States?
    Answer: Bretylium.

14. Which medication in category III within the Vaughan Williams classification system require continuous ECG monitoring postadministration for risk of developing ventricular arrhythmias?
    Answer: Ibutilide and dofetilide.

15. What is the appropriate method of administering adenosine?
    Answer: Because of its ultrashort half-life adenosine is best administered through a central line for rapid arrival at the site of action or, if given through a brachial line, the arm should be held in the upright position followed almost instantly by a saline flush.

Clinical Scenario

What are the doses of epinephrine and atropine?
Answer: Both epinephrine and atropine are given at a dose of 1 mg rapid IV push followed by a 20-ml normal saline flush.

What alternative agent could have been given instead of epinephrine?
Answer: Vasopressin at 40 units IV push may be given as a one-time dose in lieu of epinephrine.

What is the continuous infusion rate that the patient should be maintained on, to prevent the reoccurrence of ventricular fibrillation?
Answer: After administration of the 300-mg IV bolus, all patients should be started on continuous infusion, delivering amiodarone at a rate of 1 mg/min for 6 hours and then decreased to 0.5 mg/min for 18 hours, and eventually converted to the oral formulation.

What are the baseline parameters that need to be obtained prior to starting chronic amiodarone therapy?
Answer: Amiodarone is considered the culprit in a number of serious adverse effects such as pulmonary fibrosis, fulminant liver failure, hypo- and hyperthyroidism, optic neuritis, and Q-T interval prolongation. Therefore, a radiograph chest X-ray and an ECG should be obtained at baseline and then annually. The following monitoring parameters should be performed at baseline and then biennially: thyroid function tests, liver function tests, ophthalmic examination (more frequently if ocular symptoms occur), and pulmonary function tests (more frequently if dyspnea occurs). Serum creatinine and electrolytes are obtained to ensure adequate renal function, because the setting of renal insufficiency may cause electrolyte abnormalities potentiating ECG changes.

CHAPTER 20

Self-Assessment Questions

1. List the adverse effects associated with angiotensin-converting enzyme inhibitors (ACEIs).
   Answer: The most common ACEI-induced adverse effect is a persistent nonproductive dry cough, with an incidence of 20% to 30%. ACEI-induced adverse effects include rash, dysgeusia, hyperkalemia, orthostatic hypotension, blood dyscrasias, angioedema, and proteinuria.

2. Which of the β blockers possess intrinsic sympathomimetic activity (ISA)?
   Answer: The β blockers with ISA are acebutolol, carteolol, penbutolol, and pindolol.

3. Which of the β blockers possess selective β_1-blocker activity?
   Answer: Acebutolol, atenolol, betaxolol, bisoprolol, metoprolol

4. List the adverse effects associated with α_1-adrenergic antagonists?

   Answer: α_1-Adrenergic antagonist adverse effects include orthostatic hypotension, dizziness, syncope, reflex tachycardia, palpitations, and headaches. These adverse effects are generally a manifestation of the first-dose phenomenon.

5. What are the most common side effects of nitrates?

   Answer: The most common side effects of nitrates include tachycardia, palpitations, headaches, dizziness, and flushing.

6. List the metabolic effects associated with thiazide diuretics.

   Answer: The metabolic effects of thiazide diuretics include hypokalemia, hypomagnesemia, hypercalcemia, hyperuricemia, and hyperglycemia.

7. List five medications that may cause drug-induced increases in blood pressure.

   Answer: Five drugs that may cause drug-induced increases in blood pressure are venlafaxine, cyclosporine, ma huang, ibuprofen, and rofecoxib.

8. Which calcium channel blocker is most likely to cause constipation?

   Answer: Verapamil is the calcium channel blocker most likely to cause constipation.

9. What is the best parameter available to monitor the effects of warfarin?

   Answer: The international normalized ratio is the best parameter available to monitor the effects of warfarin.

10. What is the antidote for heparin?

    Answer: Protamine is the antidote for heparin.

11. What is the mechanism of action of warfarin?

    Answer: Warfarin exerts its effect by interfering with the hepatic synthesis of vitamin K–dependent clotting factors II, VII, IX, and X.

12. Name the pharmacological class responsible for inhibiting the final pathway in platelet aggregation.

    Answer: The glycoprotein IIb/IIIa inhibitors are responsible for inhibiting the final pathway in platelet aggregation.

13. Which thrombolytic is recommended for patients greater than 75 years of age who present with ST segment elevation myocardial infarction?

    Answer: Streptokinase is the thrombolytic recommended for patients greater than 75 years of age who present with ST segment elevation myocardial infarction.

14. Name the only ACEI that is available in a parenteral dosage form.

    Answer: Enalaprilat is the only ACEI that is available in a parenteral dosage form.

15. What is the best parameter available to monitor the effects of heparin?

    Answer: Activated partial thromboplastin time (APTT) is the best parameter available to monitor the effects of heparin.

16. Is clopidogrel or ticlopidine superior to aspirin for stroke prevention?

    Answer: Clopidogrel has no demonstrated superiority to aspirin, except for patients who have peripheral vascular disease. Both clopidogrel and aspirin are first-line therapy for stroke prevention. Ticlopidine has demonstrated superiority to aspirin; however, because of its deleterious side effect profile, ticlopidine is a second-line therapy for stroke prevention. Stroke prevention pharmacotherapy is lifelong.

Clinical Scenario

Is this patient a candidate for immediate administration of a glycoprotein IIb/IIIa inhibitor?

Answer: Yes, considering the significant role of platelets in non–ST segment elevation myocardial infarction, glycoprotein IIb/IIIa inhibitors would provide benefit by inhibiting platelet aggregation and thrombus formation after an atherosclerotic plaque rupture. The use of glycoprotein IIb/IIIa inhibitors reduces the risk of death or nonfatal myocardial infarction.

Is this patient a candidate for immediate administration of thrombolytic therapy?

Answer: No. This patient does not have ST segment elevation myocardial infarction and therefore is not a candidate for thrombolytic therapy. Immediate reperfusion of the infarcted artery is indicated in patients with persistent ST segment elevations. Whether thrombolytics are beneficial in non–ST segment elevation myocardial infarction has not been well elucidated and studies are being conducted in this area.

CHAPTER 21

Self-Assessment Questions

1. What is a diuretic?

   Answer: A diuretic is any substance that increases urine output.

2. Identify the five major groups of diuretics used clinically.

   Answer: Osmotic, carbonic anhydrase inhibitors, thiazide, loop, and potassium sparing.

3. If an agent such as one of the loop diuretics causes a loss of potassium, how will this lead to a metabolic alkalosis?

Answer: Sodium that is still reabsorbed will exchange for either potassium or hydrogen. Low potassium, resulting from excretion, forces reabsorbed sodium to exchange for hydrogen, depleting hydrogen ions and raising pH. Hydrogen is also excreted as a result of the diuretic, adding to the alkalosis. Potassium replacement is usually necessary to prevent hypokalemia.

4. Which diuretics would preserve potassium?
   Answer: The potassium-sparing agents, such as amiloride, triamterene, or spironolactone.

5. What is the potential effect of a carbonic anhydrase inhibitor on acid–base balance?
   Answer: A loss of bicarbonate, leading to metabolic acidosis.

6. Explain how a diuretic such as furosemide can be helpful in acute congestive (left ventricular) heart failure with pulmonary and vascular edema?
   Answer: A potent diuretic such as furosemide will cause excretion of volume from the circulatory system by limiting sodium and therefore water retention. This will decrease the amount of volume leaking from the vasculature both in the lung and in the periphery, as well as venous return to the heart. Reduced pulmonary edema will improve oxygenation, which will also improve oxygen available to the heart. Reduced preload also reduces the work of the myocardium. Reduced preload and improved oxygenation are beneficial to restoring heart function.

7. Which diuretic agent has a vasodilatory effect when used chronically?
   Answer: Hydrochlorothiazide (HCTZ).

8. In an otherwise healthy adult with mild hypertension, what diuretic agent should be considered as the first line of treatment?
   Answer: HCTZ.

9. Match each set of drugs on the left with the most likely interaction on the right.

Gentamicin **PLUS** furosemide	Hyperglycemia
Hydrochlorothiazide **PLUS** prednisone	Ototoxicity and nephrotoxicity
Spironolactone **PLUS** enalapril	Hyperkalemia
Hydrochlorothiazide **PLUS** carbamazepine	Hyponatremia

Clinical Scenario

True or False: In addition to oxygen and morphine sulfate 2 mg intravenously, a thiazide-type diuretic should be administered immediately.

Answer: False. Thiazide diuretics are generally relatively weak in their effect and have a slow onset of action. They are typically used when mild diuresis is needed or as a treatment for chronic hypertension. In acute pulmonary edema, more vigorous diuresis is needed. The patient should be given an intravenous diuretic that acts primarily in the loop of Henle (a loop diuretic). Any of the available loop diuretics would be acceptable. In general, because of its higher incidence of side effects, ethacrynic acid is reserved for patients who are allergic to the other loop diuretics or who fail to respond to them. This patient is currently taking furosemide 40 mg daily; thus an acceptable approach would be to double the oral dose and give it intravenously. Therefore furosemide 80 mg intravenously would be a reasonable choice.

If the patient fails to respond to furosemide 80 mg intravenously, should another loop diuretic be tried?

Answer: No. If within 30 to 45 minutes of receiving intravenous furosemide, the patient has not begun to diurese, another loop diuretic would be reasonable. However, typically the preceding dose of furosemide would be doubled, that is 160 mg, and administered. There are no substantial data supporting the superiority of one loop diuretic over another.

True or False: When the patient begins to diurese, close observation of the potassium level will be needed.

Answer: True. The patient does have mild renal insufficiency and is taking a β blocker. Both of these probably attenuate the normal potassium wasting seen with diuretics; however, with vigorous diuresis, he would most certainly become hypokalemic without potassium replacement. This can lead to dangerous arrhythmias, particularly in patients with ischemic cardiomyopathy. The potassium should be monitored closely and repleted to a level of 4.0 mEq/L or greater.

CHAPTER 22
Self-Assessment Questions

1. What is the difference between sedation and analgesia?
   Answer: Sedation—decreased response to stimuli, relaxes.
   Analgesia—relief of pain.

2. Identify the general class of each of the following agents (sedative-hypnotic, analgesic, tranquilizer, anesthetic, antipsychotic):
   Answer: Lorazepam—minor tranquilizer (antianxiety).
   Phenobarbital—sedative-hypnotic.
   Doxapram—respiratory stimulant.

Chloral hydrate—nonbarbiturate sedative-hypnotic.
Thiopental—general (intravenous) anesthetic.
Midazolam—general anesthetic.
Nitrous oxide—general anesthetic (gas).
Chlorpromazine—antipsychotic.
Halothane—general anesthetic (gas).
Morphine—narcotic analgesic.
Ibuprofen—nonsteroidal antiinflammatory drug (NSAID), analgesic.

3. You are planning to extubate and remove a patient from the ventilator. However, the nurse administers a large dose of lorazepam (Ativan) for anxiety. What problem may occur if you proceed?
   Answer: Hypoventilation, depressed ventilatory drive.

4. What is the most serious side effect of tranquilizers, sedatives, or analgesics (especially opioids)?
   Answer: Central nervous system depression resulting in respiratory depression—hypoventilation or respiratory arrest.

5. You have two patients, both of whom have overdosed on central nervous system depressants.
   Patient 1: Comatose, cyanotic, dilated pupils.
   Patient 2: Comatose, cyanotic, pinpoint pupils.
   Which patient may have taken a barbiturate and which a narcotic analgesic?
   Answer: Barbiturate—Patient 1.
   Narcotic—Patient 2.

6. Identify your initial priorities as a respiratory therapist in caring for a subject with an overdose of tranquilizers.
   Answer: (1) Maintenance or establishment of airway.
   (2) Provide ventilation.
   (3) Supplemental O_2 as needed to maintain PaO_2.

7. What is the mode of action of the benzodiazepines?
   Answer: Benzodiazepines bind to benzodiazepine receptors in the central nervous system, and facilitate the action of γ-aminobutyric acid in inhibiting neuronal transmission through increased chloride ion flow.

8. Identify an agent that can reverse the effects of benzodiazepines such as midazolam and triazolam.
   Answer: Flumazenil.

9. Will barbiturates be helpful in managing pain in a ventilator patient?
   Answer: No, unless a dose capable of producing unconsciousness is used. There is no direct effect on pain transmission.

10. Would meperidine be helpful to prevent or lessen perception of pain?
    Answer: Yes. Meperidine (Demerol) is a morphine-like narcotic and will occupy opiate receptors to block nerve transmission of pain.

11. For a patient with a bleeding disorder, such as hemophilia, or one who is taking anticoagulants such as warfarin, suggest an analgesic for minor pain.
    Answer: Acetaminophen would be the drug of choice. Aspirin and NSAIDs can both inhibit platelet aggregation and prolong bleeding times, even in normal subjects, and should be avoided in those with bleeding disorders.

12. Are there any serious side effects to use of a ventilatory stimulant such as doxapram?
    Answer: Yes—central nervous system stimulation to the point of seizures.

Clinical Scenario

What are the toxic side effects of TCAs, and what class of drugs (and what drug in particular) do they mimic in this regard?
Answer: Tricyclic antidepressants (TCAs) act to relieve depression by inhibiting the reuptake of norepinephrine or serotonin at the presynaptic junction in the central nervous system. However, these agents, including amitriptyline, have sedating, vasodilating, and anticholinergic effects. They can depress ventilatory drive and cause hypotension, particularly orthostatic hypotension. Their anticholinergic effects result in tachycardia, dry and warm or hot skin, blurred and unfocused vision (paralysis of accommodation), mydriasis, increased intraocular pressure, constipation, and possible urinary retention. Confusion or other mental changes may occur. A "quinidine-like" effect can prolong the PR, QRS, and QT intervals. Their anticholinergic effects mimic the action of atropine sulfate, and this can help in understanding the effects of an overdose of TCAs. Note many of these effects in this patient: HR, 140 beats/min; BP, 110/60 mmHg, pupillary mydriasis; very warm and dry skin; T, 39° C; absent bowel sounds; and prolonged PR and QRS intervals.

How is TCA overdose typically treated?
Answer: Instillation of activated charcoal slurry, in this case via the nasogastric tube, can reverse absorption of the drug from the gastrointestinal tract. Blood pressure is maintained with intravenous fluids. ECG monitoring is needed to detect changes in the P-QRS-T patterns and intervals. In the event of respiratory depression, the airway should be secured by endotracheal intubation to prevent aspiration pneumonitis and to provide for positive-pressure ventilation. Ventilatory support is maintained until the central nervous system depressant effects, particularly respiratory, have decreased, allowing a return to adequate spontaneous ventilation.

Why did the patient awaken and then fall back asleep in between doses of activated charcoal?

Answer: As the charcoal progresses through the gastrointestinal tract and is expelled, a favorable gradient for TCA diffusion from interstitial and adipose tissue to the bloodstream exists, causing a subsequent rise in blood levels of TCA, along with a renewed depressant effect. This continues until levels of TCA in the body are reduced to a sufficiently low level.

What implications does this phenomenon have for respiratory therapists in freeing TCA-overdosed patients from the ventilator? When would it have been deemed safe to extubate this patient?

Answer: Extubation and termination of ventilatory support levels should be delayed until the patient no longer falls asleep before the next dose of charcoal is due. If the patient is able to maintain his level of consciousness and adequate ventilation for more than 6 hours, this would indicate a low level of remaining drug. Blood levels of TCA should be checked to determine the success of charcoal treatment, but this is clinically helpful only if the results are available within a few hours of taking the sample.

What did the ABG values on T-piece imply regarding the patient's ventilatory status? Could the patient have been extubated with these particular ABG values? Why or why not?

Answer: Compared with the previous ABG values (pH, 7.43; CO_2, 40 torr), the ABG values on T-piece indicate decreased ventilation (pH, 7.36; CO_2, 48 torr). This trend, coupled with the degree of drowsiness and sedation observed, implies that the levels of TCA have not been reduced sufficiently, and the depressant effects still prevail, jeopardizing adequate ventilation. Extubation at this point would have been premature, because the ABG values indicate a trend of hypoventilation and documents continuing depressant effects of the drug. Extubation with depressed ventilatory drive could then result in respiratory or cardiac arrest.

Was supplemental oxygen ever needed for this patient? Why or why not?

Answer: No. An estimate of his $(A-a)D_{O_2}$ before placement on the T-piece shows a gradient of 35 torr on an $F_{I_{O_2}}$ of 0.35. There is no indication of impaired oxygenation, either by pulmonary history or by clinical signs. With adequate ventilation, gas exchange should be normal in this patient.

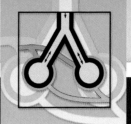

Units and Systems of Measurement

SCIENTIFIC NOTATION

Scientific notation is a method for expressing very large or very small numbers, using a single digit multiplied by a whole number power of 10.

Use of Scientific Notation

Place the decimal point of the number to the right of the first non-zero digit.

Multiply the number by 10 raised to a power equal to the number of places moved by the decimal point.

The exponent of 10 is positive for moves to the left and negative for moves to the right.

Large number, for example: 2292.0 is the same as 2.292×10^3

Small number, for example: 0.002292 is the same as 2.292×10^{-3}

METRIC SYSTEM

The metric system is based on multiples or fractions of 10.

Prefix	Scale
Kilo	10^3
Hecto	10^2
Deca	10^1
Base unit	$10^0 = 1$
Deci	10^{-1}
Centi	10^{-2}
Milli	10^{-3}
Micro	10^{-6}
Nano	10^{-9}
Pico	10^{-12}

INTERNATIONAL SYSTEM OF UNITS (SI UNITS)

(Système International d'Unités)

SI Base Units

Length:	meter, m
Mass:	kilogram, kg
Time:	second, s
Temperature:	kelvin, K
Amount of substance:	mole, mol

SI Derived Units

Area:	square meter, m^2
Volume:	cubic meter, m^3
Concentration:	mole per cubic meter, mol/m^3

TEMPERATURE SCALES AND CONVERSIONS

Scale	Absolute Zero	Freezing, Water	Boiling, Water
Kelvin	0 degrees	273 degrees	373 degrees
Centigrade	−273 degrees	0 degrees	100 degrees
Fahrenheit	−460 degrees	32 degrees	212 degrees

Conversion: Centigrade/Kelvin

To convert from Kelvin to centigrade:

$$\text{Centigrade (degrees)} = \text{Kelvin} - 273$$

To convert from centigrade to Kelvin:

$$\text{Kelvin (degrees)} = \text{centigrade} + 273$$

Conversion: Centigrade/Fahrenheit

To convert from Fahrenheit to centigrade:

$$\text{Centigrade (degrees)} = 0.55 \times (\text{Fahrenheit} - 32)$$

To convert from centigrade to Fahrenheit:

$$\text{Fahrenheit (degrees)} = (1.8 \times \text{centigrade}) + 32$$

HOUSEHOLD UNITS

In general, the metric system of measure is used for drug amounts. However, household measures such as teaspoons or tablespoons are used for administering medications in the home environment. For example, a cough syrup may have a label giving a usual adult dose as "1 teaspoon every 6 hours." Household measures are not consistent; for example, a teaspoon may vary from 3 to 5 ml. Although the metric system, which is more exact and consistent with milligrams, micrograms, and milliliters, is recommended in place of household measures, the following equivalences may be helpful. Use of household measures such as teaspoons can be very helpful in discussing amounts of substance with a patient.

1 teaspoon = 5 ml = 60 drops
1 tablespoon = 15 ml (or 3 teaspoons)
1 cup = 240 ml (or 8 fluid ounces)

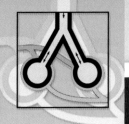

Recommendations on the Use of Aerosol Generators

USE OF TRADITIONAL SMALL VOLUME NEBULIZERS

Brands of nebulizers may differ considerably in performance capability. The following recommendations are based on average performance capability of disposable *constant-output small volume nebulizers (SVNs)*.[1,2] These specifications may not apply to newer, novel nebulizers that have greater delivery efficiency.

- *Filling volume:* Minimum of 3 ml; optimum = 5 ml at 10 L/min
- *Power gas flow rate:* 8 to 10 L/min
- *Treatment time:* 10 minutes or less
- *Pattern of inhalation:* Tidal breathing is effective; occasional slow, deep breaths with an inspiratory hold if possible
- *Inspiratory nebulization:* Power on inspiration only will increase delivery but lengthen treatment time
- *Cleaning:* Rinse after each use to prevent drug concentration; rinse with detergent and distilled water daily, and dry thoroughly

Cleaning Small Volume Nebulizers

- *After each use:* Rinse the mouthpiece, T-piece, and cup with distilled or sterile water. Tap water is discouraged[3]
- *Once a day:* Wash the mouthpiece, T-piece, and cup with mild soap and warm water. Rinse with distilled or sterile water and air dry
- *Once or twice a week:* Wash with mild soap and warm water, rinse well. Soak in solution of 1 part distilled white vinegar to 2 parts distilled water; do not reuse vinegar solution for later disinfection. Rinse well with warm running distilled or sterile water and air dry[4]

USE OF METERED DOSE INHALERS

The following instructions for the use of bronchodilator or corticosteroid aerosols with metered dose inhalers (MDIs) are written in terms that may be helpful for patient education. Package inserts on particular agents should always be checked, and these protocols should be modified as needed, especially for other drug classes.

Critical Steps in Metered Dose Inhaler Use[5]

1. Remove cap, inspect for foreign matter, and push the canister into the nozzle receptacle of the mouthpiece actuator.
2. Hold MDI in vertical position, shake the inhaler and, if not used recently, discharge a priming dose.
3. Exhale to functional residual capacity (easier for subject) or to residual volume.
4. Hold MDI about an inch in front of open mouth or, alternatively, place in mouth with teeth apart and with tongue flat.
5. Begin to breathe in slowly through mouth while actuating inhaler by pressing down on canister. Inspiration should take about 3 to 4 seconds.
6. Continue inhaling to total lung capacity, and hold breath for up to 10 seconds. (Only 1 puff for inhalation.)
7. Exhale normally, shake canister, wait 20 to 30 seconds to allow valve to refill, and repeat dose if prescribed.
8. Keep a diary of number of uses or use a counting device to keep track of number of actuations used.

NOTE: If you have trouble aiming the MDI at your open mouth, you can place the mouthpiece directly in your mouth and rest it on the lower front teeth without sealing your lips around it. If you find it hard to coordinate breathing and activating the MDI, you may wish to ask your physician to prescribe a reservoir device.

To Inhale a Corticosteroid

Use the same procedure as described previously, except for the following:

1. If you use both a bronchodilator and corticosteroid, inhale the bronchodilator first and wait 1 to 2 minutes before inhaling the corticosteroid.
2. Always use an extension or spacer device when inhaling a corticosteroid. If you do not have such a device, try to hyperextend (straighten) your head and neck as much as possible when inhaling (in other words, look at the ceiling).
3. Rinse your mouth and throat with water after finishing.

Common Errors in Use

The number of patients using MDIs incorrectly varies from 12% to 89%, according to available studies.[6]

Principal Types of Errors

- Failure to coordinate actuation of MDI with inhalation (27%)
- Too short a period of breath-hold after inhalation (26%)
- Too rapid an inspiratory flow rate (19%)
- Inadequate shaking and mixing of MDI contents before use (13%)
- Abrupt cessation of inspiration as aerosol strikes throat (cold Freon effect) (6%)
- Actuation of MDI at total lung capacity (4%)
- Firing of MDI into mouth but inhaling through nose (2%)
- Exhaling during MDI actuation
- Placing wrong end of inhaler in mouth, or holding in wrong (nonvertical) position
- Failure to take cap off before use
- Firing of MDI multiple times during a single inhalation

Cleaning Instructions: Metered Dose Inhaler

Once a day: Remove the canister, and clean the plastic actuator case in warm running water. Thoroughly dry the actuator before reinserting the canister.*

---

*Based on manufactures' recommendations

Check Canister Fullness

The best approach is to keep a patient log of use, showing date of initial use and subsequent numbers of actuations each day. If an MDI is used regularly (e.g., two actuations four times daily), the projected date of depletion can be calculated. For occasional use, tallies at the end of the day on a self-stick note kept in a convenient place, such as the bathroom, can be useful. However, counting devices can be purchased that count the number of actuations during use. Some manufacturers have a built-in counter on the actuator (e.g., Ventolin). Canister flotation in water is no longer recommended; it is imprecise, varies with different drugs, and can clog MDI nozzles.

USE OF RESERVOIR DEVICES

There is variation in the design and use of reservoir devices. The following steps are generic and are intended to describe most reservoir devices for handheld use. Specific brand instructions should be reviewed before use or instruction of patients.

1. Remove protective cap from mouthpiece if found on reservoir; inspect for foreign matter.
2. Assemble if needed for brand being used.
3. Shake MDI well; discharge if not used recently and insert into reservoir.
   - Some reservoirs (e.g., AeroChamber) accept entire mouthpiece/actuator; others accept only MDI canister nozzle.
4. Hold canister vertically, exhale normally to functional residual capacity.
5. Place mouth on mouthpiece and close lips.
6. Actuate MDI canister into reservoir.
7. Inhale through mouth (not nose) slowly and deeply to total lung capacity. If flow signal indicator sounds (usually at approximately 30 L/min), slow inspiration.
8. Hold breath for 5 to 10 seconds, if possible, and exhale (many units have an exhalation port).
9. Shake canister, wait 20 to 30 seconds, and repeat dose as prescribed.

Tips on Use[7-10]

- Use a nonelectrostatic material or prewash a nonconductive material reservoir device.
- Inhale simultaneously or right after actuating MDI, to maximize dose.
- Use a single inhalation with each MDI actuation. Multiple MDI actuations followed by a single inhalation will reduce the dose available.

- Have small children or infants inhale through device for five or six breaths to maximize emptying of the chamber.

Common Errors in Use

- Incorrect assembly
- Incorrect (nonvertical) position of MDI canister on reservoir
- Waiting too long to inhale after actuating MDI
- Inhaling too rapidly (may reduce dose?)
- Firing of multiple puffs into reservoir before inhaling
- Firing of puffs from two different MDIs before inhaling
- Failure to take mouthpiece cap off before use

USE OF DRY POWDER INHALERS

Specific instructions for use of the various dry powder inhalers (DPIs) currently available should be reviewed in the package insert before use or patient education.

Generic Recommendations That Apply to All of the Devices

1. Be sure mouthpiece is clear of all foreign matter.
2. Load the powder dose as instructed for the particular inhaler.
3. Exhale normally, *away from the inhaler* (humidity reduces dose).
4. Inhale from mouthpiece forcefully, to total lung capacity.
5. Hold breath up to 10 seconds, if possible.
6. Remove from mouth and exhale away from device.

Manufacturers' recommendations for use are summarized for the Turbuhaler, Diskus, Aerolizer, and HandiHaler. As new devices become available in the United States, package inserts will provide instructions for use.

Use of the Turbuhaler

1. Remove cover.
2. Hold inhaler upright and turn base of device completely to the right and then to the left until it clicks.
3. Exhale *away from inhaler* to functional residual capacity or residual volume.
4. Put mouthpiece between lips, holding upright or horizontally.
5. Breathe in forcefully and deeply.
6. Don't exhale; remove inhaler from mouth.
7. Hold breath according to comfort (5 to 10 seconds).

8. Exhale; wait a minimum of 20 to 30 seconds before second inhalation.
9. Rinse mouth with water when using a corticosteroid.

Use of the Diskus Inhaler

1. Push the thumbgrip away from you, to expose the mouthpiece.
2. Hold the Diskus in a level (horizontal) position, and slide the lever next to the mouthpiece away from you until it clicks.
3. Hold the Diskus level, and exhale *away from the mouthpiece.*
4. Put the mouthpiece to your lips, and inhale steadily and deeply through the Diskus.
5. Remove the Diskus from your mouth, hold your breath for about 10 seconds if possible, and breathe out slowly *away from device.*
6. Close the mouthpiece cover by sliding the thumbgrip back toward you.
7. Rinse your mouth with water when using a corticosteroid.

Do not wash any part of the device; keep it dry.

Use of the Aerolizer

1. Remove mouthpiece cover.
2. Hold base of inhaler and twist mouthpiece counterclockwise.
3. Remove capsule of medication from package and place in the base of the inhaler (only remove capsule immediately before use; do not store in inhaler).
4. Hold base of inhaler and twist clockwise to close.
5. On the sides of the inhaler are two buttons: press simultaneously to pierce capsule.
6. Exhale *away from the inhaler* to functional residual capacity or residual volume.
7. Keep head in upright position and hold the device horizontally with lips sealed around mouthpiece.
8. Breathe in as deeply as possible, holding breath for about 10 seconds if possible. Breathe out slowly, away from device.
9. Open the inhaler to expose the chamber. Examine the capsule and if powder remains, repeat inhalation.
10. Close mouthpiece and replace cover.

Use of the HandiHaler

1. Before using device, open foil package and remove capsule (only remove capsule immediately before use; do not store in inhaler).
2. Pull dust cap upward to open.

3. Open mouthpiece, place capsule in chamber.

4. Close mouthpiece firmly until you hear it click; leave dust cap open.

5. Hold device with mouthpiece up and press the piercing button once to release the medication.

6. Exhale *away from the inhaler* to functional residual capacity or residual volume.

7. Place mouthpiece into your mouth and close lips tightly around mouthpiece.

8. Breathe in slowly, at a rate sufficient to hear the capsule vibrate, until lungs are at total lung capacity, holding breath for about 10 seconds if possible. Breathe out slowly, away from device.

9. To make sure the entire dose has been inhaled, repeat steps 6–8.

10. Open the mouthpiece, tip out capsule, and throw it away.

11. Close mouthpiece and replace dust cap for storage.

Cleaning Instructions: Dry Powder Inhaler

The dry powder inhaler should not be cleaned, as moisture will decrease drug delivery. If necessary, the mouthpiece may be wiped with a dry cloth.

References

1. Rau JL, Ari A, Restrepo RD: Performance comparison of nebulizer designs: constant-output, breath-enhanced, and dosimetric, *Respir Care* 49:174, 2004.

2. Hess D, Fisher D, Williams P, Pooler S, Kacmarek RM: Medication nebulizer performance, *Chest* 110:498, 1996.

3. American Association for Respiratory Care: AARC Clinical Practice Guideline: Selection of a device for delivery of aerosol to the lung parenchyma, *Respir Care* 41:647, 1996. Available at http://www.rcjournal.com/cpgs/dalpcpg.html (accessed April 2007).

4. American Association for Respiratory Care: AARC Clinical Practice Guideline: Selection of an aerosol delivery device for neonatal and pediatric patients, *Respir Care* 40:1325, 1995. Available at http://www.rcjournal.com/cpgs/npamcpg.html (accessed April 2007).

5. Kesten S, Zive K, Chapman KR: Pharmacist knowledge and ability to use inhaled medication delivery systems, *Chest* 104:1737, 1993.

6. McFadden ER Jr.: Improper patient techniques with metered dose inhalers: clinical consequences and solutions to misuse, *J Allergy Clin Immunol* 96:278, 1995.

7. Rau JL, Coppolo DP, Nagel MW, Avvakoumova VI, Doyle CC, Wiersema KJ, Mitchell JP: The importance of nonelectrostatic materials in holding chambers for delivery of hydrofluoroalkane albuterol, *Respir Care* 51:503, 2006.

8. O'Callaghan C, Cant M, Robertson C: Delivery of beclomethasone dipropionate from a spacer device: what dose is available for inhalation? *Thorax* 49:961, 1994.

9. Rau JL, Restrepo RD, Deshpande V: Inhalation of single vs multiple metered-dose bronchodilator actuations from reservoir devices: an *in vitro* study, *Chest* 109:969, 1996.

10. Dolovich MB, Ahrens RC, Hess DR, Anderson P, Dhand R, Rau JL, Smaldone GC, Guyatt G, American College of Chest Physicians; American College of Asthma, Allergy, and Immunology: Device selection and outcomes of aerosol therapy: evidence-based guidelines: American College of Chest Physicians/American College of Asthma, Allergy, and Immunology, *Chest* 127:335, 2005.

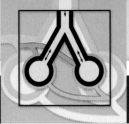

Pharmacological Management of Asthma and Chronic Obstructive Pulmonary Disease

PHARMACOLOGICAL MANAGEMENT OF ASTHMA

Definition of Asthma

Asthma is a chronic inflammatory disorder of the airways in which many cells and cellular elements play a role, in particular, mast cells, eosinophils, T lymphocytes, macrophages, neutrophils, and epithelial cells. In susceptible individuals, this inflammation causes recurrent episodes of wheezing, breathlessness, chest tightness, and coughing, particularly at night or in the early morning. These episodes are usually associated with widespread but variable airflow obstruction that is often reversible either spontaneously or with treatment. The inflammation also causes an associated increase in the existing bronchial hyperresponsiveness to a variety of stimuli.*

Stepwise Drug Therapy of Asthma for Adults and Children Older Than 5 Years

The following table summarizes levels of drug therapy for maintenance of chronic asthma. The complete National Asthma Education and Prevention Program (NAEPP) document should be consulted for details on managing asthma.

Goals of Therapy[†]
- Minimal or no chronic symptoms day or night
- Minimal or no exacerbations
- No limitations on activities; no school/work missed
- Maintain normal pulmonary functions
- Minimal use of inhaled short-acting β_2 agonist
- No or minimal adverse effects from medications

---

*National Asthma Education and Prevention Program, National Heart, Lung, and Blood Institute, National Institutes of Health: Expert Panel Report 2: *Guidelines for the diagnosis and management of asthma*, NIH Publication 97-4051. Bethesda, Md, 1997, National Institutes of Health. (Available at http://www.nhlbi.nih.gov/guidelines/asthma/asthgdln.pdf; accessed February 2007.)

[†]National Asthma Education and Prevention Program, National Heart, Lung, and Blood Institute, National Institutes of Health: Expert Panel Report: *Guidelines for the diagnosis and management of asthma—update on selected topics 2002*, NIH Publication 02-5074. Bethesda, Md, 2002, National Institutes of Health. (Available at http://www.nhlbi.nih.gov/guidelines/asthma/asthmafullrpt.pdf; accessed March 2007.)

Severity	Daily Medications
STEP 1: *Mild intermittent* Days with symptoms: ≤2 d/wk Nocturnal symptoms: ≤2 nights/mo PEF or FEV_1: ≥80% PEF variability: <20%	No daily medication is needed. Exacerbations may occur; systemic corticosteroids are recommended if exacerbation occurs. All patients should have a short-acting β_2 agonist to use as needed for symptoms for every step
STEP 2: *Mild persistent* Days with symptoms: >2/wk, but <1×/d Nocturnal symptoms: >2 nights/mo PEF or FEV_1: ≥80% PEF variability: <20%–30%	**Preferred treatment: Low-dose inhaled corticosteroid.** Alternatively: cromolyn, leukotriene modifier, nedocromil, *or* sustained release theophylline
STEP 3: *Moderate persistent* Days with symptoms: daily Nocturnal symptoms: >1 night/wk PEF or FEV_1: >60%–<80% PEF variability: >30%	**Preferred treatment: Low- to medium-dose inhaled corticosteroid and long-acting inhaled β_2 agonist.** Alternatively: inhaled corticosteroid and either leukotriene modifier or theophylline
STEP 4: *Severe persistent* Days with symptoms: continual Nocturnal symptoms: frequent PEF or FEV_1: ≤60% PEF variability: >30%	**Preferred treatment: High-dose inhaled corticosteroid and long-acting inhaled β_2 agonist** *and* systemic corticosteroids

- Review treatment every 1–6 mo to consider stepwise reduction
- If control cannot be maintained, consider stepping patient up
- Short-term bronchodilator should be used at every step for quick relief. Use of short-term bronchodilator more than twice per week may indicate a need to step up

FEV_1, forced expiratory volume in 1 second; *PEF*, peak expiratory flow.

Stepwise Therapy for Infants and Children 5 Years of Age or Younger With Acute or Chronic Asthma Symptoms

The following table summarizes levels of drug therapy for maintenance of asthma. The complete NAEPP document should be consulted for details on managing asthma.

Severity	Daily Medications
STEP 1: *Mild intermittent* Days with symptoms: ≤2 d/wk Nocturnal symptoms: ≤2 nights/mo	No daily medication is needed. All patients should have a short-acting β_2 agonist to use as needed for symptoms for every step
STEP 2: *Mild persistent* Days with symptoms: >2/wk, but <1×/d Nocturnal symptoms: >2 nights/mo	**Preferred treatment: Low-dose inhaled corticosteroid.** Alternatively: cromolyn *or* leukotriene receptor antagonist
STEP 3: *Moderate persistent* Days with symptoms: daily Nocturnal symptoms: >1 night/wk	**Preferred treatment: Low- to medium-dose inhaled corticosteroid and long-acting inhaled β_2 agonist.** Alternatively: inhaled corticosteroid and either leukotriene receptor antagonist or theophylline
STEP 4: *Severe persistent* Days with symptoms: continual Nocturnal symptoms: frequent	**Preferred treatment: High-dose inhaled corticosteroid and long-acting inhaled β_2 agonist** *and* systemic corticosteroids

- Review treatment every 1-6 mo to consider stepwise reduction
- If control cannot be maintained, consider stepping patient up
- Viral infection may constitute regular use of short-term bronchodilator
- Short-term bronchodilator should be used at every step for quick relief. This may be inhaled or oral. Use of short-term bronchodilator more than twice per week may indicate a need to step up

Management of Asthma Exacerbations: Emergency Department and Hospital-Based Care

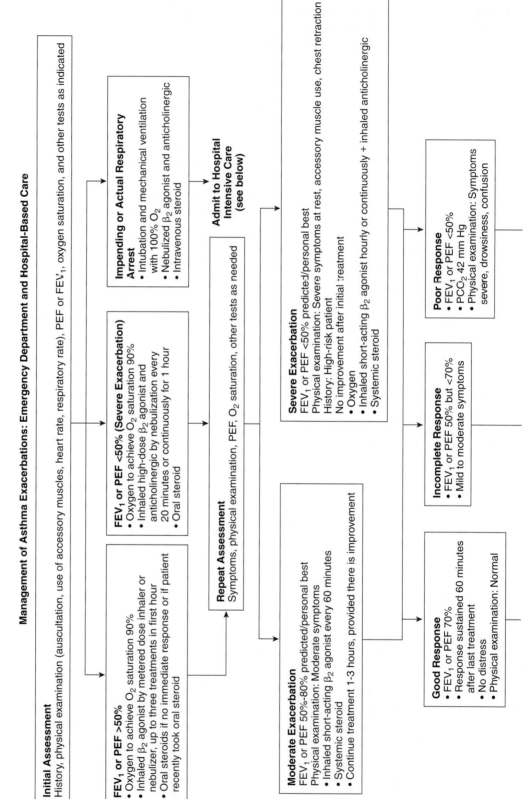

Initial Assessment
History, physical examination (auscultation, use of accessory muscles, heart rate, respiratory rate), PEF or FEV_1, oxygen saturation, and other tests as indicated

FEV_1 or PEF >50%
- Oxygen to achieve O_2 saturation 90%
- Inhaled β_2 agonist by metered dose inhaler or nebulizer, up to three treatments in first hour
- Oral steroids if no immediate response or if patient recently took oral steroid

FEV_1 or PEF <50% (Severe Exacerbation)
- Oxygen to achieve O_2 saturation 90%
- Inhaled high-dose β_2 agonist and anticholinergic by nebulization every 20 minutes or continuously for 1 hour
- Oral steroid

Impending or Actual Respiratory Arrest
- Intubation and mechanical ventilation with 100% O_2
- Nebulized β_2 agonist and anticholinergic
- Intravenous steroid

Admit to Hospital Intensive Care (see below)

Repeat Assessment
Symptoms, physical examination, PEF, O_2 saturation, other tests as needed

Moderate Exacerbation
FEV_1 or PEF 50%-80% predicted/personal best
Physical examination: Moderate symptoms
- Inhaled short-acting β_2 agonist every 60 minutes
- Systemic steroid
- Continue treatment 1-3 hours, provided there is improvement

Severe Exacerbation
FEV_1 or PEF <50% predicted/personal best
Physical examination: Severe symptoms at rest, accessory muscle use, chest retraction
History: High-risk patient
No improvement after initial treatment
- Oxygen
- Inhaled short-acting β_2 agonist hourly or continuously + inhaled anticholinergic
- Systemic steroid

Good Response
- FEV_1 or PEF 70%
- Response sustained 60 minutes after last treatment
- No distress
- Physical examination: Normal

Incomplete Response
- FEV_1 or PEF 50% but <70%
- Mild to moderate symptoms

Poor Response
- FEV_1 or PEF <50%
- PCO_2 42 mm Hg
- Physical examination: Symptoms severe, drowsiness, confusion

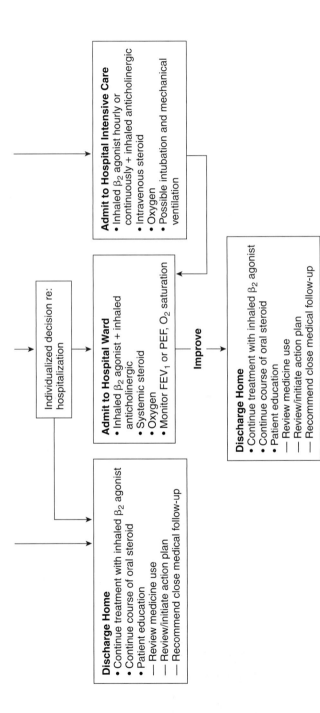

FIGURE D-1 Algorithm for management of asthma exacerbations for emergency department and hospital-based care. *FEV₁*, forced expiratory volume in 1 second; *P*co₂, carbon dioxide pressure; *PEF*, peak expiratory flow. (From National Asthma Education and Prevention Program, National Heart, Lung, and Blood Institute, National Institutes of Health: Expert Panel Report 2: *Guidelines for the diagnosis and management of asthma*, NIH Publication 97-4051. Bethesda, Md, 1997, National Institutes of Health.) (Available at http://www.nhlbi.nih.gov/guidelines/asthma/asthgdln.pdf; accessed February 2007.)

Discharge Home
- Continue treatment with inhaled β₂ agonist
- Continue course of oral steroid
- Patient education
  — Review medicine use
  — Review/initiate action plan
  — Recommend close medical follow-up

Individualized decision re: hospitalization

Admit to Hospital Ward
- Inhaled β₂ agonist + inhaled anticholinergic
- Systemic steroid
- Oxygen
- Monitor FEV₁ or PEF, O₂ saturation

Improve

Discharge Home
- Continue treatment with inhaled β₂ agonist
- Continue course of oral steroid
- Patient education
  — Review medicine use
  — Review/initiate action plan
  — Recommend close medical follow-up

Admit to Hospital Intensive Care
- Inhaled β₂ agonist hourly or continuously + inhaled anticholinergic
- Intravenous steroid
- Oxygen
- Possible intubation and mechanical ventilation

PHARMACOLOGICAL MANAGEMENT OF CHRONIC OBSTRUCTIVE PULMONARY DISEASE*

Definition of Chronic Obstructive Pulmonary Disease

Chronic obstructive pulmonary disease (COPD) is a disease that is preventable and treatable. The pulmonary component is characterized by airflow limitation that is not fully reversible. The airflow limitation is usually both progressive and associated with an abnormal inflammatory response of the lungs to noxious particles or gases.

Classification of Chronic Obstructive Pulmonary Disease by Severity

The following table summarizes the current classification of COPD.

Stage	Characteristics
Stage 1: Mild	• $FEV_1/FVC < 0.70$ • $FEV_1 \geq 80\%$ predicted
Stage 2: Moderate	• $FEV_1/FVC < 0.70$ • $50\% \leq FEV_1 < 80\%$ predicted
Stage 3: Severe	• $FEV_1/FVC < 0.70$ • $30\% \leq FEV_1 < 50\%$ predicted
Stage 4: Very severe	• $FEV_1/FVC < 0.70$ • $FEV_1 < 30\%$ predicted *or* $FEV_1 < 50\%$ predicted plus chronic respiratory failure

FEV_1, forced expiratory volume in 1 second; FVC, forced vital capacity.

The Four Components of COPD Management

1. Assess and monitor disease
2. Reduce risk factors
3. Manage stable COPD
4. Manage exacerbations

Component 1: Assess and Monitor Disease

- Review the patient's history of exposure to risk factors
- Consider a diagnosis of COPD for any patient with the following:
  - Dyspnea that is persistent, progressive, and worsens with exercise
  - Chronic cough, which may be intermittently unproductive
  - Chronic sputum production
- Confirm by spirometry

Component 2: Reduce Risk Factors

- Reduce exposure to tobacco smoke, occupational dusts and chemicals, and indoor and outdoor air pollutants
- Stop smoking

Component 3: Manage Stable COPD

- Health education, including smoking cessation
- Pharmacological management
- Exercise training programs to improve exercise tolerance and reduce symptoms of dyspnea and fatigue
- Long-term oxygen administration to patients with chronic respiratory failure

Component 4: Manage Exacerbations

- Education to prevent future exacerbations
- Pharmacological management
- Noninvasive mechanical ventilation

Pharmacological Treatment of Stable Chronic Obstructive Pulmonary Disease

None of the existing medications for COPD has been shown to modify the long-term decline in lung function. Pharmacological therapy is used to prevent and control symptoms, reduce the frequency and severity of exacerbations, and improve health status and exercise tolerance. The following table summarizes the Global Initiative for Chronic Obstructive Lung Disease (GOLD) guidelines for treatment at each stage of COPD. *The complete GOLD guidelines should be consulted for more detail in drug management of COPD.*

*Global Initiative for Chronic Obstructive Lung Disease: Executive Summary: December 2006, *Global strategy for the diagnosis, management, and prevention of COPD.* National Heart, Lung, and Blood Institute (Bethesda, Md) and World Health Organization (Geneva, Switzerland), 2006. (Available at http://www.goldcopd.org/Guidelineitem.asp?l1=2&l2=1&intId=996; accessed March 2007.)

Stage	Characteristics	Treatment
Stage 1	Mild COPD: • $FEV_1/FVC < 70\%$ • $FEV_1 \geq 80\%$ predicted • With or without chronic symptoms (cough, sputum production)	Reduction in risk factors; influenza vaccination; short-acting bronchodilator
Stage 2	Moderate COPD: • $FEV1/FVC < 70\%$ • $50\% \leq FEV1 < 80\%$ predicted • With or without chronic symptoms (cough, sputum production, dyspnea)	All the above, plus add long-acting bronchodilator and rehabilitation
Stage 3	Severe COPD: • $FEV_1/FVC < 70\%$ • $30\% \leq FEV1 < 50\%$ predicted • Increasing chronic symptoms (cough, sputum production, dyspnea)	All the above, plus add inhaled corticosteroids
Stage 4	Very severe COPD: • $FEV_1/FVC < 70\%$ • $FEV_1 < 30\%$ predicted, $FEV_1 < 50\%$ predicted plus chronic respiratory failure*	All the above, plus oxygen therapy and consider surgical options

From Global Initiative for Chronic Obstructive Lung Disease: *Executive Summary:* Global Initiative for Chronic Obstructive Lung Disease: Executive Summary: December 2006, *Global strategy for the diagnosis, management, and prevention of COPD.* National Heart, Lung, and Blood Institute (Bethesda, Md) and World Health Organization (Geneva, Switzerland), 2006. (Available at http://www.goldcopd.org/Guidelineitem. asp?l1=2&l2=1&intId=996; accessed March 2007.)
COPD, Chronic obstructive pulmonary disease; *FEV₁,* forced expiratory volume in 1 second; *FVC,* forced vital capacity.
*Respiratory failure: Pao_2 less than 8.0 kPa (60mm Hg) with or without $Paco_2$ greater than 6.7 kPa (50 mm Hg) while breathing air at sea level.

Therapy at Each Stage of Chronic Obstructive Pulmonary Disease

Patients must be taught how and when to use their treatments, and treatments being prescribed for other conditions should be reviewed. The GOLD guidelines provide the following comments on each class of drug therapy in stable COPD.

Bronchodilators

• Bronchodilator medications are central to symptom management in COPD.
• Inhaled therapy is preferred (theophylline is effective in COPD, but because of potential toxicity, inhaled bronchodilators are preferred when available).
• The choice between β_2-agonist, anticholinergic, theophylline, or combination therapy depends on availability and individual response in terms of symptom relief and side effects.
• Bronchodilators are prescribed on an as-needed or regular basis to prevent or reduce symptoms.
• Long-acting inhaled bronchodilators are more convenient.
• Combining bronchodilators may improve efficacy and decrease the risk of side effects compared with increasing the dose of a single bronchodilator.

Glucocorticoids

• Regular treatment with inhaled glucocorticosteroids is appropriate for symptomatic COPD patients with a documented spirometric response to inhaled glucocorticosteroids, or in those with an FEV_1 less than 50% of predicted and repeated exacerbations.
• Long-acting inhaled β agonist plus inhaled glucocorticosteroid is more effective than if given individually.

Other Pharmacological Treatments

• Vaccines: Influenza vaccines are recommended; pneumococcal vaccine is recommended for COPD patients 65 years and older
• α_1-Antitrypsin augmentation therapy: This therapy is recommended in young patients with severe hereditary α_1-antitrypsin deficiency and established emphysema; it is not recommended for COPD unrelated to α_1-antitrypsin deficiency.
• Antibiotics: Use of antibiotics other than to treat infectious exacerbations and other bacterial infections is not recommended.
• Mucolytic (mucokinetic and mucoregulator) agents: A few patients with viscous sputum may benefit from mucolytics, although overall benefits seem to be small; not recommended for widespread use. This

group includes agents such as ambroxol, erdosteine, carbocysteine, and iodinated glycerol.

- Antioxidant agents: Antioxidants, particularly *N*-acetylcysteine, have been shown to reduce the frequency of exacerbations and may be useful in patients with recurrent exacerbations. Additional studies are needed before recommending antioxidants in routine treatment.
- Immunoregulators: The use of immunoregulators has been shown to be effective; however, more studies are need before regular use can be recommended.
- Antitussives: Regular use of antitussives is contraindicated in stable COPD.
- Vasodilators: In stable COPD, inhaled nitric oxide can worsen gas exchange and is contraindicated.
- Narcotics: Oral and parenteral opioids are effective in treating advanced COPD. Insufficient data exist to recommend nebulized opioids. The use of opioids can have serious adverse effects, such as reduction in respiratory drive.
- Others: Nedocromil, leukotriene modifiers, or alternative healing methods (e.g., herbal medicine, acupuncture, homeopathy) have not been adequately tested in COPD patients and cannot be recommended at this time.

Nonpharmacologic Treatments

- Oxygen therapy is beneficial to patients with chronic respiratory failure.
- Ventilatory support: Noninvasive positive-pressure ventilation (NIPPV) cannot be recommended for routine treatment. The combination of NIPPV and oxygen may be of benefit to some patients.
- Surgical treatment: Bullectomy, lung volume reduction surgery, and lung transplantation may be of benefit to selected patients.

Glossary of Selected Terms

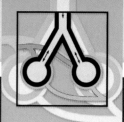

An eclectic glossary of terms encountered in pharmacology, many from the basic sciences, is offered for convenience in using the text as a study source. This glossary is not intended to substitute for a comprehensive dictionary of medical terms. Selection of terms for inclusion is based on the author's experience in reading the literature of drug actions and effects. Terms that are frequently found or used in discussing drugs but may be less well known to the practicing clinician are included.

Acetylcholine A chemical produced by the body that is used in the transmission of nerve impulses. It is destroyed by the enzyme acetylcholinesterase, also known as *cholinesterase*.

Acetylcholinesterase An enzyme that breaks down the neurotransmitter acetylcholine at the synaptic cleft so that the next nerve impulse can be transmitted across the synaptic gap.

Acid A substance that contributes hydrogen ions (protons) in solution.
Strong acid: An acid that completely dissociates in aqueous solution.
Weak acid: An acid that incompletely dissociates in aqueous solution.

Acute respiratory distress syndrome A respiratory disorder characterized by respiratory insufficiency. This may occur as a result of trauma, pneumonia, oxygen toxicity, gram-negative sepsis, and systemic inflammatory response.

Adrenal cortical hormone A chemical secreted by the adrenal cortex. An adrenal cortical hormone is also referred to as a STEROID.

Adrenergic (adrenomimetic) Refers to a drug stimulating a receptor for norepinephrine or epinephrine.

Adrenergic bronchodilator An agent that stimulates sympathetic nervous fibers, which allow relaxation of smooth muscle in the airway. Also known as a *sympathomimetic bronchodilator,* or *β₂ agonist*.

Aerodynamic diameter of a particle The diameter of a unit-density (1 g/cc) spherical particle having the same terminal settling velocity as the measured particle.

Aerosol Suspension of liquid or solid particles, between 0.001 and 100 microns (μm) in diameter, in a carrier gas.

Aerosol therapy Delivery of aerosol particles to the lungs.

Afferent Toward; in neural control, toward the central nervous system, from the periphery; for example, the sensory neural signal is an afferent impulse.

Agonist A chemical or drug that binds to a receptor and creates an effect on the body.

Airway resistance A measure of the impedance to ventilation caused by the movement of gas through the airway.

Alkaloid Any of a group of alkaline substances taken from plants, which react with acids to form salts (e.g., theophylline).

Allele One of two genes, which contain inheritable characteristics, that are paired together.

Amine A group of compounds related to ammonia (NH_3) by having one or more alkyl groups (methyl, CH_3; ethyl, CH_3CH_2; etc.) attached directly to the nitrogen atom.

Amino acid A molecule with both an amine group and a carboxyl (COOH) group.

Amnestic Having the ability to cause total or partial loss of memory.

Analgesic A drug that provides pain relief. Analgesics can be subdivided into narcotic and nonnarcotic medications. The narcotic drugs are derivatives of opium, such as morphine and codeine. The nonnarcotic medications are useful in treating pain and inflammation. They also have antipyretic activity.

Anesthetic A drug that depresses the nervous system. Anesthetics can be divided into local and general anesthetics. General anesthesia causes total loss of consciousness and reflexes, which results in the absence of pain perception. Local anesthetics are applied to a specific site and decrease pain perception at the specific site and do not affect level of consciousness. Both types of anesthetics are often used during surgical procedures.

Anion An ion with a negative charge, attracted to the anode (positive) terminal.

Antagonism   When the effect of the combination is lower than the effect expected from either agent alone (i.e., 1 + 1 < 1).

Antagonist   A chemical or drug that binds to a receptor but does not create an effect on the body; it actually blocks the receptor site from accepting an agonist.

Antiadrenergic   Refers to a drug blocking a receptor for norepinephrine or epinephrine.

Antiarrhythmic   Any of a group of cardiac medications that are classified according to mechanism of action; in some instances they may pose multiple mechanisms of action. The most common classification system of antiarrhythmics is the Vaughan Williams classification system, which is divided into four distinct categories and a miscellaneous section.

Antibiotic   Any of a group of natural compounds produced by microorganisms that either inhibit or kill other microorganisms.

Anticholinergic   Refers to a drug blocking a receptor for acetylcholine.

Anticholinergic bronchodilator   An agent that blocks parasympathetic nervous fibers, which allows relaxation of smooth muscle in the airway.

Antidepressant   Any of a group of drugs that can alter levels of certain neurotransmitters, in particular norepinephrine and serotonin, within the brain. Depending on the class of antidepressant, they can either inhibit the reuptake of neurotransmitters or decrease their degradation, ultimately allowing for increased levels of neurotransmitter at the nerve terminal.

Antihistamine   Any drug that reduces the effects mediated by histamine, a chemical released by the body during allergic reactions. Antihistamine is often administered to reduce secretions (e.g., runny nose and sneezing), but can cause drowsiness and impaired responses.

Antileukotriene   An agent that blocks the inflammatory response in asthma.

Antimicrobial   A term including both natural and synthetic compounds that either inhibit or kill microorganisms.

Antimuscarinic bronchodilator   Same as an anticholinergic bronchodilator: an agent that blocks the effect of acetylcholine at the cholinergic site.

Antipsychotic   Any of a group of drugs used to treat psychotic disorders, such as schizophrenia. These drugs affect primarily the neurotransmitter dopamine.

Antithrombotic   Drugs that prevent or break up blood clots in such conditions as thrombosis or embolism; include anticoagulants, antiplatelets, and thrombolytics.

α_1-Antitrypsin   Also known as *α_1-proteinase inhibitor (API)*. An inhibitor of trypsin that may be deficient in patients with emphysema.

API deficient: Individual has low serum levels of API possessing altered electrophoretic properties.

API dysfunctional: Individual has normal serum levels of API that does not function normally.

API normal: Individual has normal serum levels of API that functions normally.

API null: Individual has undetectable serum levels of API

Antitussive   Any of a group of drugs that suppress the cough reflex.

Anxiolytic   Any of a group of drugs used to treat several conditions, including anxiety disorders and insomnia; also known as minor tranquilizers. The most common class of anxiolytics is the benzodiazepines. They bind to the γ-aminobutyric acid receptor to increase the inhibitory actions of this neurotransmitter.

Apoptosis   A disintegration of cells into particles that can be phagocytosed by other cells. This type of cell death is not associated with signs of inflammation and is contrasted with necrosis. Also referred to as *programmed cell death*. See PHAGOCYTOSIS, PHAGOCYTE.

Arterial blood pressure (blood pressure)   Defined hemodynamically as the product of cardiac output (heart rate × stroke volume) and total peripheral resistance.

Aspiration   Refers to the accidental inhalation of food particles, fluids, or gastric contents into the lungs.

Asthma Paradox   Refers to the increasing incidence of asthma morbidity, and especially asthma mortality, despite advances in the understanding of asthma and availability of improved drugs to treat asthma.

Atrioventricular node   An area of tissue that conducts electrical impulses between the atria and ventricle.

Autocrine   Refers to secretory activity of the cell that influences only the cell itself. See PARACRINE.

Autosomal   Refers to an autosome, for example, one of the 22 non-sex chromosomes in humans.

Bioavailability   Amount of drug that reaches the systemic circulation.

Bohr effect   The presence of carbon dioxide aiding in the release and delivery of oxygen from hemoglobin.

Bradycardia   A slow heart rate, typically defined as less than 60 beats/min.

Bronchospasm   Narrowing of the bronchial airways, caused by contraction of smooth muscle.

Capsid   Protein covering around the central core of a virus particle. The capsid develops from protein units termed *protomers* and protect the nucleic acid in the core of the virus from enzymes in biological fluids; promotes attachment of virus to susceptible cells.

Capsomer   Short ribbons of protein that make up a portion of the capsid of viral particles. See CAPSID.

Cardiac output   Amount of blood that is ejected into the aorta and travels through the systemic circulation with every heartbeat.

Cardiovascular disease   Damage to the heart and blood vessels or circulation, including to the brain, kidney, and eye.

Cascade impactor   A device that uses multiple steps in determining aerosol particle sizes.

Catecholamine   Any of a group of similar compounds having sympathomimetic action; catecholamines mimic the actions of epinephrine.

Cation   An ion with a positive charge, attracted to the cathode (negative) terminal.

Central nervous system   A system that includes the brain and spinal cord, controlling voluntary and involuntary acts.

Chemical name   The name indicating the chemical structure of a drug.

Chemokine   A chemotactic cytokine that guides leukocytes from blood vessels into the tissues. Different types of leukocytes (e.g., neutrophils and eosinophils) have chemokine receptors that draw the leukocyte to chemokines in the tissues. See CYTOKINE.

Chlorofluorocarbon   A liquefied gas (e.g., Freon) propellant used to administer medication from a metered dose inhaler.

Cholinergic (cholinomimetic)   Refers to a drug causing stimulation of a receptor for acetylcholine.

Cholinesterase inhibitor   A drug that blocks the activity of cholinesterase, an enzyme that inactivates the neurotransmitter acetylcholine. Acetylcholine is found at nerve terminals in both the central and peripheral nervous systems. Cholinesterase inhibitors are used in the treatment of dementia to slow the progression of cognitive decline.

Chronic obstructive pulmonary disease   Disease process characterized by airflow limitation that is not fully reversible, is usually progressive, and is associated with an abnormal inflammatory response of the lung to noxious particles or gases. Diseases that cause this include chronic bronchitis, emphysema, asthma, and bronchiectasis.

Chronotropic   Affecting the rate of contraction of the heart.

Circadian rhythm   Human biologic variations of rhythm within a 24-hour cycle.

Clone   A group of genetically identical cells with a common ancestor.

Code name   A name assigned by a manufacturer to an experimental chemical that shows potential as a drug. An example is aerosol SCH 1000, which was the code name for ipratropium bromide, a parasympatholytic bronchodilator.

Common cold   A nonbacterial respiratory tract infection, characterized by malaise and a runny nose.

Congestive heart failure   Failure of the heart to pump the blood adequately, resulting in lung congestion and tissular edema.

Conjugate   In pharmacology, a compound resulting from the combination of drug or drug metabolite with a substrate such as glucuronic acid, by means of a catalyzing enzyme (a transferase), to form an inactive drug conjugate; this is usually a polar (water-soluble) molecule and is readily excreted.

Conscious sedation   A method of sedation used during certain invasive procedures. The goal of conscious sedation is to decrease the level of consciousness, relieve anxiety and pain, while allowing the patient to follow verbal commands. Conscious sedation is achieved through the use of several classes of drugs, including benzodiazepines and narcotic analgesics.

Creatinine clearance   Measurement of the renal clearance of endogenous creatinine per unit time; considered to be an estimate of glomerular filtration rate (GFR); overestimates GFR by 10%-15%; used for drug-dosing guidelines.

Cyclic AMP (cAMP)   Nucleotide produced by β_2-receptor stimulation; it affects many cells, but causes relaxation of bronchial smooth muscle.

Cyclic GMP (cGMP)   Nucleotide producing the opposite effect of cAMP, that is, it causes bronchoconstriction.

Cycloplegia   Flattening of the eye lens by paralysis of the ciliary muscle attached to the lens.

Cystic fibrosis   An inherited disease of the exocrine glands, affecting the pancreas, respiratory system, and apocrine glands. Symptoms usually begin in infancy and are characterized by increased electrolytes in the sweat, chronic respiratory infection, and pancreatic insufficiency.

Cytokine   A protein secreted by a variety of cells such as monocytes or lymphocytes, which regulate and control immune responses, including local and systemic inflammatory responses. Examples are interleukins, interferon, and tumor necrosis factor.

Dead volume   The amount of solution that remains in the reservoir of a small volume nebulizer once sputtering begins, causing a decrease in aerosolization.

Deposition   In respiratory pharmacology, the process by which particles deposit out of suspension to remain in the lung.

Diastolic blood pressure   Lowest pressure reached right before ventricular ejection.

***d*-(+)-Dimers**   Covalently cross-linked degradation fragments of the cross-linked fibrin polymer during plasmin-mediated fibrinolysis; the level increases after the onset of fibrinolysis, and allows for identification of the presence of fibrinolysis.

Diuretic   A drug that increases urine output.

Downregulation   Long-term desensitization of β receptors to β$_2$ agonists, caused by a reduction in the number of β receptors.

Dromotropic   Affecting the velocity of conduction at the atrioventricular node.

Drug administration   The method by which a drug is made available to the body.

Dysrhythmia/arrhythmia   Irregular (faster or slower) heart beat; the term *arrhythmia* is used more frequently than *dysrhythmia*.

Edema   Swelling due to an abnormal accumulation of fluid in intercellular spaces of the body.

Efferent   Away from; in neural control, a nervous impulse from the central nervous system to the periphery; for example, the neuromuscular fiber is an efferent fiber.

Elasticity   A rheologic property characteristic of solids; it is represented by the storage modulus *G′*.

Emitted dose   In respiratory pharmacology, the dose released by an aerosol device.

Endogenous   Refers to *inside,* produced by the body.

Enteral   Use of the intestine.

Enzyme induction   A process by which exposure to a drug induces or increases production of the enzyme responsible for metabolizing the drug.

Exogenous   Refers to *outside,* manufactured to be placed inside the body (e.g., medication).

Expectorant   Drug that increases the stimulation of mucus.

Fasciculation   Involuntary contraction or twitching of groups of muscle fibers.

Fibrillation   Quivering contractions of individual muscle fibers.

Atrial fibrillation: Extremely rapid contractions of the atria.

Ventricular fibrillation: Extremely rapid contractions of the ventricle.

Fibrin split or fibrinogen degradation products   Small peptides that result following the action of plasmin on fibrinogen and fibrin in the fibrinolytic process. Fibrinogen degradation products are anticoagulant substances that can cause bleeding if fibrinolysis becomes uncontrolled and excessive.

First-pass effect   Initial metabolism in the liver of a drug taken orally, before the drug reaches the systemic circulation.

Flu   A nonbacterial infection with rapid onset of symptoms, including fever, headache, and fatigue.

G protein   One of a family of guanine nucleotide-binding proteins, on the cytoplasmic face of the cell membrane, that links to receptors and transduces drug or neurotransmitter signals to the cell; it has a trimeric structure, designated as alpha (α), beta (β), or gamma (γ). The α subunit binds guanine nucleotides.

Gel   A macromolecular description of pseudo-plastic material having both viscosity and elasticity.

Generic name   The name assigned to a chemical by the United States Adopted Name (USAN) Council when the chemical appears to have therapeutic use and the manufacturer wishes to market the drug.

Glomerular filtration   Mechanism by which hydrostatic pressure forces fluid out of the glomerular capillaries and into the renal ducts.

Glomerular filtration rate   The volume of water filtered from the plasma by the kidney via the glomerular capillary walls into Bowman capsules per unit time; considered to be 90% of creatinine clearance, and equivalent to inulin clearance.

Glycogenolysis   Conversion of glycogen (a polysaccharide, starch formed from sugar) into glucose in tissues.

Heme   An iron-containing nonprotein portion of the hemoglobin molecule in which the iron is in the ferrous (Fe^{2+}) state.

Hemoprotein   Any protein combined with heme, a blood pigment.

Heterodisperse   In reference to the size of particles in an aerosol, meaning the particles are of different sizes.

Heterozygous   A combination of dominant and recessive alleles; two different parent genes.

Homozygous   Having similar or identical alleles (one of each pair of genes from parents).

Hydrofluoroalkane   A nontoxic liquefied gas propellant used to administer medication from a metered dose inhaler.

Hydrolysis   Chemical decomposition in which a substance is split into simpler compounds by the addition of the elements of water; for example, H_2O + salt $\leftrightarrow$ acid and base.

Hygroscopic   A tendency to absorb water.

Hypersensitivity   An allergic or immune-mediated reaction to a drug, which can be serious, requiring airway maintenance or ventilatory assistance.

Hypertensive emergency   Blood pressures above 180/120 mm Hg, when the elevation of blood pressure is accompanied by acute, chronic, or progressing target organ injury.

Hypertensive urgency   Blood pressures above 180/120 mm Hg without signs or symptoms of acute target organ complications.

Hypovolemia   Abnormally decreased volume of blood circulating in the body.

Idiosyncratic effect   An abnormal or unexpected reaction to a drug, other than an allergic reaction, as compared with the predicted effect.

IgE (immunoglobulin E)   A gamma globulin that is produced by cells in the respiratory tract.

In vitro   Mechanically simulating the clinical setting; testing in a laboratory.

In vivo   Testing done on animals or humans; clinical testing.

Infant   A child between the ages of 1 month and 1 year.

Inhalation   Taking a substance, typically in the form of gases, fumes, vapors, mists, aerosols, or dusts, into the body by breathing in.

Inhaled or delivered dose   Dose reaching the patient's mouth or artificial airway.

Inotrope   A drug affecting the strength of muscular contraction.

Intrinsic sympathomimetic activity   Having the ability to activate and block adrenergic receptors, producing a net stimulatory effect on the sympathetic nervous system.

LaPlace's Law   Physical principle describing and quantifying the relation between the internal pressure of a drop or bubble, the amount of surface tension, and the radius of the drop or bubble.

Leukotriene   Any of a group of chemical mediators that cause inflammation.

Ligand   a small molecule bound to another chemical group or molecule.

Lipocyte   A fat cell.

Lipolysis   The breakdown or decomposition of fat.

Lipophilic   Having an affinity for fat or lipids; lipid soluble.

Local effect   Limited to the area of treatment (e.g., inhaled drug to treat constricted airways).

Lung availability/systemic availability (L/T ratio)   Amount of drug that is made available to the lung out of the total available to the body.

Lung dose   Dose actually reaching the trachea and beyond.

Lymphokine   A cytokine produced by lymphocytes. See CYTOKINE.

Mast cell   A type of connective tissue cell that contains heparin and histamine.

Mast cell stabilizer   An agent used prophylactically to treat the inflammatory response in asthma; also known as a *cromolyn-like agent.*

Mean arterial pressure   Pressure that drives blood into the tissues averaged over the entire cardiac cycle.

Methylxanthine   Any of a group of drugs derived from xanthine. There are three methylated (CH_3) xanthines: caffeine, theophylline, and theobromine.

Miosis   A term describing the constriction of the circular iris muscle, causing pupillary contraction.

Monodisperse   In reference to the size of particles in an aerosol, meaning all particles are the same size.

Mood stabilizer   Any of a group of drugs used primarily to treat bipolar disorders.

Mucin   The principal constituent of mucus. The principal airway gel-forming mucins MUC2, MUC5AC, and MUC5B are proteins with attached oligosaccharide (sugar) side chains.

Mucoactive agent   A term connoting any medication or drug that has an effect on mucus secretion; includes MUCOLYTIC, EXPECTORANT, MUCOSPISSIC, MUCOREGULATORY, and MUCOKINETIC AGENTS.

Mucokinetic agent   A medication that increases ciliary clearance of respiratory mucus secretions.

Mucolytic agent   A medication that degrades polymers in secretions. *Classic mucolytics* have free thiol groups to degrade mucin and *peptide mucolytics* break pathologic filaments of neutrophil-derived DNA or actin in sputum. Classic mucolytics are ineffective for the therapy of airway disease and are not recommended, whereas dornase alfa appears to be effective for the therapy of cystic fibrosis and perhaps bronchiectasis.

Mucolytic expectorant   Agent that facilitates removal of mucus by a lysing, or MUCOLYTIC, action. *Example:* dornase alfa.

Mucoregulatory agent   A drug that reduces the volume of airway mucus secretion and appears to be especially effective in hypersecretory states such as bronchorrhea, diffuse panbronchiolitis, cystic fibrosis, and some forms of asthma.

Mucospissic agent   A medication that increases the viscosity of secretions and may be effective in the therapy of bronchorrhea.

Mucus   Secretion, from surface goblet cells and submucosal glands, composed of water, proteins, and glycosylated mucins. The glycoprotein portion of the secretion is termed MUCIN. *Mucus* (noun) is the secretion; *mucous* (adjective) is the cell or gland type.

Muscarinic   Same as cholinergic: an agent that produces the effect of acetylcholine or an agent that mimicks acetylcholine.

Myasthenia gravis   An autoimmune neuromuscular disorder characterized by chronic fatigue and exhaustion of muscles.

Mydriasis   Describes dilation of the pupil, by constriction of the radial iris muscle.

Nebulizer   A device used for making a fine spray or mist, also know as an *aerosol generator*.

Neonatal   Refers to the period of time between birth and the first month of life.

Nephrocalcinosis   Renal lithiasis in which calcium deposits form in the renal parenchyma, resulting in reduced kidney function and the presence of blood in the urine.

Nephron   The microscopic functional unit of the kidney, responsible for filtering and maintaining fluid balance. Each kidney has approximately 2 million nephrons.

Neuroeffector site   Refers to the terminal site of a nerve fiber; the target site or tissue of a nerve fiber.

Neuromuscular blocking agent   A substance that interferes with the neural transmission between motor neurons and skeletal muscles.

Neuron (nerve cell)   One of the basic functional units of the nervous system that is specialized to transmit electrical nerve impulses and carry information from one part of the body to another. A neuron consists of a cell body, axons, and dendrites.

Neurotransmitter   A chemical, such as acetylcholine or norepinephrine, that is released when the presynaptic neuron of an axon is excited, diffuses across the synapse, and attaches to postsynaptic receptors to transmit the nerve impulse.

Nominal dose   Dose in a delivery device.

Nonproprietary name   The name of a drug other than its trademarked name.

Norepinephrine   A naturally occurring catecholamine, produced by the adrenal medulla, that has properties similar to those of epinephrine. It is used as a neurotransmitter in most sympathetic terminal nerve sites.

Nosocomial pneumonia   Pneumonia that is acquired in a health care setting.

Nucleotide   A compound of phosphoric acid, a sugar, and a base group, which constitutes the structural unit of nucleic acid, either deoxyribonucleic acid (DNA) or ribonucleic acid (RNA).

Off label   Use of drugs with no U.S. Food and Drug Administration–approved labeling.

Official name   In the event that an experimental drug becomes fully approved for general use and is admitted to the United States Pharmacopeia–National Formulary, the generic name becomes the official name.

Ototoxicity   Damage to the ear, specifically the cochlea or auditory nerve and sometimes the vestibulum, by a toxin.

Paracrine   Refers to the secretion of a hormone from a source other than an endocrine gland; *paracrine control* is a general term referring to a control mechanism by which one cell secretes a substance that acts on nearby cells in the area. See AUTOCRINE.

Parasympatholytic   An agent blocking or inhibiting the effects of the parasympathetic nervous system.

Parasympathomimetic   An agent causing stimulation of the parasympathetic nervous system.

Parenteral   Administration in any way other than by the intestine; most commonly used to describe injection (e.g., intravenous, intramuscular, or subcutaneous).

Pediatric   Refers to the period of time between 1 month and 18 years of age.

Penetration   In respiratory pharmacology, refers to the depth within the lung reached by particles.

Peptide   A compound of two or more amino acids; the carboxyl group of one amino acid is linked with the amino group of another, forming a peptide bond.

Percentage   Amount of solute that is in a solution containing 100 parts.

Peripheral nervous system   Portion of the nervous system outside the central nervous system, including sensory, sympathetic, and parasympathetic nerves.

Phagocyte   A cell such as the macrophage that can ingest and digest particles such as bacteria or cell debris.

Phagocytosis   The process of ingestion and digestion of bacteria and particles by phagocytes.

Pharmacodynamics   The mechanisms of drug action by which a drug molecule causes its effect in the body.

Pharmacogenetics   The study of the interrelationship of genetic differences and drug effects.

Pharmacognosy   The identification of sources of drugs, from plants and animals.

Pharmacokinetics   The time course and disposition of a drug in the body, based on its absorption, distribution, metabolism, and elimination.

Pharmacology   The study of drugs (chemicals), including their origin, properties, and interactions with living organisms.

Pharmacotherapy   Treatment of disease by drug therapy.

Pharmacy   The preparation and dispensing of drugs.

Phenotype   Physical appearance, partially or completely determined by heredity; for example, blood groups.

Phosphodiesterase   Any of a group of enzymes that degrade the phosphodiester bond in cAMP and cGMP, thereby affecting changes in intracellular signaling.

Pneumocystis carinii (jiroveci)   The organism causing *Pneumocystis* pneumonia in humans, seen in immunosuppressed individuals such as those infected with human immunodeficiency virus.

Polar   Having positively and negatively charged sites.

Polydisperse   In reference to the size of particles in an aerosol, meaning many different particle sizes.

Polypeptide   A union of two or more amino acids.

Prodrug   A drug that exhibits its pharmacological activity once it is converted, inside the body, to its active form.

Prophylactic treatment   Prevention of respiratory distress syndrome (RDS) in very low birth weight infants, and in infants with higher birth weight but with evidence of immature lungs, who are at risk for developing RDS.

Prostaglandin   One of several hormone-type substances circulating throughout the body.

Protein   A nitrogenous compound formed by a series of amino acids.

Protonated   Having a proton, the positively charged hydrogen ion.

Pseudomonas aeruginosa   A gram-negative organism, primarily a nosocomial pathogen. It causes urinary tract infections, respiratory system infections, dermatitis, soft tissue infections, bacteremia, bone and joint infections, gastrointestinal infections, and a variety of systemic infections, particularly in patients with severe burns and in patients who are immunosuppressed (e.g., patients with cancer or acquired immunodeficiency syndrome).

Reabsorption   The return to the blood of most of the water, sodium, amino acids, and sugar that were removed during filtration; occurs mainly in the proximal tubule of the nephron.

Receptor   A cell component that combines with a drug to change or enhance the function of the cell.

α-Receptor stimulation   Causes vasoconstriction and a vasopressor effect; in the upper airway (nasal passages) this can provide decongestion.

β₁-Receptor stimulation   Causes increased myocardial conductivity and increased heart rate, as well as increased contractile force.

β₂-Receptor stimulation   Causes relaxation of bronchial smooth muscle, with some inhibition of inflammatory mediator release and stimulation of mucociliary clearance.

Recessive   Not dominant; a gene that is recessive does not express itself when paired with its dominant allele (one of two paired genes); when an individual has identical alleles, whether dominant or recessive, this is described as HOMOZYGOUS for the gene. A combination of a dominant and recessive allele is termed HETEROZYGOUS.

Renin   An enzyme also known as angiotensinogenase, released by the kidney in response to a lack of renal blood flow, and responsible for converting angiotensinogen into angiotensin I.

Rescue treatment   Retroactive, or "rescue," treatment of infants who have developed respiratory distress syndrome.

Reservoir device   Global term describing or referring to extension, auxiliary, add-on devices attached to metered dose inhalers for administration. This term could include both SPACER and VALVED HOLDING CHAMBER, defined below.

Respiratory care pharmacology   The application of pharmacology to the treatment of cardiopulmonary disease and critical care.

Respiratory syncytial virus   A virus that causes the formation of syncytial masses in cells. This leads to inflammation of the bronchioles, which may cause respiratory distress in infants.

Rheology   Study of the deformation and flow (strain) of matter.

Schedule   Amount of drug that is needed, based on a patient's weight.

Sedation   The production of a restful state of mind, particularly by the use of drugs that have a calming effect, relieving anxiety and tension.

Solute   A substance that is dissolved in a solution.

Solution   Physically homogeneous mixture of two or more substances (liquid).

Buffer solution: an aqueous solution able to resist changes of pH with addition of acid/base.

Isotonic solution: One having equal concentrations inside and outside the cell.

Normal solution: One gram-equivalent weight of solute per liter of solution.

Molal solution: One mole of solute per 1000 g of solvent.

Molar solution: One mole of solute per liter of solution.

Osmolal solution: One osmole per kilogram of solvent.

Osmolar solution: One osmole per liter of solution.

Solvent   A substance, usually a liquid, that is used to make a solution.

Somatic motor neurons   Part of the nervous system that controls muscles that are under voluntary control.

Spacer   Denotes a simple tube or extension device, with no one-way valves to contain the aerosol cloud; its purpose is simply to extend the metered dose inhaler spray away from the mouth.

Sputum   Expectorated secretions that contain respiratory tract, oropharyngeal, and nasopharyngeal secretions as well as bacteria and products of inflammation including polymeric DNA and actin. Purulent sputum contains very little mucin and is similar in composition to pus.

Stability   Describing the tendency of aerosol particles to remain in suspension.

Status asthmaticus   An exacerbation of asthma that does not respond to standard treatment.

Status epilepticus   At least 30 minutes of continuous seizure activity without full recovery between seizures.

Steroid   Also known as *glucocorticoid* or *corticosteroid,* an agent that produces an antiinflammatory response in the body.

Steroid diabetes   Hyperglycemia (e.g., increased plasma glucose levels) resulting from glucocorticoid therapy; glucocorticoids break down proteins and fats to generate building blocks for gluconeogenesis.

Stimulant   A drug that increases activity of the brain. Stimulants can be divided into two classes: the amphetamines, and respiratory stimulants. Amphetamines cause increased wakefulness, improved concentration, and appetite suppression. Respiratory stimulants include doxapram, xanthines, carbonic anhydrase inhibitors, salicylates, and progesterone.

Stimulant expectorant   Agent that increases the production and therefore presumably the clearance of mucus secretions in the respiratory tract. *Example:* guaifenesin.

Strength   In pharmacology, the amount of solute in a solution, usually expressed as a percentage.

Structure–activity relation   Relationship between a drug's chemical structure and the outcome it has in the body.

Substitute neurotransmitter   Neurotransmitter or hormone replacement that may be weaker or inert.

Substrate   The substance acted on by an enzyme.

Sudden cardiac death   An episode of ventricular fibrillation, pulseless ventricular tachycardia, pulseless electrical activity, or asystole.

Surface tension   The attraction of molecules in a liquid–air interface, such as the liquid lining in lung tissue and the air, pulling the surface molecules inward.

Surfactant   An agent that lowers surface tension.

Sympatholytic   An agent blocking or inhibiting the effect of the sympathetic nervous system.

Sympathomimetic   An agent causing stimulation of the sympathetic nervous system.

Synergism   A drug interaction that occurs from combined drug effects that are greater than if the drugs were given alone.

Synergistic effect   When the effect of two chemicals on an organism is greater than the effect of either chemical individually.

Systolic blood pressure   Peak pressure reached during ventricular ejection.

Tachycardia   An overly rapid heart beat, usually defined as greater than 100 beats/min in adults.

Tachykinin   Any of a family of small peptide mediators that stimulate a variety of neurokinin receptors on target membranes. Examples are neurokinin A and substance P.

Tachyphylaxis   A rapid decrease in response to a drug.

Target concentration   Administering a drug until a certain blood level is reached; therapeutic effects and side effects are therefore related to the drug concentration in the blood.

Target effect   Administering a drug until the desired effect is achieved or unacceptable side effects or toxicity occur.

Therapeutic index   Difference between the minimal therapeutic and toxic concentrations of a drug; the smaller the difference the greater the chance the drug will be toxic.

Therapeutics   The art of treating disease with drugs.

Tolerance   Describes a decreasing intensity of response to a drug over time.

Topical   In pharmacology, use of the skin or mucus membrane for drug administration (e.g., lotion).

Toxicology   The study of toxic substances and their pharmacological actions, including antidotes and poison control.

Transdermal   Use of the skin for drug administration (e.g., patch).

Urine output   Amount of urine produced in 24 hours. Normal urine output averages 30 to 60 ml/hr.

Valved holding chamber   Denotes a spacer device with the addition of one-way valve(s) to contain and hold the aerosol cloud until inspiration occurs.

Vasodilator   Causing dilation of the blood vessels.

Vasopressor   Causing contraction of the capillaries and arteries.

Virostatic   Stopping a virus from replicating.

Virucidal   Killing a virus.

Virus   An obligate intracellular parasite, containing either DNA or RNA, that reproduces by synthesis of subunits within the host cell and causes disease as a consequence of this replication.

Viscosity   A rheologic property characteristic of liquids and represented by the loss modulus G

Xanthine   A nitrogenous compound found in many organs and in the blood and urine.

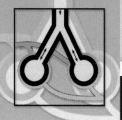

Note: Page numbers followed by "f" refer to illustrations; page numbers followed by "t" refer to table; page numbers followed by "b"refer to boxes.

Study smart…Stay ahead!

Workbook for
Rau's Respiratory Care Pharmacology, 7th Edition
ISBN: 978-0-323-04949-8

Specially designed to help you get the most out of your textbook, the **Workbook** is just what you need for in-depth study and review of the most important facts and information on respiratory care pharmacology…

- **Activities** such as labeling, defining key terms, and matching are an engaging way to reinforce what you learn.

- **Critical thinking exercises** test your understanding of key concepts.

- **Case studies** challenge you to put what you've learned into practice and apply your knowledge.

- **NBRC examination-style review questions** prepare you for certification.

Enhance your understanding of respiratory care pharmacology — get your **Workbook** today!

Order securely at **www.elsevierhealth.com**
Call toll-free **1-800-545-2522**
Visit your **local bookstore**

HP-0731